SURGICAL TECH

INTERNATIONAL™ X

INTERNATIONAL DEVELOPMENTS IN SURGERY AND SURGICAL RESEARCH

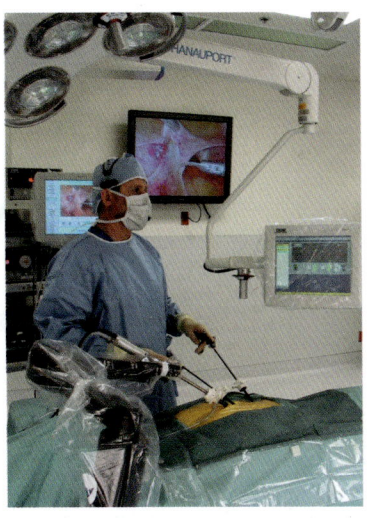

Edited by

ZOLTÁN SZABÓ, PH.D., F.I.C.S.
DIRECTOR
MICROSURGERY & OPERATIVE ENDOSCOPY TRAINING (MOET) INSTITUTE
SAN FRANCISCO, CA
MOETinst@aol.com

JAMES E. LEWIS, M.D., F.A.C.O.G.
CHIEF OF OBSTETRICS & GYNECOLOGY
KAISER PERMANENTE MEDICAL CENTER
ASSOCIATE CLINICAL PROFESSOR
UNIVERSITY OF CALIFORNIA SCHOOL OF MEDICINE
SAN FRANCISCO, CA
james.lewis@kp.org

GARY A. FANTINI, M.D., F.A.C.S.
ASSOCIATE PROFESSOR OF SURGERY
CORNELL UNIVERSITY MEDICAL COLLEGE
NEW YORK, NY
gaf@NewYorkPhysicians.com

RAGHU S. SAVALGI, M.D., PH.D.(SURG), F.R.C.S.
CHAIRMAN, DIVISION OF DISTANT MEDICINE & SURGERY
SPLAR CENTER
NEW HAVEN, CT
RSavalgi@hotmail.com

Published by

UNIVERSAL MEDICAL PRESS, INC.
ISBN: 1-890131-06-7

THOMAS F. LASZLO
PUBLISHER
info@ump.com

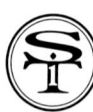

SURGICAL TECHNOLOGY INTERNATIONAL™ X

International Developments in Surgery and Surgical Research

Published annually by
UNIVERSAL MEDICAL PRESS, INC.
2443 Fillmore Street, #229, San Francisco, CA 94115, USA
Telephone: +1-415-436-9790   Fax: +1-415-436-9791
E-mail: info@ump.com   http://www.ump.com

ISBN: 1-890131-06-7; ISSN: 1090-3941

Lic. Fernando Gonzalez Vilchis	Thomas F. Laszlo	Lic. Hector Avila
General Director	*Publisher*	*Legal Counsel*

Editorial Manager: Wanda Toy
Editorial Coordinator: Kristine B. Moy, MPH
Editorial Associate: Gae O. Decker-Garrad
Sales Director: Thomas Hurd
Advertising Sales: Katrina Koller
Julian Cox
Website Engineer: Attila Horvath
Financial Controller: Marilyn P. Freeman

Reprint requests should be sent to the Editorial Department, Universal Medical Press, Inc.
2443 Fillmore Street, #229, San Francisco, CA 94115, USA. Fax: +1-415-436-9791, e-mail:info@ump.com

Front Cover Photograph: Courtesy of Karl Storz GmbH, Tuttlingen, Germany

Back Cover Photograph: Courtesy of Demetrius E. Litwin, M.D., University of Massachusetts Medical School, Worcester, MA

Section Divider Legends & Acknowledgements:

SURGICAL OVERVIEW
Gross vessel seal at 14 days using the LigaSure™ Device
Courtesy of Steven L. Peterson, D.V.M., M.D. and Ned Cosgriff, M.D.

GENERAL SURGERY
ENDOTIP™ (Karl Storz Endoscopy, Tuttlingen, Germany) cannula insertion at primary port during open laparoscopy
Courtesy of Artin M. Ternamian, M.D., F.R.C.S.C.

CARDIOVASCULAR SURGERY
Medtronic Physiologic Mitral Valve
Courtesy of W.R. Eric Jamieson, M.D., F.R.C.S.C.

TRANSPLANTATION
Intraoperative view using cardiopulmonary bypass during SLT
Courtesy of Carsten Schröder, M.D. and Paolo Macchiarini, M.D., Ph.D.

ORTHOPAEDIC SURGERY
Repositioning the hemiprosthesis into the acetabulum
Courtesy of Hans J. Erli, M.D.

PLASTIC & RECONSTRUCTIVE SURGERY
Christensen Patient-Specific™ Prosthesis
Courtesy of Robert W. Christensen, D.D.S.

Copyright © September 2002, Universal Medical Press, Inc.

All rights reserved. No part of the publication may be reproduced, stored in any retrieval system, or transmitted in any form—electronic, mechanical, photocopying, recording or otherwise—without prior consent of the Publisher. Whereas every care has been taken to ensure the data in this book are accurate, the Publisher cannot accept, and hereby disclaims, any liability to any party to loss or damage caused by errors or omissions resulting from negligence, accident or any other cause.

PRINTED AND PUBLISHED IN HONG KONG IN COOPERATION WITH MAGNUM INTERNATIONAL PRINTING CO. LTD.
Price: US $95.00

Surgical Advances for the New Millenium

- **Updates on Recent Innovations in Surgery**
- **Peer Reviewed by Expert Specialty Surgeons**
- **Indexed on MEDLINE**

"*Surgical Technology International* does a splendid job of showcasing the many aspects of recent surgical achievement and innovation that have been possible as we hurtle forward into the new millenium."
—M. David Tilson, M.D.
Professor of Surgery
Columbia University, New York

"The authors are to be congratulated on the latest edition of what is essential reading for surgeons in every discipline."
—Tom Bates, F.R.C.S.
Consultant Surgeon
The William Harvey Hospital
Ashford, Kent, England, UK

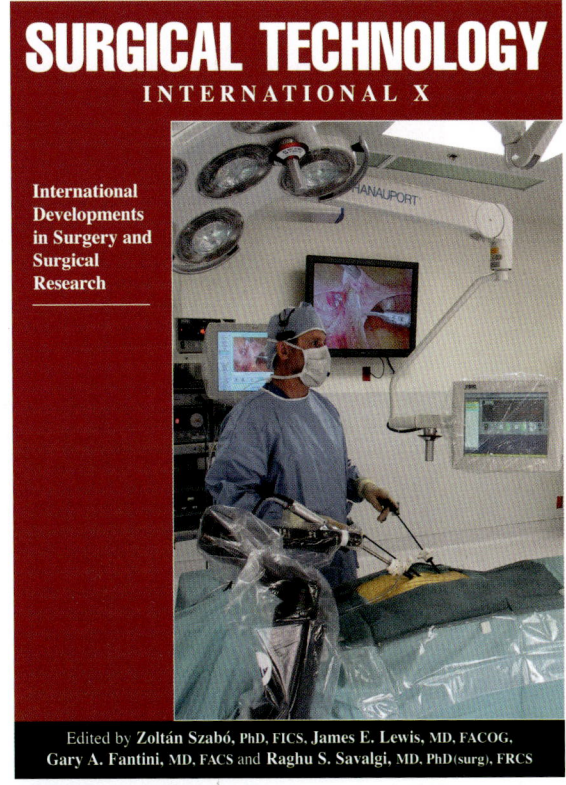

Edited by **Zoltán Szabó**, PhD, FICS, **James E. Lewis**, MD, FACOG, **Gary A. Fantini**, MD, FACS and **Raghu S. Savalgi**, MD, PhD(surg), FRCS

ISBN No. 1-890131-06-7

Order a 3-year subscription now and get 50% off the bookstore price!

Yes, please enter my subscription to Surgical Techonology International for:

☐ 3 years (6 Issues) $285   ☐ 2 years (4 Issues) $215   ☐ 1 year (2 Issues) $145   ☐ Individual Copy ($95)

Please add 10% per year for shipping & handling on U.S. orders.
Please add $46 per year for shipping & handling for international orders.   ISBN No.: 1-890131-06-7

☐ Special Back Issue Set STI III - STI X - $685 US, $755 overseas - (Includes shipping)
☐ AMEX   ☐ MasterCard   ☐ VISA   ☐ Check enclosed*   ☐ Bill me

Card Number: ☐☐☐☐☐☐☐☐☐☐☐☐☐☐☐☐

Signature: _____   Expiration Date: _____
Name: _____   Institution: _____
Address: _____
City: _____   State: _____   Zip: _____
Country: _____   Phone/Fax: _____
                            Email: _____

Please send to: Universal Medical Press, Inc., 2443 Fillmore Street, #229, San Francisco, CA 94115, USA,
or FAX YOUR ORDER TO: 1-415-436-9791. / Telephone: 1-415-436-9790 / E-mail: info@ump.com / Website: www.ump.com

* Make checks payable to **Universal Medical. Press, Inc.** California residents, please add applicable state sales tax.

SURGICAL TECHNOLOGY
INTERNATIONAL X

International Developments in Surgery and Surgical Research

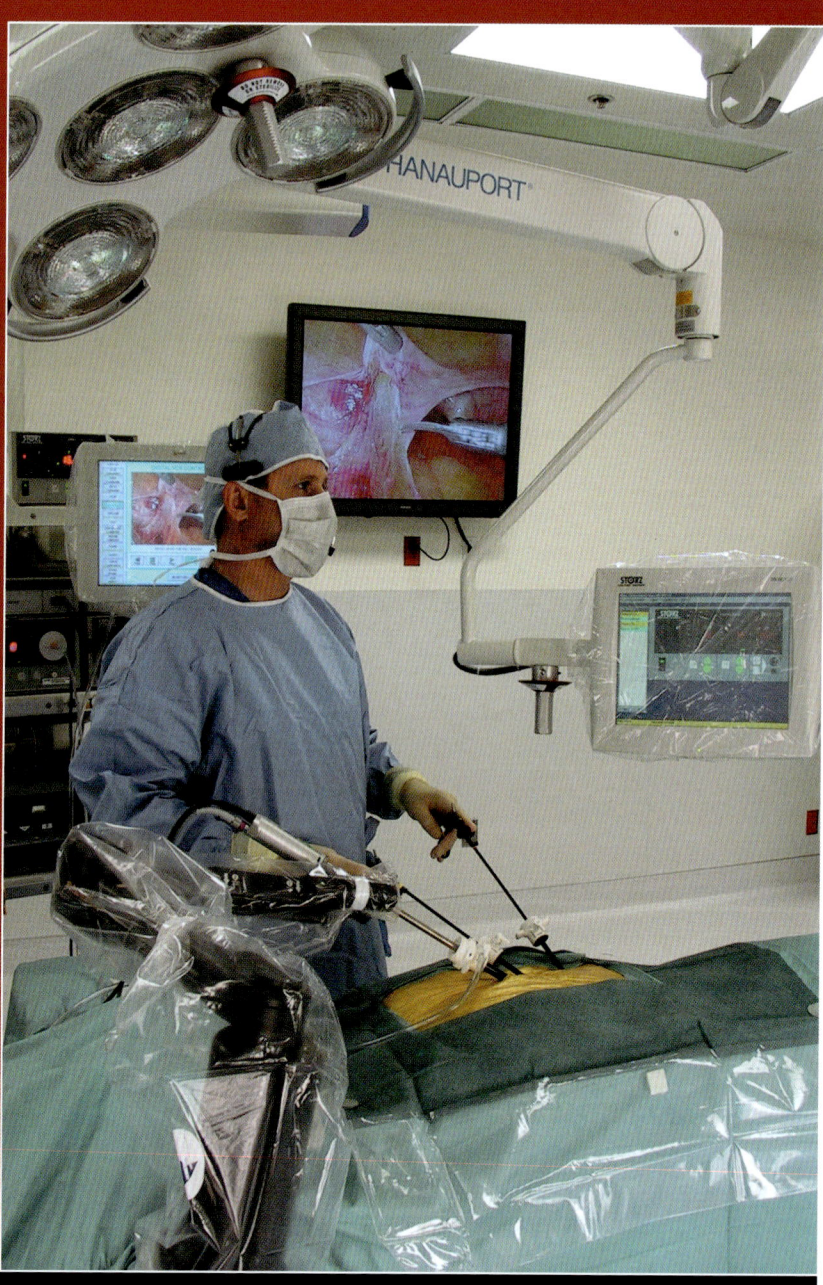

Edited by **Zoltán Szabó**, PhD, FICS, **James E. Lewis**, MD, FACOG, **Gary A. Fantini**, MD, FACS and **Raghu S. Savalgi**, MD, PhD(surg), FRCS

Editorial Board

Edited by

ZOLTÁN SZABÓ, PH.D., F.I.C.S.
DIRECTOR
MICROSURGERY & OPERATIVE ENDOSCOPY TRAINING (MOET) INSTITUTE
SAN FRANCISCO, CA
MOETinst@aol.com

JAMES E. LEWIS, M.D., F.A.C.O.G
CHIEF OF OBSTETRICS & GYNECOLOGY
KAISER PERMANENTE MEDICAL CENTER
ASSOCIATE CLINICAL PROFESSOR
UNIVERSITY OF CALIFORNIA SCHOOL OF MEDICINE
SAN FRANCISCO, CA
james.lewis@kp.org

GARY A. FANTINI, M.D., F.A.C.S.
ASSOCIATE PROFESSOR OF SURGERY
CORNELL UNIVERSITY MEDICAL COLLEGE
NEW YORK, NY
gaf@NewYorkPhysicians.com

RAGHU S. SAVALGI, M.D., PH.D.(SURG), F.R.C.S.
CHAIRMAN, DIVISION OF DISTANT MEDICINE & SURGERY
SPLAR CENTER
NEW HAVEN, CT
RSavalgi@hotmail.com

Editorial Advisory Board

MOHAN C. AIRAN, M.D., F.A.C.S., F.A.C.M.Q.
CHICAGO, ILLINOIS

TOM BATES, F.R.C.S.
ASHFORD, UK

GIORGIO BRUNELLI, M.D.
BRESCIA, ITALY

STEPHEN CHADWICK, M.S., F.R.C.S.
LONDON, UK

PROF. DR. MED. A.J. COBURG
NEUSS, GERMANY

SIR ALFRED CUSCHIERI, M.D., CH.M., F.R.C.S. ED.
DUNDEE, UK

GERGELY CSÁKY, M.D., PH.D.
MISKOLC, HUNGARY

ISTVÁN GÁL, M.D., PH.D.
GYÖNGYÖS, HUNGARY

KENNETH HANSRAJ, M.D.
NEW YORK, NEW YORK

EDWARD R. HOWARD, M.S., F.R.C.S.
LONDON, UK

W. R. ERIC JAMIESON, M.D., F.R.C.S.
VANCOUVER, BC, CANADA

STEVEN G. KAALI, M.D., F.A.C.O.G.
NEW YORK, NEW YORK

MORRIS D. KERSTEIN, M.D., F.A.C.S.
PHILADELPHIA, PENNSYLVANIA

JONATHAN KRUSKAL, PH.D.
BOSTON, MASSACHUSETTS

ADOLPH LOMBARDI, M.D.
COLUMBUS, OHIO

PAOLO MACCHARINI, M.D.
HANNOVER, GERMANY

R. UNNIKRISHNAN NAIR, M.D., F.R.C.S.
LEEDS, UK

HARRY REICH, M.D.
WILKES-BARRE, PENNSYLVANIA

ERNANE D. REIS, M.D.
NEW YORK, NEW YORK

COL. RICHARD M. SATAVA, M.D., F.A.C.S.
ALEXANDRIA, VIRGINIA

CHRISTOF SOHN, M.D.
HEIDELBERG, GERMANY

PAUL S. STRANGE, M.D., F.A.C.S.
BEECH GROVE, INDIANA

• Environmental Decontamination Systems • Equipment Management Systems • Facilities Planning Services • Field Serv

• Antimicrobial and Routine Skin Care Systems • Biohazardous Waste Management Systems • Cleaning/Decontamination Systems • Microbial Reduction Services

BactoShield® CHG 2% and 4% – Antimicrobial surgical scrub, health care personnel handwash, or pre-operative skin preparation.

Hausted® Stretchers – Patient handling and transport systems.

Amsco® 3085 SP™ Surgical Table – Multipurpose radiolucent surgical support and positioning system.

Amsco SQ240 SurgiVision™ Surgical lighting and video system.

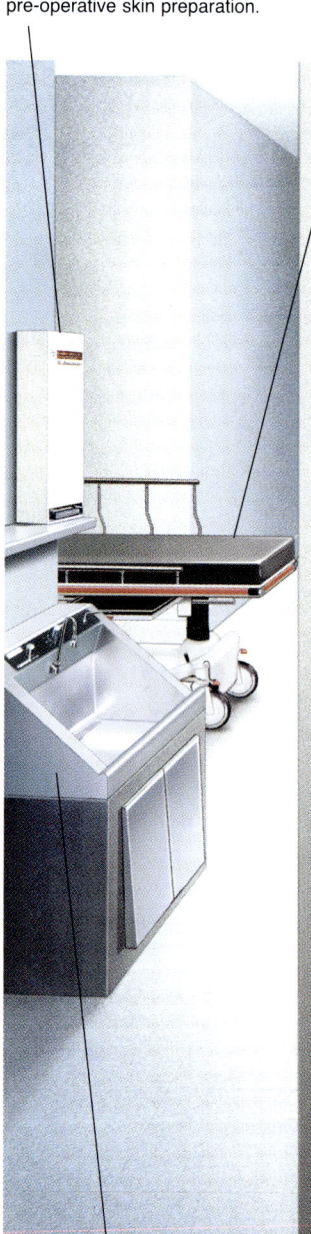

Amsco Flexmatic® – Single, dual, or triple well surgical scrub stations.

EcoCycle 10® – Site-of-use biohazardous waste collection, destruction, and decontamination system.

STERIS SYSTEM 1® with Enhanced Control – Low temperature, liquid chemical system for sterilizing heat sensitive immersible devices at or near the site-of-use.

Klenzyme® Enzymatic Detergent – One of a family of liquid presoaks and cleaners for surgical instruments, medical apparatus, and endoscopes.

• Operator Training Programs • OR Cabinetry and Cleaning Stations • Pure Water Systems • Sterile Processing Consulting Servic

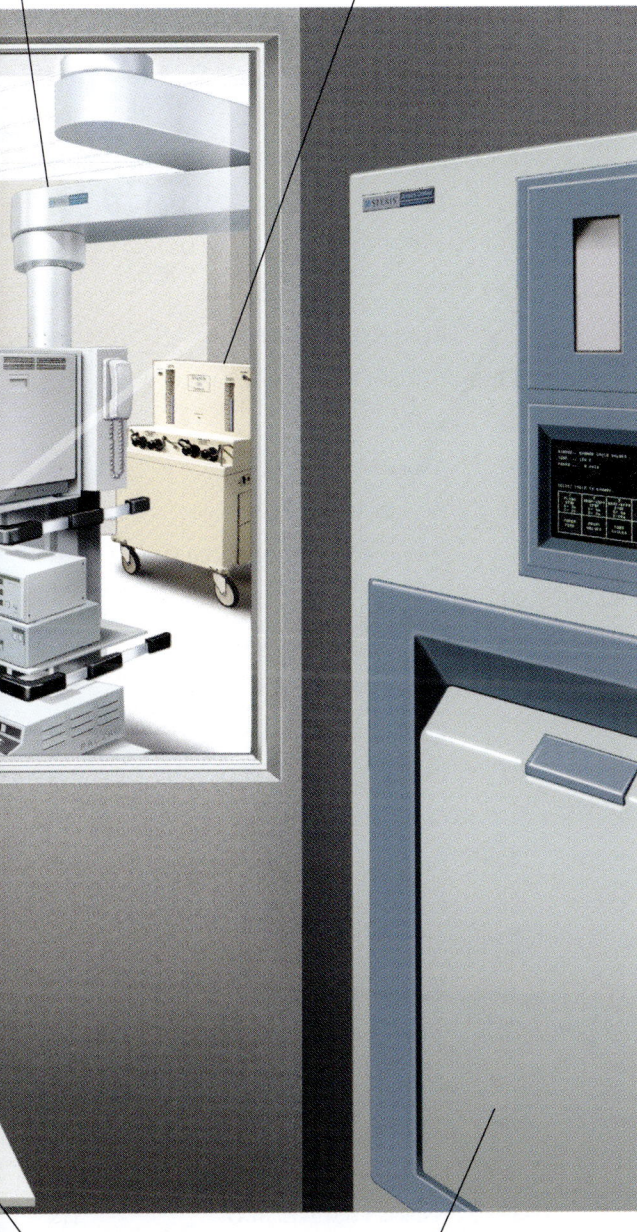

High Temperature Sterile Processing Systems • Low Temperature Sterile Processing Systems • Clinical Applications Analysis

nsco Orbiter® – Ceiling-spended equipment and ity management system.

SafeCycle® 40 – Safe, easy, and cost-effective system to collect, contain, transport, and dispose of surgical fluid waste.

overage® Spray HB – e-step environmental rmicidal detergent effective ainst HIV, HBV, VRE, d MRSA.

Millennium™ Steam Sterilization System – Sterilization system using a patented Steam Flush, Pressure Pulse cycle.

Think integrated solutions.
Think STERIS.

STERIS®

**Infection and Contamination Prevention
...Worldwide**
877-STERIS-2 (877-783-7472) • www.steris.com

Sterilants and Supplies • Continuing Education Seminars • On-Site Lunch and Learn Programs • Management Services • Contract Sterilization • Surgical Tables

Sterility Assurance Systems • Surgical Lighting Systems • Patient Positioning and Transport Systems • Validation Services

Authors Index

Author	Page
Jose Adrey, M.D.	205
Jonathan Aligbe, M.D., F.M.C.Path	71
Kaveh Alizadeh, M.D.	283
Renato Berroya, M.D., F.A.C.S.	168
Daniel Berteaux, M.D.	205
Rodger L. Bick, M.D., Ph.D., F.A.C.P.	226
Jochen Binder, M.D.	45
Marian Böttger M.D.	89
Souad Bouaichi, M.D.	151
Carrie Britton, B.S.	273
Andreas Burkart, M.D.	255
Guy-Bernard Cadiere, M.D.	109
Elie Capelluto, M.D.	109
Jordi Casas-Sabater, M.D.	212
Félix Castillo-García, M.D.	212
Younes Cheikhaoui, M.D.	151
John C. Chiu, M.D., F.R.C.S., F.A.C.S.	266
Robert W. Christensen, D.D.S.	273
Thomas J. Clifford, M.D.	266
Ned Cosgriff, M.D.	55
Marc Cots-Pons, M.D.	212
Steven A. Curley, M.D., F.A.C.S.	99
James T. Curry, D.D.S.	273
Oscar A. De Leon-Casasola, M.D.	49
Maurizio De Luca, M.D.	109
Francesco De Marchi, M.D.	109
Geoffroy Warnier De Wailly, M.D.	161
Dr. Arun Dhir, M.S., D.N.B. (Surg), F.R.C.S. Ed.	107
Yves-Marie Dion, M.D., M.Sc., F.A.C.S., F.R.C.S.C.	161
Louis Draganich, Ph.D.	201
Katrin Eichler, M.D.	89
Hans Josef Erli, M.D.	221
Gary A. Fantini, M.D., F.A.C.S.	21
Franco Favretti, M.D.	109
Victor H. Frankel, M.D., Ph.D., K.N.O.	195
Patrick Frayssinet, M.D., Ph.D.	237
Quentin Gaudissart, M.D.	109
Paul H. Gerst, M.D., F.A.C.S.	168
Hanasoge T. Girishkumar, M.D., F.A.C.S.	168
Christian Goalard, M.D.	205
Dirk J. Gouma, M.D.	61
Dominique C.R. Hardy, M.D.	237
Jacques Himpens, M.D.	109
Martin Holzner	67
Örs Peter Horváth, M.D., D.Sc.	115
Matthew J.W. Hubble, M.B., B.S., F.R.C.S. (Orth)	261
Andreas Balthasar Imhoff, M.D.	255
William B. Inabnet, M.D.	77
Francesco Izzo, M.D.	99
Jack J. Jakimovicz, M.D., Ph.D., F.R.C.S., Ed.	19
W.R. Eric Jamieson, M.D., F.R.C.S.C.	121
Rhizlene Drissi Kacemi, M.D.	151
Ihab R. Kamel, M.D., Ph.D.	186
Satish C. Khaneja, M.D., F.A.C.S.	168
Peter Klever, M.D.	221
Wolfgang Kramer, M.D.	45
Jonathan B. Kruskal, M.D., Ph.D.	186
Robert D. Kugel, M.D., F.A.C.S.	81
Dirk Lehmann-Beckow, M.D.	67
James E. Lewis, M.D., F.A.C.O.G.	21
Mario Lise, M.D.	109
Wajih Maazouzi, M.D.	151
Paolo Macchiarini, M.D., Ph.D.	178
Martin G. Mack, M.D.	89
Mohammed Messouak, M.D.	151
Carolyn Mihaichuk, M.S.	55
Kosaku Mizuno, M.D., Ph.D.	195
Christian Moisan, Ph.D.	161
James Edwin Muntz, M.D., F.A.C.P.	249
Boris A. Nasseri, M.D.	25
Christian Nourissat, M.D.	205
Michael Okobia, M.D., F.W.A.C.S.	71
Friday Okonofua, M.D., F.W.A.C.S., F.M.C.O.G.	71
Valentine Otoide, M.D.	71
Othmar Paar, M.D.	221
Andras Papp, M.D.	115
Vellore S. Parithivel, M.D., F.A.C.S.	168
Jay M. Pensler, M.D.	283
Steven L. Peterson, D.V.M., M.D.	55
Lawrence A. Pottenger, M.D., Ph.D.	201
Vassilios Raptopoulos, M.D.	186
Ernane Dodero Reis, M.D.	212
Kevin F. Reynolds, R.T.R.	186
Joaquim Rodriguez-Miralles, M.D., Ph.D.	212
Andre Roggan, M.D.	89
Francesco Rubino, M.D.	77
Raghu S. Savalgi, M.D., Ph.D. (Surg.), F.R.C.S.	21
Prof. Anton Schafmayer, M.D.	67
Dale Schmaltz, M.S.	55
Christoph Schmitz, M.D.	157
Carsten Schröder, M.D.	178
Gianni Segato, M.D.	109
Dr. Kuldip Singh, M.S.	107
Romulo Sison, O.P.A.-C., C.S.T.	266
Patricia L. Stranahan, M.D., Ph.D.	55
Ralf Straub, M.D.	89
Zoltán Szabó, Ph.D., F.I.C.S.	21, 115
Artin M. Ternamian, M.D., F.R.C.S.C.	39
Joseph P. Vacanti, M.D., F.A.C.S.	25
Rutger C.I. van Geenen, M.D.	61
Andras Vereczkei, M.D.	115
Thomas J. Vogl, M.D.	89
William Walter, M.D.	205
Gisele Warmbrand, M.D.	189
Armin Welz, M.D.	157
Dirk Woitaschek, M.D.	89
Stephan Zangos, M.D.	89

SURGICAL TECHNOLOGY INTERNATIONAL X

Table of Contents

8 Author's Index

19 Foreword – Jack J. Jakimowicz, M.D., Ph.D., F.R.C.S.(Ed)

21 Preface – Zoltán Szabó, Ph.D., F.I.C.S.; James E. Lewis, M.D., F.A.C.O.G.; Gary A. Fantini, M.D., F.A.C.S.; Raghu S. Savalgi, M.D., Ph.D.(surg), F.R.C.S.

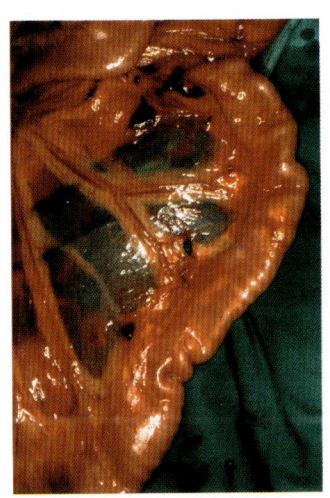

SURGICAL OVERVIEW

25 Tissue Engineering in the 21st Century
BORIS A. NASSERI, M.D.; JOSEPH P. VACANTI, M.D., F.A.C.S. - HARVARD MEDICAL SCHOOL, MASSACHUSETTS GENERAL HOSPITAL, BOSTON, MA

39 Endoscopic Threaded Imaging Port to Improve Laparoscopic Safety
ARTIN M. TERNAMIAN, M.D., F.R.C.S.C. - ST. JOSEPH'S HEALTH CENTRE, UNIVERSITY OF TORONTO, TORONTO, CANADA

45 Telerobotic Minimally Invasive Procedures in Urology — Laparoscopic Radical Prostatectomy
JOCHEN BINDER, M.D.; WOLFGANG KRAMER, M.D. - J.W. GOETHE UNIVERSITY, FRANKFURT, GERMANY

49 Using a Multi-Modal Rehabilitation Program for Patients Undergoing Open Sigmoidectomy
OSCAR A. DE LEON-CASASOLA, M.D., UNIVERSITY AT BUFFALO SCHOOL OF MEDICINE, ROSWELL PARK CANCER INSTITUTE, BUFFALO, NY

55 Comparison of Healing Process Following Ligation with Sutures and Bipolar Vessel Sealing
STEVEN L. PETERSON, D.V.M., M.D. - DENVER HEALTH TRAUMA CENTER, DENVER, CO; PATRICIA L. STRANAHAN, M.D., PH.D. - METROPOLITAN STATE COLLEGE, DENVER, CO; DALE SCHMALTZ, M.S.; CAROLYN MIHAICHUK, M.S.; NED COSGRIFF, M.D. - VALLEYLAB, BOULDER, CO

61 Impact of Hospital Volume on In-Hospital Mortality in Pancreatic Surgery
RUTGER C.I. VAN GEENEN, M.D.; DIRK J. GOUMA, M.D. - ACADEMIC MEDICAL CENTER, DEPARTMENT OF SURGERY, AMSTERDAM, THE NETHERLANDS

RIGHT TO THE POINT.

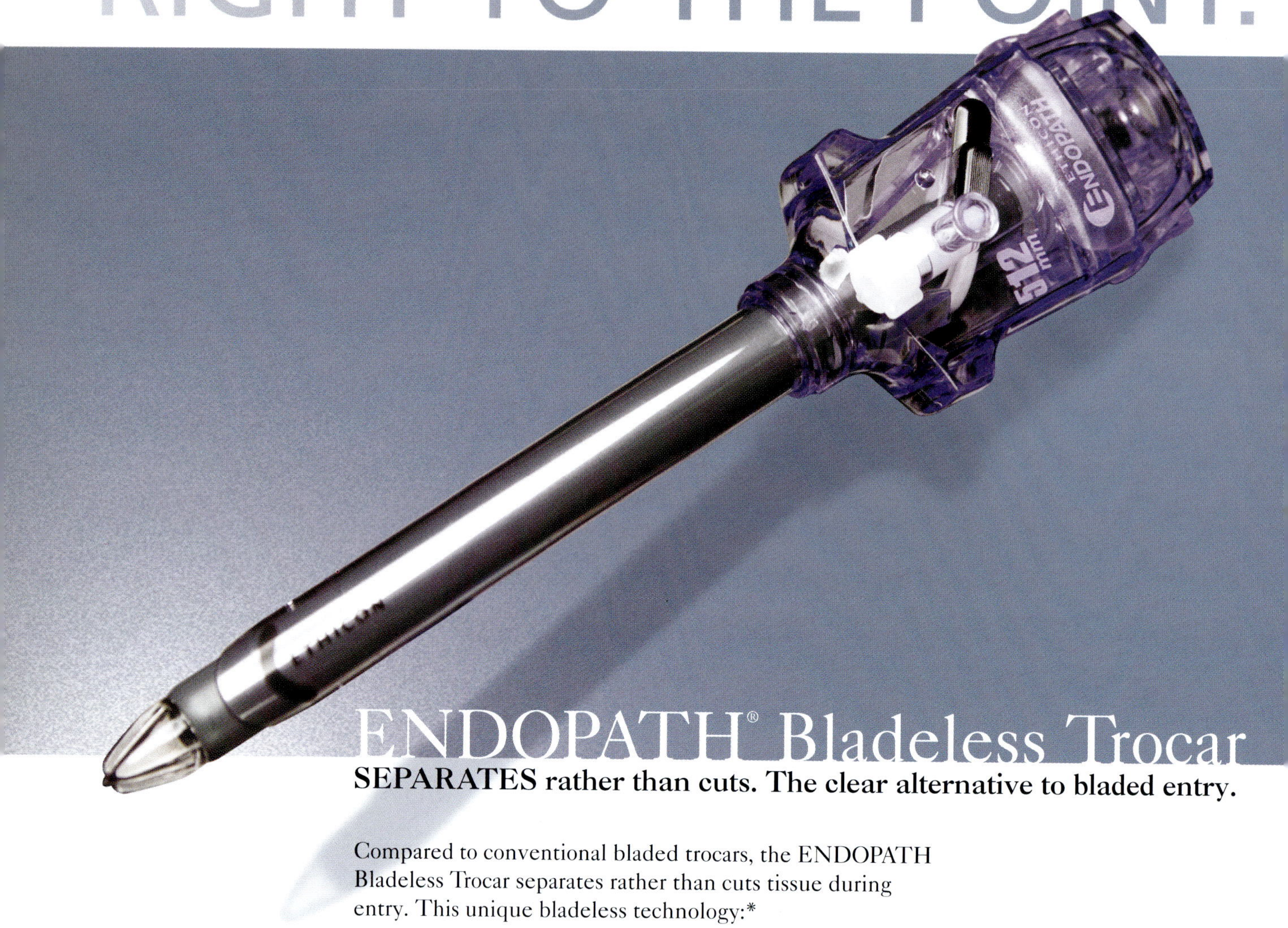

ENDOPATH® Bladeless Trocar

SEPARATES rather than cuts. The clear alternative to bladed entry.

Compared to conventional bladed trocars, the ENDOPATH Bladeless Trocar separates rather than cuts tissue during entry. This unique bladeless technology:*

- *Creates a smaller fascial defect*
- *Improves cannula retention in the abdominal wall*
- *Minimizes abdominal wall and vessel trauma*
- *May reduce the risk of port site herniation*

*Compared to conventional bladed trocars.

Rotation of the Bladeless Trocar, combined with controlled downward pressure, *separates* tissue for abdominal entry.

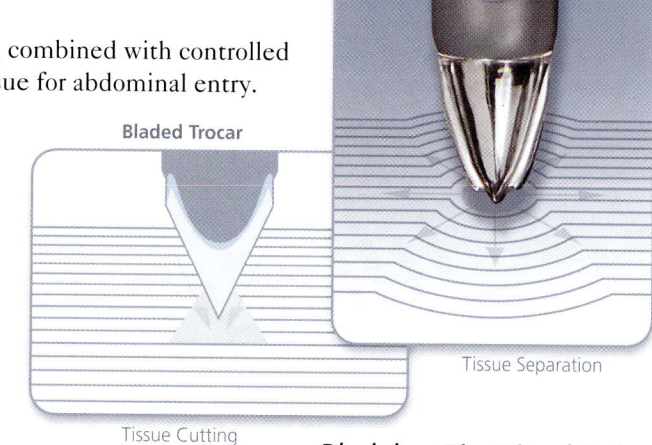

Bladeless Tip. Visual Entry.

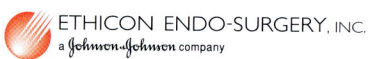

ETHICON ENDO-SURGERY, INC.
a Johnson & Johnson company

©Ethicon Endo-Surgery, Inc., 2002
ENDOPATH is a registered trademark of Ethicon Endo-Surgery, Inc.
DSL 02-0395

67 Process-Optimized Operating Room: Implementation of an Integrated OR System into Clinical Routine

PROF. ANTON SCHAFMAYER, M.D.; DIRK LEHMANN-BECKOW, M.D - SURGICAL CLINIC COMMUNITY HOSPITAL, LÜNEBURG, GERMANY; MARTIN HOLZNER - MEDICAL ENGINEERING GROUP, SIEMENS AG, ERLANGEN, GERMANY

71 Vulvar Leiomyosarcoma: A Case Report in a Nigerian Woman

VALENTINE OTOIDE, M.D.; MICHAEL OKOBIA, M.D., F.W.A.C.S. - UNIVERSITY OF BENIN TEACHING HOSPITAL, WOMEN'S HEALTH AND ACTION RESEARCH CENTER, BENIN CITY, NIGERIA; JONATHAN ALIGBE, M.D., F.M.C.PATH - UNIVERSITY OF BENIN, BENIN CITY, NIGERIA; FRIDAY OKONOFUA, M.D., F.W.A.C.S., F.M.C.O.G. - UNIVERSITY OF BENIN TEACHING HOSPITAL, WOMEN'S HEALTH AND RESEARCH CENTER, BENIN CITY, NIGERIA

GENERAL SURGERY

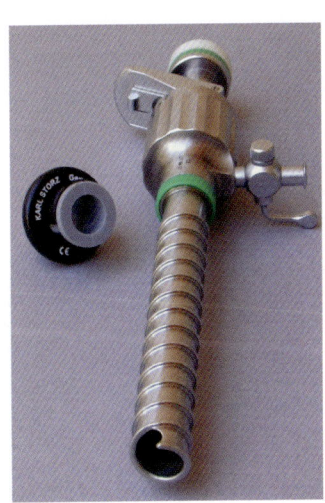

77 Ambulatory Radioguided Parathyroidectomy

FRANCESCO RUBINO, M.D.; WILLIAM B. INABNET, M.D. - THE MOUNT SINAI MEDICAL CENTER, NEW YORK, NY

81 Minimally Invasive Repair of Groin and Ventral Hernias Using a Self-Expanding Mesh Patch

ROBERT D. KUGEL, M.D., F.A.C.S. - HERNIA TREATMENT CENTER NORTHWEST, OLYMPIA, WA

89 Magnetic Resonance (MR)-Guided Percutaneous Laser-Induced Interstitial Thermotherapy (LITT®) for Malignant Liver Tumors

THOMAS J. VOGL, M.D.; MARTIN G. MACK, M.D.; RALF STRAUB, M.D.; KATRIN EICHLER, M.D.; ANDRE ROGGAN, M.D.; STEPHAN ZANGOS, M.D.; DIRK WOITASCHEK, M.D.; MARIAN BÖTTGER, M.D. - JOHANN WOLFGANG GOETHE-UNIVERSITY CLINIC, FRANKFURT AM MAIN, GERMANY

99 Radiofrequency Ablation of Primary and Metastatic Liver Tumors

STEVEN A. CURLEY, M.D., F.A.C.S - THE UNIVERSITY OF TEXAS M.D. ANDERSON CANCER CENTER, HOUSTON, TX; FRANCESCO IZZO, M.D - THE G. PASCALE NATIONAL TUMOR INSTITUTE, NAPLES, ITALY

107 Laparoscopic Cholecystectomy In Situs Inversus Totalis: A Case Report

DR. KULDIP SINGH, M.S.; DR. ARUN DHIR, M.S., D.N.B.(SURG), F.R.C.S. (ED) - DAYANAND MEDICAL COLLEGE & HOSPITAL, LUDHIANA, INDIA

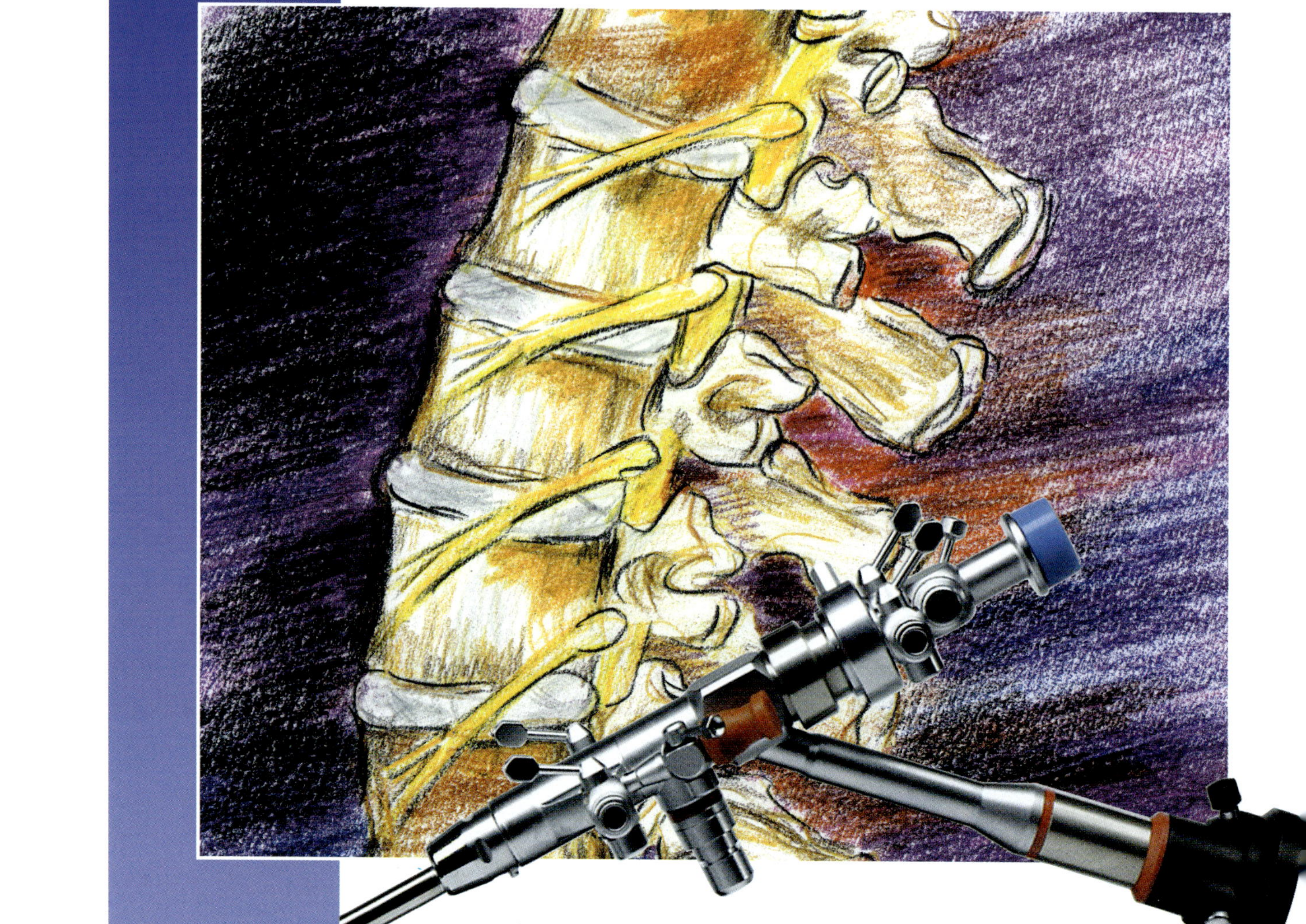

»YESS«
Yeung Endoscopic Spine Surgery System

A milestone in the therapy of disc herniations

The spine surgery instrument set by Yeung »YESS« system for arthroscopic microdiscectomy (AMD) and spinal endoscopy allows the surgeon to see anatomical structures and pathological changes in previously unimaginable quality.

The ability to perform minimally invasive interventions under vision opens up not only a broad spectrum of surgical techniques in disc herniation but also allows the evaluation of a wide range of pathological conditions.

The unique design of the endoscope system provides optimum operating conditions. One major feature is the optical irrigation system that guarantees a clear, unhindered view even in difficult situations.

Opening new dimensions

-->%

Take this opportunity to order detailed information about "YESS". Simply send this form by **fax ++49-70 43 -35 300** or by mail.

Send me:
- ❏ Further information
- ❏ Video
- ❏ Details of special courses

Your name and address: _____
_____
_____
Tel./Fax: _____

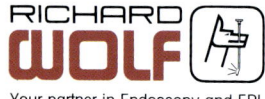
Your partner in Endoscopy and EPL

RICHARD WOLF GmbH · D-75434 Knittlingen · PF 1164 · Tel.: 0 70 43 / 35-0 · Fax: 0 70 43 / 3 53 00 · Subsidiaries in Austria · Belgium · France · Germany · Great Britain · USA

109 An Adjustable Silicone Gastric Band for Laparoscopic Treatment of Morbid Obesity—Techniques and Results

FRANCO FAVRETTI, M.D. - UNIVERSITY OF PADUA, PADUA, ITALY; GUY-BERNARD CADIERE, M.D. - FREE UNIVERSITY OF BRUSSELS, BRUSSELS, BELGIUM; GIANNI SEGATO, M.D. - UNIVERSITY OF PADUA, PADUA, ITALY; JACQUES HIMPENS, M.D. - FREE UNIVERSITY OF BRUSSELS, BRUSSELS, BELGIUM; FRANCESCO DE MARCHI, M.D. - UNIVERSITY OF PADUA, PADUA, ITALY; ELIE CAPELLUTO, M.D. - FREE UNIVERSITY OF BRUSSELS, BRUSSELS, BELGIUM; MAURIZIO DE LUCA, M.D. - UNIVERSITY OF PADUA, PADUA, ITALY; QUENTIN GAUDISSART, M.D. - FREE UNIVERSITY OF BRUSSELS, BRUSSELS, BELGIUM; MARIO LISE, M.D. - UNIVERSITY OF PADUA, PADUA, ITALY

115 A New Technique for Laparoscopic Left Adrenalectomy

ANDRAS PAPP, M.D.; ANDRAS VERECZKEI, M.D.; ÖRS PETER HORVÁTH, M.D., D.SC. - MEDICAL UNIVERSITY OF PÉCS, PÉCS, HUNGARY; ZOLTÁN SZÁBO, PH.D., F.I.C.S. - MICROSURGERY & OPERATIVE ENDOSCOPY TRAINING INSTITUTE, SAN FRANCISCO, CA

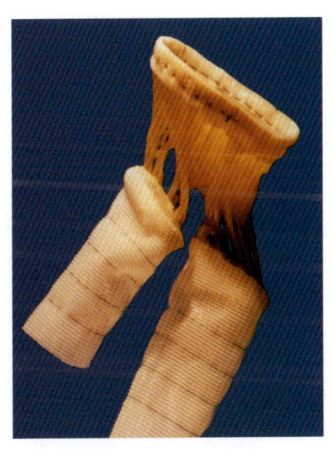

CARDIOVASCULAR SURGERY

121 Current and Advanced Prostheses for Cardiac Valvular Replacement and Reconstructive Surgery

W. R. ERIC JAMIESON, M.D., F.R.C.S. (C) - UNIVERSITY HEART CENTRE, ST. PAUL'S HOSPITAL, VANCOUVER HOSPITAL AND HEALTH SCIENCES CENTRE, VANCOUVER, CANADA

151 The Incomplete Ring with Modulated Flexibility: A New Concept of Mitral Annuloplasty

WAJIH MAAZOUZI, M.D.; YOUNES CHEIKHAOUI, M.D.; RHIZLENE DRISSI KACEMI, M.D.; MOHAMMED MESSOUAK, M.D.; SOUAD BOUAICHI, M.D. - IBN SINA HOSPITAL, RABAT, MOROCCO

157 Off-Pump Coronary Artery Bypass (OPCAB) Surgery

CHRISTOPH SCHMITZ, M.D.; ARMIN WELZ, M.D. - UNIVERSITY OF BONN, BONN, GERMANY

161 Endovascular Procedures Under Near-Real-Time MRI Guidance: Present Status and Future Perspectives

YVES-MARIE DION, M.D., M.SC., F.A.C.S., F.R.C.S.C. - QUEBEC BIOMATERIALS INSTITUTE, QUEBEC CITY, CANADA; GEOFFROY WARNIER DE WAILLY, M.D. - LAVAL UNIVERSITY, QUEBEC CITY, CANADA; CHRISTIAN MOISAN, PH.D. - ST FRANÇOIS D'ASSISE HOSPITAL, CENTRE HOSPITALIER UNIVERSITAIRE DE QUEBEC, QUEBEC CITY, CANADA

The only PEG lavage that offers your patients a choice of four fruit flavors.

- Indicated for bowel cleansing prior to colonoscopy or barium enema x-ray examination
- No significant changes in fluid and electrolyte balance
- Virtually no net absorption or excretion of salts or water

As with all PEG lavages, nausea, abdominal fullness, and bloating are the most frequent adverse reactions, occurring in up to 50% of patients. Oral medication administered within 1 hour of the start of administration of Colyte with Flavor Packs may be flushed from the gastrointestinal tract and not absorbed.

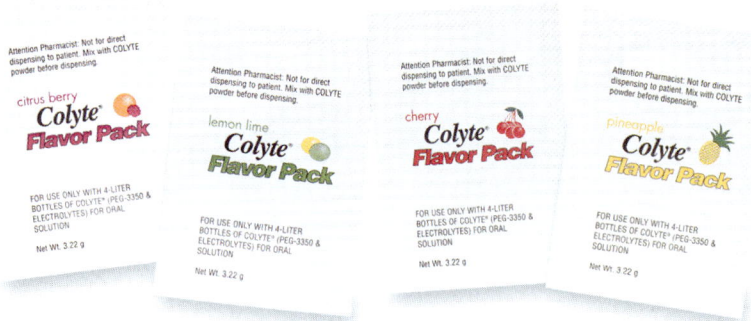

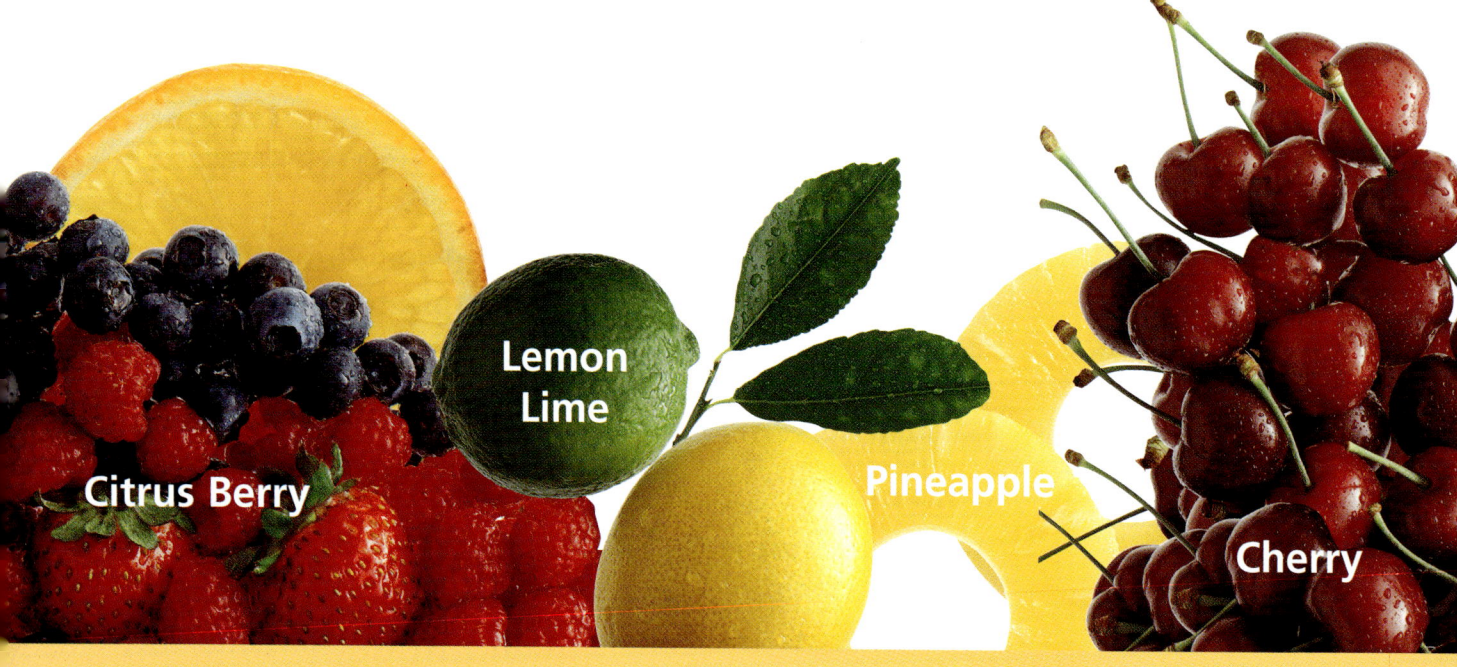

Citrus Berry · Lemon Lime · Pineapple · Cherry

Colyte with Flavor Packs
PEG–3350 and Electrolytes for Oral Solution

A tasteful solution

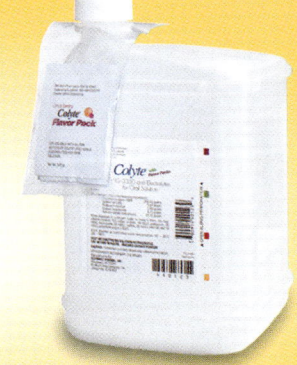

10099 9/00

© 2000 Schwarz Pharma, Inc., Milwaukee, WI 53201, USA

168 Use of Endovascular Stents in the Peripheral Circulation
HANASOGE T. GIRISHKUMAR, M.D., F.A.C.S.; VELLORE S. PARITHIVEL, M.D., F.A.C.S.; SATISH C. KHANEJA, M.D., F.A.C.S.; PAUL H. GERST, M.D., F.A.C.S. - BRONX-LEBANON HOSPITAL CENTER, BRONX, NY; RENATO BERROYA, M.D., F.A.C.S. - ST. FRANCIS HOSPITAL, ROSLYN, NY

TRANSPLANTATION

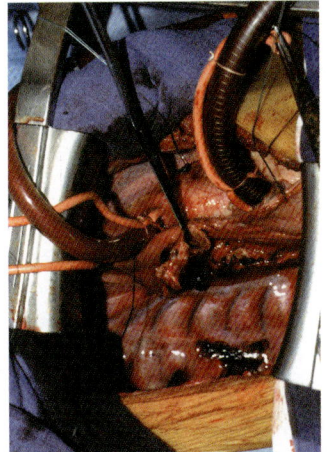

178 Human Heart, Lung, and Heart-lung Transplantation
CARSTEN SCHRÖDER, M.D.; PAOLO MACCHIARINI, M.D., PH.D. - HEIDEHAUS HOSPITAL, HANNOVER MEDICAL SCHOOL, HANNOVER, GERMANY

186 Preoperative Imaging of Donor Patients for Adult Right-Lobe Liver Transplantation
IHAB R. KAMEL, M.D., PH.D.; JONATHAN B. KRUSKAL, M.D., PH.D.; GISELE WARMBRAND, M.D.; KEVIN F. REYNOLDS, R.T.R.; VASSILIOS RAPTOPOULOS, M.D. - BETH ISRAEL DEACONESS MEDICAL CENTER AND HARVARD MEDICAL SCHOOL, BOSTON, MA

ORTHOPAEDIC SURGERY

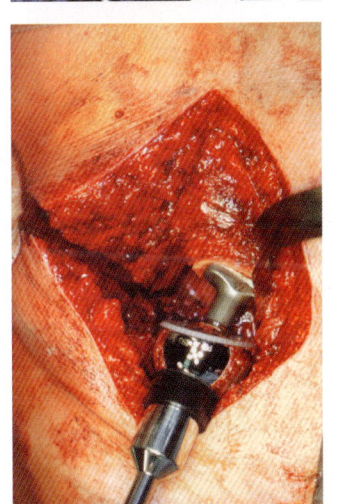

195 Management of Non-Union with Pulsed, Low-Intensity Ultrasound Therapy–International Results
VICTOR H. FRANKEL, M.D., PH.D., K.N.O. - NEW YORK UNIVERSITY, NEW YORK, NY; KOSAKU MIZUNO, M.D., PH.D. - KOBE UNIVERSITY SCHOOL OF MEDICINE, HYOGO, JAPAN

201 Prosthetic Design and Early Clinical Results of the TRAC® (Two Radii Area Contact) Knee Prosthesis
LAWRENCE A. POTTENGER, M.D., PH.D.; LOUIS DRAGANICH, PH.D. - UNIVERSITY OF CHICAGO, CHICAGO, IL

205 The ABG II Hip System Implantation Technique
CHRISTIAN NOURISSAT, M.D.; JOSE ADREY, M.D.; DANIEL BERTEAUX, M.D.; CHRISTIAN GOALARD, M.D.; WILLIAM WALTER, M.D. - MATER MISERICORDIAE HOSPITAL, SYDNEY, AUSTRALIA

212 Revision of Failed Total Hip Prosthesis with Insertion of a Hydroxyapatite-Coated Femoral Component
JORDI CASAS-SABATER, M.D.; MARC COTS-PONS, M.D.; FÉLIX CASTILLO-GARCÍA, M.D. - HOSPITAL GENERAL DE CATALUNYA, BARCELONA, SPAIN; ERNANE DODERO REIS, M.D., THE MOUNT SINAI MEDICAL CENTER, NEW YORK, NY; JOAQUIM RODRIGUEZ-MIRALLES, M.D., PH.D. - BARCELONA UNIVERSITY, BARCELONA, SPAIN

221 Bipolar Hemiarthroplasty for Treatment of Femoral Neck Fractures in Geriatric Patients–Surgical Technique and Outcome
HANS JOSEF ERLI, M.D.; PETER KLEVER, M.D.; OTHMAR PAAR, M.D. - UNIVERSITY HOSPITAL OF THE RWTH, AACHEN, GERMANY

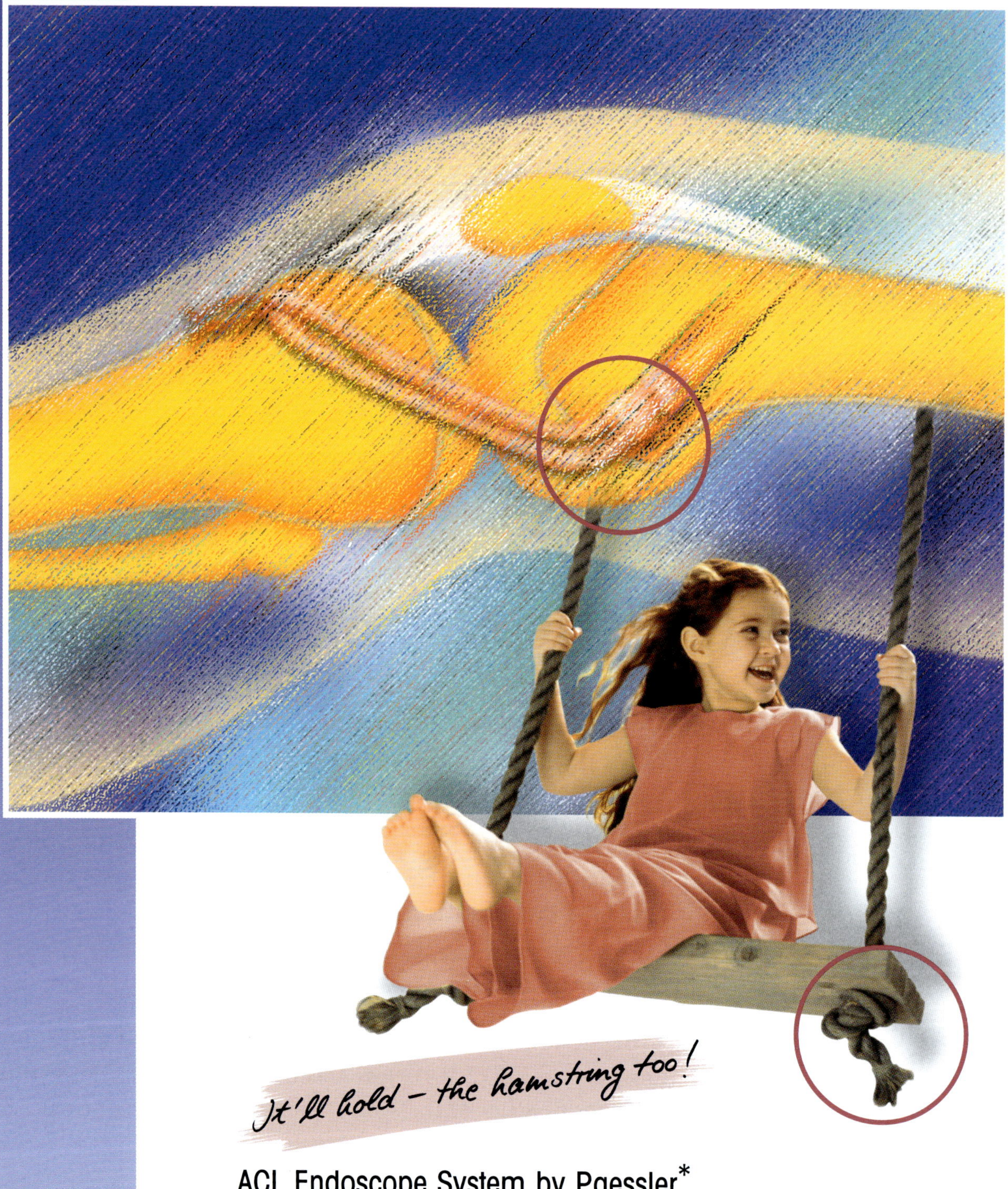

It'll hold – the hamstring too!

ACL Endoscope System by Paessler*

The innovative endoscope system from R. Wolf allows individual solutions for successful reconstruction of the anterior cruciate ligament: With the semitendinosus and gracilis tendons using the press-fit technique with bone plugs and without implants. With the patellar tendon with a bone plug using only the press-fit technique. Second look intervention following ACL an operation and renewed instability.

*Dr. med. Hans H. Paessler, ATOS-Klinik, D-69115 Heidelberg

For detailed information on the "ACL Paessler" by **Fax +49 70 43 35-300** or post.

Please send me: From: _____

❏ Further information _____
❏ Video _____
❏ CD-Rom _____
❏ Information on courses Tel./Fax: _____

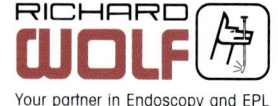
Your partner in Endoscopy and EPL

e-mail: info@richard-wolf.com · www.richard-wolf.com

RICHARD WOLF GmbH · D-75434 Knittlingen · PF 1164 · Tel.: +49 70 43 35-0 · Fax: +49 70 43 35-300 · Subsidiaries in Austria · Belgium · France · Germany · Great Britain · USA

226 Management of Venous Thrombosis and Thromboembolism: Prevention and Treatment

RODGER L. BICK, M.D., PH.D., F.A.C.P. - DALLAS THROMBOSIS HEMOSTASIS & DIFFICULT HEMATOLOGY CLINICAL CENTER, DALLAS, TX

237 Hydroxyapatite-Coated Femoral Arthroplasties: A Long-Term Study Through 29 Corail® Prostheses Explanted During a Ten-Year Survey

DOMINIQUE C.R. HARDY, M.D. - UNIVERSITY HOSPITAL SAINT-PIERRE, BRUSSELS, BELGIUM; PATRICK FRAYSSINET, M.D., PH.D. - UNIVERSITY OF TOULOUSE-RANGUEIL, TOULOUSE, FRANCE

249 Advances in Deep-Vein Thrombosis Treatment

JAMES EDWIN MUNTZ, M.D., F.A.C.P. - BAYLOR COLLEGE OF MEDICINE, HOUSTON, TX

255 Treatment of Articular Cartilage Defects with the Autologous Chondrocyte Transplantation (ACT)

ANDREAS BURKART, M.D.; ANDREAS BALTHASAR IMHOFF, M.D. - TECHNICAL UNIVERSITY OF MUNICH, MUNICH, GERMANY

261 Bone Grafts

MATTHEW J.W. HUBBLE, M.B., B.S., F.R.C.S. (ORTH) - UNIVERSITY OF BRISTOL, BRISTOL, ENGLAND, UK

266 Percutaneous Microdecompressive Endoscopic Thoracic Discectomy for Herniated Thoracic Discs

JOHN C. CHIU, M.D., F.R.C.S., F.A.C.S.; THOMAS J. CLIFFORD, M.D.; ROMULO SISON, O.P.A.-C., C.S.T. - CALIFORNIA CENTER FOR MINIMALLY INVASIVE SPINE SURGERY, THOUSAND OAKS, CA

PLASTIC & RECONSTRUCTIVE SURGERY

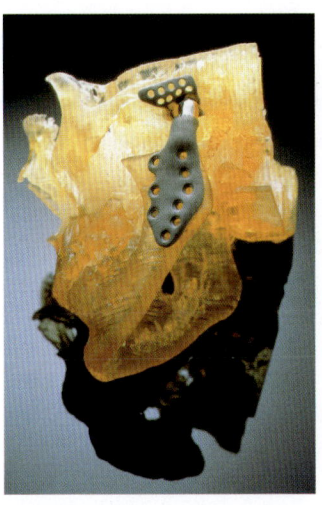

273 Use of the Christensen TMJ Fossa-Eminence Prosthesis™ System: A Retrospective Clinical Study

CARRIE BRITTON, B.S. - TMJ IMPLANTS, INC., GOLDEN, CO; ROBERT W. CHRISTENSEN, D.D.S. - CLEMSON UNIVERSITY, CLEMSON, SC; JAMES T. CURRY, D.D.S. - HIGHLAND RANCH, CO

283 Subperiosteal Rejuvenation of the Forehead

JAY M. PENSLER, M.D. - NORTHWESTERN UNIVERSITY MEDICAL SCHOOL, CHICAGO, IL; KAVEH ALIZADEH, M.D. - LONG ISLAND PLASTIC SURGICAL GROUP, GARDEN CITY, NY

Foreword

JACK J. JAKIMOWICZ M.D., PH.D., F.R.C.S.ED.

With the introduction of minimal access surgery and its steady proliferation during the past decade, medicine and particularly surgery, became strongly technology driven. A demand for early, reliable information on emerging technologies and surgical techniques resulted. *Surgical Technology International* responded to this demand by providing the medical professionals community, as well as the corporate sector, factual information on new technical developments and newly developed surgical techniques. It created a platform for exposing technological novelties, particularly those newly emerging. Furthermore, *Surgical Technology International* offered the pioneers and experts in the field an opportunity to review and exchange their experience. This current issue is a broad form of new applications and techniques. Information on new devices and concepts will not disappoint the reader; once more, *Surgical Technology International* will fulfill all expectations.

Preface

To the casual observer of medical science, surgical practice retains an ancient aura of destructive procedures aimed at removal of diseased organs and tissues. The more sophisticated student of modern surgical practice has gained an appreciation for the technological advances supporting minimally invasive procedures. Surgical Technology X explores the world of today's most forward-thinking surgical experts with an eye toward restoration of form and function.

Within this issue you will find a fascinating series of articles from the international surgical community detailing the use of new techniques and materials destined to augment and replace human components failing from age and pathology. We begin to visualize the product of interdisciplinary research as operative procedures precisely localize disease, attack with minimal lateral damage and insert highly engineered biological or inert replacement materials to heal the suffering patient.

As in prior editions, you will find reviews of common clinical problems to help the clinician prevent complications. The featured group of specialized procedures may trigger ideas for future research to develop novel approaches to cure disease and correct deformity. New instrumentation, applications of energy, manipulation of host response and implantation of devices and adjuvant materials are all displayed for possible use by today and tomorrow's advanced surgeon. The editors hope you will enjoy and comment on our latest offering, Surgical Technology International X.

Zoltán Szabó, Ph.D., F.I.C.S.
James E. Lewis, M.D., F.A.C.O.G.
Gary A. Fantini, M.D., F.A.C.S.
Raghu S. Savalgi, M.D., Ph.D.(surg), F.R.C.S.

APLIGRAF® Offers Superior Efficacy in Less Time

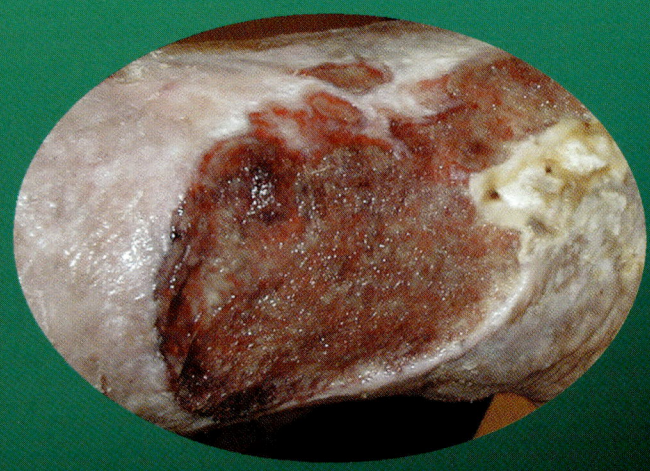

Before APLIGRAF*
80-year-old male with a venous leg ulcer
of >10 years' duration
Prior treatment: inelastic compression therapy
(Unna's boot); platelet-derived growth factor for 21 weeks

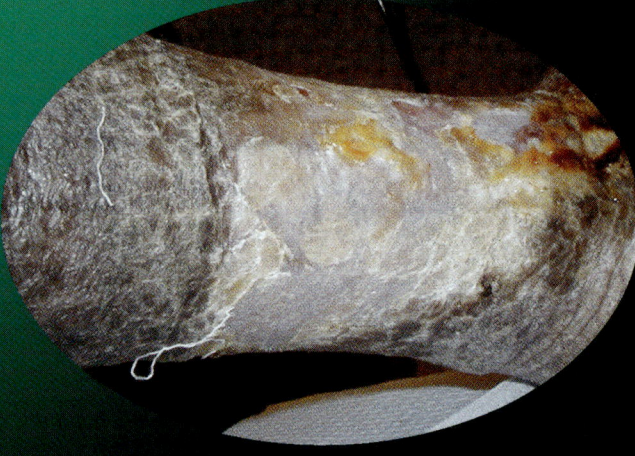

After APLIGRAF
Ulcer 100% healed by 16 weeks

For more information or to order the product, call
1-888-HEAL-2-DAY (1-888-432-5232).
Or visit our Web site at www.APLIGRAF.com

APLIGRAF should not be used on infected wounds or on patients with known hypersensitivities to any components of APLIGRAF or the shipping medium.

Please consult the complete prescribing information for a description of epidermal and dermal elements contained in APLIGRAF.

*The case presented here represents the experience of a single patient and may not be typical of all patients.

REFERENCES: 1. Wilkins LM, Watson SR, Prosky SJ, et al. Development of a bilayered living skin construct for clinical applications. *Biotechnol Bioeng* 1994;43:747-756. 2. Data on file, Novartis Pharmaceuticals Corporation and Organogenesis Inc.

INTENDED USE/INDICATION
Apligraf is indicated for use with standard therapeutic compression for the treatment of noninfected partial- and full-thickness skin ulcers due to venous insufficiency of greater than 1 month in duration and that have not adequately responded to conventional ulcer therapy.

CONTRAINDICATIONS
Apligraf is contraindicated for use on clinically infected wounds and in patients with known allergies to bovine collagen or hypersensitivity to the components of the shipping medium: agarose, L-glutamine, hydrocortisone/bovine serum albumin, bovine insulin, human transferrin, triiodothyronine, ethanolamine, O-phosphorylethanolamine, adenine, selenious acid, DMEM powder, HAM's F-12 powder.

WARNINGS AND PRECAUTIONS
Do not open and do not use Apligraf after the expiration date or if the pH is not within the acceptable range (6.8-7.7).
A clinical determination of wound infection should be made based on all of the signs and symptoms of infection.

Allergic reactions to products containing components present in the Apligraf agarose shipping medium (see CONTRAINDICATIONS section) or bovine collagen (a component of Apligraf) have been reported. Discontinue product use if a patient shows evidence of an immunological reaction. Patients should notify their physician of any symptoms of an allergic reaction. In studies with 361 patients, no allergic reactions to Apligraf were reported.

The persistence of Apligraf cells on the wound and the safety of this device in venous leg ulcers beyond one year has not been evaluated. Testing to date has not revealed a tumorigenic potential of the cells contained in the device. However, the long term potential of skin cancers from these cells is unknown.

The safety and the effectiveness of Apligraf have not been established for patients receiving greater than 5 device applications.

ADVERSE EVENTS
In the controlled clinical study conducted in patients with ulcers due to venous insufficiency of greater than 1 month in duration, the incidence of adverse events was comparable between the 2 study groups, with the exception of suspected infection, which was reported more frequently in Apligraf-treated (29.2%) than control patients (14.0%). There were 1 life-threatening and 3 severe infections in the Apligraf group and none in the control arm. Of these, two severe infections were considered related to treatment, however, one occurred one month after the last application of Apligraf and the other occurred following application on a pre-existing *Pseudomonas* infection. While the overall incidence of wound infection was higher in the Apligraf arm, the incidence of wound closure was 72/130 (55.4%) and 54/110 (49.1%) for Apligraf and control-treated patients, respectively.

HOW SUPPLIED
Apligraf is supplied in a heavy gauge polyethylene bag with a 10% CO_2/air atmosphere and agarose nutrient medium, ready for single use. To maintain cell viability, Apligraf should be kept in the sealed bag at 20°C to 31°C until use. Apligraf is supplied as a circular disk approximately 75 mm in diameter and 0.75 mm thick.

Manufactured by:
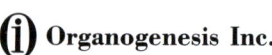

Distributed and marketed by:
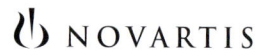
Novartis Pharmaceuticals Corporation
East Hanover, New Jersey 07936

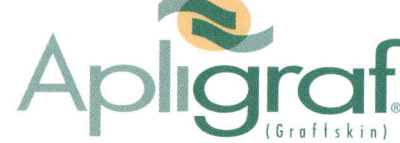

©2000 Novartis   Printed in U.S.A.   4/00   C-APG-1013   BIOENGINEERED TO CLOSE MORE WOUNDS FASTER

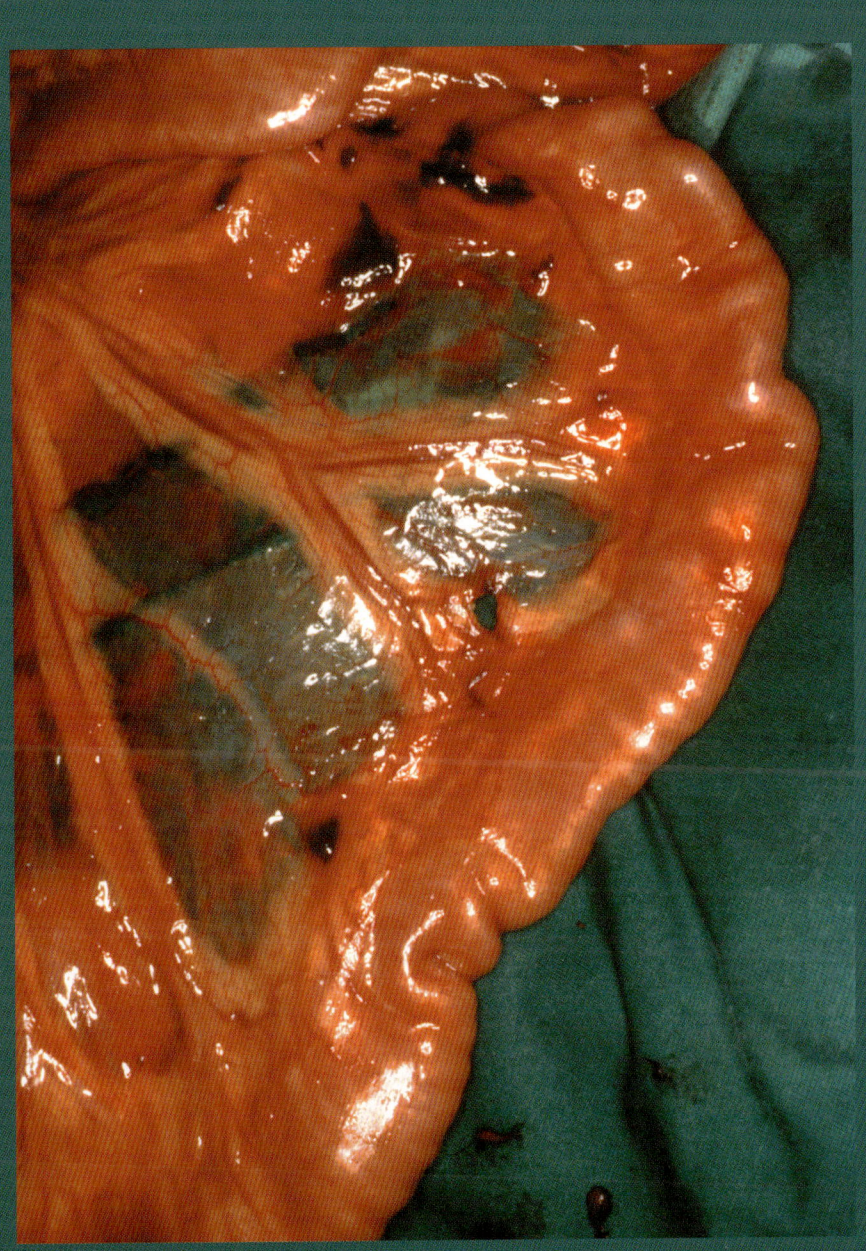

Surgical Overview

Bioengineered to Close More Wounds Faster

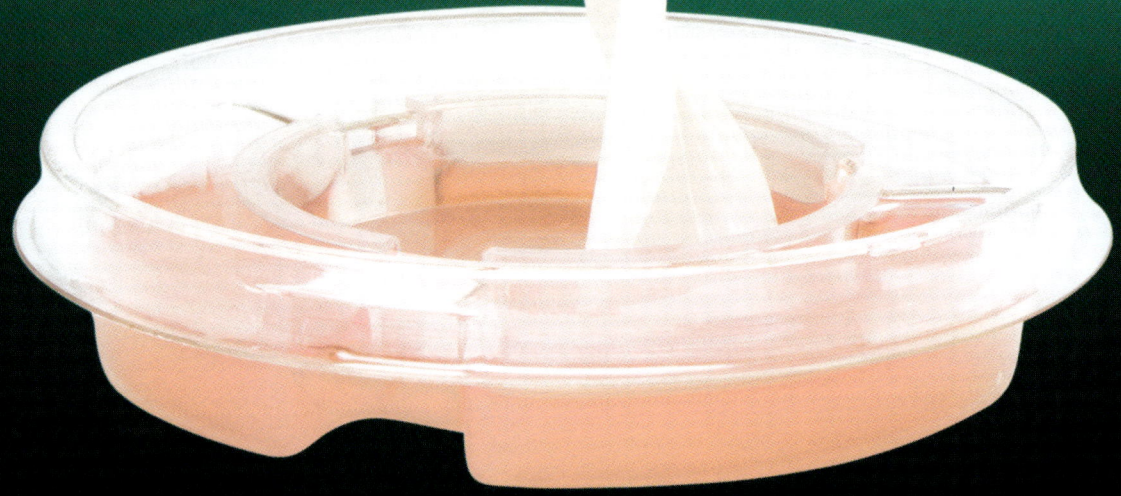

SIGNIFICANTLY MORE EFFECTIVE than compression therapy alone—APLIGRAF® achieved closure in more patients with ulcers >1 month's duration at 24 weeks than compression therapy alone (N=240, 57% vs 40%, $P=.022$)

THE ONLY BILAYERED SKIN SUBSTITUTE with a viable dermal and epidermal layer that approximates skin in structure and barrier function*[1,2]
- APLIGRAF contains matrix proteins, expresses cytokines, and prevents desiccation
- APLIGRAF does not contain melanocytes, Langerhans' cells, macrophages, and lymphocytes, or other structures such as blood vessels, hair follicles, or sweat glands

NO REJECTIONS REPORTED TO DATE in over 10,000 clinical and commercial applications[2]

The incidence and severity of adverse events both attributed and not attributed to treatment were comparable between groups with the exception of suspected wound infection, which was reported in 29% of cases in the APLIGRAF group and in 14% of cases in the control group. However, among patients with suspected wound infection, APLIGRAF-treated patients achieved an overall higher rate of complete wound closure.

*The persistence of APLIGRAF cells on the wound and the safety of this device in

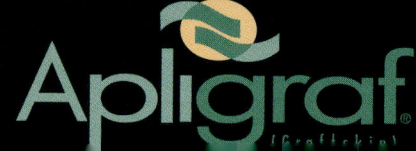

Tissue Engineering in the 21st Century

BORIS A. NASSERI, M.D.
RESEARCH FELLOW

JOSEPH P. VACANTI, M.D., F.A.C.S.
JOHN HOMANS PROFESSOR OF SURGERY

HARVARD MEDICAL SCHOOL
MASSACHUSETTS GENERAL HOSPITAL
BOSTON, MA

Traumatic and end-stage organ loss or tissue damage remains a devastating issue for everyone, and a major problem for millions of patients. It has been estimated that each year in the United States more than 8 million surgical operations are performed to solve these health problems.[1]

Therapy has improved tremendously with transplantation, reconstructive surgery, and artificial life-support systems in the second half of the last century. Murray and colleagues performed their first successful human organ transplantation in 1954, transplanting a kidney from an identical twin to his ill brother.[2] This was the first step into a new area in medicine. Just a few years later, in the early 1960s, Murray again transplanted a non-genetically identical kidney. In December 1967, Barnard performed the first heart transplantation in a man dying of heart disease.[3]

These steps and improved immunosuppression since the 1970s allowed transplantation to become a worldwide common therapeutic approach for end-stage organ failure patients. Soon thereafter, the number of patients on transplantation waiting lists far exceeded the availability of donor organs. In 1989, 19,095 patients were awaiting transplantation. In May 2000, this number had increased to 69,728 (Table 1).[4]

On April 4, 1969, Cooley and colleagues successfully bridged a patient to receive heart transplantation with a left ventricular assist device (LVAD) for 64 hours.[5] Currently, transplantation patients have an improved quality of life; patients with artificial heart devices can be bridged for more than 1000 days[6] and heart recovery with LVAD explantation is feasible.[7-9] However, limitations exist regarding organ transplantation or permanent artificial organ replacement, which include lifelong immunosuppression and anticoagulation therapy with all the disadvantages such as rejection and tumor formation, hemorrhage, and thromboembolic events. The increasing lack of donor organs is a constant problem in transplantation medicine. This lack of organs and the continuing effort of scientists to improve quality of life of transplant patients under lifelong immunosuppression, has stimulated research in tissue engineering and selective cell transplantation.

Tissue engineering is "an interdisciplinary field that applies principles and methods of engineering and the life sciences toward the development of biological substitutes that restore, maintain, and improve the function of damaged tissues and organs".[1,10,11] Tissue engineering efforts are currently being undertaken for every type of tissue and organ (Fig. 1).[12] Development and cell biologists, engineers, material scientists, and physicians are involved in the process of completing the puzzle of neoorganogenesis, which should lead to the fabrication of new, physiologic functioning tissue using living cells and matrices. To reach this goal, four strategies have been explored: 1) controlled release of soluble signals such as angiogenic factors or growth factors, 2) injection of allogenic or xenogenic isolated cells replacing lost organ function, 3) guided tissue regeneration using engineered matrices, and 4) implantation of cell-matrix-constructs.

This review focuses on the role of cell/matrix constructs.

CELL-MATRIX CONSTRUCTS

This approach is based on the following biological observations:[13] 1) every

Table 1. Transplantation Waiting List in the U.S. Data from the UNOS National Patient Waiting List.

Organ	Number of Patients Waiting for Transplantation in: 1989	May 2000
Kidney	16,294	45,273
Liver	827	15,359
Pancreas	320	917
Kidney-pancreas	0	2,278
Heart	1320	4,143
Lung	94	3,614
Heart-lung	240	209
Intestine	0	124
Total	19,095	69,728

Data from the UNOS National Patient Waiting List.

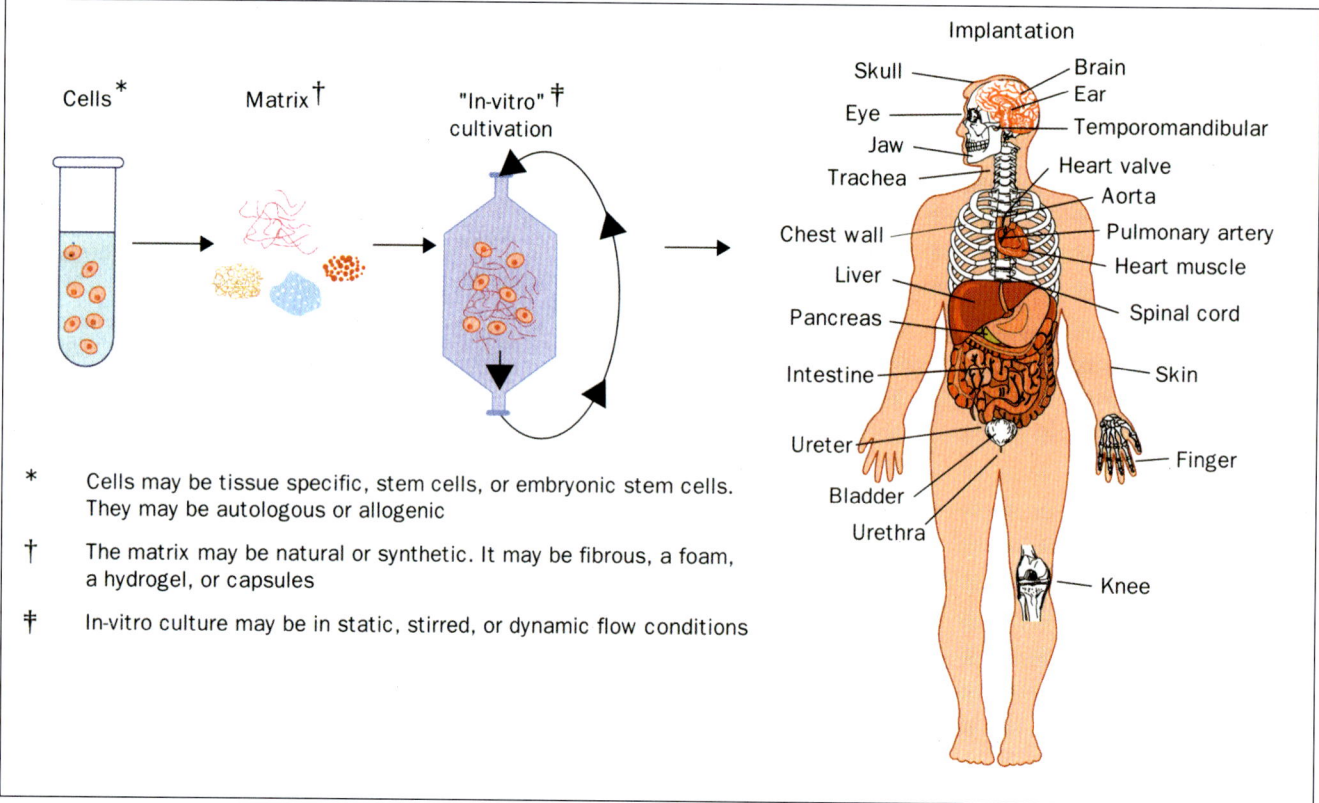

* Cells may be tissue specific, stem cells, or embryonic stem cells. They may be autologous or allogenic
† The matrix may be natural or synthetic. It may be fibrous, a foam, a hydrogel, or capsules
‡ In-vitro culture may be in static, stirred, or dynamic flow conditions

Figure 1. Principle of tissue engineering. Reproduced with permission from Lancet (1999); 354 Suppl 1:SI32-4.

living tissue in an organism undergoes constant remodeling; 2) dissociated cells tend to reform their native structures under appropriate environmental conditions;[13-15] 3) normal parenchymal cells are anchorage-dependent and require an extracellular matrix (ECM) and three-dimensional (3-D) structure to guide regulation;[13,16,17] and 4) the volume of implantable tissue is limited by requirements of nutrition, gas exchange, and removal of waste products.[13,18]

CELLS

Cells can be drawn from different sources. Tissue for cell-matrix constructs can be allogenic (from different members of the same species), xenogenic (from different species), syngeneic (genetically identical individual), or autologous (from the same person). Allogenic and xenogenic cells used in an open manner, in contrast to a closed system, are defined as cells in direct contact with the host environment;

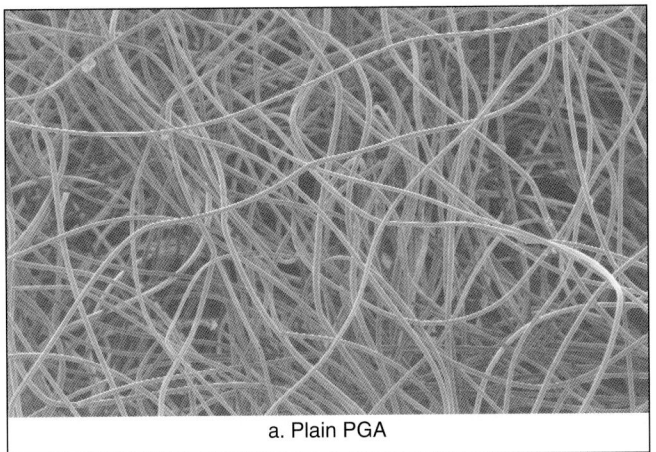
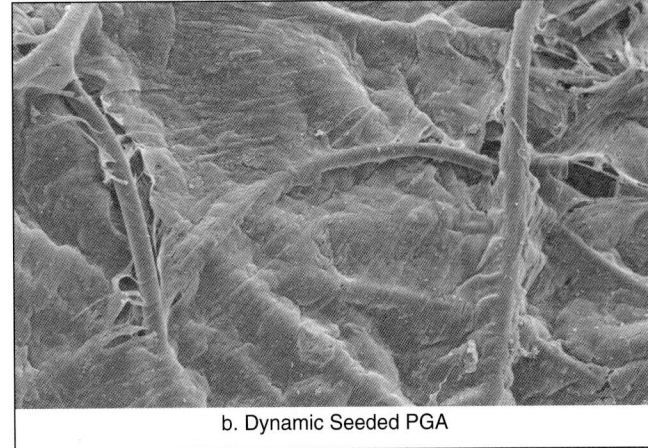

Figure 2. Scanning electron micrographs of PGA. a: Plain PGA, no cells (x62). b: PGA after 10 days, dynamic seeding with smooth muscle cells (x250).

therefore, these cells are not protected from the host immune response and immunosuppression therapy would be limiting.

The ability to isolate and expand cells in vitro is the main reason tissue-engineering approaches concentrate on autologous cells; but this ability is dependent on the cell type and can be influenced by culture conditions. Whereas endothelial cells, smooth muscle cells, and skeletal muscle satellite cells proliferate rapidly, hepatocytes in culture proliferate poorly and widely accepted is that adult cardiomyocytes do not proliferate. This observation sparked the interest in using proliferating fetal or neonatal cell sources or genetically manipulated cells. An ideal reservoir would be undifferentiated stem cells, which have the ability to differentiate into a large variety of cells.

MATRIX

An ideal matrix should fulfill certain criteria : 1) be biocompatible and bioabsorbable; 2) not be immunogenic; 3) be mechanically flexible and reproducible to bring it in different shapes and structures, and retain their shape post-implantation to provide mechanical support to maintain a space for tissue to form;[19] 4) the surface should support cell growth and function physiologically; and 5) induce angiogenesis for nutritional support of the newly formed tissue.

The most widely used polymers, fulfilling these criteria, have been the family of polylactic acid (PLA) and polyglycolic acid (PGA) (Fig. 2), as well as their copolymers (PLGA).[20,21] These polymers were first developed as absorbable suture material (PGA known as Dexon™,[22] Sherwood Medical, St. Louis, MO) and were already FDA approved for in vivo use. They proved to be readily processable into a variety of shapes and forms.[20,21] Their absorption rate depend on the design and varies from months to years.[23,24]

Other polymers are currently in use, such as the family of polyhydroxyalkanoates (PHAs) (Fig. 3), or hydrogels like Pluronic F-127 (co-polymer made from 70% ethylene oxide and 30% propylene oxide), Matrigel (a basement membrane matrix extracted from a mouse sarcoma), or Alginate (polysaccharide from species of brown algae).

LIVER

In the last 15 years, our laboratory has focused on development of 3-D polymer-hepatocyte constructs, based on biodegradable scaffolds. Successful implantation is dependent on the following conditions: 1) sufficient mass of cells must be transplanted and become engrafted after cultured *in vitro*, 2) transplanted hepatocytes must survive *in vivo*, 3) transplanted cells must remain or become functional, and 4) hepatotrophic stimulation must be provided.[25]

Different studies have shown transplantation of these constructs into the mesentery and omentum of small and large animals is feasible and effective.[17,26-29] The number of hepatocytes surviving the initial hypoxic phase after transplantation can be improved by porto-caval shunts and partial hepatectomy, which lead to increased levels of hepatic mitogens in the systemic circulation.[25,30-33] Small intestine submucosa (SIS) has been used for porto-caval shunts in rats.[34]

Other approaches to increase hepatocyte survival are co-seeding of hepatocytes with islet of Langerhans cells,

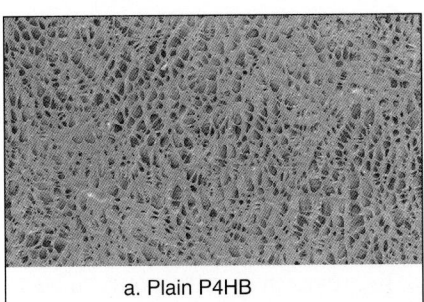
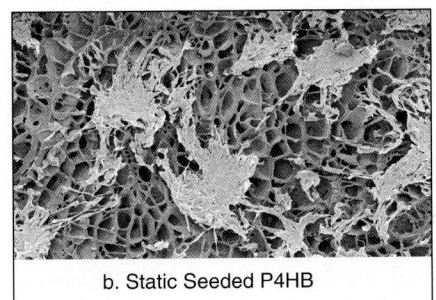
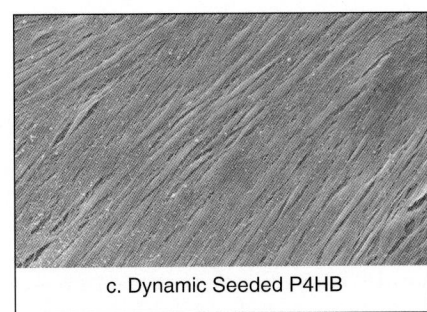

Figure 3. Scanning electron micrographs of P4HB. a: Plain P4HB, no cells (x125). b: P4HB after 3 days, static seeding with smooth muscle cells (x125). c: P4HB after 10 days, dynamic seeding with smooth muscle cells (x250).

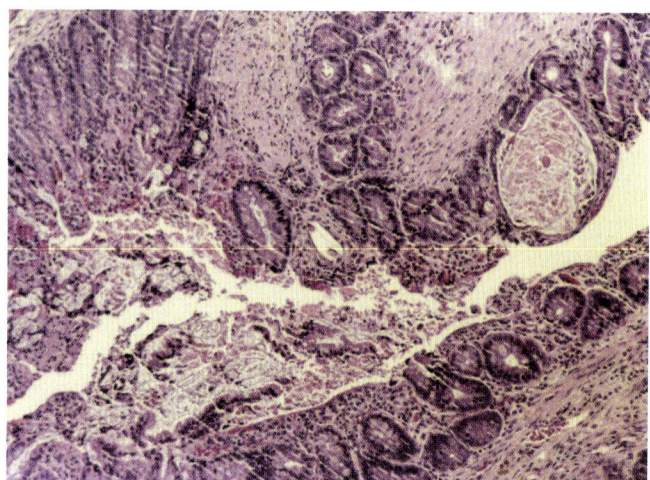

Figure 4. Tissue engineered small intestine (x100): PGA tubes (5 x 10 x 2 mm) coated with 5% PLLA and collagen, seeded with neonatal rat small intestinal organoid units. Polymer/cell constructs were then implanted into the omentum of adult rats. Animals were sacrificed after 6 weeks. Intestinal epithelium that includes a neomucosa and submucosa has organized into crypts and villi. A mucosal layer containing glands has formed. (Courtesy Dr. Kohei Ogawa).

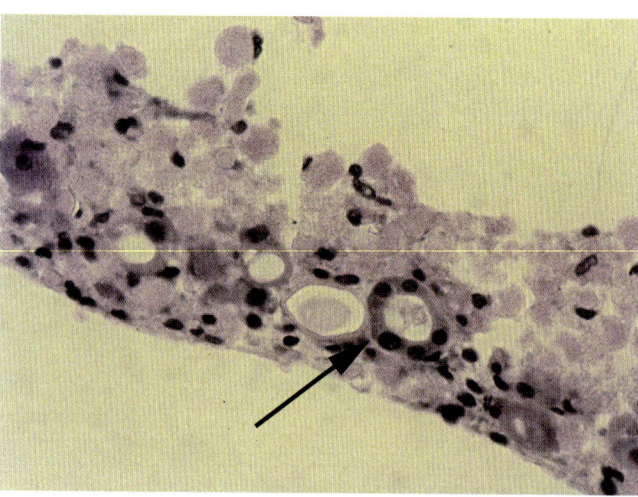

Figure 5. Tissue engineered liver (x400): PGA tubes (5 x 10 x 2 mm) coated with 5% PLLA and collagen, seeded and cultured with small hepatocytes and non-parenchymal liver cells from adolescent rats under flow conditions in a bioreactor for 3 weeks. Tubular formation was observed (see arrow). (Courtesy Dr. Kohei Ogawa).

or microspheres loaded with epidermal growth factor (EGF).[35] In a study comparing HGF-transgenic mice hepatocyte (over-expressing Hepatic Growth Factor) with wild-type mice hepatocyte transplantation on poly-L-lactic acid (PLLA), a significant improvement of hepatocyte organization and engraftment from HGF transgenic hepatocytes was present compared with wild-type hepatocytes.[36]

Flow conditions during cell culture provide a more conducive environment for hepatocyte metabolism and albumin synthesis than static conditions (Fig. 5). Co-culturing hepatocytes and sinusoidal endothelial cells under continuous flow conditions on PLLA induces spheroid formation with endothelial cells lining the outside of HEPATOCYTE spheroids.[37] Asonuma showed that as little as 12% of the whole liver mass in heterotopic partial liver transplantation (HLT) reduces serum bilirubin significantly in 24 hours in a fashion similar to whole-organ orthotopic liver transplantation (OLT).[38] Uyama and colleagues transplanted a hepatocyte mass equivalent to a whole rat liver into a 5-day prevascularized polyvinyl alcohol (PVA) sponge device. Prevascularization involved implanting the sponge devices into the mesentery or omentum. After 7 days post-transplantation, up to 18% of the hepatocytes were engrafted and functioning. Preoperative bilirubin levels could be reduced from 9.1 ± 0.46 mg/dL to 6.8 ± 0.46 mg/dL after 1 week.[30]

Using cell/polymer constructs to engineer liver tissue is encouraging, but much work remains to be done. One of our main focuses is to provide the engineered tissue with microvascular architecture. Three-dimensional printing (3-DP) is a novel approach of constructing polymers in complex geometric shapes with highly precise intrinsic architecture. PLGA in a liquid state is expelled onto a powder base from a modified ink-jet printer, computer-driven to create two-dimensional (2-D) polymer patterns. The polymer solidifies upon contact with the base. After one layer of polymer is expelled and solidified, subsequent layers are stacked on top. The powder is then removed, creating empty spaces within the polymer. Using this technology termed, "solid free form fabrication," highly complex and intricate 3-D polymers can be created.[39,40] Porous and interconnected channels formed by this technique allow blood vessels to spread into the polymer and supply tissue with oxygen and nutrients immediately after transplantation.

INTESTINE

"Short bowel syndrome," after major surgical resection, is a condition of malabsorption and malnutrition. Parental and home nutritional support has improved survival and lifestyles of patients with this disorder. However, morbidity with prolonged hyperalimentation remains significant, with complications of infections and line sepsis, progressive liver dysfunction, loss of vascular access, and pulmonary embolism.[41-43] Although intestinal transplantation has become a feasible alternative, it has serious limitations. The overall worldwide survival rate for isolated small bowel transplantation is currently 50%, and for combined small bowel and liver transplantation is 40%. Significant complications are rejection, sepsis, and lymphoproliferative disease.[44]

Tissue engineering may represent an alternative to allogenic transplantation (Fig. 4). Intestinal progenitor crypt cells isolated from Lewis rats are seeded onto a sheet of PGA fibers and rolled around a silastic stent. Transplantation of these cell/PGA constructs into the mesentery or omentum generated stratified epithelium reminiscent of fetal gut development.[45,46] However, this approach is limited by the absence of epithelial-mesenchymal cell-cell interaction, required for crypt cells to survive, proliferate, and differentiate.[47]

Small aggregates of epithelium and stroma, known as organoid units, are capable of generating the topographic signals necessary for 3-D regeneration of neomucosal after transplantation into subcutanous pockets.[48] This neomucosal layer forms crypts and villi, which contain all epithelial stem cell lineages; i.e., absorptive enterocytes, goblet cells, Paneth's cells, and enteroendocrine cells. Furthermore, the multipotent generative potential of the

Table 2. Tissue engineered skin products.

Product name/Company	Materials
Apligraf/Organogenesis	E – Living human neonatal foreskin-derived keratinocytes D – Living human neonatal foreskin-derived dermal fibroblasts and bovine tendon-derived collagen plus the fibroblast-produced matrix and growth factors N – Available in Canada for venous ulcers; pivotal trials completed for venous ulcer
AlloDerm/ Life Sciences	D – Decellularized human allogenic processed dermis N – Available in US for full-thickness burns
Biobrane (temporary wound dressing)/Dow Hickam	E – Silicone membrane D – Nylon fabric bonded with porcine-derived collagen peptides
Dermagraft/Advanced Tissue Sciences	D – Living human neonatal foreskin-derived dermal fibroblasts and the collagen and other matrix and growth factors they produce; initially grown on a bioabsorbable polyglactin mes N- Available in Canada for diabetic ulcers; pivotal trials completed for diabetic ulcers
Dermagraft TC/Advanced Tissue Sciences	E – Silicone membrane D – Nylon mesh with non-viable cultured foreskin-derived human dermal fibroblasts and their products N – Available in US for temporary covering in burns
Epical ASAProgram/Genzyme Tissue Repair	E – Living cultured self-derived (autologous) keratinocytes attached to petrolatum gauze backing N – Available for burns
Integra Artificial Skin/Integra Life Sciences	E – Polysiloxane (silicone) D – Bovine tendon collagen and shark glycosaminoglycan N – Available in US for burns

D, dermis-like component; E, epidermis-like component; N, notes.

Reproduced with permission from J Am Acad Dermatol (1998); 39(6):1007-10.

---

stem cells within these cellular aggregates is maintained with production of all progeny.[49] These organoid units can be seeded onto PGA tubes and transplanted into the omentum of rats. Organoid/polymer units survive and proliferate, and constructs demonstrated larger cysts with greater crypt-villus morphology.[50]

Kaihara, Kim, and colleagues transplanted these constructs into the omentum of Lewis rats. After 3 weeks, they anastomosed (surgically connected) the native jejunum and tissue-engineered intestine in an end-to-end fashion. Ten weeks later, the overall patency rate of the anastomosis was 78% to 100%, and, histologically, a well-developed neomucosal layer continuous with the native intestine had formed. Anastomosis had a significant impact on villus number and height, crypt number and area, and mucosal surface length compared to tubes in which no anastomosis was performed. They also showed that small bowel resection and porto-caval shunt (connecting the main liver vein with a major body vein) performed with anastomosis had a significant impact in villus number and height, crypt number and area, and mucosal surface length compared to anastomosis alone.[51-54]

These publications reflect the potential role of tissue engineering in creating small bowel for replacement of damaged or diseased native intestine. An interesting observation consistent across other organ tissues is that mixed populations of cells have the tendency to "self sort" and form histologically appropriate tissue.

UROLOGIC TISSUES

Tissues and organs in urology, such as the bladder, clitoris, corpus cavernosum (erectile tissue of the penis), kidney, testes, ureter, and urethra, have been created in the laboratory, with varying degrees of functionality. This section concentrates on the most advanced urologic tissue and probably the first internal organ implanted into a human: the bladder.

One of the first steps was done with seeding in vitro expanded uroepithelial cells on PGA meshes and implanting these cell vehicles, again, into the mesentery, omentum, or retroperitoneum of athymic mice. After 10 days post-implantation, isolated single-cell layers were seen lining the polymer fibers. Twenty and 30 days after transplantation, PGA degradation was evident, and continuous wall thickening with multilayer urothelium-associated cytokeratin cells were observed.[55] PGA also supports the proliferation and survival of human urothelial and bladder muscle cells in situ.[56]

Data from Cilento and colleagues demonstrated that primary cultures of autologous human bladder epithelial cells can be expanded extensively in vitro without changing chromosomal complement, and therefore, can be used for urologic reconstruction.[57] In 1998, Yoo and colleagues showed that allogenic bladder submucosa seeded with muscle cells on one side and urothelial cells on the opposite side appears to be an excellent option as a biomaterial for bladder augmentation. Compared with cell-free submucosa, the cells seeded onto submucosa showed a 99% increase in capacity.[58] One year later, Oberpfenning and colleagues constructed an autonomous hollow bladder and performed the first replacement of native bladder with the tissue-engineered neo-organ in a canine model. They used urothelial and smooth muscle cells from canine native bladder biopsies, which they seeded onto preformed bladder-shaped polymers. After 11 months, the bladder neo-organs demonstrated normal elastic properties, normal capacity to retain urine, and normal histologic architecture.[59]

Trials of bladder replacement using tissue-engineering techniques are currently being arranged. Recent progress suggests engineered urologic tissues may have clinical applicability in the future.[60]

SKIN

Skin represents the body's first tissue-engineered organ to receive Food and Drug Administration (FDA) approval for clinical application. Approximately 1.25 million burn injuries occur each year in the United States.[61] Approximately 15.7 million patients suffer from diabetes mellitus in the United States, and many of these patients have chronic skin ulcers. These patients already benefit from tissue-engineered skin.[62]

Currently, skin products made of 1) ECM materials alone, 2) cells alone, or 3) a combination of cells and matrices, have been referred to as tissue-engineered skin (Table 2).[63] This section provides a summary of cell/matrix products.

All currently available tissue-engineered skin (Epicel®, GenzymeTissue Repair, Cambridge, MA; Dermagraft®, Advanced Tissue Sciences, La Jolla, CA; and Apligraf®, Graftskin, Organogenesis Inc., Canton, MA, USA, which contain living cells) does not appear to function as permanent replacements, but these constructs do not seem to induce classic immunologic rejection;[64] perhaps because these skin products contain neonatal foreskin-derived dermal fibroblasts and do not contain antigen-presenting Langerhans cells or endothelial cells. Over time, these skin constructs are believed to be replaced by the recipient's own tissue ("silent rejection").[65,66] Skin products containing cells on a matrix are known as "smart tissue," perhaps because they have the ability to sense the environment in which they are placed and take "corrective actions." It is believed that they can do so by producing ECM or signaling factors, such as collagen or cytokines.[62,63] Tissue-engineered skin has reached the United States market. Originally, these engineered skin grafts were principally matrix materials; however, tissue-engineered grafts containing living cells are currently entering the market. Some of them are FDA approved, whereas others are in pre-market studies.

CARTILAGE

Joint pain due to cartilage degeneration caused by injury, chronic damage, or diseases is a common and serious problem, affecting people of all ages. Spontaneous repair of injured or damaged cartilage is limited,[67] and variables of focal cartilage defects have not been defined precisely.[68-69] Over 1 million surgical procedures in the United States each year involve cartilage replacement.[1] Although many surgical procedures are currently used to treat this affliction (transplantation, artificial polymer implantation, or metal prostheses), none have had complete success.

The avascular nature of articular cartilage is responsible for its necrosis in response to injury, but the inflammatory phase is almost absent. Therefore, if the damage is limited to the cartilage layer and does not involve the subchondral bone, no recruitment of undifferentiated cells is present to effect the repairing process.

Articular cartilage contains chondrocytes embedded in an ECM composed primarily of type II collagen, proteoglycans, and other collagens and noncollagenous proteins.[70]

Ideally, engineered cartilage should be indistinguishable from native articular cartilage with respect to zonal organization, biochemical composition, and mechanical properties.[71] Tissue-engineering techniques have indicated that new cartilage can be formed from isolated chondrocytes in nude mice.[72,73]

Light microscopy and immunohistochemistry biopsies after autologous chondrocyte transplantation in humans showed zonal heterogeneity on the structural organization and hyaline-like articular cartilage on the biochemical composition throughout the repair tissue after 12 months.[74]

Tissue-engineering concepts have been applied to a variety of biomaterials to design chondrocyte-seeded or cell-free implants for cartilage repair. Among the materials in these engineered devices are PLA,[75] PGA,[76] PGA/PLA and PGA/PLGA co-polymer,[71,77] alginate gel,[78] fibrin glue,[79-82] collagen gels,[83-91] collagen fibers,[92,93] and others. Some of these polymers have been implanted successfully with good results on the repair of cartilage. Special interests in this particular problem arise, because complete repair of partial cartilage defects implies side-to-side joining of matrices.[81,82,94,95]

The chondrocyte donor shortage has led to use of alternative cell sources. "Mesenchymal stem cells" (MCS) have also been tested as grafts. These osteochondral progenitor cells, from either bone marrow or periosteal tissue, have been used to repair articular cartilage defects.[91] These cells were isolated from either tissue, cultured in collagen gel, and transplanted into rabbits with femoral condyle defects. Similar results were seen with both types of progenitor cells. By 2 weeks, the autologous MSCs had differentiated into chondrocytes. At 12 weeks, the subchondral bone was restored completely and defects were filled with hyaline-like cartilage. By 24 weeks, however, the repair tissue showed thinning. Both groups had areas of incomplete integration of the repair and host cartilage. Mechanically, the repair tissue was more compliant than normal cartilage.[91]

Other cartilage tissue has been engineered in the configuration of the human ear[96,97] (Fig. 6), nasoseptal

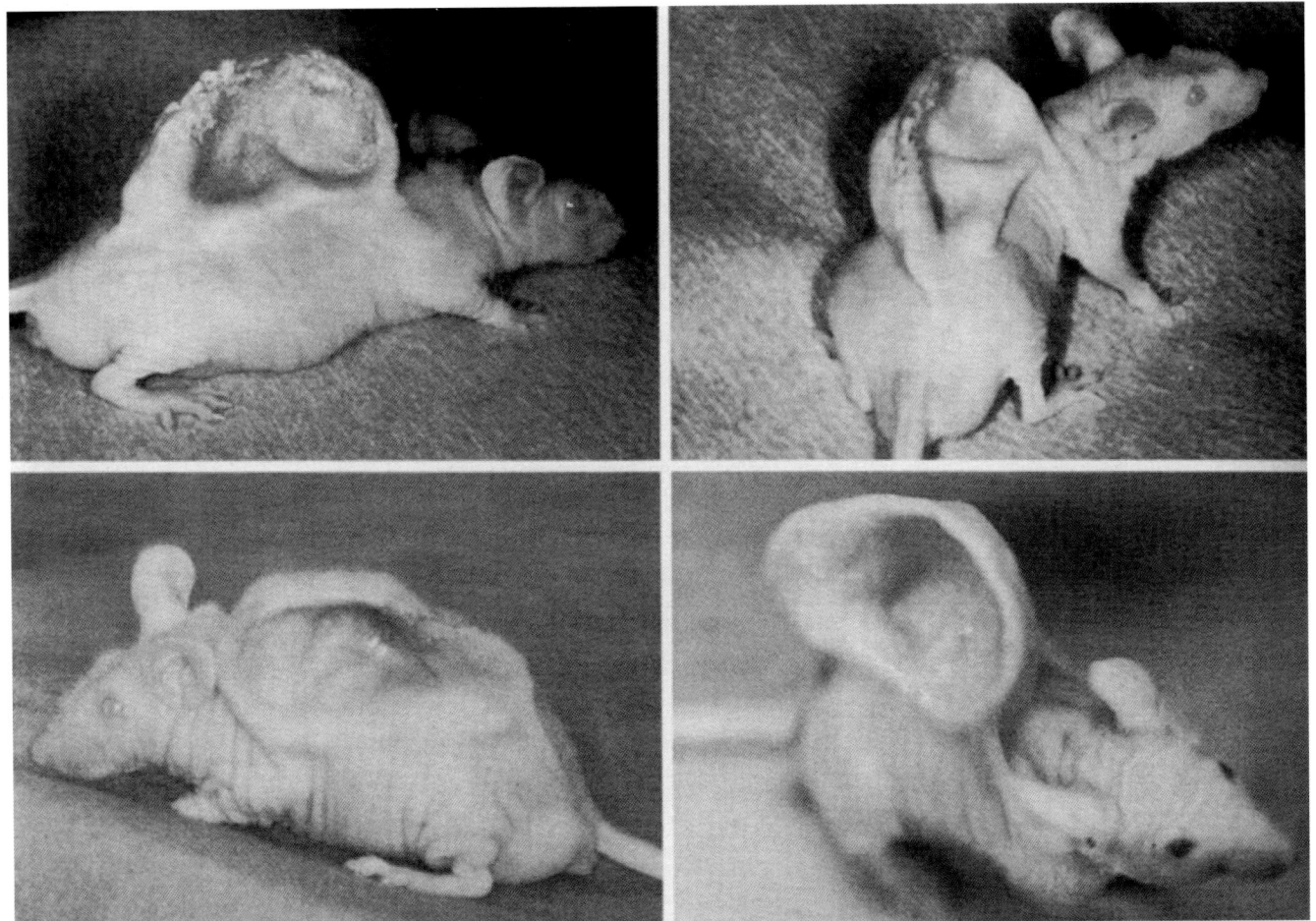

Figure 6. Gross appearance of construct 12 weeks after subcutaneous implantation into a nude mouse. Note the three-dimensional shape that is almost identical to that of a human ear. Reproduced with permission from Plast Reconstr Surg (1997); 100(2):297-302; discussion 303-4.

implants [98] and temporomandibular joint disk.[99]

Tissue-engineered cartilage constructs have also been used in non-native sites. Chondrocytes in hydrogels have been injected into vesicoureteral tissue to prevent vesicoureteral reflux,[100] or have been used to create artificial nipple mounds in pig.[101] Chondrocyte seeded PGA tubes or meshes were used to create ventriculoperitoneal shunts for treatment of hydrocephalus[102] or close full-thickness cranial defects.[103]

BONE

Loss of bone tissue occurs due to injury or disease. Current therapies include replacement of damaged bone with foreign materials (e.g., total hip or knee replacement) or bone autografts and allografts. Secondary damage to autograft sides, limited allograft availability, and host response to allografts, as well as the risk of transfectious disease, are limiting factors.

Tissue-engineered cell/matrix constructs are potentially osteoinductive in addition to being osteoconductive. Again, these constructs should ideally be indistinguishable from native bone, or other autologous tissue such as bone marrow, with respect to zonal organization, biochemical composition, and mechanical properties. The ability of bone marrow-derived osteoprogenitor cells to promote repair of critical-size tibial gaps upon autologous transplantation on a hydroxyapatite ceramic (HAC) carrier was tested in a sheep model by Kon and colleagues. They showed that sheep bone marrow stromal cell (BMSC) implantation in immunocompromised mice led to extensive bone formation. They compared cell-loaded HAC with cell-free HAC cylinders implanted into sheep tibial gaps over a 2-month period. Their data suggest the use of autologous BMSC in conjunction with HAC-based carriers results in faster bone repair compared to HAC alone.[104]

Gazil and colleagues used "genetically engineered pluripotent mesenchymal cells" (GEPMC), which carry "recombinant human bone morphogenetic protein" (rhBMP-2 has been used as a bone substitute) and "beta-galactosidase" (LacZ used as a cell marker), to show *in vitro* differentiation into osteogenic cells expressing alkaline phosphatase and *in vivo* differentiation into osteoblasts. Analysis of new bone formation disclosed that at 4 to 8 weeks post-transplantation, these GEPMC enhanced segmental defect repair significantly. With this study, they showed that cell-mediated gene transfer can be used for growth-factor delivery to signaling receptors of transplanted cells (autocrine effect) and host mesenchymal cells (paracrine effect), suggesting the ability of GEPMC to engraft, differentiate, and stimulate bone growth.[105]

Lee and colleagues isolated, cultured, and seeded fetal rat calvarial osteoblastic cells onto biodegradable chitosan/tricalcium phosphate (TCP) sponges and showed that these sponges have the potential to support the proliferation and differentiation of osteoblastic cells *in vitro*. This potential was

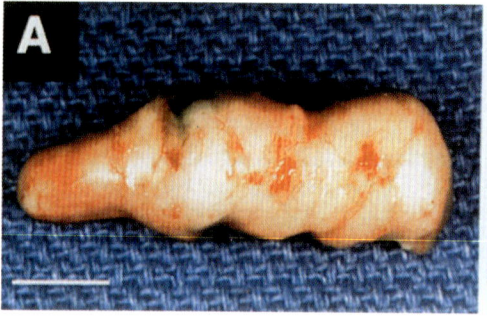 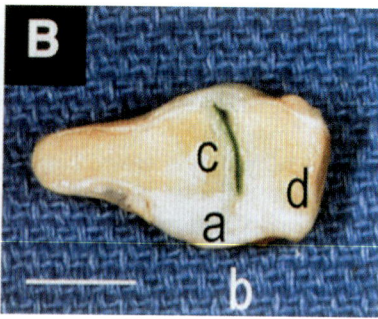

Figure 7. Photographs showing a tissue-engineered distal interphalangeal joint (Group III) at twenty weeks. Articular chondrocyte-polymer sheets were sutured separately to the periosteum-polymer constructs of the distal and middle phalanges to create articular surfaces. The joint then was fabricated by wrapping these two composites with additional polyglycolic acid polymer sheets seeded with tenocytes.
A: Macroscopic view showing considerable vascularity over the surface (x1.5; bar = one centimeter).
B: Longitudinal section of portion of the construct, demonstrating that the tenocapsule of the joint was well formed from the tenocyte-polymer construct. The joint space is green (x1.65; bar = one centimeter). (Regions a through d are enlarged in Fig. 8) Reproduced with permission from J Bone Joint Surg Am (1999); 81(3):306-16.

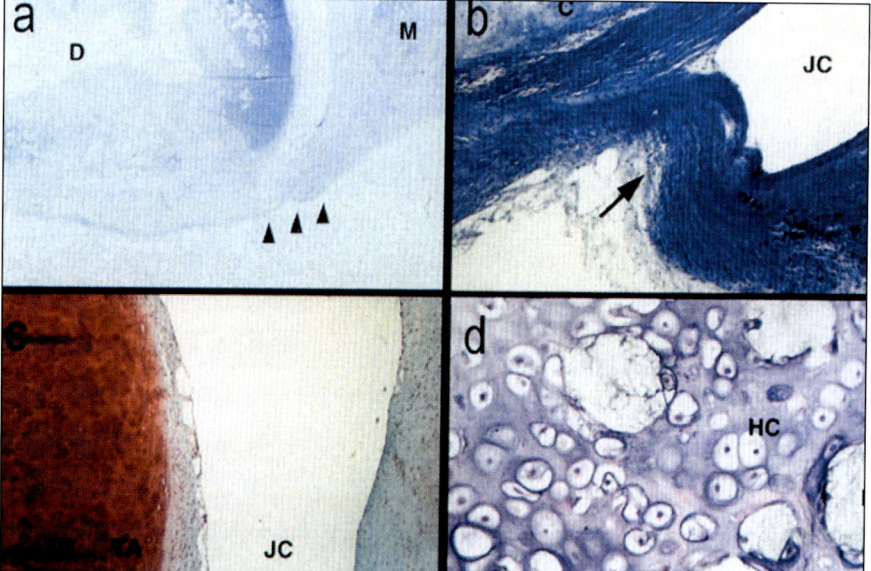

Figure 8. Light photomicrographs of specimens from the tissue-engineered joint.
a: The tenocapsule region (arrowheads) corresponding to regions a and b in Fig. 7, B, is intact between the distal (D) and middle (M) phalanges of the composite. The adjacent cartilaginous articular surfaces are visible on staining with hematoxylin and eosin (x12).
b: Enlarged view of a, showing the insertion of tendon into the bone model as in Fig. 6, c; a joint cavity (JC); and a portion of the joint capsule (arrow). Articular cartilage (C) adjacent to the joint capsule is apparent on staining with Masson's trichrome (x80).
c: Staining with safranin O shows that the tissue-engineered articular surface corresponding to region c in Fig. 7, B, and also seen in a may be separated into superficial tangential (TA) and transitional zones (TR) along the joint cavity (JC). A narrow layer of fibrous tissue (blue) lines the articular cartilage (x80).
d: The interior spaces of the diaphyseal shaft, such as those corresponding to region d in Fig. 7, B, are seen to contain numerous hypertrophic chondrocytes (HC) as well as remnants of residual polymer (P)(hematoxylin and eosin, x330).
Reproduced with permission from J Bone Joint Surg Am (1999); 81(3):306-16.

indicated by high alkaline phosphatase (ALPase) activity and deposition of mineralized matrices by the cells. Small bone-like spicules had formed and were observed on the sponge matrix.[106]

Other polymers have been used to build 3-D bone tissue. The most common are: porous hydroxyapatite (HA),[107,108] PGA/PLA co-polymer,[109-111] and hyaluronan-gelatin.[112] Isogai and colleagues wrapped bovine periosteum around the central portion of phalanges constructed from PGA/PLLA co-polymers. Calf chondrocyte-seeded PGA sheets were then sutured to the proximal end of distal phalanges and distal end of middle phalanges to create opposing articular surfaces. These phalanges were wrapped with additional PGA-mesh sheets seeded with calf tenocytes, which created a distal interphalangeal joint. Constructs were implanted into the dorsal subcutaneous space of athymic nude mice and examined after 20 weeks. Constructs retained their original shape and formed a phalangeal joint resembling their normal counterparts. The periosteum-polymer composite had developed into bone tissue, and the articular chondrocyte-polymer construct had developed into cartilage. The tendocyte-polymer composite formed a teno-capsule around the joint distinguishable from the surrounding connective tissue. After 40 weeks, the entire construct arrangement showed further improvement compared to the 20-week constructs. Vascularization occurred, Haversian channels were noted in areas of lamellar bone formation, intact junction had formed between articular cartilage and the subchondral bone, subchondral bone contained bone spicules and cartilage, and a growth plate similar to those seen *in vivo* had formed (Fig. 7 and Fig. 8).[109]

CARDIOVASCULAR TISSUE

Cardiovascular disease (CVD) is the number one killer of women and men of all ages, all races, worldwide; 59,700,000 Americans are suffering from CVD.[113] CVD claimed 953,110 lives in the United States in 1997. In 1996, $26.1 billion in payments were made to Medicare beneficiaries for hospital expenses due to cardiovascular problems; that amount represented 33.3% of all hospitalization expenditures. The cost of CVD and stroke in the United States in 2000 is estimated to be $326.6 billion.[114] The following sections discuss the different parts of the cardiovascular system regarding tissue-engineering efforts: valves, small and large vessels, and myocardium.

HEART VALVES

Approximately 32,000 babies are born each year with cardiovascular defects,[115] many of which involve one or more valves. During 1997, 78,000 valve replacements were performed in the United States.[116] Currently, heart valve replacement with mechanical prosthesis, xenografts, and homografts, or valve repairs are effective therapies. Unfortunately, these therapies have limitations including inability of these structures to grow, repair, or remodel, as well as susceptibility to both thrombogenesis and infection. These charac-

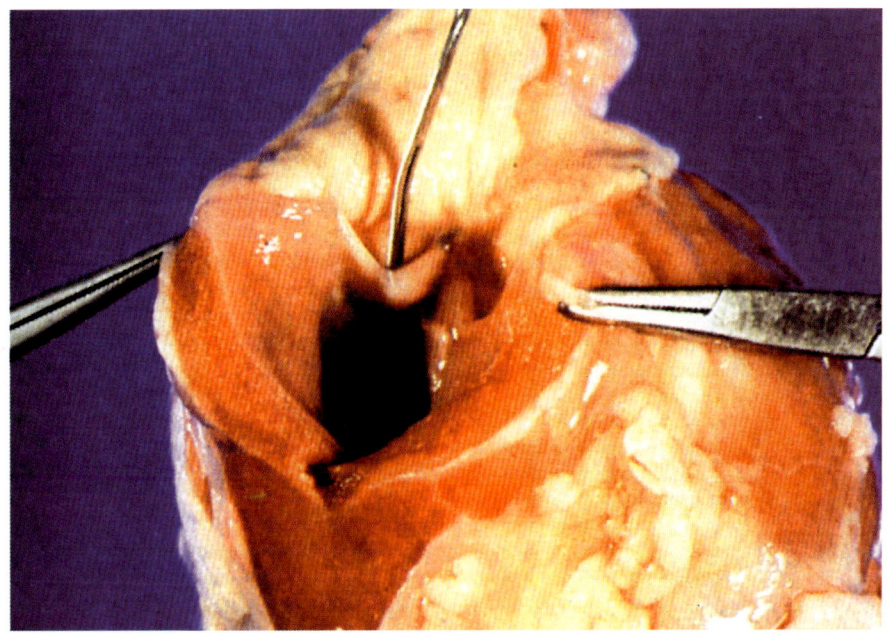

Figure 9. The gross morphology of the tissue-engineered leaflet (probe) 11 weeks after implantation (magnification x100). Reproduced with permission from Circulation (1996); 94(9 Suppl):II164-8.

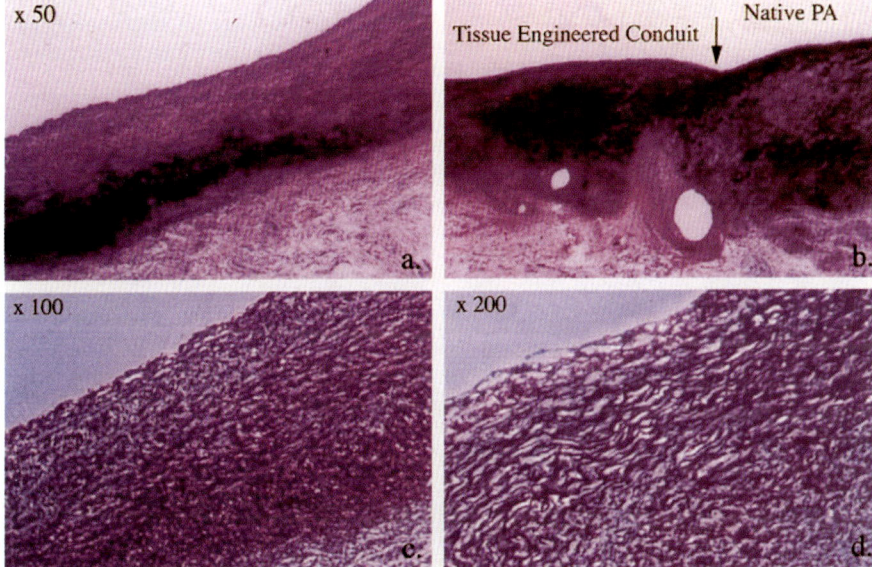

Figure 10. Miller's elastic staining confirmed the presence of elastic fibers (black staining material) and collagen fibers in the constructed conduit. a, Tissue-engineered conduit after 4 months of implantation in group A (original magnification x50). b, Junction between tissue-engineered conduit and native pulmonary artery (PA) (original magnification x50). c, Tissue-engineered conduit in group V (original magnification x100). d, Tissue-engineered conduit in group V (original magnification x200). Reproduced with permission from J Thorac Cardiovasc Surg (1998); 115(3);536-45; discussion 545-6.

teristics have limited their durability and longevity significantly. Furthermore, complications such as bleeding from life-long anticoagulation and foreign-body reactions may occur.

These complications opened the field for tissue-engineered heart valves with autologous cells. The first step was to engineer one leaflet. Shinoka and colleagues constructed 7 leaflets by seeding PGA meshes with fibroblast and endothelial cell isolated from ovine arteries. These constructs were implanted as right posterior leaflets into the pulmonary position. They showed the feasibility of replacing a single leaflet with a tissue-engineered one, and that these constructs are functional in the pulmonary position. Furthermore, ECM develops and appropriate cellular architecture forms (Fig. 9).[117,118] These remodeling processes continue for at least 6 months.[119]

Myofibroblasts for creation of tissue-engineered leaflet seems preferable to dermal fibroblasts with current tissue culture conditions.[120] Supplementation with ascorbic acid to myofibroblast cultures increases collagen content, crucial for mechanical stability of cardiovascular structures.[121, 122] Sodian and colleagues postulated that hemodynamic stress in a bioreactor might direct tissue formation to greater mechanical strength.[123] Bader and colleagues isolated endothelial cells from human saphenous vein, expanded them *in vitro*, and seeded them onto acellularized (by a non-tanning detergent extraction procedure) aortic porcine valves. The xenogenic matrix was acellularized successfully and reseeded with human endothelial cells.[124] Other materials are currently under evaluation for tissue-engineering heart valves: PGA/PHA,[123,125] and PGA/poly-4-hydroxybutyrate (P4HB).[126]

BLOOD VESSELS

Repair of many congenital cardiac defects requires the use of conduits. Homografts or prosthetic conduits lack growth potential. Calcification or tissue ingrowth can obstruct these vessel repairs, leading to the need for multiple conduit replacements.

Current expanded polytetrafluorethylene (PTFE) and textile prostheses do not perform satisfactorily when their diameters are reduced to less than 6 mm. For the small-diameter prostheses, it is necessary to develop less thrombogenic materials and design the structure of the prostheses to match more closely the mechanical properties of natural arteries.

In 1986, Weinberg and Bell were the first to construct a completely biological tissue-engineered blood vessel (TEBV) from bovine-cultured endothelial cells, fibroblast, smooth muscle cells, and animal collagen gels. Their constructs failed to exhibit the required burst strength and mechanical properties for *in vivo* implantation, even after reinforced with Dacron® meshes.[127]

Human collagen gel and endothelial, fibroblast, and smooth muscle cells put together in the same manner, showed similar results.[128] L'Heureux and colleagues grew human smooth muscle cells and fibroblast into cohesive cellular sheets. They wrapped the smooth muscle cells around a tubular support to produce a media and then wrapped the fibroblast sheet around the media to provide an adventitia. The tubular sup-

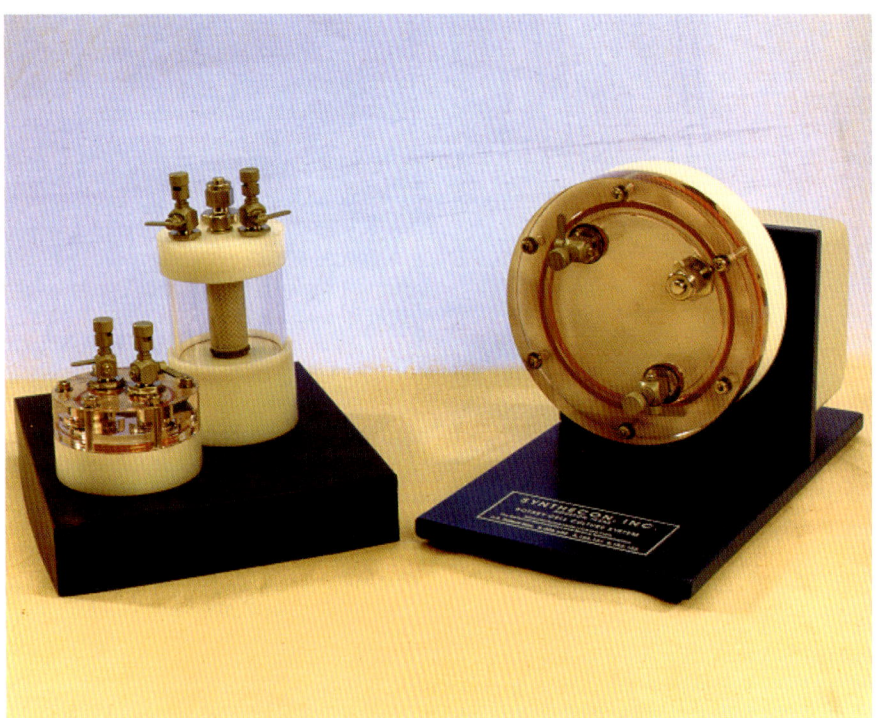

Figure 11. Bioreactor: Rotary cell culture system. (Courtesy of Synthecon Inc.)

port was then removed and human endothelial cells were seeded intraluminally. With this method, they created a TEBV with well-defined, three-layered organization and numerous ECM proteins, including elastin. This vessel had a burst strength of over 2000 mmHg. Non-endothelialized TEBVs were implanted as arterial xenografts into immunosuppressed mongrel dogs (n=6) in the femoral position. After 7 days, 50% of the TEBVs were patent.[129]

Niklason and colleagues trained their small vessel constructs with pulsatile flow. After 8 weeks, the PGA polymer had degraded substantially and was replaced by a dense smooth muscle cell medial layer and an inner endothelial lining. The construct demonstrated many of the physiologic and mechanical characteristics of native arteries, including burst pressures of more than 2000 mm Hg. TEBVs implanted in the femoral artery position were patent after 4 weeks.[121]

Shinoka and colleagues replaced a 2-cm pulmonary artery segment in lambs with a polyglactin/PGA tubular construct seeded with in vitro expanded autologous arterial or venous cells. The animals were euthanized after 11 and 24 weeks. All 7 grafts were patent and demonstrated a nonaneurysmal increase in diameter suggesting growth. Calcium content was elevated, but was not detected macroscopically. Endothelial lining and ECM, including collagen and elastic fibers, developed (Fig. 10).[130] The same constructs used in the systemic circulation resulted in aneurysmal formation.

PGA/PHA was used successfully to replace abdominal aortas in lamb. Tissue contents and mechanical properties approached that of a native vessel after 5 months.[131]

MYOCARDIUM

In 1998, 2340 heart transplants were performed in the United States in about 272 transplant centers. Each year, between 20,000 and 40,000 Americans are estimated to benefit from a heart transplant.[132] Although artificial hearts help to bridge patient with end-stage heart failure to allogenic heart transplantation, and total artificial hearts are being evaluated for permanent replacement, the American Heart Association (AHA) considers "the artificial heart to be an experimental device."[133]

In contrast to skeletal muscle, in which capacity for tissue repair is attributed to the presence of satellite cells, myocardium lacks the ability to regenerate following an injury. An increase in cardiomyocyte or cardiomyocyte-like cell number in diseased hearts could improve function. Cell transplantation is a potential alternative.

Different cell sources are under investigation: fetal,[134,135] neonatal,[136] and adult cardiomyocytes,[137] immortalized atrial cells, myogenic cell lines, adult skeletal myoblasts,[138-140] embryonic stem cells,[141] genetically altered fibroblasts, smooth muscle cells, and bone marrow-derived cells.[142] Allogenic cell transplantation—even fetal or neonatal—is dependent on immunosuppression therapy. Adult cardiomyocytes do not proliferate, hence making in vitro cell expansion infeasible. To perform autologous cardiomyocyte transplantation with any benefit to the patient, sufficient cells should be transplanted. To harvest enough autologous cardiomyocytes, biopsies from healthy myocardium must be of sufficient size; however, this would cause damage and scar formation to the biopsy side, decreasing myocardial function.

Myogenic progenitor cells and bone marrow stem cells are especially intriguing because of their potential ability to differentiate into myocardium.

LOOKING INTO THE FUTURE

Just 50 years ago, organ transplantation and open-heart surgery were unachievable. In a short time, these treatments became standard life-saving procedures. With the increasing understanding of our immune system, development of better immunosuppression therapies, and more accurate organ-matching post-transplantation, survival and quality of life continue to improve. Donor shortage leads us to investigate new organ sources, such as xenoransplantation, but further research is necessary to bring this strategy into clinical use.

Tissue engineering is a relatively new approach with the attempt to reproduce organogenesis. In the last 20 years, tremendous steps toward neoorganogenesis have been made in different subspecialties. Developmental, molecular, and cell biologists help one understand more about the mechanisms of organ development, cell-cell interaction, and signaling. With this knowledge, engineers create new biomaterials that can specifically signal cell behavior and gene expression.[143]

Autologous cells are an ideal source for transplantation; but organ specific-cell isolation has disadvantages: 1) cells are fully differentiated; and 2) it requires an invasive procedure to access the cells, with potential damage to the organ. Although most organs tolerate the procedure well, fully differentiated cells can have weak proliferative abilities; therefore, the ideal autologous cell source would be a non-differentiated pluripotent cell—the stem cell. To our knowledge, these stem cells are rare or non-existent in most organs. Bone marrow stem cells and circulating progenitor cells have the ability to differentiate under the right conditions into a variety of tissues. New markers to identify these cells are under investigation; therefore, these cells would be easily accessible. Another interesting observation has come from the space sciences. Mechanical forces, such as shear stress, produced in microgravity bioreactors have a positive input on cell seeding and culturing, as well as tissue growth (Fig. 11). Although we have made great strides toward neo-organogenesis, we still have a long way to go. One major barrier in growing thick, complex tissue is vascularization. We are focusing our work on micromachining technologies to generate complete vascular systems.[144]

Tissue engineering unites scientists from many specialized areas of expertise. The scientific era at hand promises to be an exciting one as advances in biotechnology in genomics, ECM construction, and graft versus host events (the latter described in the article by Spack and and Borrows in this issue) meet the surgeon's hands in the clinic.

REFERENCES

1. Langer R, Vacanti JP. Tissue engineering. Science 1993; 260(5110): 920-6.
2. Murray JE, Merrill JP, Harrison JH. Renal hemotransplantation in identical twins. Surg Forum 1955; 6: 432-6.
3. Barnard CN. Human cardiac transplantation. An evaluation of the first two operations performed at the Groote Schuur Hospital, Cape Town. Am J Cardiol 1968; 22(4): 584-96.
4. http://www.unos.org/frame_Default.asp?Category=Newsdata.
5. Cooley DA, Liotta D, Hallman GL, et al. Orthotopic cardiac prosthesis for two-staged cardiac replacement. Am J Cardiol 1969; 24(5): 723-30.
6. Dohmen PM, Laube H, de Jonge K, et al. Mechanical circulatory support for one thousand days or more with the Novacor N100 left ventricular assist device. J Thorac Cardiovasc Surg 1999; 117(5): 1029-30.
7. Hetzer R, Muller J, Weng Y, et al. Cardiac recovery in dilated cardiomyopathy by unloading with a left ventricular assist device. Ann Thorac Surg 1999; 68(2): 742-9.
8. Loebe M, Hennig E, Muller J, et al. Long-term mechanical circulatory support as a bridge to transplantation, for recovery from cardiomyopathy, and for permanent replacement. Eur J Cardiothorac Surg 1997; 11 Suppl: S18-24.
9. Muller J, Wallukat G, Weng YG, et al. Weaning from mechanical cardiac support in patients with idiopathic dilated cardiomyopathy [see comments]. Circulation 1997; 96(2): 542-9.
10. Skalak R, Fox CF. Tissue Engineering. Liss, NY, 1988.
11. Nerem RM. Cellular engineering. Ann Biomed Eng 1991; 19(5): 529-45.
12. Ferber D. Tissue engineering. Growing human corneas in the lab [news; comment]. Science 1999; 286(5447): 2051, 2053.
13. Vacanti JP. Beyond transplantation. Third annual Samuel Jason Mixter lecture. Arch Surg 1988; 123(5): 545-9.
14. Folkman J, Haudenschild C. Angiogenesis in vitro. Nature 1980; 288(5791): 551-6.
15. Morse MA, Vacanti JP. Time-lapse photography: a novel tool to study normal morphogenesis and the diseased hepatobiliary system in children. J Pediatr Surg 1988; 23(1 Pt 2): 69-72.
16. Folkman J, Moscona A. Role of cell shape in growth control. Nature 1978; 273(5661): 345-9.
17. Vacanti JP, Morse MA, Saltzman WM, et al. Selective cell transplantation using bioabsorbable artificial polymers as matrices. J Pediatr Surg 1988; 23(1 Pt 2): 3-9.
18. Folkman J, Hochberg M. Self-regulation of growth in three dimensions. J Exp Med 1973; 138(4): 745-53.
19. Mooney DJ, Langer RS. Engineering biomaterials for tissue engineering:the 10-100 micron size scale. The Biomedical Engineering Handbook, Bronzino JD, ed. Boca Raton, FL: CRC Press, 1995.
20. Cima LG, Langer R, Vacanti JP. Polymers for tissue and organ culture. J Bioactive Compat Polymers 1991; 6: 232-40.
21. Langer RS, Vacanti JP. Artificial organs. Sci Am 1995; 273: 100-3.
22. Frazza EJ, Schmitt EE. A new absorbable suture. J Biomed Mater Res 1971; 5(2): 43-58.
23. Cima LG, Vacanti JP, Vacanti C, et al. Tissue engineering by cell transplantation using degradable polymer substrates. J Biomech Eng 1991; 113(2): 143-51.
24. Wong W, Mooney D. Synthesis and properties of biodegradable polymers used as synthetic matrices for tissue engineering. In: Atala A, Mooney D, eds. Synthetic Biodegradable Polymer Scaffolds, Boston: Birkhauser, 1997. p 51-82.
25. Sano K, Cusick RA, Lee H, et al. Regenerative signals for heterotopic hepatocyte transplantation. Transplant Proc 1996; 28(3): 1857-8.
26. Takeda T, Kim TH, Lee SK, et al. Hepatocyte transplantation in biodegradable polymer scaffolds using the Dalmatian dog model of hyperuricosuria. Transplant Proc 1995; 27(1): 635-6.
27. Mooney DJ, Kaufmann PM, Sano K, et al. Transplantation of hepatocytes using porous, biodegradable sponges. Transplant Proc 1994; 26(6): 3425-6.
28. Mooney DJ, Park S, Kaufmann PM, et al. Biodegradable sponges for hepatocyte transplantation. J Biomed Mater Res 1995; 29(8): 959-65.
29. Johnson LB, Aiken J, Mooney D, et al. The mesentery as a laminated vascular bed for hepatocyte transplantation. Cell Transplant 1994; 3(4): 273-81.
30. Uyama S, Kaufmann PM, Takeda T, et al. Delivery of whole liver-equivalent hepatocyte mass using polymer devices and hepatotrophic stimulation. Transplantation 1993; 55(4): 932-5.
31. Cusick R, Sano K, Lee H, et al. Heterotopic fetal rat hepatocyte transplantation on biodegradable polymers. Surg Forum, 1995.
32. Kaufmann PM, Sano K, Uyama S, et al. Heterotopic hepatocyte transplantation: assessing the impact of hepatotrophic stimulation. Transplant Proc 1994; 26(4): 2240-1.
33. Kaufmann PM, Sano K, Uyama S, et al. Heterotopic hepatocyte transplantation using three-dimensional polymers: Evaluation of the stimulatory effects by portacaval shunt or islet cell cotransplantation. Transplant Proc 1994; 26(6): 3343-5.
34. Kim SS, Kaihara S, Benvenuto MS, et al. Small intestinal submucosa as a small-caliber venous graft: A novel model for hepatocyte transplantation on synthetic biodegradable polymer scaffolds with direct access to the portal venous system. J Pediatr Surg 1999; 34(1): 124-8.
35. Kaufmann PM, Sano K, Uyama S, et al. Evaluation of methods of hepatotrophic stimulation in rat heterotopic hepatocyte transplantation using polymers. J Pediatr Surg 1999; 34(7): 1118-23.
36. Kim TH, Lee HM, Utsonomiya H, et al. Enhanced survival of transgenic hepatocytes expressing hepatocyte growth factor in hepatocyte tissue engineering. Transplant Proc 1997; 29(1-2): 858-60.
37. Pollok JM, Kluth D, Cusick RA, et al. Formation of spheroidal aggregates of hepatocytes on biodegradable polymers under continuous-flow bioreactor conditions. Eur J Pediatr Surg 1998; 8(4): 195-9.
38. Asonuma K, Gilbert JC, Stein JE, et al. Quantitation of transplanted hepatic mass necessary to cure the Gunn rat model of hyperbilirubinemia. J Pediatr Surg 1992; 27(3): 298-301.
39. Kim SS, Utsunomiya H, Koski JA, et al. Survival and function of hepatocytes on a novel three-dimensional synthetic biodegradable polymer scaffold with an intrinsic network of channels [see comments]. Ann Surg 1998; 228(1): 8-13.
40. Park A, Wu B, Griffith LG. Integration of surface modification and 3D fabrication techniques to prepare patterned poly(L-lactide) substrates allowing regionally selective cell adhesion. J Biomater Sci Polym Ed 1998; 9(2): 89-110.
41. Dudrick SJ, Latifi R, Fosnocht DE. Management of the short-bowel syndrome. Surg Clin North Am 1991; 71(3): 625-43.
42. Gambarara M, Goulet O, Bagolan P, et al. Long-term parenteral nutrition in the management of extremely short bowel syndrome. Transplant Proc 1998; 30(6): 2539-40.
43. Vanderhoof JA, Langnas AN, Pinch LW, et al. Short bowel syndrome. J Pediatr Gas-

troenterol Nutr 1992; 14(4): 359-70.
44. Brook G. Quality of life issues: Parenteral nutrition to small bowel transplantation—a review. Nutrition 1998; 14(10): 813-6.
45. Organ GM, Mooney DJ, Hansen LK, et al. Transplantation of enterocytes utilizing polymer-cell constructs to produce a neointestine. Transplant Proc 1992; 24(6): 3009-11.
46. Organ GM, Mooney DJ, Hansen LK, et al. Enterocyte transplantation using cell-polymer devices to create intestinal epithelial-lined tubes. Transplant Proc 1993; 25(1 Pt 2): 998-1001.
47. Haffen K, Kedinger M, Simon-Assmann P. Mesenchyme-dependent differentiation of epithelial progenitor cells in the gut. J Pediatr Gastroenterol Nutr 1987; 6(1): 14-23.
48. Evans GS, Flint N, Somers AS, et al. The development of a method for the preparation of rat intestinal epithelial cell primary cultures. J Cell Sci 1992; 101(Pt 1): 219-31.
49. Tait IS, Flint N, Campbell FC, et al. Generation of neomucosa in vivo by transplantation of dissociated rat postnatal small intestinal epithelium. Differentiation 1994; 56(1-2): 91-100.
50. Choi RS, Vacanti JP. Preliminary studies of tissue-engineered intestine using isolated epithelial organoid units on tubular synthetic biodegradable scaffolds. Transplant Proc 1997; 29(1-2): 848-51.
51. Kaihara S, Kim S, Benvenuto M, et al. End-to-end anastomosis between tissue-engineered intestine and native small bowel. Tissue Eng 1999; 5(4): 339-46.
52. Kaihara S, Kim SS, Benvenuto M, et al. Anastomosis between tissue-engineered intestine and native small bowel. Transplant Proc 1999; 31(1-2):661-2.
53. Kim SS, Kaihara S, Benvenuto MS, et al. Effects of anastomosis of tissue-engineered neointestine to native small bowel. J Surg Res 1999; 87(1): 6-13.
54. Kim SS, Kaihara S, Benvenuto MS, et al. Regenerative signals for intestinal epithelial organoid units transplanted on biodegradable polymer scaffolds for tissue engineering of small intestine. Transplantation 1999; 67(2): 227-33.
55. Atala A, Vacanti JP, Peters CA, et al. Formation of urothelial structures in vivo from dissociated cells attached to biodegradable polymer scaffolds in vitro. J Urol 1992; 148(2 Pt 2): 658-62.
56. Atala A, Freeman MR, Vacanti JP, et al. Implantation in vivo and retrieval of artificial structures consisting of rabbit and human urothelium and human bladder muscle. J Urol 1993; 150(2 Pt 2): 608-12.
57. Cilento BG, Freeman MR, Schneck FX, et al. Phenotypic and cytogenetic characterization of human bladder urothelia expanded in vitro. J Urol 1994; 152(2 Pt 2): 665-70.
58. Yoo JJ, Meng J, Oberpenning F, et al. Bladder augmentation using allogenic bladder submucosa seeded with cells. Urology 1998; 51(2): 221-5.
59. Oberpenning F, Meng J, Yoo JJ, et al. De novo reconstitution of a functional mammalian urinary bladder by tissue engineering [see comments]. Nat Biotechnol 1999; 17(2): 149-55.
60. Atala A. Tissue engineering of artifical organs [In Process Citation]. J Endourol 2000; 14(1): 49-57.
61. (NHIS) NHIS. Based on data from: National Ambulatory Medical Care Survey, National Hospital Ambulatory Medical Care Survey, National Medical Expenditure Survey. 1997
62. Naughton G, Mansbridge J, Gentzkow G. A metabolically active human dermal replacement for the treatment of diabetic foot ulcers. Artif Organs 1997; 21(11): 1203-10.
63. Eaglstein WH, Falanga V. Tissue engineering for skin: an update. J Am Acad Dermatol 1998; 39(6): 1007-10.
64. Eaglstein WH, Iriondo M, Laszlo K. A composite skin substitute (graftskin) for surgical wounds. A clinical experience. Dermatol Surg 1995; 21(10): 839-43.
65. Hefton JM, Amberson JB, Biozes DG, et al. Loss of HLA-DR expression by human epidermal cells after growth in culture. J Invest Dermatol 1984; 83(1): 48-50.
66. Burt AM, Pallett CD, Sloane JP, et al. Survival of cultured allografts in patients with burns assessed with probe specific for Y chromosome. BMJ 1989; 298(6678): 915-7.
67. Meachim G. The effect of scarification on articular cartilage in the rabbit. J Bone Joint Surg 1963; 45B: 150-61.
68. Mankin HJ. Nontraumatic necrosis of bone (osteonecrosis). N Engl J Med 1992; 326(22): 1473-9.
69. Brittberg M, Lindahl A, Nilsson A, et al. Treatment of deep cartilage defects in the knee with autologous chondrocyte transplantation [see comments]. N Engl J Med 1994; 331(14): 889-95.
70. Buckwalter JA, Mow VC, Ratcliffe A. Restoration of injured or degenerated articular cartilage. J Am Acad Orthop Surg 1994; 2(4): 192-201.
71. Freed LE, Martin I, Vunjak-Novakovic G. Frontiers in tissue engineering. In vitro modulation of chondrogenesis. Clin Orthop 1999(367 Suppl): S46-58.
72. Sims CD, Butler PE, Cao YL, et al. Tissue engineered neocartilage using plasma derived polymer substrates and chondrocytes. Plast Reconstr Surg 1998; 101(6): 1580-5.
73. Paige KT, Cima LG, Yaremchuk MJ, et al. Injectable cartilage. Plast Reconstr Surg 1995; 96(6): 1390-8; discussion 1399-400.
74. Richardson JB, Caterson B, Evans EH, et al. Repair of human articular cartilage after implantation of autologous chondrocytes. J Bone Joint Surg Br 1999; 81(6): 1064-8.
75. Chu CR, Coutts RD, Yoshioka M, et al. Articular cartilage repair using allogeneic perichondrocyte-seeded biodegradable porous polylactic acid (PLA): A tissue-engineering study. J Biomed Mater Res 1995; 29(9): 1147-54.
76. Vacanti CA, Kim W, Schloo B, et al. Joint resurfacing with cartilage grown in situ from cell-polymer structures. Am J Sports Med 1994; 22(4): 485-8.
77. Freed LE, Vunjak-Novakovic G, Biron RJ, et al. Biodegradable polymer scaffolds for tissue engineering. Biotechnology (N Y) 1994; 12(7): 689-93.
78. van Susante JL, Buma P, van Osch GJ, et al. Culture of chondrocytes in alginate and collagen carrier gels. Acta Orthop Scand 1995; 66(6): 549-56.
79. Hendrickson DA, Nixon AJ, Grande DA, et al. Chondrocyte-fibrin matrix transplants for resurfacing extensive articular cartilage defects. J Orthop Res 1994; 12(4): 485-97.
80. Homminga GN, Buma P, Koot HW, et al. Chondrocyte behavior in fibrin glue in vitro. Acta Orthop Scand 1993; 64(4): 441-5.
81. Peretti GM, Randolph MA, Caruso EM, et al. Bonding of cartilage matrices with cultured chondrocytes: An experimental model. J Orthop Res 1998; 16(1): 89-95.
82. Silverman RP, Bonasser L, Passaretti D, et al. Adhesion of tissue-engineered cartilage to native cartilage. Plast Reconstr Surg 2000; 105(4): 1393-8.
83. Fujisato T, Sajiki T, Liu Q, et al. Effect of basic fibroblast growth factor on cartilage regeneration in chondrocyte-seeded collagen sponge scaffold. Biomaterials 1996; 17(2): 155-62.
84. Hansen AL, Foster BK, Gibson GJ, et al. Growth-plate chondrocyte cultures for reimplantation into growth-plate defects in sheep. Characterization of cultures. Clin Orthop 1990(256): 286-98.
85. Mizuno S, Glowacki J. Chondroinduction of human dermal fibroblasts by demineralized bone in three-dimensional culture. Exp Cell Res 1996; 227(1): 89-97.
86. Nixon AJ, Sams AE, Lust G, et al. Temporal matrix synthesis and histologic features of a chondrocyte-laden porous collagen cartilage analogue. Am J Vet Res 1993; 54(2): 349-56.
87. Sams AE, Nixon AJ. Chondrocyte-laden collagen scaffolds for resurfacing extensive articular cartilage defects. Osteoarthritis Cartilage 1995; 3(1): 47-59.
88. Sams AE, Minor RR, Wootton JA, et al. Local and remote matrix responses to chondrocyte-laden collagen scaffold implantation in extensive articular cartilage defects. Osteoarthritis Cartilage 1995; 3(1): 61-70.
89. Grande DA, Pitman MI, Peterson L, et al. The repair of experimentally produced defects in rabbit articular cartilage by autologous chondrocyte transplantation. J Orthop Res 1989; 7(2): 208-18.
90. Wakitani S, Kimura T, Hirooka A, et al. Repair of rabbit articular surfaces with allograft chondrocytes embedded in collagen gel. J Bone Joint Surg [Br] 1989; 71(1): 74-80.
91. Wakitani S, Goto T, Pineda SJ, et al. Mesenchymal cell-based repair of large, full-thickness defects of articular cartilage. J Bone Joint Surg Am 1994; 76(4) :579-92.
92. Pachence JM. Collagen-based devices for soft tissue repair. J Biomed Mater Res 1996; 33(1): 35-40.
93. Toolan BC, Frenkel SR, Pachence JM, et al. Effects of growth-factor-enhanced culture on a chondrocyte-collagen implant for cartilage repair . J Biomed Mater Res 1996; 31(2): 273-80.
94. Wolohan MJ, Zaleske DJ. Hemiepiphyseal reconstruction using tissue donated from fetal limbs in a murine model. J Orthop Res 1991; 9(2): 180-5.
95. Reindel ES, Ayroso AM, Chen AC, et al. Integrative repair of articular cartilage in vitro: Adhesive strength of the interface

region. J Orthop Res 1995; 13(5): 751-60.

96. Cao Y, Vacanti JP, Paige KT, et al. Transplantation of chondrocytes utilizing a polymer-cell construct to produce tissue-engineered cartilage in the shape of a human ear [see comments]. Plast Reconstr Surg 1997; 100(2): 297-302; discussion 303-4.

97. Rodriguez A, Cao YL, Ibarra C, et al. Characteristics of cartilage engineered from human pediatric auricular cartilage. Plast Reconstr Surg 1999; 103(4): 1111-9.

98. Puelacher WC, Mooney D, Langer R, et al. Design of nasoseptal cartilage replacements synthesized from biodegradable polymers and chondrocytes. Biomaterials 1994; 15(10): 774-8.

99. Puelacher WC, Wisser J, Vacanti CA, et al. Temporomandibular joint disc replacement made by tissue-engineered growth of cartilage. J Oral Maxillofac Surg 1994; 52(11): 1172-7; discussion 1177-8.

100. Atala A, Cima LG, Kim W, et al. Injectable alginate seeded with chondrocytes as a potential treatment for vesicoureteral reflux. J Urol 1993; 150(2 Pt 2): 745-7.

101. Cao YL, Lach E, Kim TH, et al. Tissue-engineered nipple reconstruction. Plast Reconstr Surg 1998; 102(7): 2293-8.

102. Lee IW, Vacanti JP, Taylor GA, et al. The living shunt: a tissue engineering approach in the treatment of hydrocephalus. Neurol Res 2000; 22(1): 105-10.

103. Lee IW, Vacanti JP, Yoo J, et al. A tissue engineering approach for dural and cranial grafts. Congress of Neurological Surgeons, New Orleans, LA, 1997.

104. Kon E, Muraglia A, Corsi A, et al. Autologous bone marrow stromal cells loaded onto porous hydroxyapatite ceramic accelerate bone repair in critical-size defects of sheep long bones. J Biomed Mater Res 2000; 49(3): 328-37.

105. Gazit D, Turgeman G, Kelley P, et al. Engineered pluripotent mesenchymal cells integrate and differentiate in regenerating bone: A novel cell-mediated gene therapy. J Gene Med 1999; 1(2): 121-33.

106. Lee YM, Park YJ, Lee SJ, et al. Tissue engineered bone formation using chitosan/tricalcium phosphate sponges [In Process Citation]. J Periodontol 2000; 71(3): 410-7.

107. Yoshikawa T, Ohgushi H. Autogenous cultured bone graft—bone reconstruction using tissue engineering approach. Ann Chir Gynaecol 1999; 88(3): 186-92.

108. Yoshikawa T, Ohgushi H, Nakajima H, et al. In vivo osteogenic durability of cultured bone in porous ceramics: A novel method for autogenous bone graft substitution. Transplantation 2000; 69(1): 128-34.

109. Isogai N, Landis W, Kim TH, et al. Formation of phalanges and small joints by tissue-engineering. J Bone Joint Surg Am 1999; 81(3): 306-16.

110. Murphy WL, Kohn DH, Mooney DJ. Growth of continuous bonelike mineral within porous poly(lactide-co- glycolide) scaffolds in vitro. J Biomed Mater Res 2000; 50(1): 50-8.

111. Zhang R, Ma PX. Poly(alpha-hydroxyl acids)/hydroxyapatite porous composites for bone- tissue engineering. I. Preparation and morphology. J Biomed Mater Res 1999; 44(4): 446-55.

112. Angele P, Kujat R, Nerlich M, et al. Engineering of osteochondral tissue with bone marrow mesenchymal progenitor cells in a derivatized hyaluronan-gelatin composite sponge [In Process Citation]. Tissue Eng 1999; 5(6): 545-54.

113. AHA-web-site. 1 Source: Phase I, National Health and Nutrition Examination Survey III (NHANES III), 1988-91, CDC/NCHS and the American Heart Association. 2 Source: National Health and Nutrition Examination Survey III (NHANES III), 1988-94, CDC/NCHS and the American Heart Association.
3 Source: National Health and Nutrition Examination Survey II (NHANES II), 1976-80, CDC/NCHS and the American Heart Association. .

114. AHA-web-site. Health Care Financing Administration [HCFA]. .

115. AHA-web-site. http://www.americanheart.org/Heart_and_Stroke_A_Z_Guide/conghds.html.

116. AHA-web-site. http://www.americanheart.org/Heart_and_Stroke_A_Z_Guide/openh.html.

117. Shinoka T, Breuer CK, Tanel RE, et al. Tissue engineering heart valves: Valve leaflet replacement study in a lamb model. Ann Thorac Surg 1995; 60(6 Suppl): S513-6.

118. Shinoka T, Ma PX, Shum-Tim D, et al. Tissue-engineered heart valves. Autologous valve leaflet replacement study in a lamb model. Circulation 1996; 94(9 Suppl): II164-8.

119. Stock UA, Nagashima M, Khalil PN, et al. Tissue-engineered valved conduits in the pulmonary circulation [In Process Citation]. J Thorac Cardiovasc Surg 2000; 119(4 Pt 1): 732-40.

120. Shinoka T, Shum-Tim D, Ma PX, et al. Tissue-engineered heart valve leaflets: Does cell origin affect outcome? Circulation 1997; 96(9 Suppl): II-102-7.

121. Niklason LE, Gao J, Abbott WM, et al. Functional arteries grown in vitro [see comments]. Science 1999; 284(5413): 489-93.

122. Hoerstrup SP, Zund G, Ye Q, et al. Tissue engineering of a bioprosthetic heart valve: Stimulation of extracellular matrix assessed by hydroxyproline assay. Asaio J 1999; 45(5): 397-402.

123. Sodian R, Sperling JS, Martin DP, et al. Tissue engineering of a trileaflet heart valve-early In vitro experiences with a combined polymer [In Process Citation]. Tissue Eng 1999; 5(5): 489-94.

124. Bader A, Schilling T, Teebken OE, et al. Tissue engineering of heart valves—human endothelial cell seeding of detergent acellularized porcine valves. Eur J Cardiothorac Surg 1998; 14(3): 279-84.

125. Williams SF, Martin DP, Horowitz DM, et al. PHA applications: Addressing the price performance issue: I. Tissue engineering. Int J Biol Macromol 1999; 25(1-3): 111-21.

126. Sodian R, Hoerstrup SP, Sperling JS, et al. Evaluation of biodegradable, three-dimensional matrices for tissue engineering of heart valves. Asaio J 2000; 46(1): 107-10.

127. Weinberg CB, Bell E. A blood vessel model constructed from collagen and cultured vascular cells. Science 1986; 231(4736): 397-400.

128. L'Heureux N, Germain L, Labbe R, et al. In vitro construction of a human blood vessel from cultured vascular cells: A morphologic study. J Vasc Surg 1993; 17(3): 499-509.

129. L'Heureux N, Paquet S, Labbe R, et al. A completely biological tissue-engineered human blood vessel [see comments]. Faseb J 1998; 12(1): 47-56.

130. Shinoka T, Shum-Tim D, Ma PX, et al. Creation of viable pulmonary artery autografts through tissue engineering. J Thorac Cardiovasc Surg 1998; 115(3): 536-45; discussion 545-6.

131. Shum-Tim D, Stock U, Hrkach J, et al. Tissue engineering of autologous aorta using a new biodegradable polymer. Ann Thorac Surg 1999; 68(6): 2298-304; discussion 2305.

132. AHA-web-site. http://www.americanheart.org/Heart_and_Stroke_A_Z_Guide/htrans.html.

133. AHA-web-site. http://www.americanheart.org/Heart_and_Stroke_A_Z_Guide/arthertv.html.

134. Leor J, Patterson M, Quinones MJ, et al. Transplantation of fetal myocardial tissue into the infarcted myocardium of rat. A potential method for repair of infarcted myocardium? Circulation 1996; 94(9 Suppl): II332-6.

135. Li RK, Jia ZQ, Weisel RD, et al. Cardiomyocyte transplantation improves heart function. Ann Thorac Surg 1996; 62(3): 654-60; discussion 660-1.

136. Li RK, Mickle DA, Weisel RD, et al. In vivo survival and function of transplanted rat cardiomyocytes. Circ Res 1996; 78(2): 283-8.

137. Li RK, Yau TM, Weisel RD, et al. Construction of a bioengineered cardiac graft. J Thorac Cardiovasc Surg 2000; 119(2): 368-75.

138. Marelli D, Desrosiers C, el-Alfy M, et al. Cell transplantation for myocardial repair: An experimental approach. Cell Transplant 1992; 1(6): 383-90.

139. Taylor DA, Atkins BZ, Hungspreugs P, et al. Regenerating functional myocardium: improved performance after skeletal myoblast transplantation [published erratum appears in Nat Med 1998 Oct;4(10): 1200]. Nat Med 1998; 4(8): 929-33.

140. Van Meter CH Jr, Claycomb WC, Delcarpio JB, et al. Myoblast transplantation in the porcine model: A potential technique for myocardial repair. J Thorac Cardiovasc Surg 1995; 110(5): 1442-8.

141. Klug MG, Soonpaa MH, Koh GY, et al. Genetically selected cardiomyocytes from differentiating embronic stem cells form stable intracardiac grafts. J Clin Invest 1996; 98(1): 216-24.

142. Tomita S, Li RK, Weisel RD, et al. Autologous transplantation of bone marrow cells improves damaged heart function. Circulation 1999; 100(19 Suppl): II247-56.

143. Maheshwari G, Brown G, Lauffenburger DA, et al. Cell adhesion and motility depend on nanoscale RGD clustering. J Cell Sci 2000; 113(Pt): 1677-86.

144. Kaihara S, Borenstein J, Koka R, et al. Silicon micromachining to tissue engineer branched vascular channels for iver fabrication. Tissue Engineering 2000; 6(2): 105-17.

Introducing a New Spin on Laparoscopy
EndoTIP®

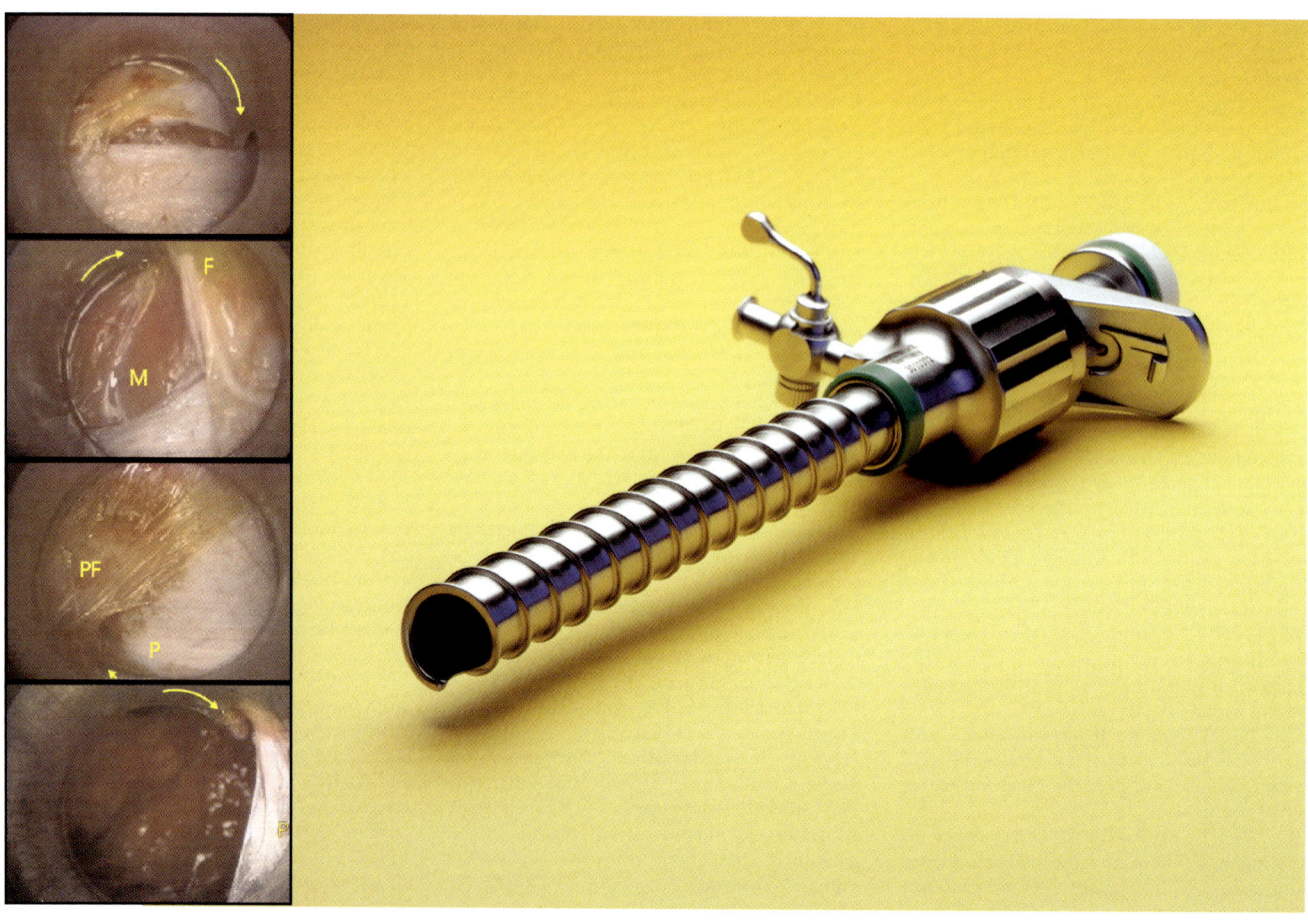

Karl Storz now offers a twist on the usual methods of port insertion. EndoTIP®, Endoscopic Threaded Imaging Port, is a reusable visual entry instrument that makes blind, uncontrolled access of trocars a thing of the past. The unique threadlike design of EndoTIP® separates muscle and tissue fibers, pulling the next level of tissue onto the cannula and away from vital organs.

The EndoTIP® radially dilates the individual tissue layers of the abdominal wall, as opposed to the forward force of pushing in a traditional trocar, reducing the chance of injury or accidental perforation.

As a result, no tissue is transected at entry and no tissue is trapped at exit. This helps to preserve the fascial shutter mechanism, reducing the need for fascial suturing.

Contact your Karl Storz representative today or call us at **(800) 421-0837** for a free demonstration.

KARL STORZ GmbH & Co. KG
Mittelstraße 8, D-78532 Tuttlingen, Germany
Postfach 230, D-78503 Tuttlingen, Germany
Telefon: (07461) 70 80
Telefax: (07461) 70 81 05

KARL STORZ Endoscopy-America, Inc.
600 Corporate Pointe
Culver City, CA 90230-7600
Telephone: (310) 338-8100
            (800) 421-0837
Telefax: (310) 410-5530

KARL STORZ Endoscopy-Canada, Ltd.
438 University Avenue, Suite 1800
Toronto, Ontario, Canada M5G 2K8
Telephone: (416) 596-9900
            (800) 268-4880 (English)
            (800) 361-7388 (Francais)
Telefax: (416) 596-9333

KARL STORZ Endoscopia Latino America
815 N.W. 57th Ave., Ste. No. 480
Miami, FL 33126-2042, USA
Telefono: (305) 262-8980
Telefax: (305) 262-8986

E-mail: karlstorz-marketing@karlstorz.de
Internet: http://www.karlstorz.de
            http://www.karlstorz.com

STORZ
KARL STORZ ENDOSCOPY
THE DIAMOND STANDARD

© 2000 Karl Storz Endoscopy-America, Inc.

Endoscopic Threaded Imaging Port to Improve Laparoscopic Safety

ARTIN M. TERNAMIAN, M.D., FRCSC
DIVISION OF GYNECOLOGIC ENDOSCOPY
ST. JOSEPH'S HEALTH CENTRE
UNIVERSITY OF TORONTO, CANADA

President Clinton's Advisory Commission report on Consumer Protection & Quality in the Health-Care Industry, identified *medical error prevention* as an important issue in health-management. Patient safety is finally being institutionalized due to growing concern over the increasing cost of human error. Medicine's punitive perfectibility model in dealing with unintended injury is slowly evolving to accept error during operations as an inevitable, yet manageable, reality of surgery.[1]

Congress recently passed legislation ordering the Agency for Health-Care Policy and Research to identify strategies to reduce medical error in all fields where "human error" may lead to serious injury. Laparoscopic surgery presents a unique and complex safety challenge compared to conventional surgery, as it is a more dynamic and technology-dependent specialty with complex applications.

Laparoscopists are expected to perform flawlessly in a distorted proprioceptive environment, where pattern recognition, depth perception, tactile feedback, and other important intuitive fundamentals of conventional surgery are lacking.

Fortunately, the incidence of serious laparoscopic injury is rare; however, the reported frequency of access mishaps appears to remain unchanged.[2,3] Surgeons are aware of the potential dangers of endoscopy, especially those associated with laparoscopic port creation using conventional blind push-through trocar systems.[4-6]

In a large prospective study by Jansen and colleagues, the overall complication rate was 5.7/1000 laparoscopic procedures.[7] The authors acknowledged that access injury accounts for up to half the incidence of reported serious laparoscopic complications.[8,9]

The increasing number of procedures performed globally, growing laparoscopic applications in different surgical fields, and increasing frequency of repeat laparoscopies performed on the same patients necessitate serious study and urgent redesign of existing access systems.

The Medical Device Reports (FOI Services Inc., Gaithersburg, MD) data have registered more than 400 serious laparoscopic injuries and 20 deaths for the period of 1994 to 1997, related directly to use of conventional push-through access trocars. Furthermore, laparoscopic mishaps are now less tolerated and most injuries proceed to litigation with an attempt at financial compensation.[10]

When the recent Physician Insurers Association of America statistics are reviewed, laparoscopic injuries appear to be significantly more severe, resulting in higher mean compensation values. Technical limitation and unavoidable surgical complications are clearly part of the laparoscopic approach. Absolute prevention of technical misadventures, whereas desirable medico-legally, may be clinically unachievable, given our current knowledge and technology.[11]

Access systems that use the trocar and cannula design have been described as *First Generation*, as they require application of perpendicular Penetration Force at port site, through a sharp or pointed trocar, to propel the trajectory blindly into body cavities.[12] More importantly, they are unable to offer the surgeon an interactive, error-tolerant access environment where error is anticipated, avoided, or at least, recognized when injury occurs.[13,14]

The ability to introduce safer port methods and intuitive access designs has been limited, because most of our conventional *First-Generation* access systems are blind. Investigators have been unable to observe tissue dynamics at port site during insertion and removal of access cannulas. Consequently, little significant change has occurred in our understanding of port competence, port toilet, and accident causation.

To prevent error recurrence and introduce a laparoscopic port creation system that allows error recovery, detailed *Failure Analysis* should be conducted.[15] This process requires three steps that should be undertaken: (1) review of published frequency and incident reports of access complications; (2) critical analysis of error dynamics; and (3) introduction of innovative system changes that not only avoid error, but also discourage error from progressing to injury.[16]

Detailed observational studies are required to identify weaknesses of conventional *First-Generation* access systems and help determine specific *Performance Shaping Factors* (PSF) that underlie laparoscopic errors and contribute to their resultant surgical complications.[17]

Conventional push-through trocar and cannula design access systems require application of considerable axial Penetration Force to a sharp or pointed trocar. Insertion of the trajectory is usually blind and uncontrolled where the anterior abdominal wall is tented toward the viscera.

The compilation of these PSFs during port insertion render the process more error-prone and sets the stage for inadvertent injury—an accident waiting to happen. Accessing becomes a perilous first step during laparoscopy, even in the best-trained hands, using contemporary instruments and methods.[18] In a large Finnish study, risk of entry-related injury was higher in operative compared to diagnostic laparoscopy.[19]

Surgeons are often reminded that most serious access injuries are operator error-related, implying that inexperience, lack of surgical judgment, or failure to adhere to strict insertion techniques are the principle causative factors.[20,21] However, in complex safety-critical domains other than health, where error-prone tasks are performed by a team of humans, it has been proved that punishment of people, training, and motivation are *ineffective* means of preventing further adverse events.[22]

Possibly, rather than instigating accidents, endoscopic surgeons are often the victims of unreasonable patient expectations, poor access system design, and sub-optimal laparoscopic instrument ergonomics. This important shift in position from "blaming the human," allows one to reexamine the taxonomy of port insertion objectively, and understand tissue dynamics and port competence issues. It can then be appreciated that port insertion and removal is more complex than accepted previously.

Second-Generation Visual Port System: ENDOTIP™

A *Second-Generation* port insertion system (Endoscopic Threaded Imaging Port [ENDOTIP™], Karl Storz, Tuttlingen, Germany) has been developed that attempts to buffer error, through system redesign and ergonomic instrument changes that avoid incorporation of the previously identified PSFs. Trocar entry lacerations can be reduced considerably when port insertion is visual.[23,24]

A port system, to be truly interactive, must incorporate an error-anticipation feature, where the image-capture mechanism visualizes port tissue-dynamics, as it evolves in real-time, ahead of the advancing cannula. Visual control is an important safety factor during laparoscopic ancillary port placement as well. The importance of visual port removal is also recognized, as it relates to long-term port-competence and port-contamination issues.

In this article, the visual laparoscopic *Second-Generation* access system is described and different applications of the new device are illustrated, which, by design, renders port creation more forgiving.

INSTRUMENT DESIGN

Collaboration between surgeon and design engineers, using sophisticated simulation computer software, produced several ergonomic working prototypes for evaluation. Cycles of system design, instrument design, evaluation, and redesign resulted in several prototypes. Additional important considerations included avoidance of moving parts, ease of sterilization, compatibility with currently used equipment, ease of assembly and storage, minimal maintenance and no sharpening required, safety of Operating Room personnel, and gender-related issues.

The final *Second-Generation* access system, introduced the ENDOTIP™ method as an embodiment of our deliberations and trials. ENDOTIP™ has a proximal valve section and distal stainless steel cannula section with a single thread winding diagonally on its outer surface. The thread ends distally in a blunt tip and is available in several lengths and diameters for different surgical applications. It may be used at primary or ancillary ports and can be applied with or without pre-insufflation during closed or open laparoscopy. The cannula also allows extra- or retro-peritoneal laparoscopic operations.[25]

The plastic locking ring (*telescope stopper*), is mounted ahead of the cannula onto the laparoscope to maintain the monitor picture in focus during insertion and removal of the cannula. These reusable rings come in different sizes to fit telescopes of different diameters (Fig. 1).

SURGICAL TECHNIQUE

When performing sophisticated endoscopic operations, surgeons must be knowledgeable in the open conventional methods as well as laparoscopic approach. The decision to pre-insufflate (*closed laparoscopy*) or apply the primary port first and then insufflate (*Hasson's open laparoscopy*) depends on the surgeon's training and other clinical considerations.

An umbilical skin incision is made using a round-tipped, 15-mm surgical blade to allow the cannula to enter the wound. Ribbon retractors and peanut sponges are used to expose the anterior rectus fascia. A small, 8-mm anterior rectus fascial incision is then made under direct vision.

ENDOTIP™ Cannula Insertion At Primary Port During Closed Laparoscopy

The Veress needle is inserted through the anterior fascial incision in the usual way. During insufflation, a 0° laparoscope is defogged and white-balanced, then the telescope stopper followed by the cannula is mounted. The telescope stopper is locked to keep the laparoscope's end 2 cm short of the cannula's distal end. The camera is focused to the cannula's blunt end, and laparoscope held vertical to the patient's supine abdomen using the surgeon's non-dominant hand. When insufflation is complete, the Veress needle is removed, and cannula lowered into the umbilical well with the carbon dioxide (CO_2) stopcock in the ***closed*** position. The cannula is rotated clockwise, using the wrist muscles of the dominant hand while keeping the forearm horizontal to the patient's abdomen, with the surgeon's shoulders square in a resting position facing the monitor.

The blunt tip engages the anterior fascial window, stretches radially, and then lifts to transpose the different tissue layers sequentially onto the cannula's outer thread. Further rotation of the cannula engages the *white* anterior rectus fascia, *red* rectus muscle, then *pearly white* posterior fascia are pulled sequentially up along the outer pitch until the *yellowish* pre-peritoneal space is reached (Fig. 2).

The laparoscope's intense light rays traverse the thin tented peritoneal membrane without reflection, when parietal peritoneal adhesions are absent. The CO_2-filled peritoneal cavity appears *grayish-blue* and vessels, bowel, or adhesions are recognized, avoiding inadvertent injury.

Further rotation of the ENDOTIP™ parts the peritoneum incrementally, under direct visual control, without use of pointed or sharp trocars or application of perpendicular Penetration Force. The cannula must be kept perpendicular to the tissues at all times to avoid tunneling.

When the pre-peritoneal layer is reached, if intra-peritoneal adhesions are present, intense light rays of the laparoscope are reflected off the adherent scar tissue and the area looks white instead of the typical translucent *grayish-blue*. Most post-surgical parietal peritoneal adhesions are linear and the involved tissue may hang vertically in the insufflated abdominal cavity. The surgeon often finds a clear grayish-blue adhesion-free segment through which entry is achieved safely.

The cannula is lifted slightly to disengage the blunt tip and free-rotated to a clear sector where the tip is re-engaged and clockwise rotation resumed. The cannula's blunt tip parts the peritoneal membrane, starting from an adhesion-free clear sector. During clockwise rotation, the adherent tissues tend to move radially out of harm's way, allowing safe and visual placement of the primary cannula.

ENDOTIP™ Cannula Insertion At Primary Port During Open Laparoscopy

When inserting the cannula at the primary port without pre-insufflation, a pair of anterior rectus fascial absorbable stay-sutures are applied at 3 and 9 o'clock and held on a pair of clamps. Ribbon retractors could be applied to

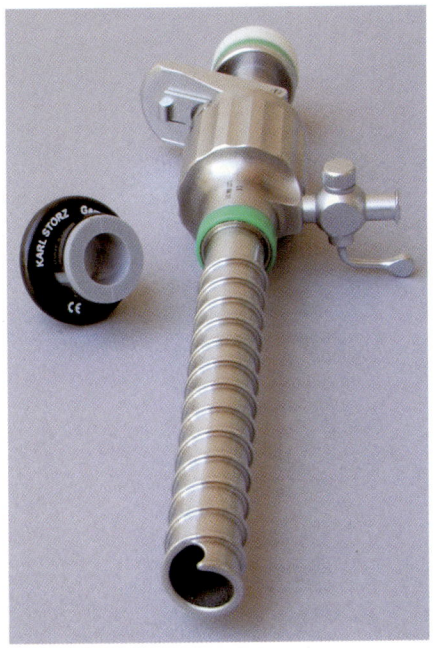

Figure 1. ENDOTIP™ (Karl Storz, Tuttlingen, Germany) cannula and telescope stopper.

better expose the anterior rectus fascia by holding the retractors apart. An 8-mm anterior rectus fascial incision is made using a round-tipped, 15-mm surgical blade (Fig. 3).

The laparoscope is defogged and camera white-balanced, after which the telescope stopper and cannula are mounted. The telescope stopper is then locked to keep the laparoscope's end 2 cm short of the cannula's distal end. The camera is focused to the cannula's blunt end and laparoscope held vertical to the patient's supine abdomen using the surgeon's non-dominant hand.

The ENDOTIP™ cannula, with the CO_2 stopcock in the *open* position, is then lowered into the umbilical well and rotated clockwise, using the wrist muscles of the dominant hand while keeping the forearm horizontal and shoulders square in the resting position.

The cannula's tip engages the anterior fascial window, stretches radially, then lifts to transpose the successive tissue layers on the cannula's outer thread. The *white* anterior rectus fascia, *red* rectus muscle, then *pearly white* posterior fascia are pulled up along the outer pitch to the *yellowish* pre-peritoneum. At this level, given the intense light and magnification of the laparoscope, bowel or omentum may be observed on the monitor, moving across the transparent peritoneal membrane with the respiratory movements of the patient. After a peritoneal opening is created, room-air streams through the cannula's open CO_2 stopcock, into the vacuum-sealed peritoneal cavity and the peritoneal edge is clearly recognized.

During closed pre-insufflated laparoscopy, the CO_2-filled buffer zone is interposed between the access device and intra-abdominal organs. In open laparoscopy, the visual access cannula encounters the abdominal contents directly upon peritoneal entry. Consequently, it is very important not to push the cannula axially towards the abdomen while rotating, once the peritoneal cavity is entered.

When a fixed intra- or retroperitoneal organ is encountered upon entering the abdominal cavity, such as large bowel or a large pelvic mass, room air streams in between the organ's surface and partially parted peritoneal membrane. Clockwise rotation is then stopped, and CO_2 insufflation initiated under direct visual control (Fig. 4).

If loose, freely mobile intra-peritoneal organs such as omentum or small bowel are encountered at the access site, upon entering the abdominal cavity, part of the omentum or small bowel may balloon into the cannula, given the open CO_2 stopcock. Rotation is then stopped and CO_2 insufflation initiated. The inflowing CO_2 gas recedes the ballooned tissues back into the peritoneal cavity as the abdominal wall rises with insufflation (Figs. 5 & 6).

During retro- or extra-peritoneal laparoscopic procedures, such as para-aortic lymph node dissection, extraperitoneal hernia repair or uro-suspension procedures, the cannula's rotation is stopped when the desired tissue layer is reached. A virtual cavity is then created under direct vision by blunt dissection and CO_2 insufflation. As the dissection is monitored visually, inadvertent perforation of the peritoneal membrane is avoided. At ancillary ports, especially where the skin incision is small, the cannula is anchored securely at port site by the outer thread. The snug fit discourages CO_2 loss. The retro-peritoneal approach is preferred by several onco- and uro-laparoscopists, as it is believed to cause less pain and less risk for inadvertent bowel or vascular injury.[26] Although safe to be used in any body weight, overweight patients and those who have had previous abdominal surgery could require a

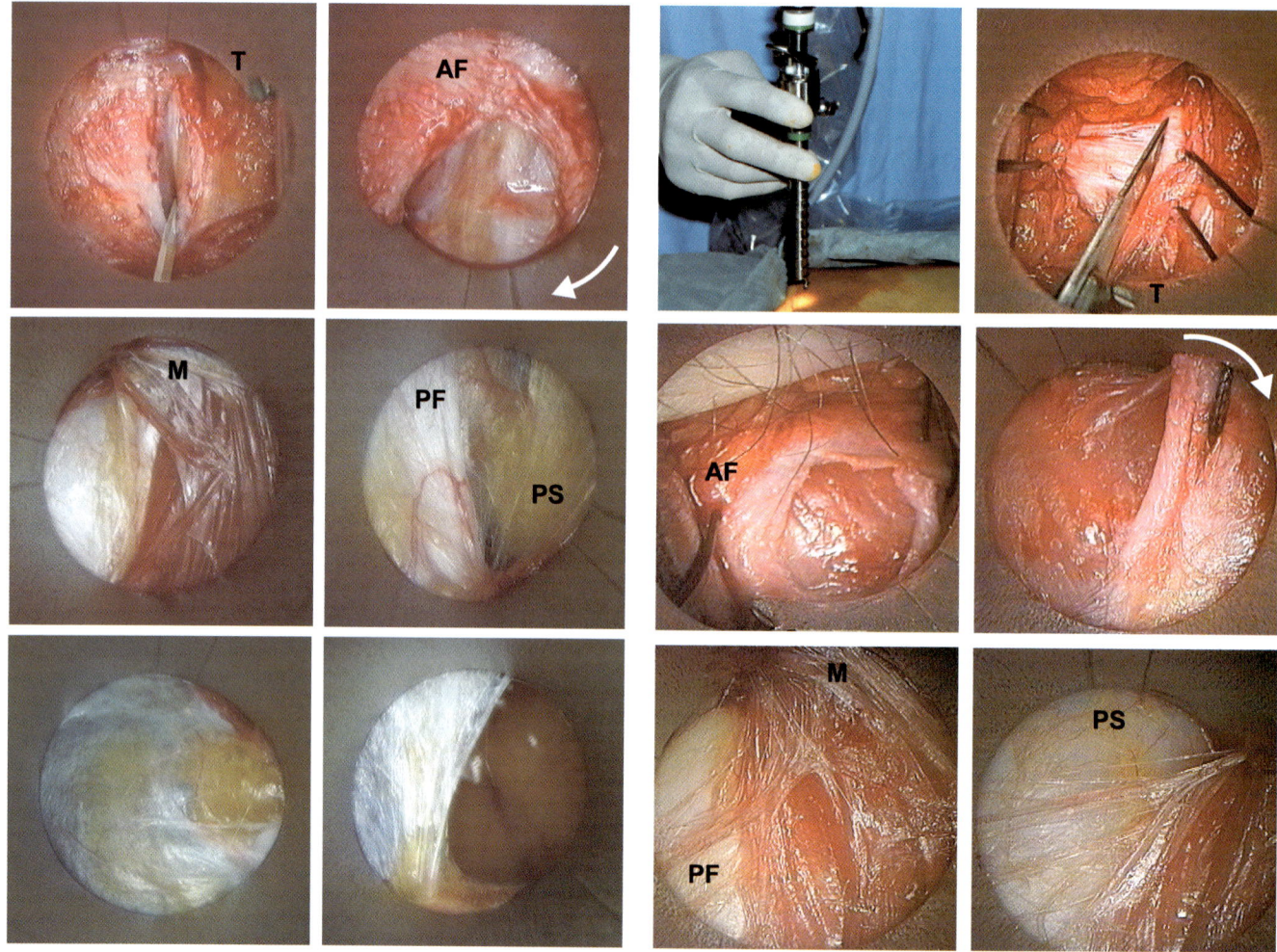

Figure 2. ENDOTIP™ (Karl Storz, Tuttlingen, Germany) cannula insertion at primary port during closed laparoscopy (carbon dioxide [CO_2] stopcock in closed position). Clockwise rotation lifts, white anterior rectus fascia (AF), *red* rectus muscle (M), *pearly-white* posterior fascia (PF) up along outer thread until *yellowish* pre-peritoneal space (PS) is reached. CO_2-filled, adhesion-free peritoneal cavity looks *grayish-blue*.

Figure 3. ENDOTIP™ (Karl Storz, Tuttlingen, Germany) cannula insertion at primary port during open laparoscopy (carbon dioxide [CO_2] stopcock in open position). Anterior rectus fascia incised using 15-mm scalpel. Blunt cannula tip (T). *White* anterior rectus fascia (AF), *red* rectus muscle (RM), *pearly-white* posterior fascia (PF) are pulled up along outer thread until *yellowish* pre-peritoneal space is reached. Pre-peritoneal space (PS).

longer insertion time.[27]

ENDOTIP™ Cannula Insertion At Ancillary Port

During ancillary port insertion, only a skin incision and dissection of the subcutaneous tissue is needed; an anterior rectus fascial incision and ancillary telescope are not necessary. As with all ancillary port insertions, the ENDOTIP™ cannula must also be introduced under direct visual control through the primary port.

The cannula is held perpendicular to the skin surface and rotated clockwise with the dominant hand. To avoid peritoneal tunneling, insertion must remain at a right angle to the skin surface until the abdominal cavity is entered. Vessels encountered along the cannula's path gravitate radially out of harm's way and are not transected (Fig. 7).

The position of the *superficial epigastric vessels* and *inferior epigastric vessels* should also be determined before insertion. The urinary bladder must be emptied before insertion of suprapubic ports. If the obliterated umbilical artery is encountered, a peritoneal opening can be created using an L-hook cautery through the partly inserted ancillary port. The cannula is then threaded through the peritoneal opening.

ENDOTIP™ Cannula Removal

When the operation is completed, the CO_2 stopcock is closed, tubing disconnected, laparoscope's end retracted 2 cm into the cannula, telescope stopper locked in position, and camera focused to the cannula's end. The laparoscope is held perpendicular to the patient's abdomen with the non-dominant hand, and cannula rotated counterclockwise with the surgeon's dominant hand (Fig. 8).

The CO_2 is released through an ancillary cannula to avoid spraying of body fluids onto the telescope's lens. The anterior abdominal wall layers disengage in sequence off the cannula's outer thread to regain their natural grid-iron orientation and restore the shutter mechanism at the access site.

The threaded cannula is gradually rotated counterclockwise, with the laparoscope mounted in the cannula until removed completely. Removal is visual, incremental, and controlled.

Rapid cannula removal is discouraged; rather, the surgeon can identify the compromised or at-risk port sites visually, and take appropriate measures to reinforce the fascial area in question

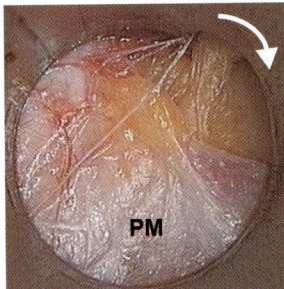 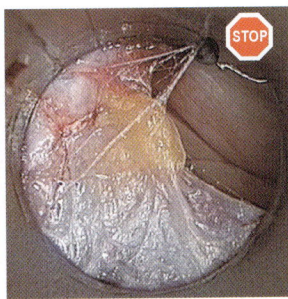 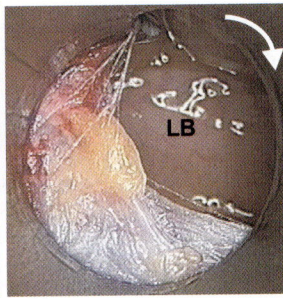

Figure 4. When peritoneal cavity is entered, rotation is stopped and insufflation initiated under visual control. When retro- or extra-peritoneal organs present, such as large bowel (LB), air streams underneath peritoneal membrane (PM), and peritoneal edge seen clearly.

to avoid hernia formation, although port-site fascial closure does not appear to necessarily avoid hernia formation. Tissue injury or entrapment along the cannula's tract is also avoided.[28]

Closure of fascial defects is important when cannulas with a diameter of more than 10 mm are used, the fascia at port-site is extended for surgical tissue retrieval, port-site tissues are inflamed or thin, infection is suspected, patient has chronic cough or asthma, following long laparoscopic operations, and/or tissue integrity appears compromised.

CONCLUSION

Creation of ports has always been considered a critical first step in laparoscopy. In the past, newer port systems and devices have been introduced to improve safety, with no real change in the conventional push-through trocar design.

First-generation port systems require considerable, uncontrolled axial Penetration Force at port-site to thrust the trajectory blindly toward the peritoneum. This access method is unable to avoid, or recognize error when it occurs, and has no redundancy.

A new *Second-Generation* port system and access instrument is described to render laparoscopic port insertion and removal error-tolerant. This system effectively buffers inevitable surgical error through access system redesign, where perpendicular Penetration Force is avoided by realigning the direction of entry force from axial to radial. Sharp or pointed trocars are not required and visual, incremental, and interactive port creation is possible.

Surgeons can visualize tissue dynamics at port site and have an opportunity to better address port toilet and port

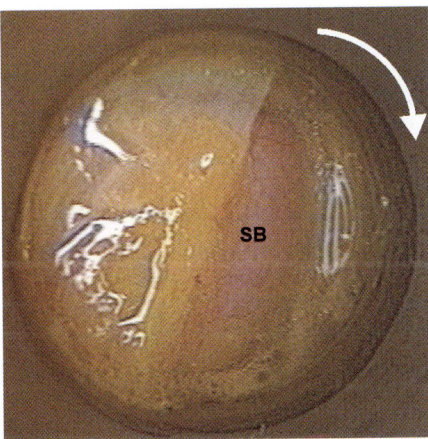 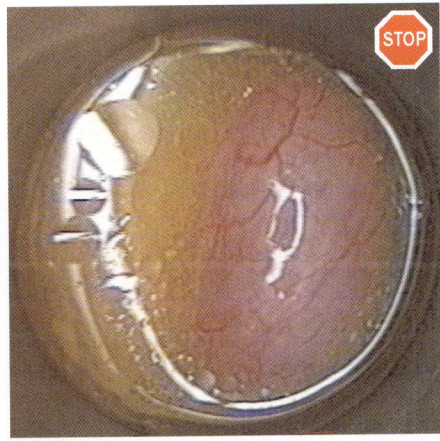 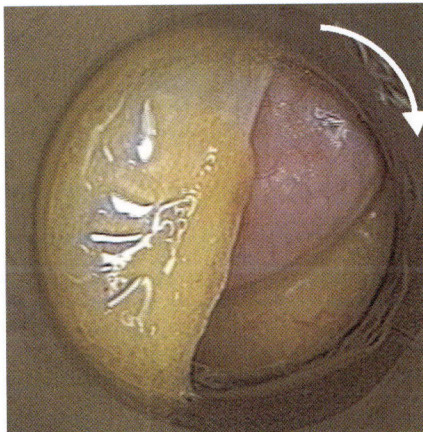

Figure 5. When presenting organ is freely mobile in peritoneal cavity, such as small bowel (SB), after peritoneal cavity is entered, room-air streams in through open carbon dioxide (CO_2) stopcock. Small bowel balloons into cannula. Rotation is stopped and insufflation initiated under visual control.

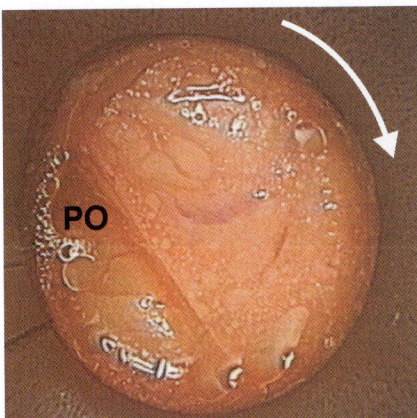 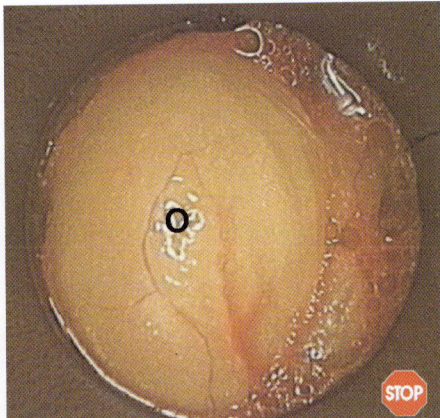 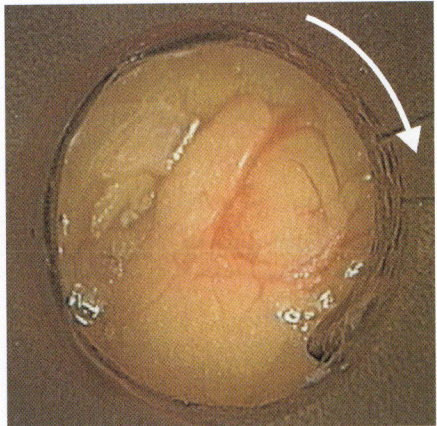

Figure 6. After peritoneal layer is reached, thin peritoneal membrane transilluminates. Omentum or bowel is recognized and inadvertent injury avoided. When peritoneal opening (PO) is created, room air streams in through open carbon dioxide (CO_2) stopcock. Omentum (O) balloons into cannula. Rotation is stopped, and insufflation initiated under vision. Omentum falls back into peritoneal cavity. Clockwise rotation is resumed to complete insertion.

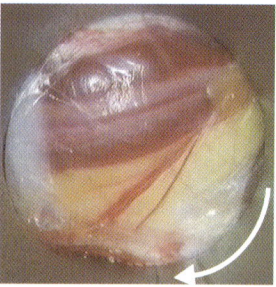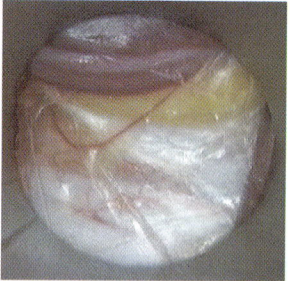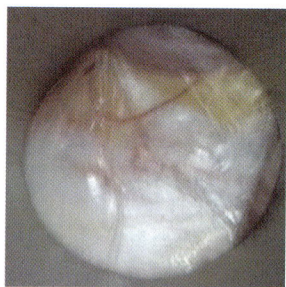

Figure 7. Vessels encountered along cannula's tract are not transected, they are moved radially out of cannula's path.

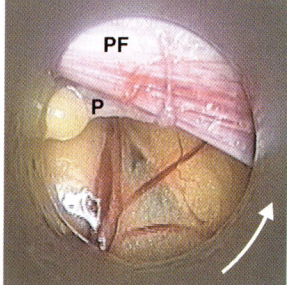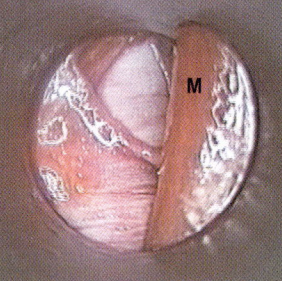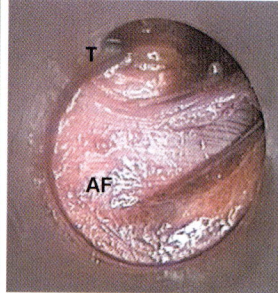

Figure 8. Anterior abdominal wall layers disengage in sequence off cannula's outer thread to regain their natural grid-iron orientation and restore shutter mechanism at access site. Peritoneum (P), posterior rectus fascia (PF), rectus muscle (M), cannula tip (T), anterior rectus fascia (AF).

competence concerns. By recognizing error in real-time, when mishaps occur, the surgeon has a timely error-recovery opportunity that prevents error from progressing to harm.

Given the visual and intuitive nature of *Second-Generation* access systems, it is anticipated that our understanding of the etiology of laparoscopic access complications and safety will improve. Rather than blaming surgical performance or instrument design, instituting tolerant laparoscopic *access systems* can improve patient safety and reduce the probability of recurrent access error.

Given Congress aiming at a 50% reduction of unintended medical error over the next five years, patient-safety initiatives such as safer laparoscopic access methods and instruments are urgently needed to render minimally invasive surgery a truly patient-friendly and safer-operative method.

REFERENCES

1. Leap LL. Error in medicine. Special Communication. JAMA 1994; 272: 1851-7.
2. Jackimowicz JJ. Current state and trends in minimal access surgery in Europe. J R Coll Surg Edin 1995; 40: 397-406.
3. Querleu D, Chapron C. Complications of gynecologic laparoscopic surgery. Curr Opin Obstet Gynecol 1995; 7: 257-61.
4. Hashizume M, Sugimachi K. Needle and trocar injury during laparoscopic surgery in Japan. Study group of endoscopic surgery in Kyushu, Japan. Surg Endosc 1997; 11: 1198-201.
5. Mac Cordick C, Lecuru F, Rizk E, et al. Morbidity in laparoscopic gynecological surgery. Surg Endosc 1999; 13: 57-61.
6. Nuzzo G, Giuliante F, Tebala G D, et al. Routine use of open technique in laparoscopic operations. J Am Coll Surg 1997; 184: 58-62.
7. Jansen FW, Kapiteyn K, Trimbos-Kemper T, et al. Complications of laparoscopy: a prospective multicentre observational study. Br J Obstet Gynaecol 1997; 104: 595-600.
8. Deziel DJ. Avoiding laparoscopic complications. Int Surg 1994; 79: 1-4.
9. Chandler J, Bartholomew L. Complications of cholecystectomy. J Gastrointest Surg 1997; 1(2): 138-45.
10. Garry R. Towards evidence-based laparoscopic entry techniques: clinical problems and dilemmas-Editorial. Gynae Endosc 1999; 8: 315-26.
11. Kern K A. Malpractice litigation involving laparoscopic cholecystectomy. Cost, cause, and consequences. Arch Surg 1997; 132: 392-8.
12. Ternamian AM. A second-generation laparoscopic port system: ENDOTIP™. Gynae Endosc 1999; 8: 397-401.
13. Chapron CM, Querleu D, Bruhat M-A, et al. Surgical complications of diagnostic and operative gynaecological laparoscopy: a series of 29 966 cases. Eur Soc Hum Reprod Embryol 1998; 13: 867-72.
14. Soderstrom R. Bowel injury litigation after laparoscopy. J Am Assoc Gynecol Laparosc 1993; 1: 74-7.
15. Troidl H, Bäcker B, Langer B, et al. Fehleranalyse-Evaluierung und Verhütung von Komplikationen; ihre juristische Implikation. Langenbeck Arch Chir Suppl 1993: 59-72.
16. Troidl H, Eypasch E, Spangenberger W, et al. Schonendes Operieren. Verfahrenswahl und Strategie. Invasives versus minimal invasives Operieren. Langenbeck Arch Chir Suppl 1991: 48.
17. Joice P, Hanna GB, Cuschieri A. Errors enacted during laparoscopic surgery—a human reliability analysis. Applied Ergonomics 1998; 29: 409-14.
18. Ternamian AM. Laparoscopy without trocars. Surg Endosc 1997; 11: 815-8.
19. Härkki-Sirén P, Sjöberg J, Kurki T. Major complications of laparoscopy: a follow-up Finnish study. Obstet Gynecol 1999; 94: 94-8.
20. Marret H, Harchaoui Y, Chapron C, et al. Trocar injuries during laparoscopic gynaecological surgery. Report from the French Society of Gynaecological Laparoscopy. Gynae Endosc 1998; 7: 235-41.
21. Chapron C M, Pierre F, Lacroix S, et al. Major vascular injuries during gynecologic laparoscopy. J Am Coll Surg 1997; 185: 461-5.
22. Reason J. Human Error. Cambridge, Mass: Cambridge University Press; 1992.
23. Marret H, Pierre F, Chapron C, et al. Complications of laparoscopy caused by trocars. Preliminary study from the national registry of the French Society of Gynaecologic Endoscopy. J Gynécol Obstét Biol Repro 1997; 26 (4): 405-12.
24. Mettler L, Ibrahim M, Vu Quang V, et al. Clinical experience with an optical access trocar in gynecological laparoscopy-pelviscopy. J Soc Laparo Surg 1997; 1: 315-8.
25. Ternamian AM. A trocarless reusable visual-access cannula for safer laparoscopy; an update. J Am Assoc Gynecol Laparosc 1998; 5: 197-201.
26. Kuenkel M, Schaller G, Korth K. Retroperitoneoscopy-the approach to urological minimal invasive surgery. J Endouro 1993; 7: (Suppl 1): S224.
27. Ternamian A, Deitel M. Endoscopic threaded imaging port (ENDOTIP) for laparoscopy: Experience with different body weights. Obestet Surg 1999; 9: 44-7.
28. Montz FJ, Holschneider CH, Monro MG. Incisional hernia following laparoscopy: a Survey of the American Association of Gynecological Laparoscopists. Obstet Gynecol 1994; 84: 881-4.

Telerobotic Minimally Invasive Procedures in Urology — Laparoscopic Radical Prostatectomy

JOCHEN BINDER, M.D.
UROLOGIST, PRIV. DOZ.

WOLFGANG KRAMER, M.D.
UROLOGIST, PRIV. DOZ.

DEPT. OF UROLOGY AND PEDIATRIC UROLOGY
J. W. GOETHE UNIVERSITY
FRANKFURT, GERMANY

A telerobotic device, the daVinci Surgical System (Intuitive Surgical, Inc., Mountain View, CA) is one of the recently developed, remotely operated systems for laparoscopic surgical procedures.[1] This telemanipulation system consists of two components: a control console operated by the surgeon, and the surgical arm cart that holds a three-dimensional (3-D) 30° laparoscope and two detachable laparoscopic surgical tools. The instruments are equipped with a wrist — a unique feature that provides additional dexterity. Since its clinical introduction in Europe in early 1999, this system has opened up a new era in minimally invasive surgery enhancing endoscopic vision and anastomosis suturing.[2] For the first time, cardiac surgeons were able to perform a totally endoscopic coronary bypass procedure on a beating heart.[3]

To our knowledge, no information exists regarding the applicability of this novel telerobotic device in standard and advanced laparoscopic procedures in the field of urology. Before introduction of this telerobic system, standard laparoscopic procedures at our institution included nephrectomies for benign conditions and pelvic lymphadenectomies. However, complex urologic operations were performed routinely by way of the standard open surgical approach.

Specifically, for radical prostatectomy, the method of choice was the open retropubic technique. The feasibility of laparoscopic radical prostatectomy had been established initially by Schuessler et al. in 1992.[4] However, only in the past two years has the technique of laparoscopic radical prostatectomy been standardized by Guillonneau and Vallancien as well as others and, by the year 2001, has replaced the open retropubic approach in some centers.[5-7]

This telerobotic system has been developed to facilitate adaptation of laparoscopic surgery for the conventionally trained surgeon. The Endowrist instrument technology introduces additional ranges of freedom and, thereby, a high degree of articulation of the laparoscopic tools, whereas the 3-D vision system provides the surgeon full control over the laparoscope, as well as an excellent magnified view. As urologic surgeons without experience with

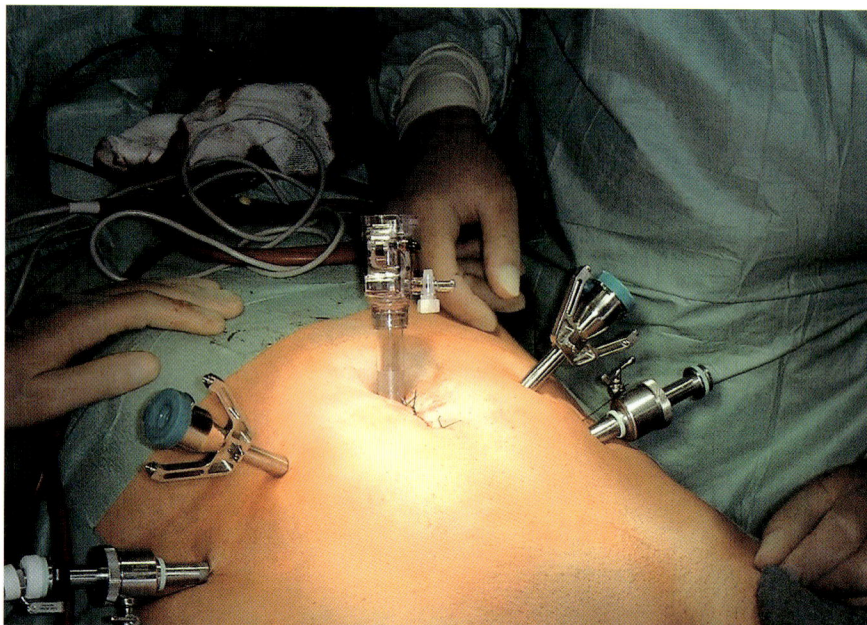

Figure 1. The patient is placed supine with arms at the sides and legs parted on spreader bars. A 2.5- to 3.0-cm midline laparotomy is made subumbilically, and all trocars inserted under digital guidance: two 8-mm special trocars for the robotic-assisted tools are positioned pararectally bilaterally, and two 10-mm standard trocars just medial to the iliac crest. Laparotomy is closed temporarily around the 12-mm camera trocar to prevent gas leakage from the pneumoperitoneum.

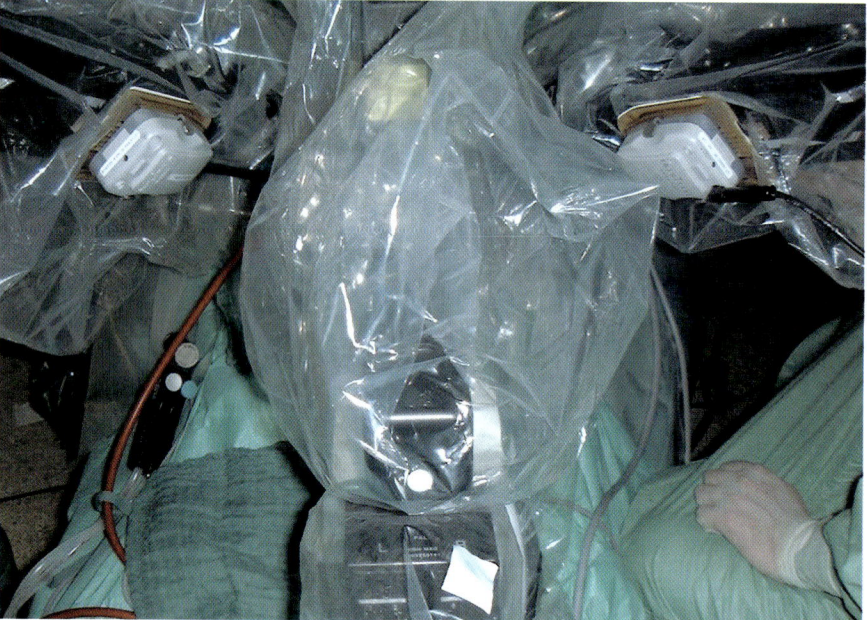

Figure 2. Intraoperative external view. The surgical arm console is positioned at the foot of the operation table, and three-dimensional 30° laparoscope inserted into the subumbilical trocar and connected to the middle robotic arm. Special laparoscopic tools are inserted into the two pararectally placed trocars and attached to the two lateral robotic arms by the assistant at the patient site.

complex laparoscopic procedures, our objective was to test the usefulness of this telerobotic system in introduction of laparoscopic radical prostatectomy.

OPERATIVE TECHNIQUE

The patient is placed supine with arms at the sides and legs parted on spreader bars. A 2.5- to 3.0-cm midline laparotomy is made subumbilically and all ports are inserted under digital guidance. Two 8-mm special trocars for the robotic-assisted tools are positioned pararectally bilaterally, and two 10-mm standard trocars just medially to the iliac crest. The laparotomy is closed temporarily around the 12-mm camera trocar to prevent gas leakage from the pneumoperitoneum (Fig. 1). The surgical arm console is positioned at the foot of the operation table, and the 3-D 30° laparoscope inserted into the subumbilical trocar and connected to the middle robotic arm (Fig. 2)

Having completed these preparations at the patient site, the urologist sits comfortably at the console, head tilted forward and eyes peering down through binoculars (Fig. 3). The urologist views a high-resolution, 3-D video image and can adjust the position of the laparoscope mounted on a robotic arm for the best view of the magnified operative field. A variety of different laparoscopic tools is inserted into the two pararectally placed trocars and attached to the two lateral robotic arms by his assistant at the patient site; from these, the surgeon chooses two of them. The surgeon's hands are held in a comfortable position in front of his body and his fingers are inserted into the system's master interfaces that monitor, in minute detail, the position of his hands as he performs the surgery. Every move the surgeon makes is replicated precisely and simultaneously by tiny, electromechanically driven surgical tools inside the patient's body. By the system's motion-scaling capability, the urologist's hand movements are translated into small movements at the operating site, while effects of hand tremors are filtered out.

When viewing the surgical field through the console, the urologist can see the ends of the robotic arms (the instrument tips) as they move under his direction. In addition, a certain haptic sense, a force feedback, is reproduced. When the instrument arm encounters resistance inside the patient, that resistance is transmitted back to the console, where it can be felt by the urologist.

A primary component of this telerobotic system is the EndoWrist technology (Fig. 4). It allows the urologist to roll, pitch, yaw, and grip his laparoscopic tools, providing a total of seven degrees of freedom for each hand. The instruments used most frequently are a cautery hook, short-tip grasper, bipolar hemostatic grasper, and two needle holders. These tools are all equipped with EndoWrist articulations.

The entire laparoscopic procedure including bilateral pelvic lymph node dissection, radical prostatovesiculectomy, and urethrovesical anastomosis was performed by the operating urologist from the remote console. A urologic assistant and operating room nurse remained at the patient site and used the two lateral 10-mm ports, which allowed access for conventional laparoscopic instruments as clip applier, large grasper, and a suction device.

The operative technique is essentially a combined retrograde and anterograde prostatectomy procedure. Most operative steps resemble those used for open retropubic radical prostatectomy at our institution. In brief, it includes bilateral pelvic lymphadenectomy and frozen section examination of lymph tissue; dissection of the urachus to open up Retzius space; preparation and lateral incision of the endopelvic fascia; dissection of the puboprostatic ligaments and preparation of the prostatic apex; ligation of the venous plexus with vicryl 2-0; dissection of the urethra; incision of Denonvilliers' fascia and ascending preparation of the dorsal aspect of the prostate; dissection of the bladder neck, descending dissection of ducts and seminal vesicles; parking of the prostate in an organ bag; reconstruction of the bladder neck; and vesicourethral anastomosis with eight interrupted sutures PDS 3-0 (Fig. 3); transurethral insertion of a 20-Fr Foley catheter; insertion of a silicone drain; removal of the organ bag through the midline laparotomy; closure of the rectus fascia; and, finally, wound closure (Fig. 5).

EARLY CLINICAL RESULTS

The first urologic applications of the daVinci Surgical System were performed at our institution between May and September 2000, in patients eligible for laparoscopic radical prostatectomy (n=20).[8]

Median patient age was 60.5 (range: 57-72) years; clinical tumor stage was T1b, T1c, T2a, or T2b, and median prostate-specific antigen (PSA) concentration was 6.0 ng/mL (range: 0.5-22.4). Two patients had a previous transurethral resection of the prostate; six had a neoadjuvant hormone ablative therapy prescribed elsewhere. All operations were performed by one of the two authors. In 18 of 20 patients, the planned operative procedure was completed after a median laparoscopy time of 9 (range: 7.5-11) hours. After 42 patients, operating time was reduced to 4 hours (240 minutes). Laparoscopy was abandoned in one patient due to

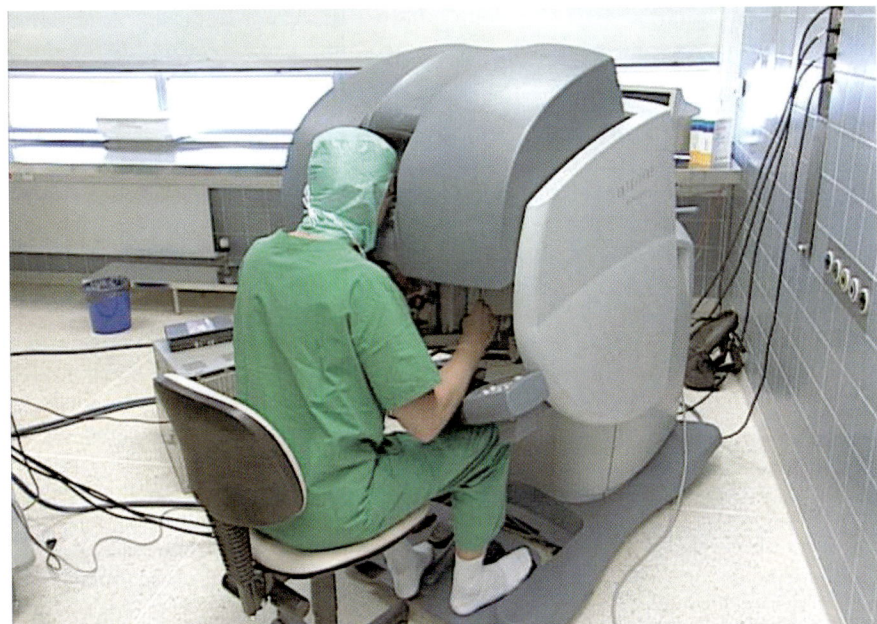

Figure 3. Control console. The urologist sits at the console, head tilted forward and eyes peering down through binoculars. The surgeon's hands are held in a comfortable position in front of his body and his fingers are inserted into the system's master interfaces that monitor, in minute detail, the position of his hands as he performs the surgery.

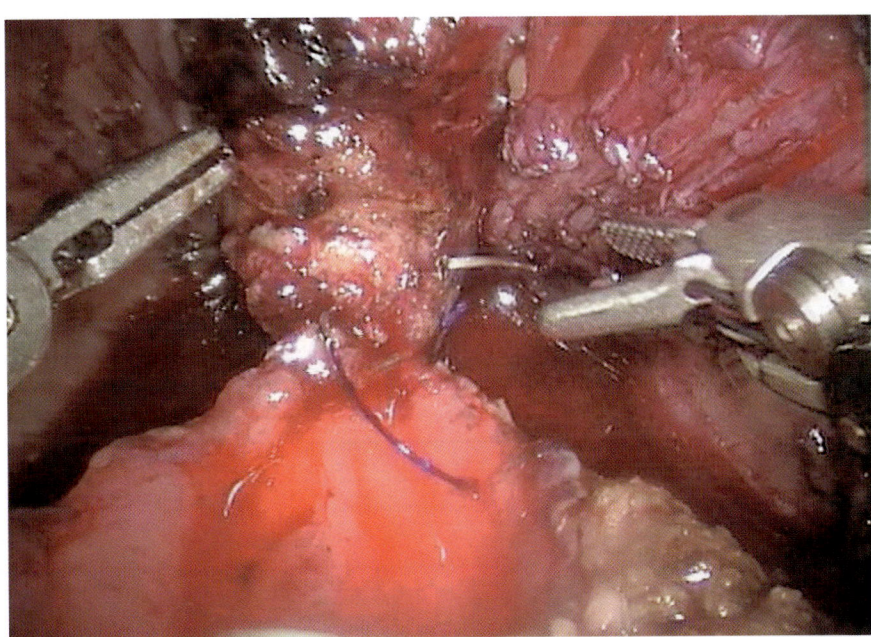

Figure 4. Intraoperative endoscopic view. Anastomosis of the bladder neck with the urethral stump using two needle holders. EndoWrist technology allows the urologist to roll, pitch, yaw, and grip the laparoscopic tools, providing a total of seven degrees of freedom for each hand.

difficulties in controlling hemostasis (case number 1) after completion of prostatectomy, and in one due to loss of a tool fragment between the small bowel (case number 14). Intraoperative complications occurred in 3 (15%) patients: profuse bleeding from the venous plexus in one, an epigastric artery laceration in one, and a partial and reversible obturator nerve injury in one. The reoperation rate was 5% (ligation of epigastric artery). The transfusion rate was 40% (n=8), with a median transfusion of two units of blood. All patients recovered quickly after surgery. The transurethral Foley catheter was removed after a median of 14 (range: 5-23) days. When discharged one to three days after catheter removal, most patients complained of mild-to-moderate stress incontinence.

The final pathologic examination of

the specimen disclosed 4 to 12 pelvic lymph nodes, with no evidence for regional lymph node metastases in 19 of 20 patients. In one patient with a preoperative PSA value of 3.3 ng/mL, however, small lymph node metastases had been missed by frozen section. Prostate histology showed adenocarcinomas of the prostate, classified as: pT2a (n=5), pT2b (n=10), pT3a (n=3), pT3b (n=2); positive resection margins (R1) were noted in five patients (1/15 pT2 tumors, 4/5 pT3 tumors).

DISCUSSION

In this article, the feasibility of laparoscopic radical prostatectomy using a remotely operated surgical system is demonstrated. The daVinci Surgical System provides not only provide a hardware interface but, more importantly, a computer interface between the surgeon's hands and its robotic arms. In addition to high-resolution 3-D visualization and a relaxed working position at the console with harmonious control of two surgical instruments and camera position, the Endowrist instrument technology empowers the surgeon to dissect, suture, and tie knots endoscopically much as he does in open surgery. In many ways, laparoscopic surgery with this telerobotic system resembles open surgery under a dome.

From our initial experience with 20 patients, we expect the functional and oncologic results with this operative technique should be equally as good, or better than, with our standard open retropubic prostatectomy technique. The long operative time reflects the learning process, as our experience with telemanipulation and with complex laparoscopy has been rather limited. Despite its broader dissemination in the last two years, laparoscopic radical prostatectomy is still regarded as a difficult and complex procedure.[9] In addition to perfect knowledge of the topographic anatomy and broad conventional surgical experience, it demands training of specific laparoscopic skills such as endoscopic suturing and intracorporeal knotting within a limited space below the symphysis on the pelvic floor. The learning curve for the individual urologist has been estimated to require experience of approximately 50 cases.[10] As has been seen with other laparoscopic techniques (i.e., cholecystectomy), the operative time can be expected to decrease substantially with increasing routine.[11] In fact, after a series of 42 patients, the operating time has been reduced by more than half, to 4 hours (240 minutes).

The potential of the presented novel technique is definitely its great surgical accuracy. Moreover, introducing computer technology to bridge the surgeon's hands with robotic tools may well lead to an expansion of the surgeon's capabilities beyond the limitations of conventional surgery. Our initial experience leads us to believe urologic patients may be among those profiting from this development. In the case of radical prostatectomy, nerve-sparing surgery may become more reliable without taking a risk concerning the oncologic result.

REFERENCES

1. Stoianovici D. Robotic surgery. World J Urol 2000; 18:289-95.
2. Loulmet D, Carpentier A, d'Attellis N, et al. Endoscopic coronary artery bypass grafting with the aid of robotic assisted instruments. J Thorac Cardiovasc Surg 1999; 118:4-10.
3. Falk V, Diegeler A, Walther T, et al. Total endoscopic computer enhanced coronary artery bypass grafting. Eur J Cardiothorac Surg 2000; 17:38-45.
4. Schuessler WW, Kavoussi LR, Clayman RV, et al. Laparoscopic radical prostatectomy: Initial case report. J Urol 1992; 147:246A.
5. Guillonneau B, Vallancien G. Laparoscopic radical prostatectomy: The Montsouris-technique. J Urol 2000; 163:1643-9.
6. Abbou C, Hoznek A, Salomon L, et al. Laparoscopic radical prostatectomy. J Urol 1999; 161:17A.
7. Rassweiler J, Sentker L, Seemann O, et al. Laparoscopic radical prostatectomy: Technique and early experience. [in German] Akt Urol 2000; 31:237-45.
8. Binder J, Kramer W. Robotically-assisted laparoscopic radical prostatectomy. BJU International 2001; 87:408-410.
9. Janetschek G, Marberger M. Laparoscopic surgery in urology. Curr Opin Urol 2000; 10:351 7.
10. Thüroff JW. Laparoscopic radical prostatectomy: Feasibility studies or the future-standard technique? Editorial comment. Curr Opin Urol 2000; 10:363-4.
11. Guillonneau B, Vallancien G. Laparoscopic radical prostatectomy: The Montsouris experience. J Urol 2000; 163:418-22.

Using a Multi-Modal Rehabilitation Program for Patients Undergoing Open Sigmoidectomy

OSCAR A. DE LEON-CASASOLA, M.D.
PROFESSOR OF ANESTHESIOLOGY
VICE-CHAIRMAN FOR CLINICAL AFFAIRS
UNIVERSITY AT BUFFALO SCHOOL OF MEDICINE
CHIEF OF PAIN MEDICINE
ROSWELL PARK CANCER INSTITUTE
BUFFALO, NEW YORK

Postoperative ileus, a temporary inhibition of gastrointestinal function, is a universal complication after major abdominal surgery. Treatment for ileus is supportive, and has changed little since Wangensteen's 1932 report.[1] Nasogastric suction could delay or replace operative management of bowel obstruction, thereby reducing mortality. Gastric decompression, together with intravenous (IV) hydration and electrolyte replacement, remains the only proven therapy for ileus.[2,3]

Liu and colleagues[4] suggested that epidural analgesia may shorten the duration of postoperative ileus significantly. The benefits of a reduction in ileus include decreased patient morbidity and, potentially, substantial cost-savings, as prolongation of hospital stay in the United States due to ileus has been estimated to cost $1,500 per patient, or $750 million dollars annually.[3] However, clinical guidelines currently promulgated by some consulting firms continue to state that "while epidural analgesia is effective for thoracic surgery and certain major musculoskeletal procedures, it has often been associated with prolonged ileus, delayed oral nutrition, and discharge in patients with gastrointestinal surgery (Milliman and Robertson, Inc., Actuaries and Consultants, Seattle, WA, written communication, 1996).

In this article, the pathophysiology of postoperative ileus is reviewed, and a framework for recognizing the theoretical basis for an effect of epidural anesthesia, especially thoracic epidural anesthesia, and a multi-modal rehabilitation program implemented in the first two postoperative days, on ileus is provided. The major focus of this article is to review the results of a recent study that has been published applying this concept. Comments are also included regarding our experience in using this protocol for management of patients.

PATHOPHYSIOLOGY

Nearly 100 years ago, Canon and Murphy[5] demonstrated that opening the peritoneal cavity and manipulating the intestines resulted in a striking inhibition of contractile activity in the gastrointestinal tracts of dogs. The same authors also reported ileus associated with an extra-abdominal procedure (crushing the testicles) in cats, whereas Meltzer and Auer[6] noted that ileus may follow various, less-noxious stimuli in rabbits.

Parasympathetic stimulation increases gastrointestinal motility, but tonic inhibitory sympathetic control normally predominates. Thus, blockade of the splanchnic nerves or spinal anesthesia

Table 1. Factors that alter gastrointestinal motility in humans or animals

Increased Motility	Decreased Motility
Parasympathetic stimulation	Sympathetic Stimulation
Splanchnic nerve blockade	Pain
Spinal anesthesia	Opioids
Epidural anesthesia	Nitrous Oxide
Alpha-adrenergic blockade	Inhalation anesthetics
Beta-adrenergic blockade	Vasopression
Cholinergic agonists	Catecholamine administration
Anticholinesterase agents	Increased endogenous catecholamines
Local anesthetics (IV)	

results in increased motility or inhibits development of ileus, whereas thoracotomy has little apparent effect. Although the autonomic nervous system has a major role in regulating gastrointestinal transit, other factors also must be involved. Factors that alter gastrointestinal motility in humans or animals are listed in Table 1.

Typically, uncomplicated postoperative ileus is associated with restoration of motility in the stomach and small bowel within 24 hours, whereas the colon recovers over 48 to 72 hours.[7,8] Neely[9] suggested that duration of postoperative ileus was related to severity of the surgical procedure, but other authors' findings do not confirm these data. Other authors used the term, paralytic or adynamic ileus, to refer to more severe, prolonged inhibition of bowel function, as differentiated from the usual type of uncomplicated postoperative ileus that lasts no more than three days.

The duration of postoperative ileus is increased by opioids.[10] The dose-dependent inhibitory effects of morphine and other opiates on motility suggest a possible contributory role for endogenous opioids in the pathogenesis of postoperative ileus. However, the lack of effect of naloxone on postoperative bowel function in rats does not support this notion.[11]

Inhaled anesthetics may decrease gastrointestinal motility, but motility consistently recovers within a matter of minutes after cessation of anesthesia in multiple animal studies. Thus, it is unlikely that inhaled anesthetics are responsible for diminished gastrointestinal motility lasting much beyond the immediate postoperative period.

Nitrous oxide may have longer lasting deleterious effects on motility than do the volatile anesthetics. In a study of 40 patients undergoing elective major large-bowel surgery under general anesthesia with isoflurane and fentanyl, Scheinin and colleagues[12] noted significantly earlier return of bowel function, as assessed by the passage of flatus and feces, in the 20 patients randomly allocated to compare with the 20 patients allocated to intraoperative nitrous oxide. The groups were comparable with respect to demographics and surgical procedures. The duration of postoperative hospital stay was significantly shorter for the air group (mean +/- SD; 10 +/- 1.3 vs. 11.7 +/- 2.5 days, P 0.05).

IV infusion of lidocaine shortens the duration of postoperative ileus in humans.[13] In a double-blind study of patients undergoing cholecystectomy, the passage of radio-opaque markers through the colon was significantly faster in the 15 patients who received IV lidocaine (100 mg bolus before anesthesia, continuous infusion at 3 mg/min for 24 hours) than in the 15 patients who received IV saline. The authors speculated that systemic lidocaine may reduce postoperative peritoneal irritation, thereby suppressing inhibitory gastrointestinal reflexes. However, patients in the lidocaine group received significantly less postoperative opioids, providing another explanation for the more rapid resolution of the ileus.

LOCATION OF EPIDURAL CATHETER AND BOWEL FUNCTION

Steinbrook[14] reviewed 16 studies published since 1977 comparing epidural anesthesia/analgesia with general anesthesia/systemic analgesia with regard to the postoperative recovery of bowel function. In all eight studies, with the epidural catheter placed above T-12, the bowel function recovered significantly more rapidly when epidural anesthesia/analgesia was used. In the studies in which the epidural catheter was placed at T-12 or below, or when the location was not specified, the studies were equally likely to show faster recovery of bowel function with either technique of analgesia. In no study was the return of bowel function faster with systemic opioid analgesia. Thus, location of the epidural catheter and its placement before surgery is a crucial detail in determining postoperative outcome, at least as far as bowel function is concerned.

Thoracic placement of the epidural catheter and postoperative infusion of a local anesthetic are apparently necessary elements to accelerate return of bowel function after abdominal surgery, compared to either systemic or epidural morphine alone. There are two obvious possible explanations. One possibility is that use of intra- and postoperative local anesthetics allows the avoidance of intraoperative opioids, and decreases the requirements for postoperative opioids,[15] which can slow the recovery of bowel function.

The other possibility is that epidural local anesthetics may decrease the sympathetic tone of the bowel, increasing the relative parasympathetic tone, thus increasing blood flow to the bowel resulting in earlier and more effective bowel motility.[14] If the epidural catheter is not placed at the spinal level, close to the dermatomes affected by surgical pain (and to the dermatomes providing sympathetic innervation to the bowel), the postoperative local anesthetic solution (less concentrated than the solution used intraoperatively) cannot reach the appropriate dermatomes to have the necessary effects. Thus, it makes no sense to place a lumbar epidural catheter in a patient undergoing abdominal surgery, at least as far as bowel function and control of dynamic pain are concerned (Table 2).

Table 2. Mechanisms by which thoracic epidural anesthesia and analgesia may promote gastrointestinal motility.

Blockade of Nociceptive Afferent Nerves
Blockade of cervicolumbar efferent nerves
Unopposed parasympathetic efferent nerves
Reduced need for postoperative opioids
Increased gastrointestinal blood flow
Systemic absorption of local anesthetics

RATIONALE FOR A MULTIMODAL REHABILITATION PROGRAM AFTER OPEN SIGMOIDECTOMY

Colonic surgery usually requires a postoperative hospital stay that ranges from five to seven days with a morbidity rate that oscillates between 10% and 15%.[16,17,18,19,20,21] Limiting factors for early discharge include pain, nausea, vomiting and ileus, stress-induced organ dysfunction, postoperative fatigue syndrome, and durational hardware such as nasogastric tubes, surgical drains, etc. All these factors may retard rehabilitation and contribute to a prolonged intrahospital morbidity. Single modality intervention with laparoscopically assisted operation has only partially improved the outcome.[18,19,21] In contrast, multimodal intervention with laparscopically assisted surgery, preoperative patient information, epidural anesthesia and analgesia, and enforced early oral nutrition and mobilization have been reported to reduce hospital stay to about two days in high-risk patients.[22] However, a recent study has evaluated the recovery and hospital stay of patients undergoing open sigmoidectomy with a multimodal rehabilitation program. These results are in accord with our pilot study, and have used the same methods we are currently using.[23]

THERAPEUTIC PLAN FOR THE MULTIMODAL THERAPY

1) No premedication
2) Preoperative teaching of the patient.
3) Epidural anesthesia at T9-T10-T11 level. A bolus of preservative free morphine with 2 mg in the epidural space in patients of less than 70 years of age, and 1 mg in those more than 70 years of age.
4) Ropivacaine (1%) was then injected in amounts that varied from 8 mL to 12 mL in 2- to 4-mL aliquots to achieve a T5-T6 sensory level. Propofol was used for induction of anesthesia and a laryngeal mask airway inserted without the use of muscle paralysis. For maintenance of anesthesia, a propoful infusion at 4-8 mg per kilo per hour was administered. No IV opioids were given preoperatively or intraoperatively. For maintenance of epidural anesthesia, a ropivacaine (1%) infusion was started at a rate of 6-8 mL per hour and titrated to maintain an adequate sensory block. Hypotension was treated with ephedrine boluses of 5-10 mg at a time.
5) Surgical incision: curved transverse on the left iliac fossa.
6) Avoid use of a nasogastric tube.
7) Postoperative epidural analgesia with ropivacaine 0.2% + morphine 0.05 mg per mL at a rate of 8-10 mL per hour to produce adequate sensory analgesia at the site of surgery. Additionally, a nonsteroidal antiinflammatory agent was used, typically Keterolac 15 mg IV q 6 h for 48 hours.
8) Patients were mobilized on the afternoon or evening after surgery.
9) Patients were then fed with a chicken or a beef bouillon soup.
10) Cisapride 20 mg every 12 h and magnesium 1 mg every 12 h were administered po.
11) On the first postoperative day, patients were mobilized 6-8 hours they were taken out of bed and encouraged to ambulate as much as they tolerated. Free fluid intake was allowed for all patients. A protein drink containing 1 g per kilo of body weight; i.e., 60-80 g of protein a day, and a total of 3,500 kcal in 24 hours was administered. Typically, three to four protein drinks are currently available on the market for regular consumption.
12) The urinary bladder catheter was removed 24 hours after surgery.
13) Patients were mobilized 8-12 hours on postoperative day two.
14) Patients were discharged to home on full diet, and oral non-steroidal inflammatory agent, which up to the advent of the COX-2 inhibitors was Ketoprofen, but at this point we switched to rofecoxib 25-50 mg po q 24 h, and magnesium 1-2 g q 24 hours, and a mild opioid such as hydrocodone q 4 hours prn.

RESULTS

With this protocol, patients underwent surgery for a median time of more or less 100 (range: 70-180) minutes. The median blood loss was 150 (range: 50-300) m/L. The median hospital stay, including the day of surgery, was 2 (range: 2-6) days. Patients ambulated a mean of 13 hours on the first postoperative day, and fluid intake was at the goal level in 14 of 16 (88%) patients in the Kehlet study, and remained on goal in approximately 85% of our patients. Defecation occurred in 15 to 16 patients within 48 hours in the Kehlet study,[23] and occurred in approximately 90% of our patients within the first 48 hours as well. Two of the 16 (13%) patients had urinary retention requiring catheterization on the first postoperative day in the Kehlet study, and is our study one in ten (10%) required catheterization without reinsertion of a Foley catheter. No readmissions to the hospital occurred within one month after surgery in the Kehlet study; we have followed up our patients for two months, and none of them have developed any complications in the postoperative period.

ANALYSIS OF THE FINDINGS

These preliminary results suggest elective sigmoid resection in unselected patients with malignant or non-malignant disease can be performed with a short (2-3 days) postoperative hospital stay, when using a multimodal rehabilitation program with perioperative epidural local anesthesia continuously for 48 hours, including a local anesthetic and opioid in reduced amounts, plus a non-steroidal antiinflammatory agent together with early enforced oral nutrition and mobilization. When a two-day discharge regimen plan before the operation is in place, the majority of patients are able to leave the hospital with no complications. If confirmed in a large-scale study and by other centers, these results represent a considerable improvement compared with traditional care programs in the colonic surgery literature. The perioperative use of epidural anesthesia and analgesia to achieve short-term recovery of various body organs' function was based on previous findings that the combination of these drugs given by an epidural catheter can reduce the afferent neural nociceptive input that may be deleterious in recovery of high-risk patients. Future studies are needed to clarify whether the additional use of oral adjuvant drugs would be of further benefit. One of the most impressive findings in the Kehlet study, and in our experience, was the short duration of postoperative ileus—several days shorter than in previous observations. The explanation for this is probably the multimodal effort with omission of gastrointestinal tubes and institution of early oral nutrition and mobilization, as well as the beneficial effects of epidural anesthetic techniques administered in the thoracic epidural space with a local anesthetic. Finally, use of a transverse curve incision may have contributed to the smooth postoperative course, as transverse incisions result in less pain than midline incisions. Exposure of the surgical field with this incision is excellent, and may be extended left upwards, if required.

The current descriptive uncontrolled studies represent the first efforts to assess the potential value of an accelerated recovery program in patients undergoing open colonic resection. Obviously, important limitations exist in such initial uncontrolled observations, which may be considered as generating of hypothesis before one embarks on randomized trials. With these provisions, the present results suggest there may be no major differences compared with laparoscopically assisted resection, in which a similar shorter stay was achieved with enforced rehabilitation. This study needs to be repeated by others and, if the results are confirmed, large-scale, multi-center prospective or randomized trials should be performed, to document safety and expected reduction of morbidity compared with traditional care. Such data are of major relevance because colonic operations represent one of the most common abdominal operations and are often performed in elderly, high-risk patients with significant morbidity, and with a considerable cost for the healthcare system.

REFERENCES

1. Wangensteen OH. The early diagnosis of acute intestinal obstruction with comments on pathology and treatment: with a report on successful decompression of three cases of mechanical small bowel obstruction by nasal catheter siphonage. WJ Surg Obstet Gynecol 1932;40:1-17.
2. Heimbach DM, Crout JR. Treatment of paralytic ileus with adrenergic neuronal blocking drugs. Surgery 1971;69:582-7.
3. Livingston EH, Passaro EP. Postoperative Ileus. Dig Dis Sci 1990;35:121-32.
4. Liu S, Carpenter RL, Neal JM. Epidural anesthesia and analgesia: The role in postoperative outcome. Anesthesiology 1995; 82:1474-506.
5. Canon WB, Murphy ST. The Movement of the stomach and intestine in some surgical conditions. Ann Surg 1906:43:512-36.
6. Meltzer SJ, Auer J. Peristaltic movement of the rabbit's cecum and their inhibition, with demonstration. Proc Soc Exp Biol Med 1907; 4:37-40.
7. Wells C, Rowlingson K, Tinckler L, et al. Ileus and postoperative intestinal motility. Lancet 1961;2:136-7.
8. Woods JH, Ericsson, LW, Condon N, et al. Postoperative ileus: a colonic problem? Surgery 1978;84:527-33.
9. Neely J. The effects of analgesic drugs on gastrointestinal motility in man. Br J Surg 1969;56:925-9.
10. Yukioka H, Bogod DJ, Rosen M. Recovery of bowel motility after surgery: detection of time of first flatus from carbon dioxide concentration and patient estimate after nalbuphan and placebo. Br J Anesthesiol 1997;59:581-4.
11. Howd RA, Avamovics J, Palekar A. Naloxone and intestinal motility. Experientia 1978;34:1310-1.
12. Scheinin B, Lindgren L, Scheinin TM. Perioperative nitrous oxide delays bowel function after colonic surgery. Br J Anaesthesiol 1990;64:154-8.
13. Rimback G, Cassuto J, Tolleson P-O. Treatment of postoperative paralytic ileus by intravenous lidocaine infusion. Anesth Analg 1990;70:414-9.
14. Steinbrook RA. Epidural anesthesia and gastrointestinal motility. Anesth Analg 1998;86:837-44.
15. Stevens RA, Mikait-Stevens M, Flanagan R, et al. Does the choice of anesthetic technique affect the recovery of bowel function after radical prostatectomy? Urology 1998;52:213-8.
16. Retchin SM, Pinberthy L, Desch C, et al. Perioperative management of colonic cancer under Medicare risk programs. Arch Intern Med 1997;157:1878-84.
17. Schoetz DJ Jr, Bockler M, Rosenblatt MS, et al. "Ideal" length of stay after colectomy: whose ideal? Dis Colon Rectum 1997;40:806-10.
18. Lacy AM, Garcia-Valdecasas JC, Pique JM, et al. Short term outcome analysis of a randomized study comparing laparoscopic vs. open colectomy for colon cancer. Surg Endosc 1995;9:1101-5.
19. Franklin ME Jr, Rosenthal D, Abrego-Medina, D, et al. Prospective comparison of open vs laparoscopic colon surgery for carcinoma. Five-year resutls. Dis Colon Rectum 1996;39 (10 Suppl):s36-6.
20. Bokey EL, Chapuis PH, Fung C, et al. Postoperative morbidity and mortality following resection of the colon and rectum for cancer. Dis Colon Rectum 1995;38:480-7.
21. Stage JG, Schulze S, Moller P, et al. Prospective randomized study of laparoscopic versus open colonic resection for adenocarcinoma. Br J Surg 1997;84:391-5.
22. Bardram L, Funch-Jensen P, Jensen P, et al. Recovery after laparoscopic colonic surgery with epidural analgesia, and early oral nutrition and mobilization. Lancet 1995;345: 763-4.
23. Kehlet H, Mogensen T. Hospital stay of two days after open sigmoidectomy with a multimodal rehabilitation programme. Br J Surg 1999;86:227-30.

Laparoscopic Surgery Skills Training

- **Laparoscopic Suturing Focus**
- **Intracorporeal Knot Tying**
- **Anastomosis Techniques**

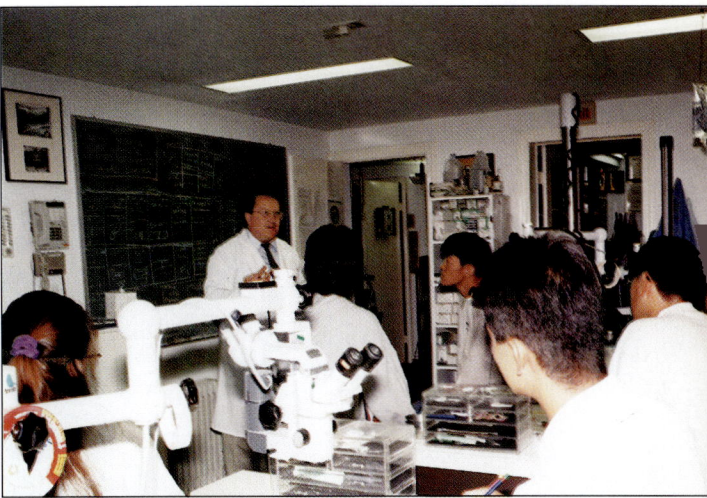
Lecture on principles of magnified surgery

EMPHASIS:

Principles of set-up
Effective use of magnification (camera control)
Hemostatic dissection, proper exposure and retraction

Economy of motion principle
Magnified eye-hand coordination
Two-handed ambidextrous technique

Overall surgical strategy
Common pitfalls & difficulties
Technical nuances ("tricks of the trade")

Precision suturing and anastomotic techniques
Choreographed intracorporeal knotting techniques
Needle control and suture handling

Skill Evaluation: performance and time standards

- **Personalized tutorials**
- **Intensive Hands-on sessions**
- **Small class size**
- **Sole use of training stations**

Accreditation and Approvals:
The Microsurgery & Operative Endoscopy Training (MOET) Institute is accredited by the Accreditation Council for Continuing Medical Education (ACCME) to provide continuing medical education programs for physicians.

CME Credits:
Category 1 AMA (ACCME)
Category 1 Cognates (ACOG)
SAGES approved

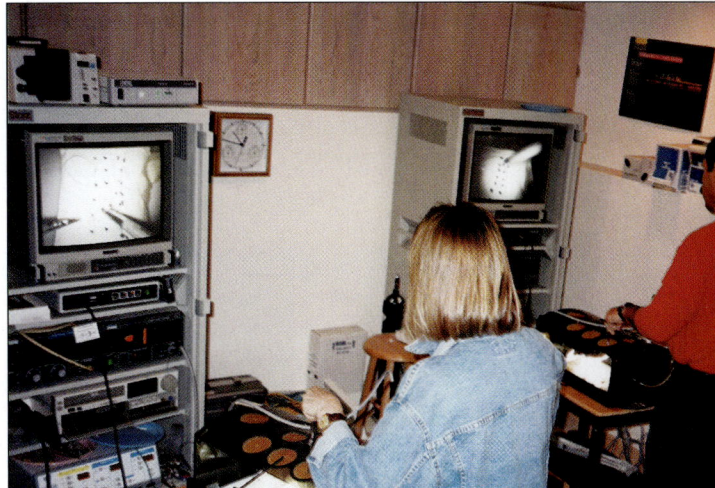
Laparoscopic training stations

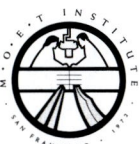 **M·O·E·T INSTITUTE**
Microsurgery & Operative Endoscopy Training

Zoltan Szabo, Ph.D., F.I.C.S.
Director

Course Location: M.O.E.T. Institute, San Francisco
These programs are also taught at hosting institutions in other US cities and international locations. Please contact MOET Institute for further information.

Frequency: available year-round by arrangement

For information please contact:

Wanda Toy, Program Administrator
M.O.E.T. Institute
153 States Street
San Francisco, CA 94114

Fax (415) 626-3444
Tel. (415) 626-3400

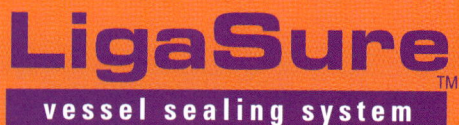

LigaSure™
vessel sealing system

When Edison invented the lightbulb, it revolutionized the way we see.

The LigaSure™ System Will Revolutionize The Way You Operate

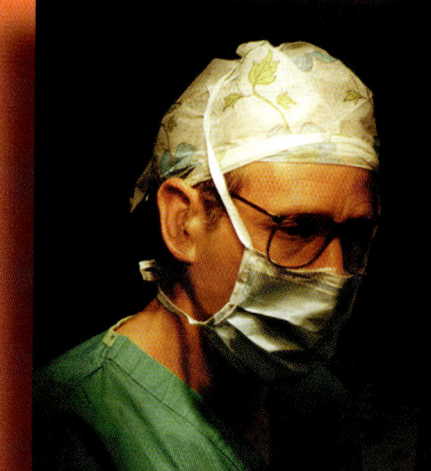

The LigaSure™ Vessel Sealing System gives you something no other electrosurgical tool can — permanent vessel occlusion. The LigaSure™ System's revolutionary technology replaces almost all other hemostatic tools because it doesn't just ligate vessels, **it actually fuses vessel walls to create a permanent seal.**

The LigaSure™ System reliably and permanently seals any vein, artery, and tissue bundle you're likely to encounter in surgery.

The LigaSure™ System:

- Seals vessels up to 7 mm in diameter and tissue bundles
- Provides potential time savings compared to suturing
- Has significantly reduced thermal spread compared to standard bipolar
- Creates seals that withstand a minimum of 3 times normal systolic pressure

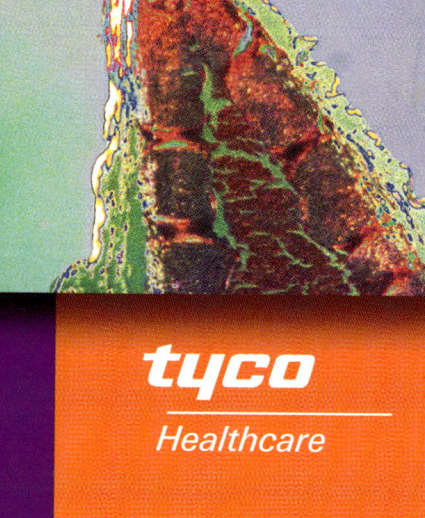

tyco
Healthcare

Valleylab™

1.800.255.8522
©2000 Valleylab

www.valleylab.com

Comparison of Healing Process Following Ligation with Sutures and Bipolar Vessel Sealing

STEVEN L. PETERSON, D.V.M., M.D.
CHIEF, DIVISION OF PLASTIC SURGERY
DENVER HEALTH TRAUMA CENTER
DENVER, COLORADO

PATRICIA L. STRANAHAN, M.D., PHD.
PROFESSOR AND CHAIRMAN, DEPARTMENT OF BIOLOGY
METROPOLITAN STATE COLLEGE
DENVER, COLORADO

DALE SCHMALTZ, M.S.
ENGINEERING MANAGER

CAROLYN MIHAICHUK, M.S.
ENGINEER

NED COSGRIFF, M.D.
MEDICAL DIRECTOR
VALLEYLAB
BOULDER, CO

Local hemostasis is critical for successful surgical intervention and may be accomplished with a variety of techniques ranging from direct pressure to lasers. Critical assessment of the clinical situation is required to determine the appropriate technology necessary to achieve effective hemostasis. As a general rule, ligatures remain the mainstay for effecting hemostasis in all but the smallest isolated vessels. Although ligatures have been in use since the first century AD, both the applications as well as their sophistication have increased dramatically. As sutures are foreign material to the human body, tissue reaction is unavoidable. This response may be mitigated, but not eliminated completely, through the use of non-absorbable sutures. The body's inflammatory response triggers a complex cascade of cellular and biochemical events that lead to fibrinogenesis and coagulation. This process, in turn, results in an increased deposition of collagen that may result in formation of adhesions.

As an alternative, heat may be used to achieve hemostasis by denaturing the proteins in tissue. Energy-based thermal coagulation devices have been in use since Cushing and Bovie's work with electrocautery in 1928.[1] Today's systems for electrosurgical coagulation use alternating high-frequency current to deliver the energy necessary to achieve hemostasis. The two primary electrosurgical delivery methods are monopolar and bipolar. In monopolar electrosurgery, current flows from the electrode at the surgical site, through the patient's body, and back to the generator by way of a

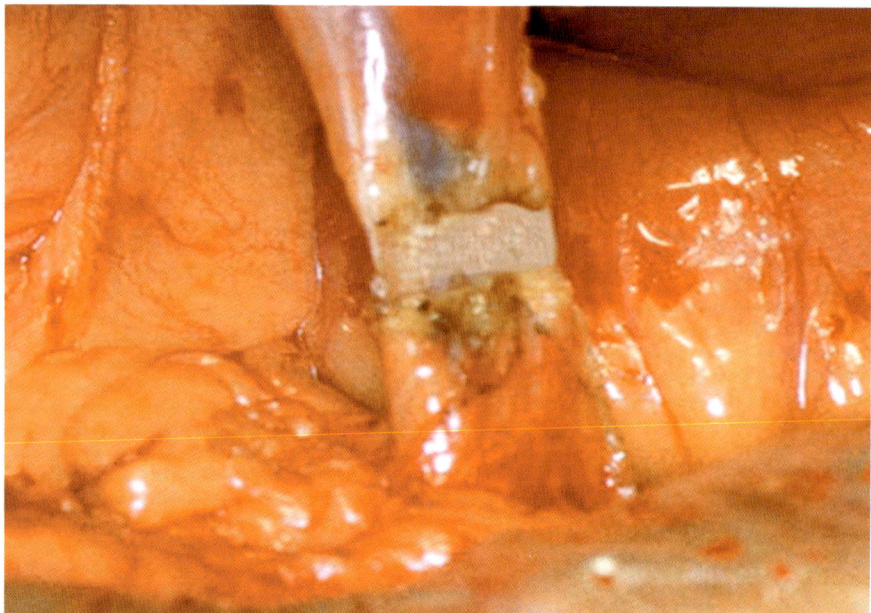

Figure 1. Close-up of sealed vessel.

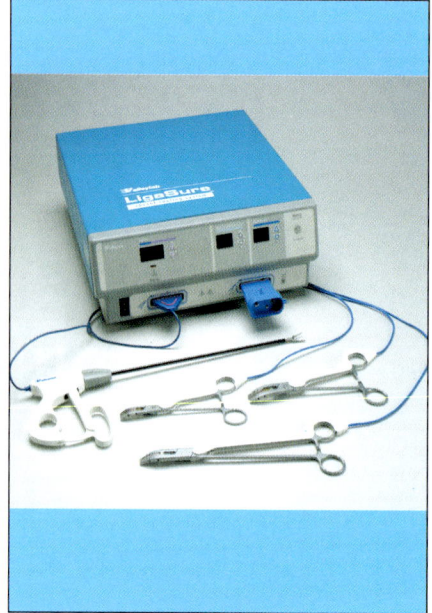

Figure 2. Vessel sealing system.

return electrode located at a distant site on the patient's body. In bipolar electrosurgery, current flows between two electrode poles positioned on either side of the target tissue.

Monopolar electrosurgery can be used to effectively coagulate small vessels <1.5 mm in diameter. Whereas bipolar electrosurgery can coagulate vessels up to 2 mm in diameter, reliability of the application decreases dramatically with an increase in vessel size. Although in bipolar electrosurgery the energy delivery is confined to the tissue between the electrodes, the thermal tissue effect extends much further. Despite bipolar electrosurgery's ability to coagulate larger vessels, the sticking, charring, and thermal spread associated with traditional bipolar limit its effectiveness in many surgical applications.

VESSEL SEALING TECHNOLOGY

A new technology for surgical hemostasis in 1 to 7 mm diameter vessels has been developed recently: LigaSure™ (Valleylab, a division of Tyco International Healthcare, Boulder, CO). This new technology provides an alternative to standard ligation methods: ligatures, clips, staples, electrosurgical instruments, as well as other energy-based technologies (e.g. ultrasonic coagulators). This system uses an enhanced form of bipolar electrosurgery to achieve permanent vessel wall fusion by denaturing the collagen and elastin in vessel walls and reforming them into a hemostatic seal (Fig. 1). As reflected in the seal burst strength, performance of this new technology depends on the application of mechanical energy, in the form of pressure, in conjunction with delivery of electrical energy. The simultaneous delivery of mechanical and electrical energy remodels the vessel tissue to form a desiccated absorbable collagen seal out of native vessel protein.

The mechanical and electrical energy necessary to create the seal is delivered through an instrument that resembles a

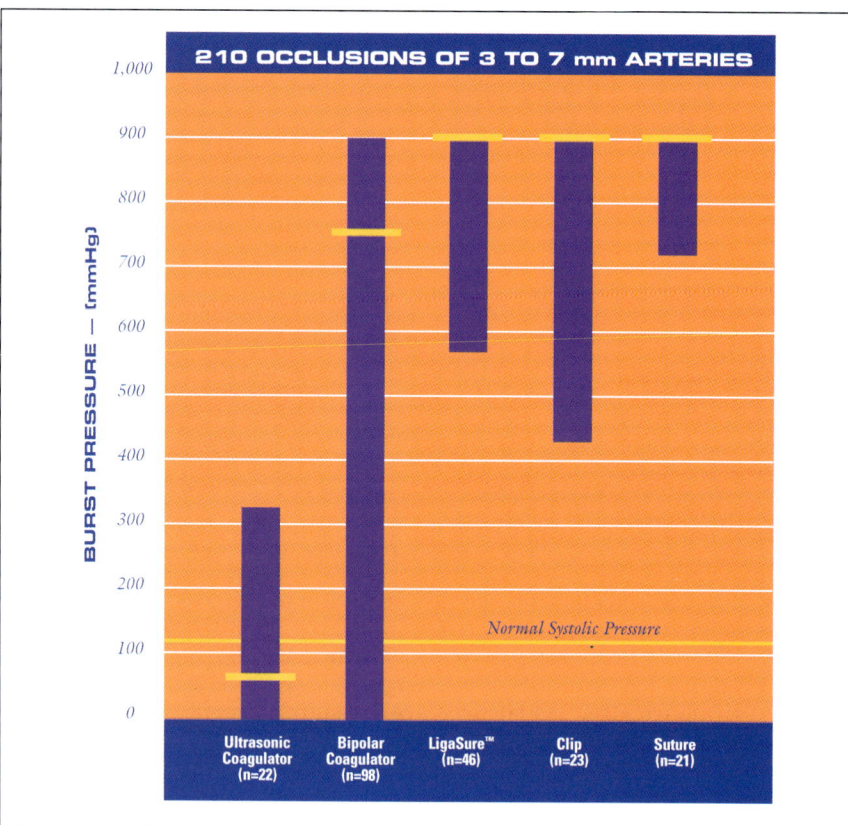

Figure 3. Burst pressure graph.

surgical hemostat (Fig. 2). The instrument's power source is an electrosurgical generator, which delivers radio-frequency bipolar current at 470 kHz with a maximum open circuit voltage of 120 V_{rms} and a maximum short circuit current of 4.00 A_{rms} at a maximum of 150 Watts. The current is conducted to the instrument through an insulated cable connected to the instrument's ring handles.

Through measurements of both voltage and current, the LigaSure™'s bipolar generator control algorithm monitors tissue response. A final cool cycle, during which no power is delivered, is maintained for a short time while the tissue is held in tight apposition. When the cooling period is finished, an audio signal from the generator indicates to the surgeon the cycle is complete. The entire process from start to finish takes an average of 5 seconds.

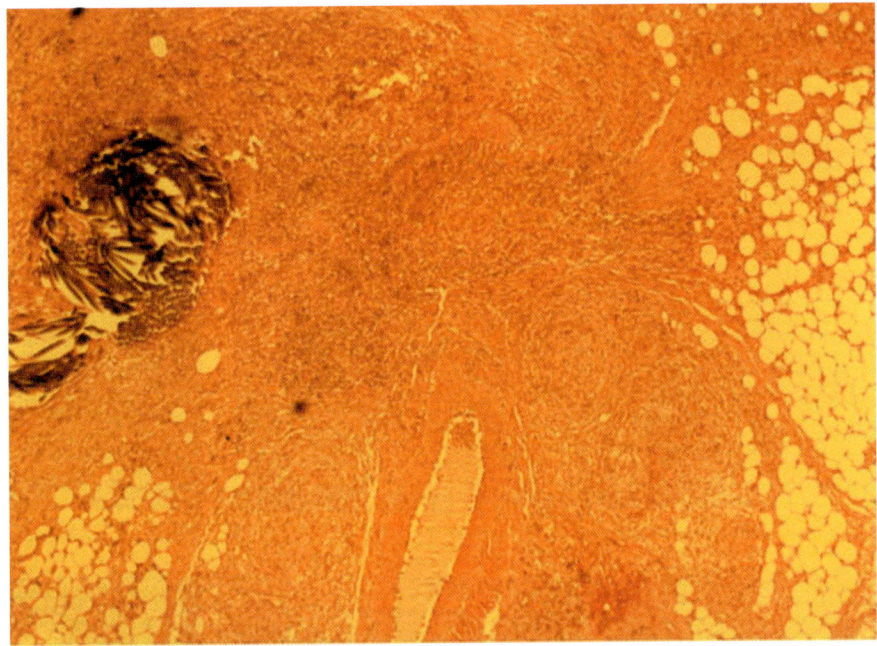
Figure 4a. Suture, hematoxylin & eosin (H&E), 7 days.

OBJECTIVE

Prior studies have demonstrated the effectiveness of the seals created by the LigaSure™ System. Reduced charring, sticking, and limited thermal spread characterized the tissue response associated with application of this new vessel sealing system. The seal quality, as reflected in burst strength, was determined to be comparable to existing mechanical-based techniques such as clips and suture. In these studies, seal-burst pressures were determined using an angiocath to deliver saline to the seal site while recording the pressure with a digital transducer. Mean burst pressures in excess of 900 mmHg were obtained for vessels of 3 to 7 mm in diameter, is comparable to results obtained using surgical clips and suture on vessels in the same size range (Fig. 3). To help further elucidate the differences between suture ligation and vessel sealing, a comparison of the associated healing process was undertaken in the canine model.

Early canine studies demonstrated a normal healing process for seals made with the LigaSure™ System. Thermal spread was measured histologically and noted to extend on average less than 2 mm beyond the seal site.[2] In this study, we compared the gross and histologic results obtained from vessels and tissue bundles ligated using 3.0 silk suture with similar vessels and tissue bundles ligated using the new system.

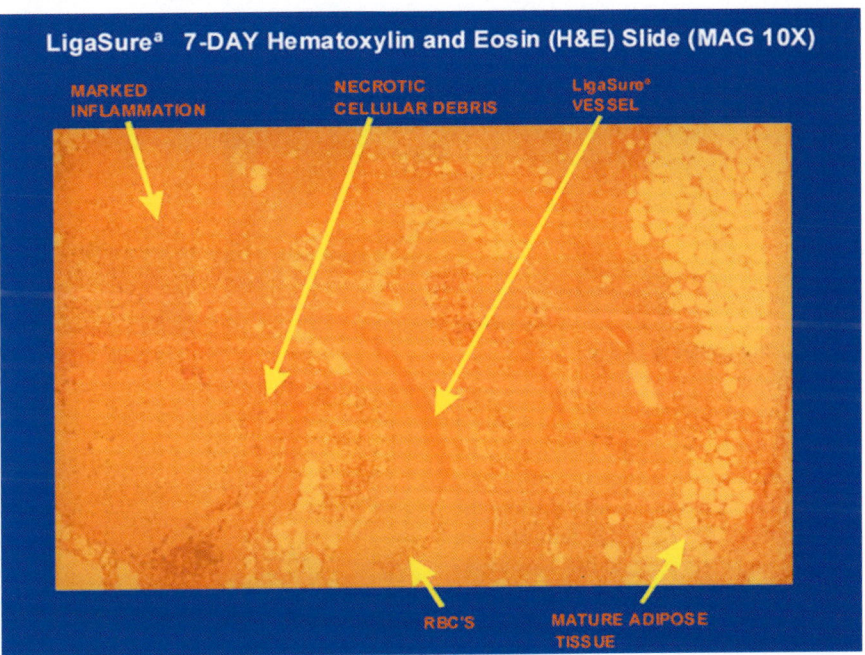
Figure 4b. Vessel seal H&E, 7 days.

MATERIALS AND METHODS

This study was performed in compliance with the Food and Drug Administration (FDA) mandated Guide for the Care and Use of Laboratory Animals. All protocols were approved by the Animal Research Committee at the University of Colorado Health Sciences Center. Three adult female dogs (15 to 20 kg) received no food or water the night before surgery and were treated with atropine (0.05 mg/kg) and actyl-promazine (3 mg) before surgery. Surgical anesthesia was induced with intravenous thiopental (10-15 mg/kg) followed by intubation and respirator ventilation with isoflorane.

On the day of the initial surgery, all three dogs underwent midline laparotomies. The small bowel was inspected for adhesions and ileocolic junction identified. Beginning from the distal ileum, the mesenteric arcades visualized and ten target vessels were identified and ligated using 3.0 silk suture.

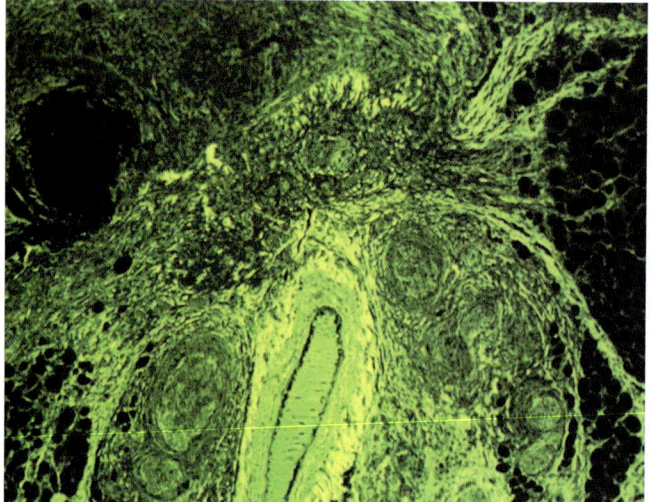
Figure 4c. Suture florescence, 7 days.

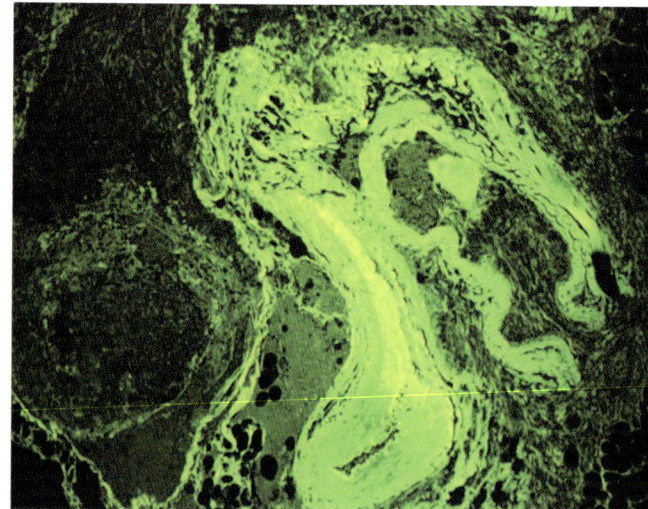
Figure 4d. Vessel seal floresence, 7 days.

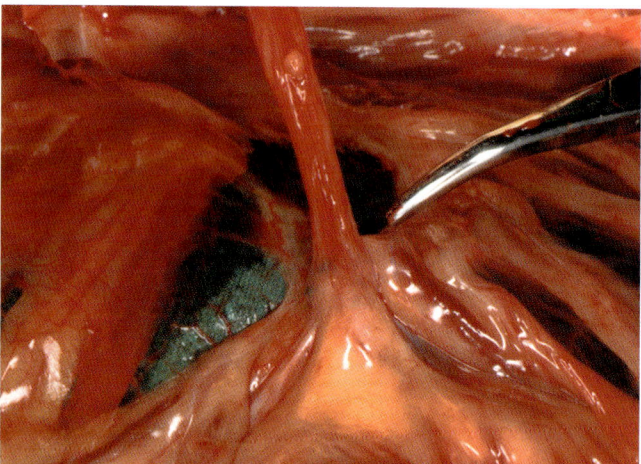
Figure 5a. Gross suture at 14 days.

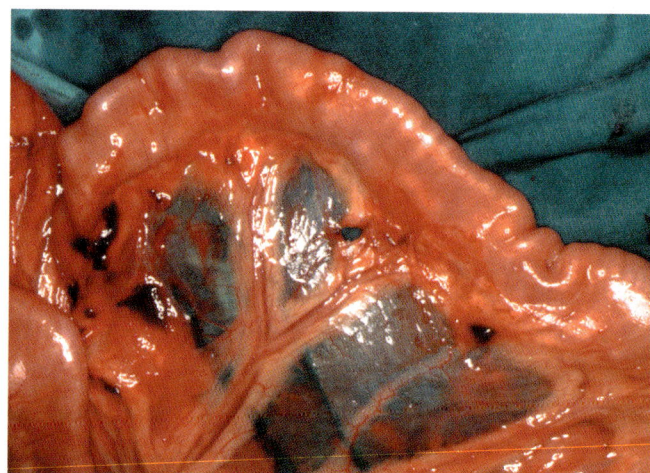
Figure 5b. Gross vessel seal at 14 days.

Sutures were placed approximately 24 cm apart with care being taken to ligate only vessels with adequate collateral circulation to avoid compromising the small bowel. In a similar fashion, ten vessels were ligated using the Liga-Sure™ vessel-sealing device beginning approximately 24 cm proximal to the final suture ligation.

Splenectomies were then performed on all three animals using ten 3.0 silk ligations followed by ten applications of the new system on the splenic arcade. The spleen was removed and animals closed with nylon suture and skin staples. Animals were recovered and monitored on a daily basis.

SPECIMEN COLLECTION AND EVALUATION

At each of the necropsy dates (7, 14, and 28 days after the initial surgery), one dog underwent re-operation. The

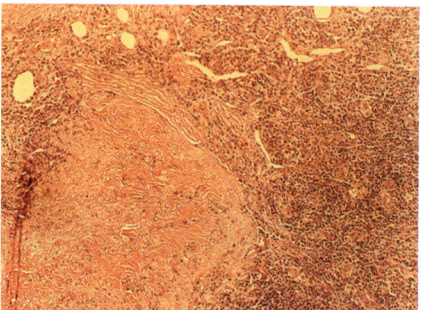
Figure 5a. Suture H&E, 14 days.

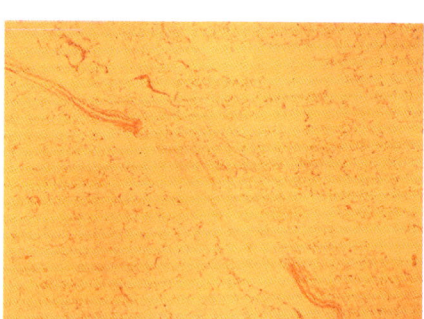
Figure 5b. Vessel seal H&E, 14 days.

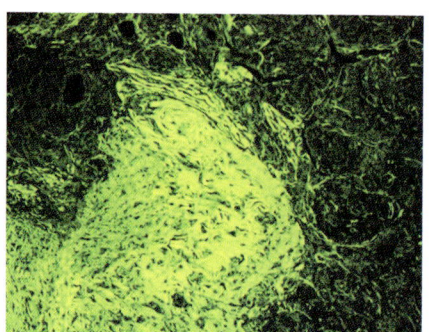
Figure 5c. Suture florescence, 14 days.

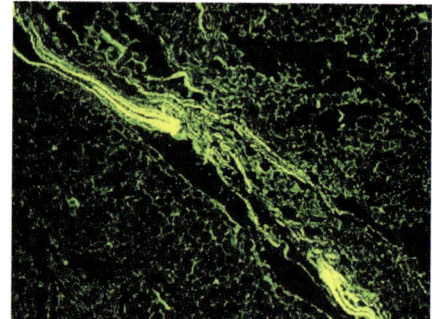
Figure 5d. Vessel seal floresence, 14 days.

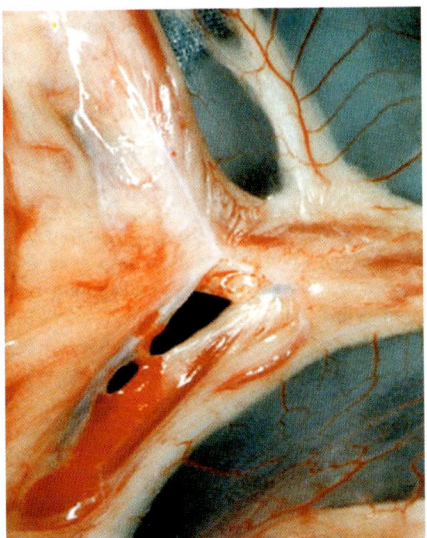
Figure 6a. Gross suture at 28 days.

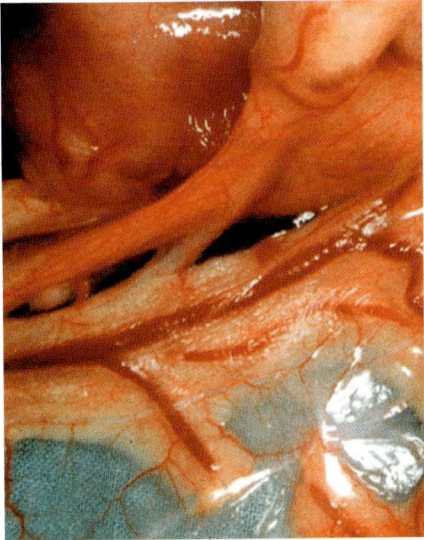
Figure 6b. Gross vessel seal at 28 days.

At 28 days numerous evolved adhesions were present at the suture sites. The coagulated seal sites were difficult to locate, with the tissue involved appearing essentially normal to the unaided eye (Figs. 6a,b). Tissue samples indicated that the sutured vessels continued to be involved in formation of a tremendous granulomatous infiltrate. Numerous reactive fibroblasts, foreign-body giant cells, macrophages, and dense irregular connective tissue surrounded the suture. The LigaSure™ sites displayed thin ribbons of connective tissue with only rare appearances of the remnant vessels. Newly laid down adipose tissue was associated with the ribbons of connective tissue. No granulomatous reaction was noted and no

sites of the suture and vessel-sealing ligations were identified and photographed for gross assessment of inflammation. The suture and seal sites were then harvested and placed in 10% buffered formalin for histologic evaluation. A total of 60 ligations with silk and 60 ligations using the LigaSure™ System were placed during the study on tissue bundles, and vessels ranging from 1 to 4 mm in diameter. All gross and microscopic evaluations were made by a board certified pathologist.

RESULTS

The suture sites and seals made with the LigaSure™ System were located for visual and histologic inspection throughout the study. No postoperative complications or bleeding occurred in any of the animals. A normal healing process was noted in all three animals.

At seven days, both electrothermal-coagulated and suture sites exhibited gross signs of inflammation. Microscopically, both specimens disclosed the usual changes associated with acute inflammation and repair. Vessel adventitia was associated with numerous reactive fibroblasts, many polymorphonuclear leukocytes, and degenerating fibrous connective tissue (Figs. 4a,b,c,d).

At 14 days, the LigaSure™ sites demonstrated far less gross inflammation than the corresponding suture sites. Numerous adhesions were noted at the suture sites whereas the LigaSure™ seals did not affect any of the surrounding tissue (Figs. 5a,b).

Microscopically, the sutured vessels

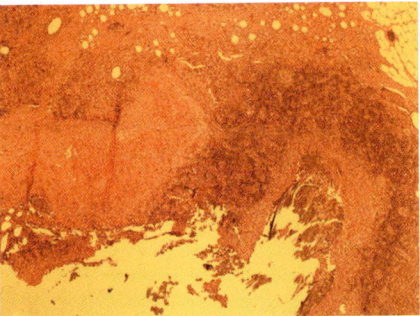
Figure 6a. Suture H&E, 28 days.

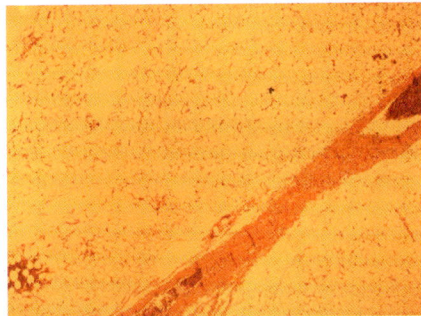
Figure 6b. Vessel seal H&E, 28 days.

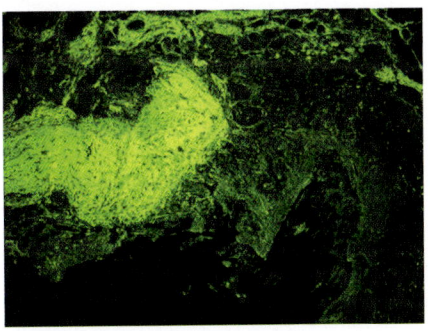
Figure 6c. Suture florescence, 28 days.

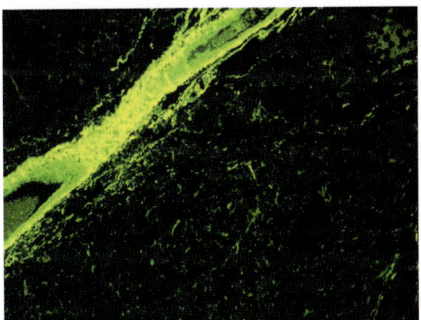
Figure 6d. Vessel seal floresence, 28 days.

appeared within masses of reactive fibroblasts, foreign body giant cells, macrophages, and lymphocytes. The vascular intima, media, and adventitia were involved in the evolving chronic inflammatory response. Conversely, the LigaSure™ ligation sites were associated with foci of reactive fibroblasts and newly developed fibro-adipose tissue. The vascular intima, media, and adventitia contained fibrous connective tissue and occasional nests of lymphocytes. No evolution of the tremendous chronic inflammatory infiltrate was present as noted in the suture-ligated vessels (Figs. 5a-d).

foreign body giant cells or islands of lymphocytes were present in the electrothermally-coagulated specimens (Figs.6a-d).

DISCUSSION

The new electrothermal vessel system proved to be a viable alternative to suture ligatures for ligating vessels encountered commonly in surgery. To date, more than 6,000 surgical procedures have been performed using the LigaSure™ System. Ease of use, combined with a decrease in time per application, have resulted in reports of time savings in the performance of hemorrhoidectomies,[2] vaginal hysterectomies,[3] prostatectomies,[4] and a wide range of open and laparoscopic general surgical procedures.[5]

As this system gains more widespread use, other benefits related to vessel sealing are being reported. The ability to ligate vessels effectively up to 7 mm in diameter without the introduction of a foreign body has been shown to be an advantage in the performance of laparoscopic nephrectomies.[6] Pediatric surgeons have determined the laparoscopic handpiece of the LigaSure™ system to be effective in a wide variety of surgical procedures.[7] Cardiovascular surgeons have experienced the ease of use and limited thermal spread in saphenous vein harvesting,[8] and transplant surgeons have recently incorporated its use in living donor liver transplants.

The ability to seal large vessels quickly and effectively, combined with an associated decrease in needle passes on the operating field, suggest benefits directly associated with the use of electrothermal vessel sealing system. Perhaps a more promising finding lies in the shorter duration associated with the inflammatory response. The potential for seals composed of the patient's native tissue to reduce the inflammatory response may translate to a decrease in post-surgical adhesions. Clinical studies are currently in progress to quantify the relationship between seals made with the LigaSure™ Vessel Sealing System and the incidence of post-surgical adhesions.

REFERENCES

1. Kennedy J.S.; Stranahan P.L.; Buysse S.P.; Ryan T.P.; Pearce J.A.; Thomsen S. "Large Vessel Ligation Using Bipolar Energy: A Chronic Animal Study and Histological Evaluation", Seventh International Meeting of the Society for Minimally Invasive Therapy, 1995.

2. Johnson C.J.;Cosgriff N.;"Use of a New Energy Source for Vessel Sealing in Hemorrhoidectomy", (Manuscript in Progress).

3. Levy B., Use of the LigaSure™ System in Vaginal Hysterectomy. Association of American Gynecologic Laparoscopists Meeting, Las Vegas, NV., November 1999.

4. Crawford E.D.;Kennedy J.S.;Sieve V."Use of the LigaSure™ Vessel Sealing System in Urologic Cancer Surgery"; Grand Rounds in Urology, Fall 1999.

5. Heniford B.T.;Sing R.;Matthews B.;Greene F.; "Initial Results with an Electrothermal Bipolar Vessel Sealer", Society of American Gastrointestinal Endoscopic Surgeons, Atlanta, GA, March 2000.

6. Chan D.Y.;Bishoff J.T.; Kavoussi L.R.;Jarrett T.W.; "Endovascular Gastrointestinal Stapler Device Malfunction During Laparoscopic Nephrectomy: Early Recognition and Management";Journal of Urology, (In Press).

7. Rothenberg S.S.; Bealer J.F.; "Experience with a New Energy Source for Tissue Sealing in Minimally Invasive Surgery In Children"; IPEG Congress, March 2000, (Manuscript in Progress).

8. Godge O. Koukal C. Hannekum A.; "Electrical Vessel Sealing with the LigaSure™ System-First Results in Saphenous Vein Harvesting"; The Thoracic and Cardiovascular Surgeon, Supp Vol. 48, Feb 2000, 8.

Impact of Hospital Volume on In-Hospital Mortality in Pancreatic Surgery

RUTGER C.I. VAN GEENEN, M.D.
DIRK J. GOUMA, M.D.
ACADEMIC MEDICAL CENTER, DEPARTMENT OF SURGERY
AMSTERDAM, THE NETHERLANDS

Pancreaticoduodenectomy, mostly performed for pancreatic cancer, has been associated with considerable morbidity rates (40%-60%) and mortality rates (20%-30%). Even after resection, the prognosis is poor, and as a result some physicians have kept a nihilistic approach; Gudjonsson concluded in his review that pancreatic resections are a waste of resources.[1] During the last decade, mortality rates have decreased dramatically to less than 5% in centers with experience, and have led to a more optimistic view in favor of resection.

Another development of importance is increasing knowledge of the effect of hospital volume and surgeon experience (surgeon volume) on patient outcome. For many different major surgical procedures such as colorectal resections,[2] oesophagectomy,[3,4] hepatic resection,[4] coronary bypasses,[5] and pancreaticoduodenectomy,[6-8] during the past years data have shown that a high hospital volume or surgeon volume was associated with low mortality rates. These findings lead to a plea for centralization of major surgery including pancreatic surgery;[9] however, nuances have to be made. The patient population of the high- and low-volume hospitals could be different and factors other than the surgeon or hospital volume also might influence mortality rates. Expertise of the other disciplines involved in treatment of patients who undergo pancreatic surgery has been suggested to be of great importance. In this article, different aspects of centralization are described. First, the effect of hospital volume on outcome of pancreatic resections nationwide in the Netherlands are summarized. Second, the impact of surgeon experience versus hospital volume on patient outcome after pancreatic resection, as studied in our center (AMC, Amsterdam), is described. Finally, the literature on these subjects was reviewed and are summarized.

PANCREATICODUODENECTOMY IN THE NETHERLANDS

A recent study in the Netherlands described the relation between hospital volume and in-hospital mortality.[10] Data were obtained from, and recorded by, an independent central nationwide registration system (Landelijke Medische Registratie). A population-based cohort of 1126 patients underwent pancreaticoduodenectomy between 1994 and 1998. During this period, the annual mortality rate was approximately 10%, much higher than expected, and did not decrease significantly in time (1994: 13%; 1998: 10%). Furthermore, the study demonstrated that centralization is not generally accepted in the Netherlands; 49% of the pancreatoduodenectomies were performed in small-volume hospitals (<5 resections/year) in 1994, which resulted in a mortality rate of 18% compared to 0% in high-volume centers. At the end of the study period (1998), this pattern remained virtually unchanged; 32% of the patients was treated in low-volume hospitals, with 15% mortality rates versus 0% in high-volume hospitals (Fig. 1). A clear relation existed between hospital volume and in-hospital mortality, with a relative and absolute risk reduction of 94% and 15% for the high-volume compared to low-volume centers, respectively (Table 1). Nevertheless, several low-volume hospitals had little or no mortality after pancreaticoduodenectomy (Fig. 2).

SURGEON VOLUME VERSUS HOSPITAL VOLUME: A MULTIDISCIPLINARY APPROACH

Due to data recruitment of the previous study, analysis according to the impact of surgeon volume versus hospital volume could not be made. Therefore, the authors analyzed 463 consecutive pancreaticoduodenectomies performed at the AMC during the period of 1983-1999.[10] The series was separated into three different periods, and the mean number of resections per year increased from 17 in the first period to 50 during the last period, with a decrease in mortality rates from 5% to 0.7% (Table 2). Morbidity rates decreased from 60% to 41%, and the median hospital stay decreased from 24 to 15 days during this period. The influence of the surgeon experience was evaluated in a risk-factor analysis for complications in the last 300 patients (period: 1993 to 1999). No significant difference was noted between fellows and the experienced staff surgeons. Remarkably, the three deaths after surgery occurred after resection by different experienced staff surgeons. During the study period, a staff member was always present during surgery when the fellow was operating. Not only the experience of surgeons but also hospital volume, and by that experience of other specialties in management of complications of these patients after resection, is of great importance. Pancreaticoduodenectomy is a complicated procedure with a high risk of complications. Major complications such as anastomotic leakage of the pancreaticojejunostomy or hepaticojejunostomy and bleeding are the most serious complications associated with high mortality. Adequate management of complications depends on early detection and "aggressive" multidisciplinary treatment. Well-trained personnel at the

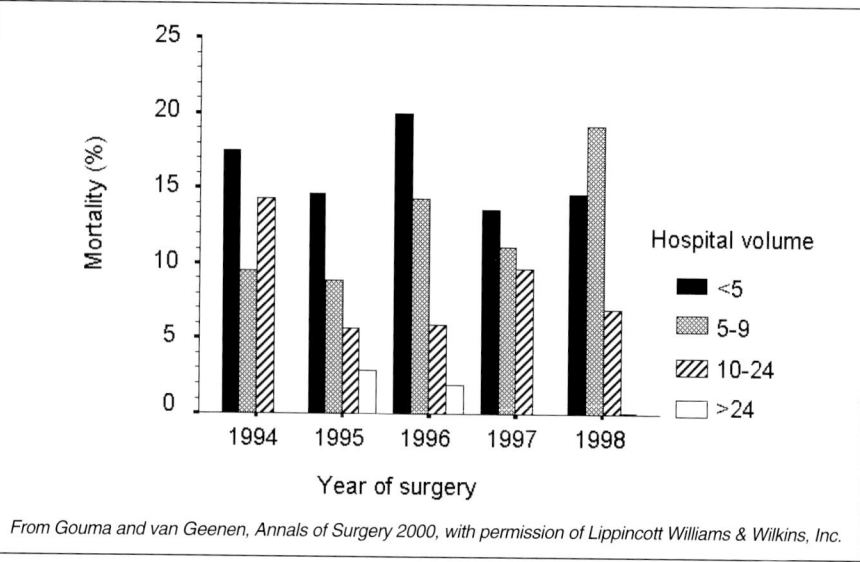

From Gouma and van Geenen, Annals of Surgery 2000, with permission of Lippincott Williams & Wilkins, Inc.

Figure 1. Hospital mortality rates versus hospital volume after pancreatic resection in the Netherlands, 1994-1996.

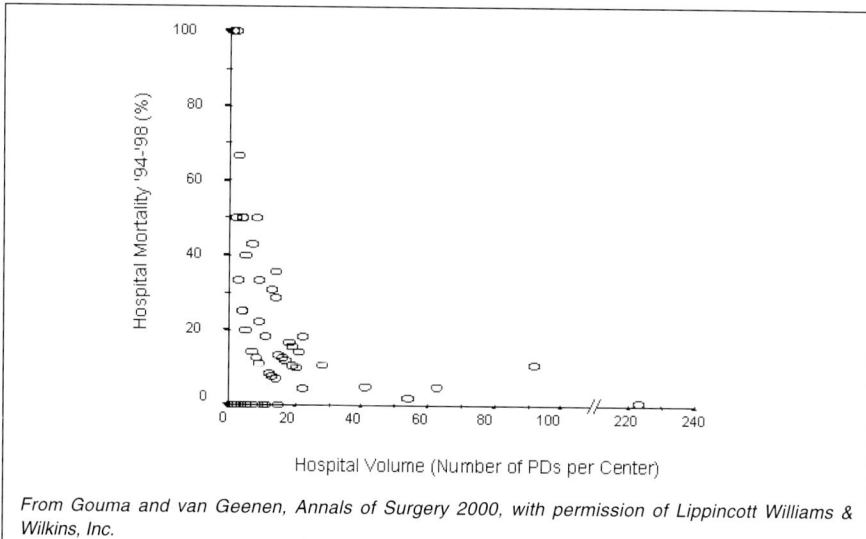

From Gouma and van Geenen, Annals of Surgery 2000, with permission of Lippincott Williams & Wilkins, Inc.

Figure 2. Percentage of pancreaticoduodenectomies in hospitals classified by annual hospital volume in the Netherlands.

Table 1. Relative risk (RR) with 95% confidence interval (95% CI), relative risk reduction (RRR), and absolute risk reduction (ARR) of surgery of different hospital volumes compared with low-volume hospitals (<5 resections/year) of 1126 patients in the period between 1994 and 1998 in the Netherlands.

Hospital Volume	No. of resections	Death rate (%)	RR	95% CI	RRR (%)	ARR (%)
< 5	463	16	1.00	-	-	-
5 - 9	205	13	0.79	0.52-1.20	21	3
10 - 24	235	8	0.48	0.29-0.78	52	8
≥25	223	1	0.06	0.01-0.23	94	15

ARR = absolute risk reduction; CI, confidence interval; RR relative risk; RRR, relative risk reduction.

From Gouma and van Geenen, Annals of Surgery 2000, with permission of Lippincott Williams & Wilkins, Inc.

Table 2. The number of subtotal pancreatoduodenectomies per year, postoperative morbidity, mortality, and hospital stay in 300 patients who underwent subtotal pancreatoduodenectomy between October 1992 and 1999, and the historical reference group (n=163).

Variables	1983 - Oct. 1992 n=163	Oct. 1992-1996 n=149	1997- Dec.1999 n=151
No. of resections/year	17	35	50
No. of patients with complications	97 (60) ‡	81 (54) ‡	62 (41) ¶†
Relaparotomy	22 (13)	25 (17) ‡	12 (8) †
Median hospital stay (range)	24 (5-293) †‡	18 (7-222) ¶‡	15 (6-167) ¶†
Hospital mortality	8 (4.9) ‡	2 (1.3)	1 (0.7) ¶

P<0.05 compared with: ¶Historical reference group (1983-1992), †period Oct.1992-1996, ‡period 1996-Dec.1998

Adapted from Gouma and van Geenen, Annals of Surgery 2000, with permission of Lippincott Williams & Wilkins, Inc.

Intensive Care Unit (ICU) and clinical wards, as well as experts in different fields such as radiology, gastroenterology, intensive care, and surgery, are mandatory for successful management of these patients. These demands and benefits of an experienced multidisciplinary setting are illustrated clearly with the following case history.

CASE HISTORY

A 73-year-old man with a severe kyphoscolioses, but without other contraindications or comorbidity, underwent a pylorus preserving pancreaticoduodenectomy for a small (2 cm) ampullary adenocarcinoma. On the second postoperative day, the drain located in the foramen of Winslow produced bile, and a percutaneous transhepatic drainage procedure under ultrasound guidance was performed for leakage of the hepaticojejunostomy (Fig. 3). The patient received Gelofusine® (B. Braun Medical SA, Crissier, Switzerland) because of low blood pressures (70/30 mm Hg) due to sepsis, after which an anaphylactic shock occurred. The patient had to be resuscitated and was transferred to the ICU. After five days, a re-laparotomy was performed because of persistent sepsis, and leakage of the pancreaticojejunostomy and necrosis of the pancreatic corpus were noted. The anastomosis was broken down, jejunal blind loop was closed, and pancreatic corpus was resected. A small (3 cm) remnant of the pancreatic tail was left in situ to maintain the endocrine pancreatic function. A drainage catheter was left behind to prevent pancreatic abscess formation. In the absence of clinical improvement, a second re-laparotomy was performed at a later stage and the pancreatic remnant also was resected. Respiratory insufficiency after closing the open abdomen a few weeks later, also increased by the kyphoscoliosis, resulted in long-term intubation and a prolonged ICU stay. After 88 days (the day before return to the normal ward), rectal blood loss and blood loss through the nasogastric tube occurred. Gastroscopy showed old blood in the stomach without an actual bleeding focus. The focus was suspected in the proximal jejunum and because of recurrent blood loss, an angiography was performed the next day. A pseudoaneurysm at the site of a branch of the hepatic artery was identified as the

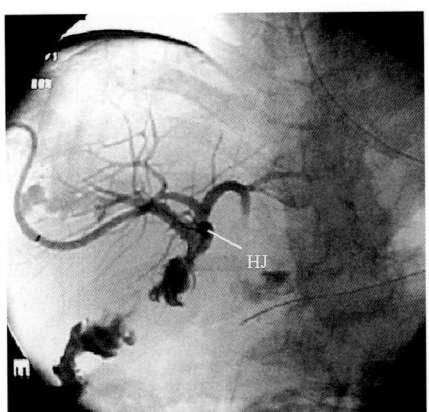

Figure 3. Leakage of the hepaticojejunostomy (HJ), treated successfully by percutaneous transhepatic cholangiography without leakage during control cholangiography five days later.

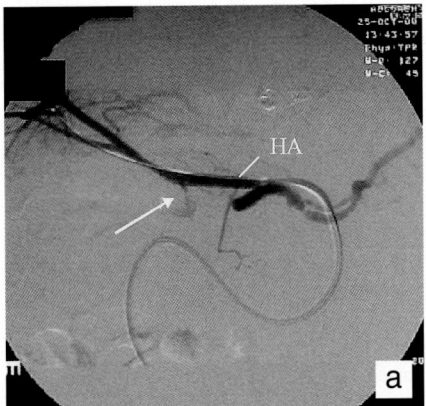 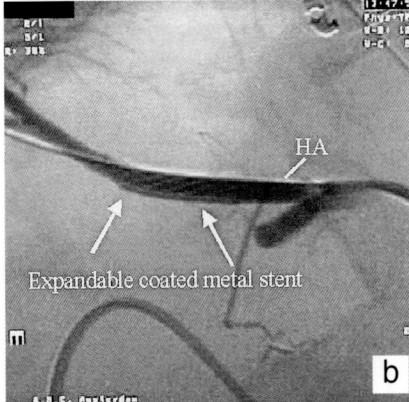

Figure 4. Bleeding from a branch (arrow) of the hepatic artery (HA) demonstrated by angiography. a) Bleeding focus, b) Occlusion by insertion of an expandable coated metal stent (arrows).

Table 3. Studies between 1990 and 2001 addressing mortality of pancreatic resection in relation to hospital volume or surgeon volume.

Author	Year	Setting	Resection type	No. pts	No. of resections/yr low vs. high volume			No. of high volume hosp.	In-hospital mortality low vs. high volume			Statistical significance	Case mix high-volume hospitals	statistical significance of surgeon volume
Edge et al[12]	1993	University hs	PD/TP	223	≤5	vs.	≥14	10	7.4	vs.	5.1	no	not analyzed	no
Lieberman et al[6]	1995	New York	PD/TP	1972	<1.3	vs.	>10.1	?	18.9	vs.	5.5	yes	not analyzed	no
Gordon et al[7]	1995	Maryland	PD	502	local	vs.	referral hosp.	1	13.5	vs	2.2	yes	> whites, >Hypertension < pulmonary disease = age, = gender	not analyzed
Glasgow et al[8]	1996	California	PD	1705	<2	vs.	>50	2	14	vs.	3.5	yes	= comorbidity	not analyzed
Wade et al[13]	1996	DOD hosp.	PD	130	<1	vs.	>2	3	6	vs.	9	yes	not analyzed	not analyzed
Neoptolemos et al[11]	1997	UK	PD/TP	1026	logistic regression with individual hospital data							yes	not analyzed	not analyzed
Begg et al[4]	1998	USA	PD	742	≤5	vs.	≥11	10	12.9	vs.	5.8	yes	> comorbidity = cancer stage = age	not analyzed
Gorden et al[15]	1998	Maryland	PD	795	<20	vs.	≥20	1	'84:19.5 '95:12.4	vs. vs.	3.2 1	yes yes	= gender, = age > whites < complexity	not analyzed
Birkmeyer et al[14]	1999	USA	PD	7229	<1	vs.	≥5	40	16.1	vs.	4.1	yes	> comorbidity = age, = gender	not analyzed
Gouma et al[10]	2000	Netherlands	PD/TP	1126	<5	vs.	≥25	1	16	vs.	1	yes	not analyzed	not analyzed

DOD hosp. = Department of Defense hospitals

bleeding focus (Fig. 4), and an expandable coated metallic stent was placed that stopped the bleeding (Fig. 4b). Eventually, the patient recovered and 139 days after resection was discharged. Close cooperation between different specialties (intesivist, radiologist, gastroenterologist, vascular radiologist, and surgeons) enabled successful management of the complications of these patients, illustrating the impact of hospital volume on a well-trained team of different specialists.

REVIEW OF THE LITERATURE

In recent years, articles have been published that describe the relation between hospital volume or surgeon volume and mortality after pancreatic resection. In an attempt to obtain an overview of the data available, a Medline search was conducted using the following keywords: pancreatic neoplasm or pancreaticoduodenectomy combined with mortality, and experience, hospital volume, case load, regionalization, or centralization. This data set was limited to the English language and human studies in the period between 1990 and January 2001; the search provided 151 hits. All studies were analyzed, and only ten described adequately the relation between hospital volume or surgeon volume and mortality after pancreatic resection (Table 3). The following variables were investigated: setting, type of resection, number of patients included in the studies, definition of high and low volume and their related in-hospital mortality, number of high-volume centers, case mix, and impact of surgeon volume on in-hospital mortality rates.

The majority of the studies were performed in the USA, and two were performed in European countries.[10,11] All studies described patients who underwent subtotal pancreaticoduodenectomy or total pancreatectomy, and generally included large numbers of patients. Only two studies included less than 250 patients.[12,13] The definition of low- and high-volume centers varies greatly, and is based on personal preference in most studies. Only one study used approximate quartiles to divide the hospital into different volume categories.[14] In three of the ten studies, the high-volume category contained only one high-volume center.

Most studies described a clear inverse relation between hospital volume and in-hospital mortality. Only one study described an opposite relation between hospital volume and in-hospital mortality,[13] and one reported no relation between hospital volume and mortality. In these studies, relatively limited numbers of patients were included (130 and 223 patients, respectively),[8,12] and the definition of high volume (>2/year)[8] was low-volume when compared with most other studies. Data on case mix were available in only four studies and showed that gender and age were divided equality among the hospital-volume categories. Two studies[4,14] showed that patients included in high-volume centers had more co-morbidity compared to low-volume hospitals. In one study, co-morbidity appeared to be higher in high-volume hospitals because of a higher prevalence of hypertension; however, pulmonary disease was more frequent at low-volume centers.[7] Patient complexity was measured using the All Patient Refined DRG Grouper (3M Health Information Systems, Provo, Utah, USA) in one study[15] and was less in high-volume centers.

Two studies[6,12] analyzed the influence of surgeon volume and one showed that high-volume surgeons, who performed more than 41 resections in seven years, had significantly less mortality than low-volume surgeons, who performed less than nine resections (6.0 vs. 13.0, respectively).[6] But in a logistic regression analysis, no relation was noted between surgeon volume and hospital mortality.

The data from this review strongly suggest centralization of pancreatic surgery could further decrease mortality. State-wide regionalization of pancreaticoduodenectomy appears to be responsible for a great part of the mortality reduction rate (61%) in Maryland, USA.[15] In other countries, such as the Netherlands, such an impact was not noted.

However, controversy remains regarding the scientific value of these studies. Some large studies[7,10,15] describe only one high-volume center, and the authors are from that center; therefore, outcome might be biased. Many studies used national or regional health-care databases. These databases are not conclusive and contain limited data. As a result, in some studies case mix cannot be identified and might partially be responsible for the relation between hospital volume and mortality.[6,10-13] Referral patterns can result in higher prevalence of co-morbidity in high-volume centers,[4,14] whereas others reported less patient complexity in high- volume centers.[15] No evidence exists of case mix for gender and age,[4,7,8,14] and the inverse relation of hospital volume and mortality cannot be explained by case mix, however, nor can it be excluded.

Although centralization appears to be beneficial, there are some downsides to this concept. In rural areas, centralization would lead to increasing travel distance for patients with malignant disease in poor condition and need the support of relatives and friends. Therefore, not surprisingly, a recent study[16] demonstrated that many patients prefer to undergo surgery in local centers, even when travel to a regional center would result in a lower operative mortality. The majority of patients with pancreatic cancer are not candidates for resection, and palliative procedures that do not prolong their limited survival time may as well be provided in the patients' own environment. Yet, some studies demonstrated that palliative procedures such as bypass surgery or stent insertion performed at high-volume centers result in less mortality compared to low-volume centers.[17] Others stated that centralization could endanger the financial viability of smaller hospitals and their ability to recruit general surgeons.[18]

To date, pancreaticoduodenectomy can be performed with limited morbidity and mortality provided patients are selected carefully, and the resection is performed in a high-volume center with sufficient support of other experienced disciplines involved in treatment of postoperative complications. Palliative treatment is merely non-surgical and preferably can be performed in the patient's own environment, or in one-day referrals to central hospitals (stent insertion). These insights have the potential to further improve the outcome of management of pancreatic cancer.

REFERENCES

1. Gudjonsson B. Carcinoma of the pancreas: critical analysis of costs, results of resections, and the need for standardized reporting [see comments]. [Review] [350 refs]. J Am Coll Surg 1995;181:483-503.
2. Harmon JW, Tang DG, Gordon TA, et al. Hospital volume can serve as a surrogate for surgeonbvv volume for achieving excellent outcomes in colorectal resection. Ann Surg 1999;230:404-11.
3. Matthews HR, Powell DJ, McConkey CC. Effect of surgical experience on the results of resection for oesophageal carcinoma. Br J Surg 1986;73:621-3.
4. Begg CB, Cramer LD, Hoskins WJ, et al. Impact of hospital volume on operative mortality for major cancer surgery [see comments]. JAMA 1998;280:1747-51.
5. Hannan EL, Kilburn HJ, Bernard H, et al. Coronary artery bypass surgery: the relationship between inhospital mortality rate and surgical volume after controlling for clinical risk factors. Med Care 1991;29:1094-107.
6. Lieberman MD, Kilburn H, Lindsey M, et al. Relation of perioperative deaths to hospital volume among patients undergoing pancreatic resection for malignancy. Ann Surg 1995;222:638-45.
7. Gordon TA, Burleyson GP, Tielsch JM, et al. The effects of regionalization on cost and outcome for one general high-risk surgical procedure [see comments]. Ann Surg 1995;221:43-9.
8. Glasgow RE, Mulvihill SJ. Hospital volume influences outcome in patients undergoing pancreatic resection for cancer. West J Med 1996;165:294-300.
9. Gouma DJ, Obertop H. Centralization of surgery for periampullary malignancy. Br J Surg 1999;86:1361-2.
10. Gouma DJ, van Geenen RCI, van Gulik ThM, et al. Rates of complications and death after pancreaticoduodenectomy: risk factors and the impact of hospital volume. Ann Surg 2000;232:786-94.
11. Neoptolemos JP, Russell RC, Bramhall S, et al. Low mortality following resection for pancreatic and periampullary tumours in 1026 patients: UK survey of specialist pancreatic units. UK Pancreatic Cancer Group [see comments]. Br J Surg 1997;84:1370-6.
12. Edge SB, Schmieg REJ, Rosenlof LK, et al. Pancreas cancer resection outcome in American University centers in 1989-1990. Cancer 1993;71:3502-8.
13. Wade TP, Halaby IA, Stapleton DR, et al. Population-based analysis of treatment of pancreatic cancer and Whipple resection: Department of Defense hospitals, 1989-1994. Surgery 1996;120:680-5.
14. Birkmeyer JD, Finlayson SR, Tosteson AN, et al. Effect of hospital volume on in-hospital mortality with pancreaticoduodenectomy [see comments]. Surgery 1999;125:250-6.
15. Gordon TA, Bowman HM, Tielsch JM, et al. Statewide regionalization of pancreaticoduodenectomy and its effect on in-hospital mortality. Ann Surg 1998;228:71-8.
16. Finlayson SR, Birkmeyer JD, Tosteson AN, et al. Patient preferences for location of care: implications for regionalization. Med Care 1999;37:204-9.
17. Sosa JA, Bowman HM, Gordon TA, et al. Importance of hospital volume in the overall management of pancreatic cancer. Ann Surg 1998;228:429-38.
18. Birkmeyer JD. Should we regionalize major surgery? Potential benefits and policy considerations. J Am Coll Surg 2000;190:341-9.

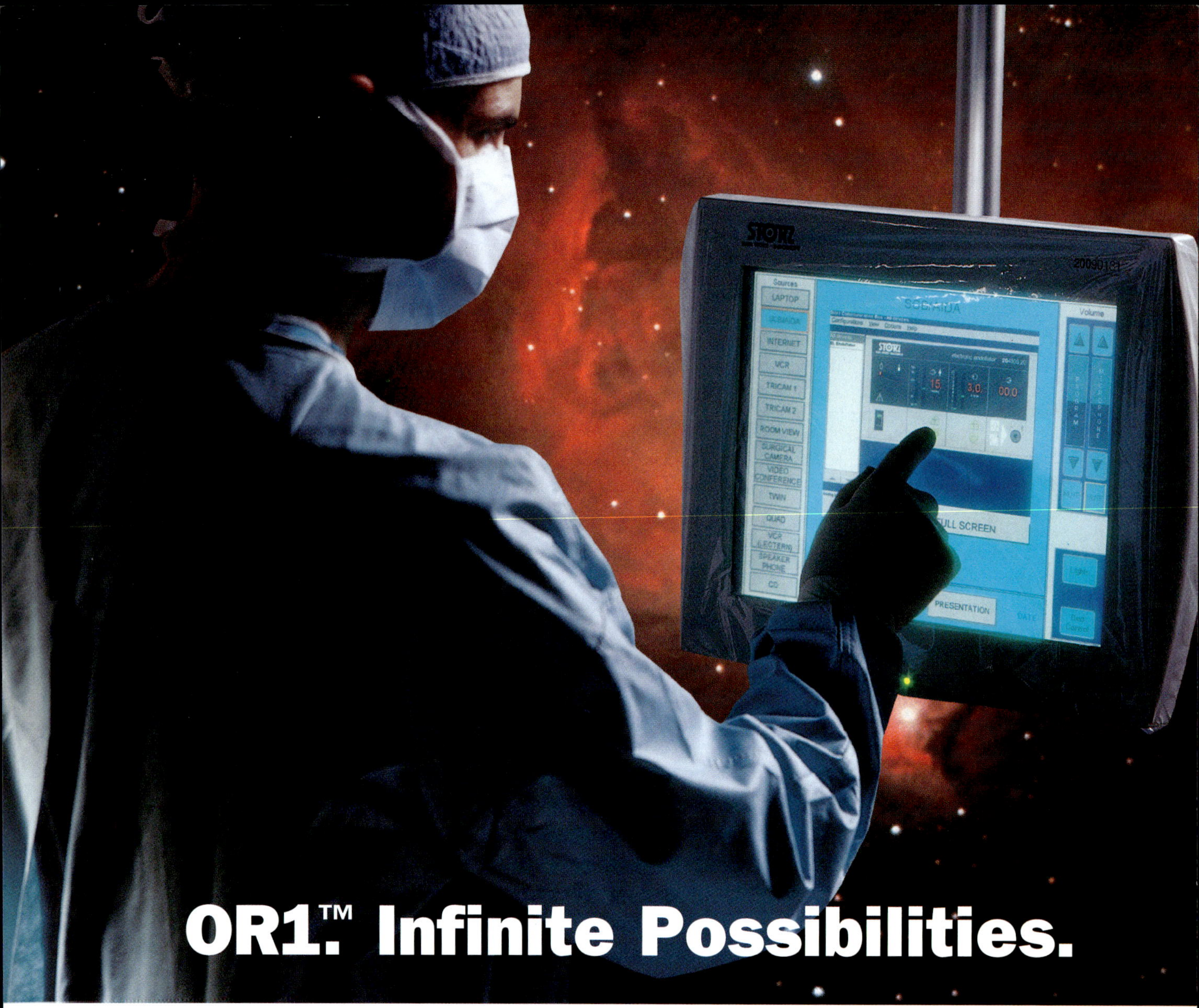

OR1.™ Infinite Possibilities.

The Future Of Endoscopy Starts With One.

Imagine everything you want in an OR. Then imagine more. That's the promise of Karl Storz and OR1.™

OR1™ gives you the power to integrate virtually every OR component into a single, optimized system. The power to control medical devices, teleconferencing, hospital computers, room and surgical lighting is yours—all from a centralized station—inside or outside the sterile field.

What's more, OR1™ places no limits on the way you configure your surgical suite. Karl Storz will custom build it to your specifications, including the latest technological advances. And with its PC-based architecture, your OR1™ suite can be easily upgraded with future software updates.

Learn how infinite possibilities can become your reality. Just call **1-800-421-0837**. And discover the power of one.

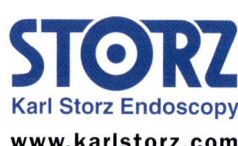

STORZ
Karl Storz Endoscopy
www.karlstorz.com

Process-Optimized Operating Room: Implementation of an Integrated OR System into Clinical Routine

PROF. ANTON SCHAFMAYER, M.D.
MEDICAL SUPERINTENDENT
SURGICAL CLINIC COMMUNITY HOSPITAL
LÜNEBURG, GERMANY

DIRK LEHMANN-BECKOW, M.D.
SURGICAL CLINIC COMMUNITY HOSPITAL
LÜNEBURG, GERMANY

MARTIN HOLZNER
MEDICAL ENGINEERING GROUP
SIEMENS AG
ERLANGEN, GERMANY

The surgeon's working environment has changed continuously in recent years regarding the technical complexity of the components in use in the operating room (OR). Parallel to this development, demands for process-optimized procedures have also grown constantly. The impetus for these changes was the beginning of use of minimally invasive techniques in surgery. In contrast, overall development of the OR itself has been slight or nonexistent. What we are typically confronted with currently is an OR outfitted with high-tech medical equipment, whereas only to a limited extent can the design of the OR itself be regarded as ergonomic or holistic. This situation has spread to related specialties as well, and represents a general tendency. Whereas dentists, for example, already enjoy the benefits of a centralized management and operation workplace, this development has not yet reached a satisfactory level for surgeons.

The tremendous potential for improvement in this area has not gone unnoticed. Some time ago, Siemens resolved to develop an integrated OR system with the objective of optimizing pre-, intra-, and postoperative processes, which includes a new room design that contributes to more efficient use of space available in the OR (Fig. 1).

INTEGRATED OR SYSTEM FOR USE IN MULTIFUNCTIONAL ORS

Development began with extensive analyses of OR processes; conducted with valuable input from users, these analyses provided essential information regarding the individual sub-processes where optimization was possible. The result is the Siemens Integrated OR System (SIOS). Intense cooperation between Siemens and other industry and clinical partners has enabled development of a system with opportunities for centralized operation and control to meet the essential requirements of various surgical disciplines (general surgery, gynecology, urology, orthopedics)

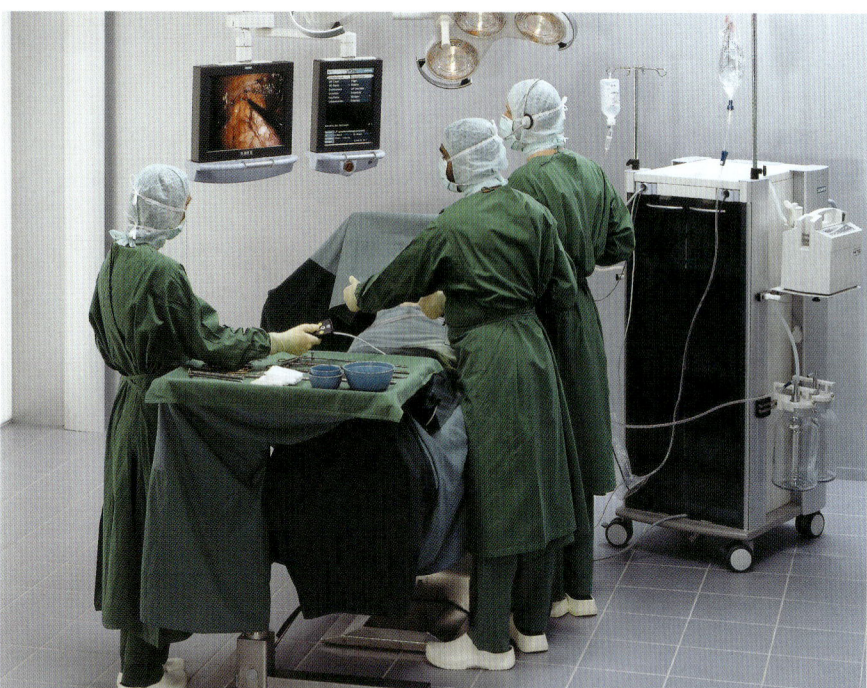

Figure 1. Typical Siemens Integrated OR System (SIOS) configuration.

currently and in the future. The new system design incorporates control of vital OR components directly from the sterile area (OR lights, table, endo light, endo camera, insufflator, X-ray, ultrasound, video recorder, telephone, video printer, etc.). As a prerequisite for the central control of OR components from different manufacturers, a proven interface standard was adapted for communication, which resulted in an optimized workflow and increased overall efficiency of OR processes.

NEW INTERFACE STANDARD CREATES THE BASIS FOR PROCESS OPTIMIZATION IN THE OR

Communication between SIOS and the individual components is based on CANopen BUS technology, an internationally recognized industry standard that has proved itself over the years, and has been implemented successfully in a wide variety of business fields. Siemens adapted this standard for use with SIOS and now makes it available to all its partners, with the goal of establishing this type of communication as a new "interface standard" for integrated OR solutions. The advantage of a BUS system of this type is that a nearly unlimited number of OR components can be connected to SIOS, with stable and reliable data transmission.

CENTRALIZED DISPLAY OF VARIOUS LIVE IMAGES ON A FLATSCREEN MONITOR

SIOS features a ceiling-mounted monitor system that comprises an image monitor and control monitor, both of which are flatscreen Thin Film Transistor (TFT) monitors of the newest generation. The monitors are light and positioned easily, so they can always be placed ergonomically for optimal visibility by the surgeon, regardless of application. The image monitor displays images from the selected live-image source-endo camera, X-ray, or ultrasound-to the user. The control monitor shows the operating menus of the selected OR components and important status information, such as CO_2 consumption. A special emphasis was placed on unified and ergonomic design of the user interfaces of the individual system menus-the prerequisite for integration of components from different manufacturers in one system with simple, user-friendly operation.

UNIFIED OPERATION OF IMPORTANT OR COMPONENTS DIRECTLY FROM THE STERILE FIELD

SIOS permits the OR team to completely control all integrated OR components. Individual control functions are activated or changed with a steriliz-able remote or voice control, typically done by the scrub nurse or surgeon. The voice control is independent of the speaker; it uses a headset, and has the decisive advantage that the surgeon has both hands free at all times so she or he can concentrate solely on handling the OR instruments. Clearly defined, standardized command inputs, in conjunction with a unified operating philosophy for all components (visually displayed on the second flatscreen monitor) ensure optimal, efficient operation of the entire system. The components selected determine which function changes are affected in the corresponding operating menus on the monitor. The open system architecture of SIOS enables integration of future technologies and new SIOS-compatible OR components from additional manufacturers.

NEW ROOM DESIGN CENTRALIZES CONTROL OF ESSENTIAL OR COMPONENTS

The new room design mentioned above means components previously spread randomly around the OR can now be combined with one mobile device box and one electronics cabinet. A single documentation unit can now be provided covering all integrated imaging systems. The risk of tripping over a thicket of cables can be eliminated by one central cable routing for the power supply, CO_2, compressed air, vacuum, and video signals. Process optimization is primarily the result of integration of different OR components into one system, permitting central operation from the sterile field, which satisfies the prerequisites for control of all important systems by surgeons, surgical nurses, or both. The non-sterile nurse previously responsible for these tasks can now attend to other responsibilities even outside the OR, and can be recalled to the OR when needed at any

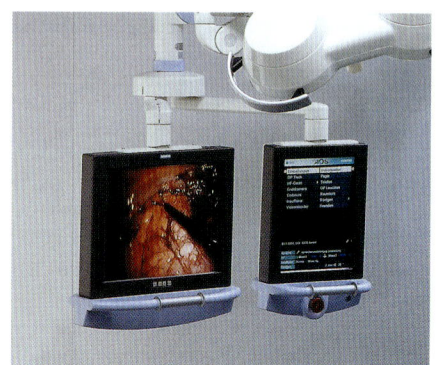

Figure 2. SIOS image and control monitor (right).

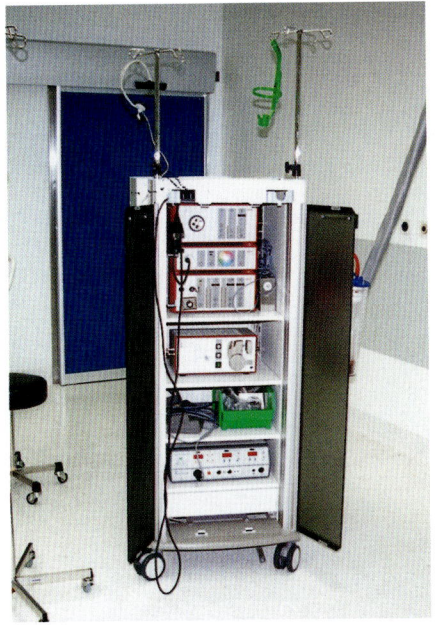
Figure 3. Open device box with central routing of supply cables.

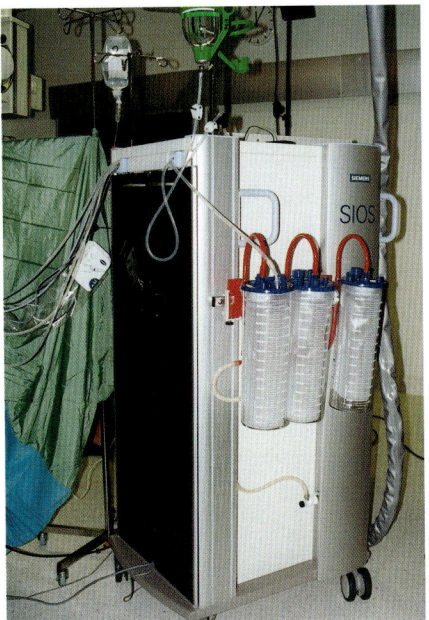
Figure 4. Device box with doors closed.

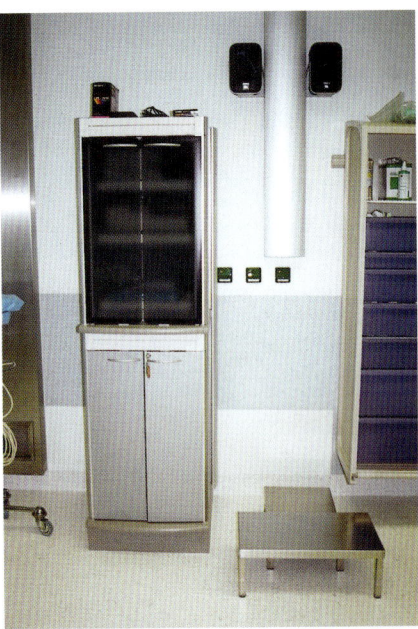
Figure 5. Central Siemens Integrated OR System (SIOS) control unit.

time by way of the SIOS pager. This process directly effects the time required for surgical interventions, reduced by elimination of wait times for execution of commands by the "non-sterile" circulating nurse.

SIMPLE, INTUITIVE SYSTEM OPERATION

The first SIOS worldwide was installed as part of a pilot project in the OR of the Community Hospital in Lüneburg, Germany. Following start-up in June 2000, surgeons, OR staff, and technicians were able to test the system's performance together. The original expectation was that the system would be extremely complicated and technical, as well as suitable for use of only a few surgeons and nurses with experience in endoscopic surgery. However, it was a pleasant surprise to discover how simple and clear the menu-guided control provided by the Typical SIOS configuration system (Fig. 1) for all technical components used in endoscopic surgery was: no user manual or detailed explanations were needed from the manufacturers. Work with the new equipment commenced after no more than half an hour's introduction, most of which related to explanations of a few system components (camera, light source, insufflator) not familiar to the users. SIOS itself was nearly invisible in the OR; the only indication of its presence was the two flatscreen monitors suspended from the ceiling (Fig. 2) and a device box with central power cable routing (Figs. 3 & 4). The heart of the system, the computer unit, was concealed in an electronics cabinet outside the sterile field (Fig. 5). The result was a neat and orderly landscape without the tangle of cables that too often accompanies technical progress.

Everyone involved harbored some skepticism regarding the voice control. Previous experience with voice-recognition programs, and discouraging reports regarding other voice-controlled operating equipment, did not raise the hopes of those who would be working with SIOS in their daily routine. A number of unanswered questions existed: Is voice control practical? What will the accuracy rate be? Could there be fatal malfunctions? Will the noise level be disruptive? How many commands are there to learn, and how long will it take to learn them? Will the staff members issuing the voice commands have to adjust to SIOS, or will SIOS adjust to the speakers? Most of these concerns were overcome during the first demonstration, and efficiency and safety of the SIOS voice control were confirmed in practical use. Within a few weeks, all surgeons and surgical nurses involved in endoscopy—including the interns—were familiar with SIOS. The system was adopted enthusiastically by everyone, and was also used by staff members on call.

RELIABLE PERFORMANCE OF THE VOICE CONTROL

During the introductory phase, 50 endoscopic surgeries (cholecystectomy, hernioplasty, appendectomy, thoracoscopies, diagnostic interventions) were performed in the presence of Siemens engineers. Recognition rate of the voice control was tested with a questionnaire that documented the commands issued by the surgeon. The frequency of unrecognized commands was also recorded. The recognition rate of the specially developed Siemens voice program was rated as high. On average, SIOS recognized 9 of 10 commands, regardless of the speaker who issued them. No differences were present in the recognition of male and female voices. No malfunctions occurred as a result of an incorrectly identified command. When the voice command was not recognized, the function concerned was not executed. It is not necessary to learn the voice commands before using the system; the commands are displayed legibly on the control monitor (Figs. 6 & 7) when a system menu is selected from the main menu (Fig. 8). Thus, the surgeon simply reads the appropriate command, learning the voice commands during the operation. Even in the introductory phase, most surgeons were able to control device functions without reading commands from the monitor, thus saving additional time. An additional advantage of this

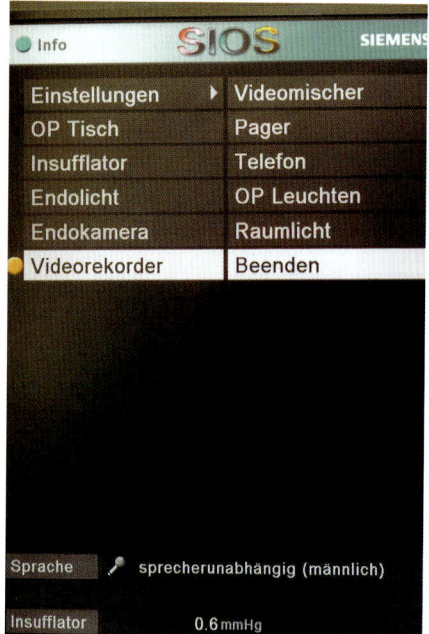

Figure 6. Control menu for Operating Room (OR) table.

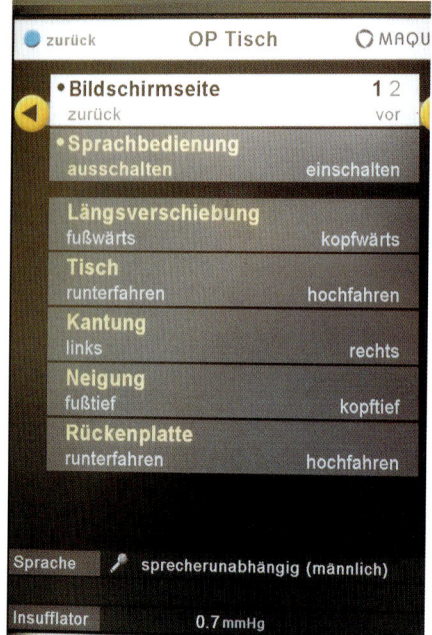

Figure 7. Control menu for endo camera.

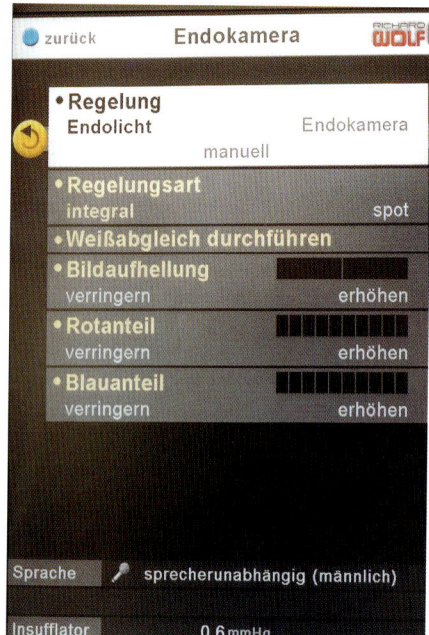

Figure 8. Main menu with list of integrated components.

system was the use of flatscreen monitors that could be swivelled to be visible from anywhere in the OR. Monitor positions could be changed during a procedure without time-consuming changes to system connections and without endangering the sterility of the surgical area.

The need to wear a headset to ensure accurate speech recognition was not perceived as disruptive (Fig. 9). Alternatively, the system can also be controlled manually with an autoclavable remote control (Fig. 10), a system standard. No difficulty was encountered in voice-controlled operation of the OR table. For larger travel distances, commands must be repeated several times, as the extent of movement per command issued is limited to small increments for safety reasons. Future options to optimize table positioning with selectable pre-defined table positions will be considered.

SAVING TIME, INCREASING EFFICIENCY

One vital advantage is the already-mentioned control of all components in the OR unit from the sterile field, which can reduce the burden on the "non-sterile" circulating nurse noticeably. Currently, the presence of a "non-sterile" circulating nurse in the OR is required for only 10% of the total surgical time; in the time saved, the nurse can attend to other tasks in and outside the OR. When needed, the nurse can be recalled at any time by way of the SIOS pager. Average operation times had already been reduced after only 50 surgical procedures. The results obtained for process optimization with SIOS up to this point will have to be supplemented by data from additional operations before a final evaluation can be prepared. Future plans include integrating SIOS into the hospital's IT solutions, making it possible, for example, to call up X-ray and CT exposures in the OR at any time by way of the video monitor and a "picture-in-a-picture" system.

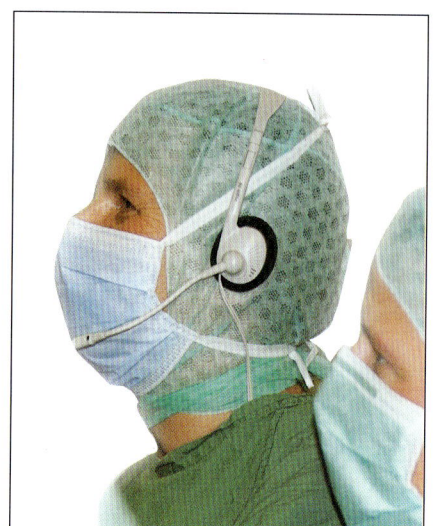

Figure 9. Surgeon with headset.

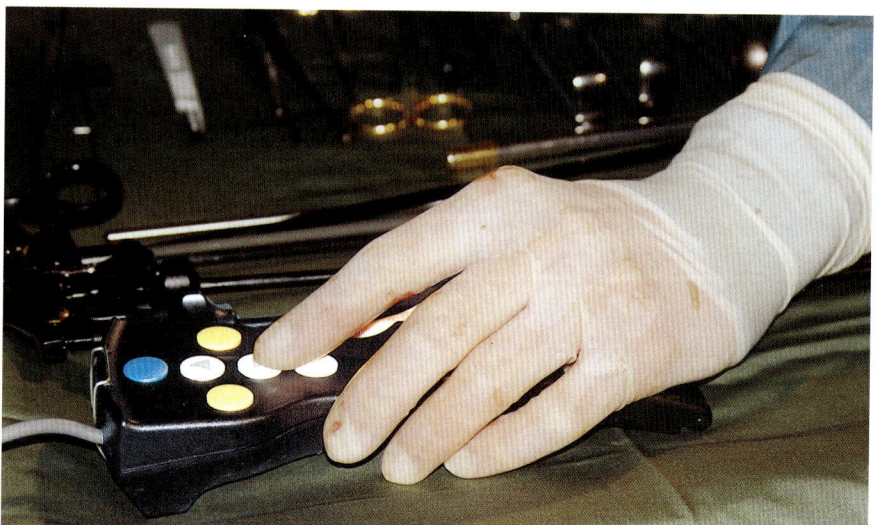

Figure 10. Autoclavable remote control.

Vulvar Leiomyosarcoma: A Case Report in a Nigerian Woman

VALENTINE OTOIDE, M.D.
SENIOR REGISTRAR
PROGRAM COORDINATOR
DEPARTMENT OF OBSTETRICS AND GYNAECOLOGY

MICHAEL OKOBIA, M.D., F.W.A.C.S.
CONSULTANT SURGEON & ASSOCIATE
DEPARTMENT OF SURGERY

UNIVERSITY OF BENIN TEACHING HOSPITAL
WOMEN'S HEALTH AND ACTION RESEARCH CENTRE
BENIN CITY, NIGERIA

JONATHAN ALIGBE, M.D., F.M.C.PATH
CONSULTANT PATHOLOGIST
DEPARTMENT OF PATHOLOGY
UNIVERSITY OF BENIN
BENIN CITY, NIGERIA

FRIDAY OKONOFUA, M.D., F.W.A.C.S., F.M.C.O.G.
PROFESSOR OF OBSTETRICS AND GYNAECOLOGY
UNIVERSITY OF BENIN
DEAN, FACULTY OF MEDICINE AND DIRECTOR
WOMEN'S HEALTH AND ACTION RESEARCH CENTRE
DEPARTMENT OF OBSTETRICS AND GYNAECOLOGY
UNIVERSITY OF BENIN TEACHING HOSPITAL
WOMEN'S HEALTH AND ACTION RESEARCH CENTER
BENIN CITY, NIGERIA

Leiomyosarcoma of the vulva is a rare gynaecological malignancy. To date, only few cases have been reported in the literature, the majority of which are from Western countries.[1-3] Although leiomyosarcoma is classically regarded as a malignant tumor, the generally favorable prognosis following surgical treatment, as well as its reduced propensity for widespread metastasis, makes it one of the most enigmatic malignancies in the medical literature. In addition, the tumor may attain enormous morphological proportions, a situation unusual in many malignant tumors.

To the best of our knowledge, there has been no reported case of vulvar leiomyosarcoma in any African population. Malignant growths of the vulvar in African women are, in themselves, rare with the majority being vulvar carcinomas occurring in older women. Available evidence suggests not more than one to two cases of vulvar carcinomas are seen each year, even in the most busy gynaecologic oncology units of tertiary hospitals in Africa. Due to the rarity of vulvar cancers in African women, we report here a case of a giant vulvar leiomyosarcoma that occurred in a 45-year-old Nigerian woman. The case was managed with simple wide excision followed by adjuvant chemotherapy, and

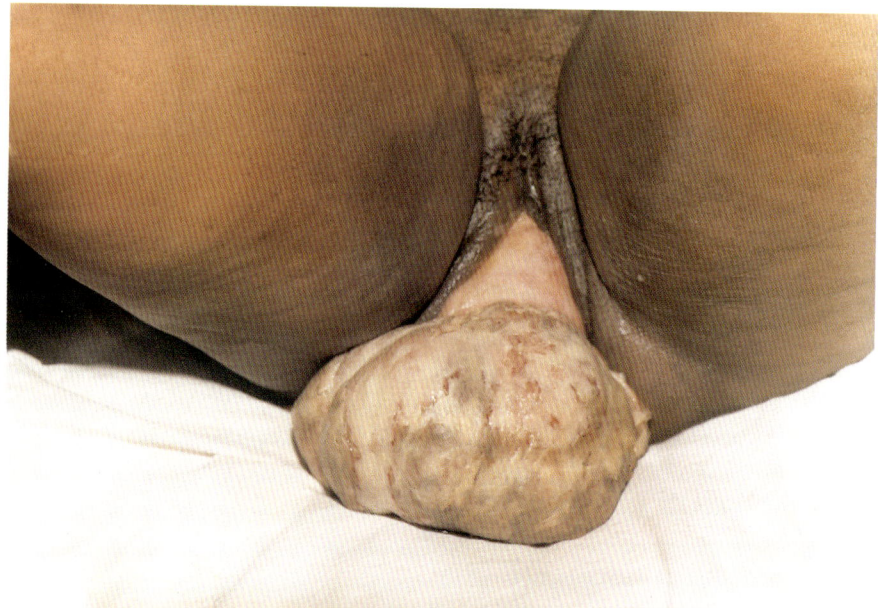

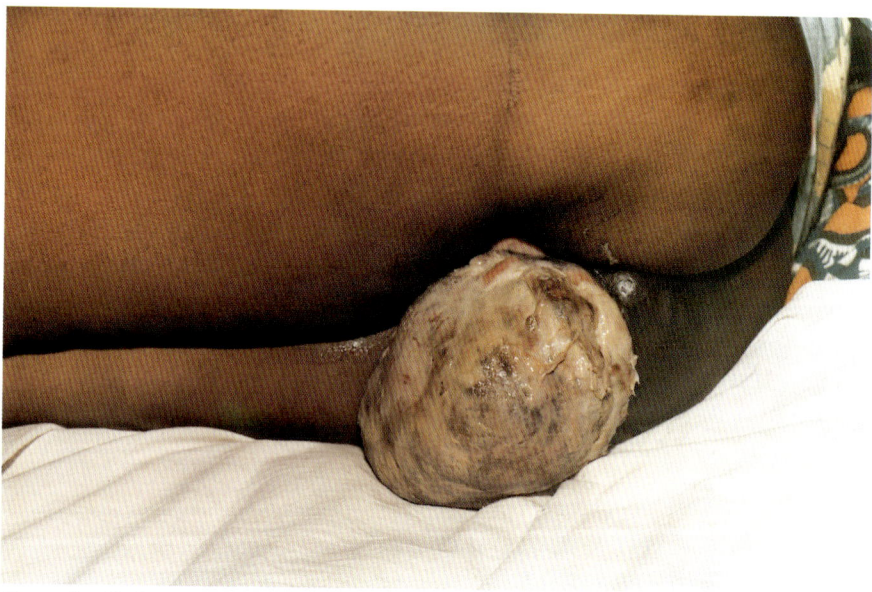

Figures 1a, 1b. Preoperative vulva mass (12 cm by 14 cm).

no recurrence has been seen after six months of follow up. The peculiar features of clinical presentation and management of the case are described.

CASE REPORT

The woman, a 45-year-old para 4, was admitted at the University of Benin Teaching Hospital (Nigeria) in September 1998, with the history of a painful fungating vulvar mass of six months' duration. The mass had increased gradually in size and had recently started to exude an offensive discharge. She complained of persistent weight loss but she had no vaginal discharge, vaginal bleeding, or abdominal symptoms. She also did not have symptoms relating to the urinary, cardiovascular, respiratory, or central nervous systems.

On physical examination, the patient weighed 54 kg, and had a height of 163 cm. She had marked conjunctival pallor but was not jaundiced or febrile. Her vital signs were normal, respiratory and cardiovascular systems were normal, and she had no palpable peripheral lymphadenopathy. Her abdomen was normal and spleen, liver, and kidneys were not palpably enlarged.

Examination of her external genitalia disclosed a huge, fungating, and lobulated mass arising deep within the right labium majus that measured 12 x 14 cm (Fig. 1). A diffuse necrotic part in the inferior edge of the mass emitted a profuse, offensive sero-sanguineous discharge. The inguinal lymph nodes were not palpably enlarged. The rectal mucosa was normal. However, a bimanual vaginal and pelvic examination could not be carried out because the mass completely occluded the vaginal introitus.

Preliminary investigations showed a haematocrit of 24%; normal electrolytes, urea, creatinine, and liver function tests; a normal chest x-ray; and normal intravenous pyelogram. Her human immunodeficiency virus (HIV) sero-status was negative.

She was transfused with two units of compatible blood and given broad-spectrum antibiotics. Subsequently, an examination under anaesthesia was carried out followed by a tissue biopsy of the mass. During this examination, a bimanual pelvic examination was done, which showed a normal uterus and normal pelvic adnexa. Specifically, we were able to confirm the mass had not extended beyond the immediate external vulvar and perineal organs.

Thereafter, a histological examination of the extirpated specimen was carried out, which suggested a diagnosis of vulvar leiomyosarcoma (see histological report below). The patient was transfused with two units of blood and counseled for a wide surgical excision of the tumor.

SURGICAL MANAGEMENT

Surgical excision of the tumor was carried out under balanced general anaesthesia. First, the extent of the mass was defined as involving the entire length of the right labium majus, burying deep into its musculature and occluding the vaginal introitus. A cleavage point was identified at its infero-medial edge where the tumor merged with the vaginal mucosa. A gentle dissection was initiated at this point and extended superiorly to expose the entire medial plane of the right vulva. The major bleeding points along the route were identified and tied. Thereafter, the superior edge of the tumor was determined to extend underneath a healthy-looking vulvar tissue.

The dissection was then carried 2 cm beyond this portion to not leave behind any residual tumor mass. The dissection was carried out through the tumor bed from its medial part to the lateral area, occluding all large vessels that formed the bed. At the lateral wall, a 2-cm portion of normal tissue was resected along with the tumor, leaving a wide raw area.

Further examination of the vulvar showed a complete removal of the tumor. The area was then closed in layers and a corrugated drain left *in situ* to maintain a dry operation site. Her estimated blood loss was 200 mL.

POSTOPERATIVE/ADJUVANT MANAGEMENT

The patient was given broad-spectrum parenteral antibiotics in the immediate postoperative period. She had intravenous ampicillin, 1 g every six hours, and intravenous metronidazole, 500 mg every eight hours for 48 hours, followed by oral treatment for an additional three days. She also had gentamicin, 80 mg every eight hours for five days. She was commenced on daily dressing with an antiseptic lotion, as well as daily sitz baths. Subsequently, the vulva wound healed slowly, and was healed completely by three weeks after surgery (Fig. 2).

One week after surgery, the patient was commenced on parenteral cyclophosphamide, 200 mg daily for five days. This course of chemotherapy was repeated at intervals of three to four weeks following satisfactory haematological, liver, and renal investigations. Six months after surgery, there has been no evidence of local recurrence of the tumor, and has not demonstrated any evidence of widespread metastasis. She has gained weight progressively, with her most recent weight being 62 kg.

PATHOLOGICAL EXAMINATION

Grossly (Fig. 3a), the tumor consisted of a huge, poorly encapsulated, firm, brownish yellow mass with attached Negroid skin; it weighed 800 g and measured 20 x 15 x 10 cm. The transected surface showed whorled-like appearance with yellowish mucoid areas (Fig. 3b). Histologically, a well-circumscribed pseudo-encapsulated neoplasm was covered by smooth muscle and skin. It consisted of alternating areas of hypercellularity and hypocellularity. The hypercellular areas were composed of pleomorphic spindle cells having variable amounts of cytoplasm and nuclei arranged in fascicles. The cytoplasm was eosinophilic and lacked fibrillar sub-structure, whereas the nuclei were irregular and had prominent vesiculation and mitotic figures. Dispersed throughout this sarcomatous proliferation were variable amounts of myomatous changes and tracts of tumor necrosis (Figs. 4a, b).

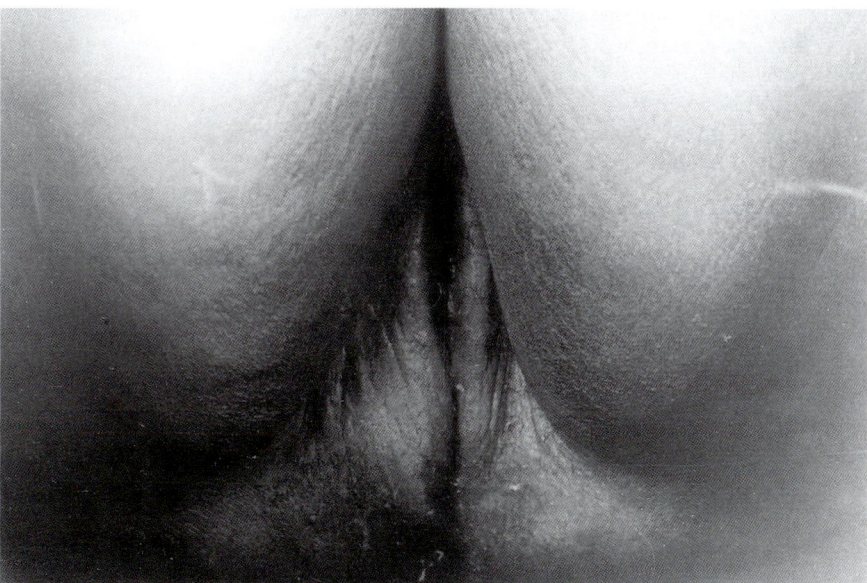

Figure 2. Completely healed vulva 3 weeks (post-surgery).

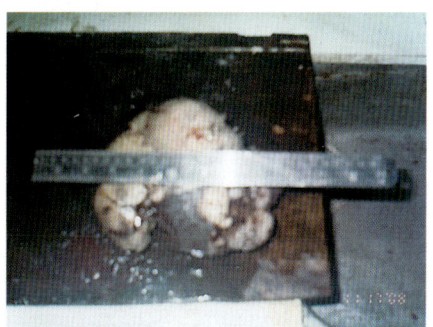

Figure 3a. Excised specimen of the tumor; huge lobulated brownish yellow mass covered at the lower portion by Negroid skin.

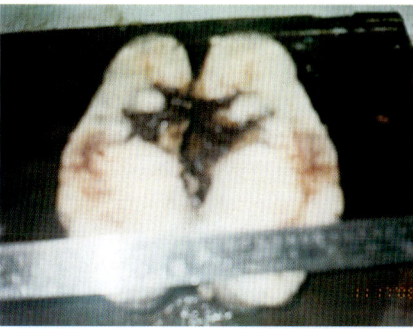

Figure 3b. Excised tumor mass bisected; cut surface is uniformly white with areas of haemorrhage at the periphery and Negroid skin at the midline of the upper portion.

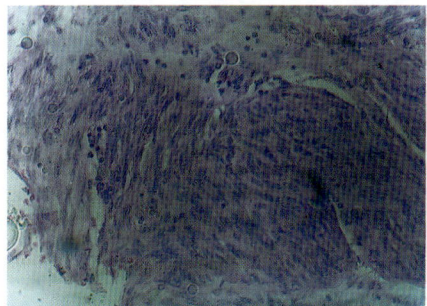

Figure 4a. The tumor is hypercellular with spindle cells arranged fascicles with notable mitotic activity (magnification x 120).

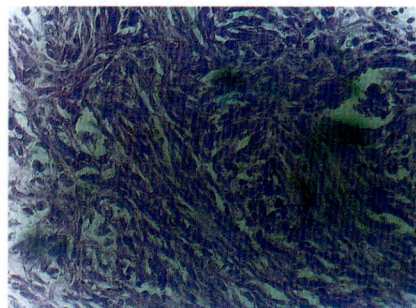

Figure 4b. Another portion of tumor; hypercellular with spindle cells arranged in whorl-pattern with notable mitotic activity (magnification x 200).

DISCUSSION

Contribution of the vulva to the body surface is only 1% to 2%.[4] Nevertheless, it gives rise to a wide variety of tumors originating from its skin and surrounding appendages. In Africa, vulvar malignancies are uncommon, with the majority being carcinomas originating from epithelial tissues.

Leiomyosarcoma is a solid tumor of the vulva that accounts for approximately 40% of vulvar sarcomas.[5] The majority of leiomyosarcomas develop on the labia majora, perineal body, or Bartholin's gland.[5] The origin of the tumor in this reported case was not clearly discernible, as the tumor spanned a wide area encompassing the Bartholin gland, labia majora and minora, and the perineal body. Generally, the growth of vulvar sarcoma tends to begin as a small lump from within the deep sub-epithelial tissue elements.[6] This mode of presentation often leads patients to delay in seeking treatment, as the disease may not be symptomatic at the onset. In this case, the tumor attained a large proportion before the patient presented in hospital.

The major challenge in management of vulvar leiomyosarcoma is the differential diagnosis. The usual criteria for tissue malignancy are not easily comprehensible, resulting in great difficulties with pathological interpretation. In this patient, no additional evidence of local or distant metastasis could be identified, further compounding the problem of histological diagnosis. Such difficulties have often been resolved by electron microscopy.[5-8] However, as a result of lack of this modality of diagnosis in our centre, we have relied on high-resolution light microscopy to confirm the diagnosis.

Surgical removal is the primary method for treatment of vulvar leiomyosarcoma. The advocated surgical methods have ranged from wide local excision,[3] to simple vulvectomy and radical vulvectomy.[1,2] A more radical approach is often adopted when clear evidence of widespread metastasis beyond the lymph node of cloquet is present. The authors decided to manage the patient with conservative surgery, as a result of the lack of evidence of widespread metastasis and low hypercellularity pattern of the tumor histology. In addition, we were wary about indulging in an extensive operative in a chronically ill, malnourished patient who had little resources for follow-up care.

Recurrence of leiomyosarcoma following primary surgical excision has been reported. To reduce this possibility, we provided adjuvant postoperative chemotherapy. In view of the rarity of this tumor, the effectiveness of such treatment is currently unknown. However, any benefit will likely improve the clinical outlook for the patient in resource-poor settings.

In conclusion, a case of leiomyosarcoma has been reported in a Nigerian woman. The major associated problem was late presentation of the patient in hospital. Considering most vulvar tumors have better prognosis when treated early, the need exists to provide health education on genital tract malignancies to women in developing countries.

REFERENCES

1. Patel IS, Kapadia A, Desia A, et al. Leiomyosarcoma of the vulva. Eur J Gynaecol Oncol 1993;14(5):406-7.
2. Krag-Moller LB, Nygaard N, Trolle M. Leiomyosarcoma vulvae. Acta Obstet Gynecol Scand 1990;69 (2):187-9.
3. Kuller JA, Zucker PK, Peng TC. Vulvar leiomyosarcoma in pregnancy. Am J Obstet Gynecol 1990;160(1):164-6.
4. Woodruff JD, Buscema J. Surgical conditions of the vulva. In: Thompson JN, Rock JD eds). Te linde operative gynaecology, 7th edition. Philadelphia: JB Lippincott Company; 1992. p 1065-124.
5. Townsend ED. Malignant melanoma, paget's disease and sarcoma of the vulva. In: Williams CJ, Krikorian JG, Green MR, et al (eds). Textbook of uncommon cancer. Chichester: John Wiley and Sons; 1988. p 211-22.
6. Hall DJ, Grimes MM, Goplend DR. Epithelioid sarcoma of the vulva. Gynecol Oncol 1980;9:237-9.
7. Ulbright TM, Brokaw SA, Stehman FB, et al. Epithelioid sarcoma of the vulva. Cancer 1983;52:1462-8.
8. Gaffney EF, Bhagirath M, Bryan JA. Nodular fascitis (pseudosarcomatous fascitis) of the vulva. Int J Gynecol Pathol 1982;1:307-9.

On the Forefront of New Technologies

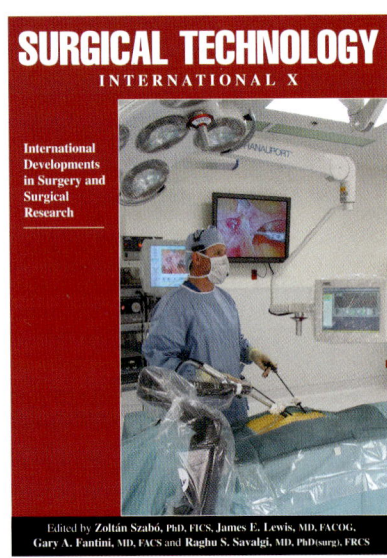

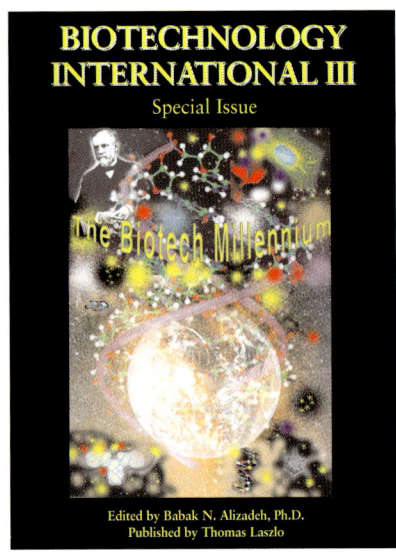

Find what is new in Surgery, Medicine & Biotechnology

Visit our Website at **www.ump.com**

Universal Medical Press, Inc., San Francisco, USA

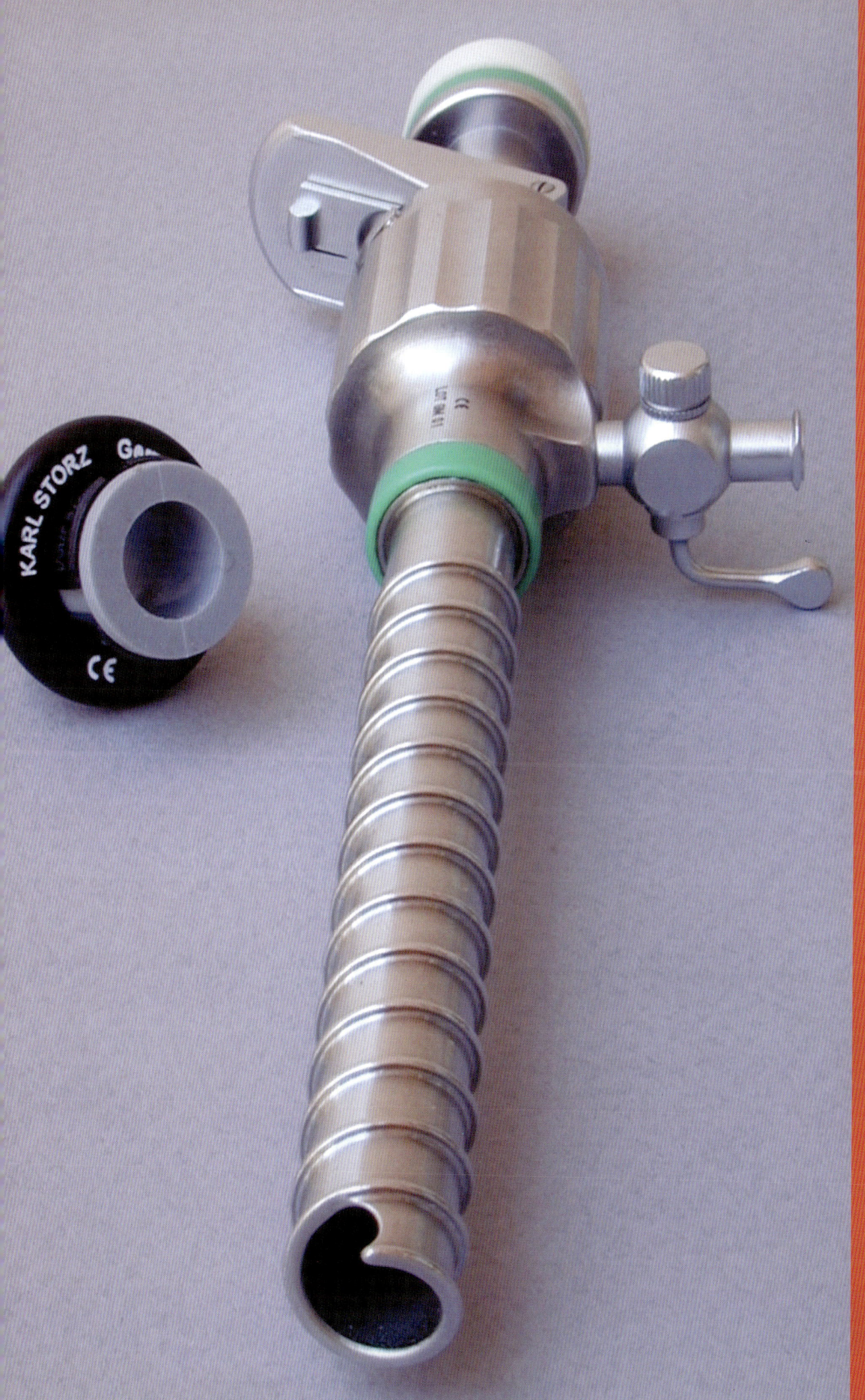

General Surgery

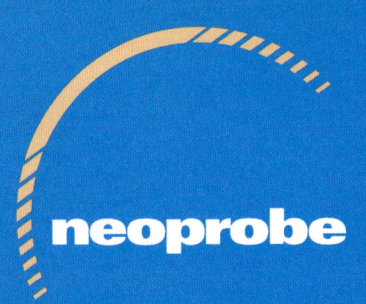

neo2000®
gamma detection system

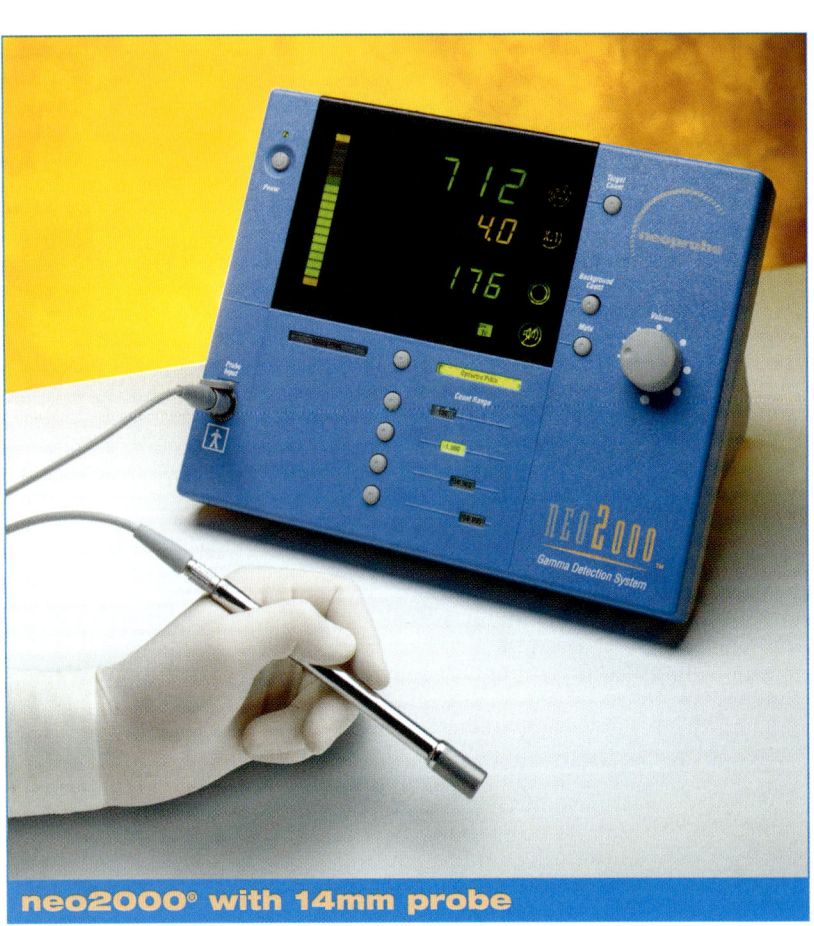

neo2000® with 14mm probe

Simplified Operation

- Fixed 10 second count
- Auto-ranging for audio feedback
- Automated windowing
- No field calibration
- Easy to read, illuminated display
- Continuous & fixed time counts
- AC power
- Lightweight design
- Symphonic quality sound modes
- Field software upgradeable

State-of-the-art system for radio-guided surgical applications

Distributed by:
Ethicon Endo-Surgery, Inc
4545 Creek Rd
Cincinnati, OH 45242
1-800-USE ENDO (873-3636)
www.breastcareinfo.com

Manufacturer:
Neoprobe Corporation
425 Metro Place North, Suite 3
Dublin, OH 43017 USA
1-800-876-4656
614-793-7500 Fax: 614-793-7
www.neoprobe.com

Innovators in Gamma Guided Surgery

Ambulatory Radioguided Parathyroidectomy

FRANCESCO RUBINO, M.D.
FELLOW IN LAPAROSCOPIC SURGERY

WILLIAM B. INABNET, M.D.
ASSISTANT PROFESSOR OF SURGERY
THE MOUNT SINAI MEDICAL CENTER
NEW YORK, NY

Primary hyperparathyroidism (HPT) is a common disease that occurs in one of 500 women and one of 2000 men over the age of 40.[1] In 85% to 90% of patients, primary HPT is caused by a solitary parathyroid adenoma. Recent advances in evaluation and surgical management of HPT, including improved localization techniques and intraoperative parathyroid hormone (PTH) monitoring, have permitted a more targeted approach to parathyroid surgery.

The use of sestamibi scanning and high-resolution ultrasonography, which have a sensitivity ranging from 85% to 90% and 70% to 80%, respectively, have greatly improved the ability to localize solitary parathyroid adenomas.[2,3] Accordingly, patients who have had successful localization of a solitary adenoma are candidates for minimally invasive parathyroidectomy.

The quick PTH assay, popularized by Irvin and Deriso in the early 1990s, also has an integral role in minimally invasive parathyroidectomy.[4] Using this assay, PTH levels can be measured during surgery, which provides the surgeon with immediate feedback on the adequacy of parathyroidectomy. A decrease in the PTH of more than 50% of the baseline value accurately predicts cure.[5]

Recently, radioguided parathyroidectomy (RGP), a technique that uses intraoperative nuclear mapping in patients with a positive sestamibi scan, has been popularized.[6] This report describes the technique of RGP, placing an emphasis on patient selection and surgical technique.

MATERIAL AND METHODS

Patient Selection

The most important factor in patient selection for RGP is successful localization of a solitary parathyroid adenoma, which can be obtained with a high-quality sestamibi scan—with or without ultrasonography—in the majority of patients with sporadic primary HPT. Selection criteria for RGP include absence of co-existing thyroid disease requiring surgical therapy, and no history of familial HPT or multiple endocrine neoplasia.[3]

Patients with laboratory confirmation of primary HPT and a preoperative sestamibi scan, showing a solitary parathyroid adenoma, represent the most common patient group selected for RGP. Radioguidance can facilitate the identification of glands located in deep or unusual locations, such as in the tracheoesophageal groove. RGP also can also be helpful in patients who have had prior neck surgery, especially in persistent or recurrent HPT.[7,8] In this patient population, the incidence of operative

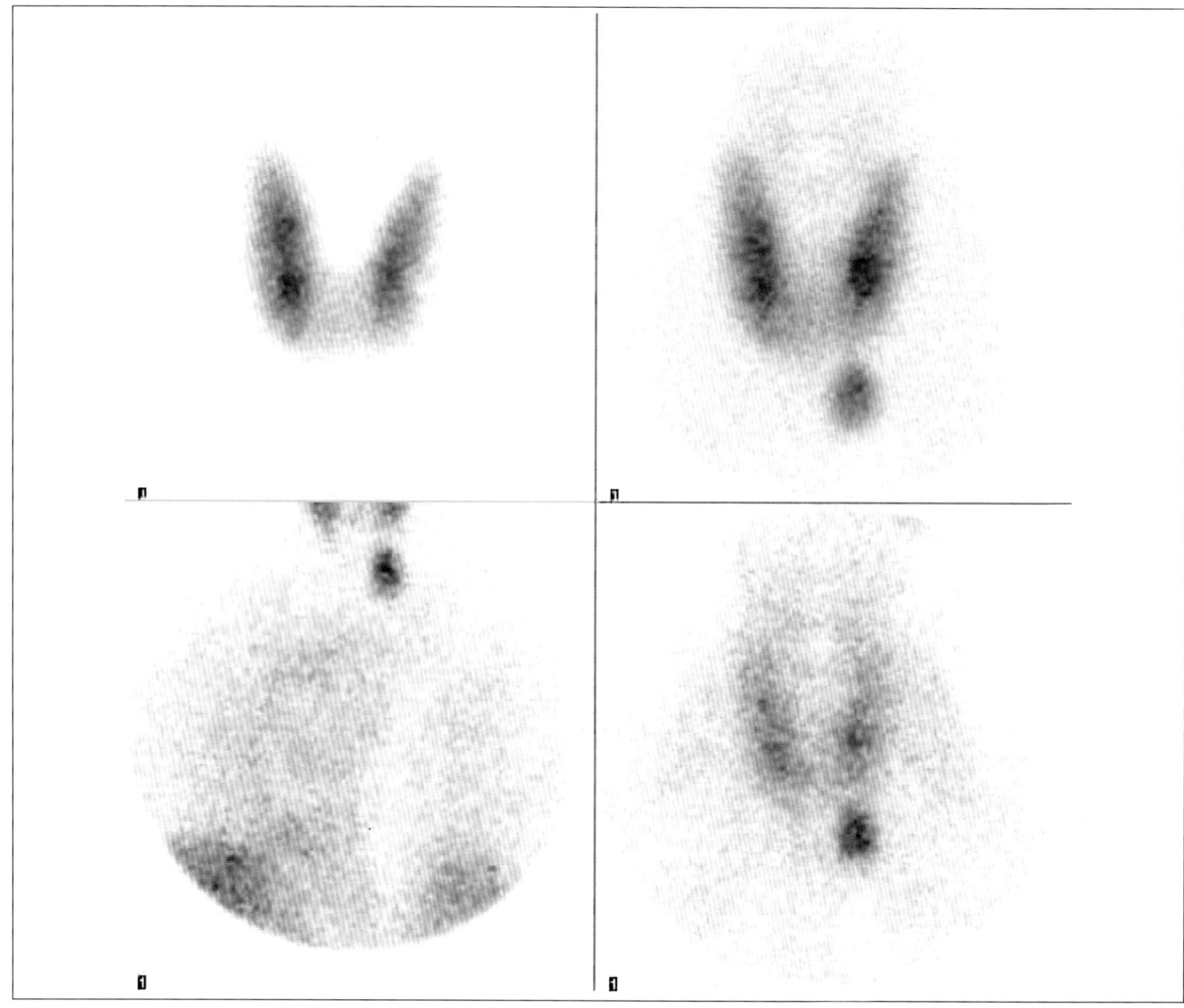

Figure 1. Sestamibi scan demonstrating preferential retention in an enlarged left inferior parathyroid gland.

failure and complications is significantly higher than with first-time parathyroid operations.[8] RGP can provide precise intraoperative guidance, thereby minimizing unnecessary surgical dissection.

RGP is not indicated in patients with unsuccessful preoperative localization or in those with parathyroid hyperplasia. Use of technetium-99m-sestamibi is contraindicated in pregnancy.

Preoperative Localization

Significant improvements in parathyroid imaging have been obtained with technetium-99m-sestamibi scanning.[6] Since the initial report by Coackley and colleagues,[9] several reports have clearly established the superiority of sestamibi scanning among noninvasive parathyroid imaging techniques, especially for solitary adenomas.[10] Sestamibi is absorbed by tissues rich in mitochondria, which have a high blood flow. For this reason, sestamibi is concentrated initially by both thyroid and parathyroid tissue, but is retained preferentially by enlarged parathyroid glands, which contain a greater number of mitochondria. A recent meta-analysis determined that the sensitivity and specificity of sestamibi scanning was 91% and 99%, respectively.[11]

At our institution, the dual-phase technique of technectium-99m-sestamibi scanning is performed as follows. The patient is given an oral dose of I123 to allow early visualization of the thyroid gland, followed by an intravenous dose of 0.3 mCi/kg of 99Tc-labeled sestamibi (18 to 25 mCi). Patients are scanned 15 minutes and 2 hours after injection. Straight antero-posterior images are obtained at both early and delayed time points, one of which includes a mediastinal view (Fig. 1). Single photon emission computerized tomography (SPECT) is performed routinely to provide precise anatomic information regarding the location of abnormal parathyroid glands. Alternatively, left and right lateral oblique views can be obtained to help differentiate abnormal parathyroid glands from adjacent or superimposed structures.[10]

Intraoperative PTH Monitoring

The quick PTH assay (Nichols Diagnostics, San Capistrano, CA) is an important tool in directing unilateral cervical exploration, especially when used in conjunction with preoperative localization.[12,13,14] Several studies have reported a shortened operative time,

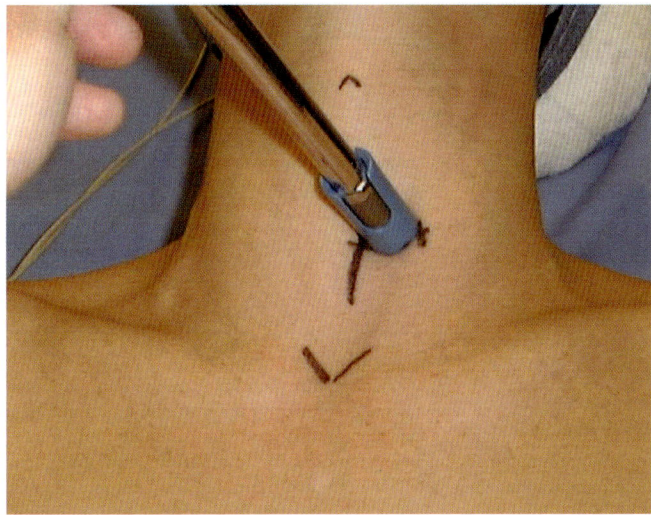
Figure 2. The gamma probe is used to localize the maximal area of radioactivity.

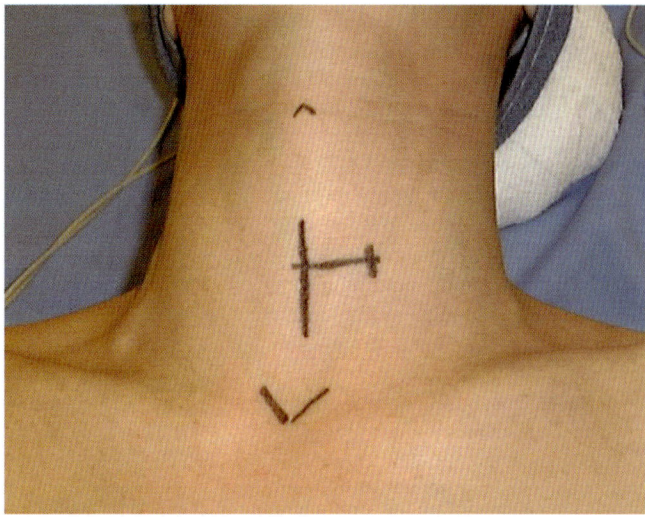
Figure 3. Marking the incision site and administration of local anesthesia.

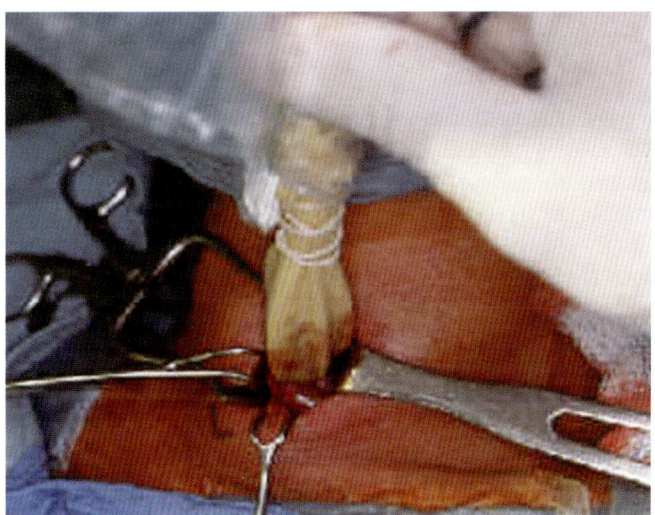
Figure 4. Use of the gamma probe to guide the surgical dissection.

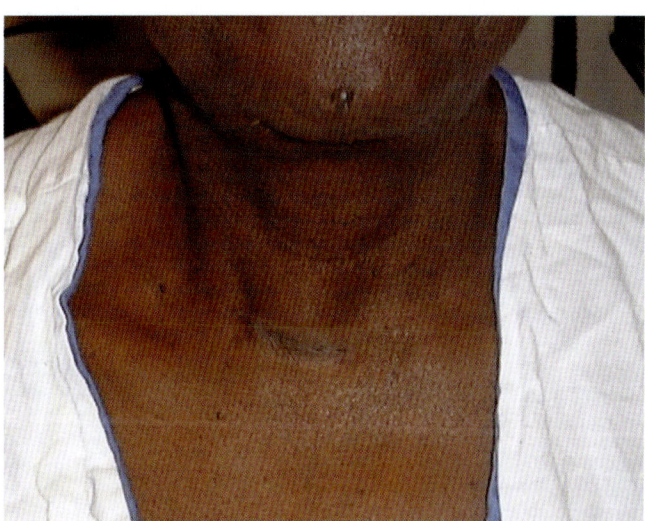
Figure 5. Cosmetic appearance two weeks after parathyroidectomy.

decreased costs, and ability to perform outpatient procedures while maintaining success rates similar to conventional parathyroidectomy. When using the quick PTH assay, peripheral blood samples are collected after administration of anesthesia and at 0, 10, and 20 minutes after parathyroidectomy. A 50% decline 10 minutes following parathyroidectomy correlates accurately with excision of all hyperfunctioning parathyroid tissue.

Technique of RGP Under Local Anesthesia

Approximately 2 hours before surgery, the patient is given 18 mCi of technetium-99m-sestamibi. After positioning the patient on the operating room table, an 11-mm, hand-held gamma counter (Neoprobe Corp., Dublin, OH) is used to measure radioactivity in the neck, including the isthmus (background) and four quadrants of the neck that correspond to the superior and inferior parathyroid glands. A marking pen is used to identify the point of maximal radioactivity (Figs. 2 and 3). The patient is then positioned, prepped, and draped in the usual manner.

At our institution, intraoperative PTH monitoring is used in all parathyroid operations, regardless of the approach. After obtaining a blood sample to determine the baseline PTH level, 1% lidocaine (Xylocaine) is administered in the skin and subcutaneous tissue. A 2- to 3-cm incision is made in the region over the parathyroid adenoma, as determined by both sestamibi scanning and measurements of gamma emissions with the probe. Light intravenous sedation is administered (midazolam or propofol). A small window is made in the strap muscles in the longitudinal plane to gain access to the thyroid bed. The strap muscles are never divided; alternatively, a lateral approach may be used for deeply located adenomas (i.e., retroesophageal).

If additional exposure is needed, the thyroid capsule can be infiltrated with 0.5 mL of local anesthesia and a Babcock clamp used to retract the thyroid lobe medially. Dissection is directed precisely by repeatedly placing the gamma probe in the wound to localize the highest source of radioactivity, which allows a much smaller operative field than would ordinarily be necessary (Fig. 4). After the adenoma has been identified, it is carefully mobilized and the vascular pedicle is isolated and ligated with small clips. When the adenoma is located in a deep position, an attempt is made to identify the recurrent laryngeal nerve.

After the parathyroid adenoma has been excised, the degree of radioactivity of the specimen is measured ex vivo. Any tissue emitting more than 20% of background neck activity can be considered a successful excision of parathyroid adenoma. As shown by Murphy and Norman, lymph nodes, normal parathyroid glands, and fat never contain more than 2% of background radioactivity, whereas thyroid and hyperplastic parathyroids contain 6% and 8%, respectively.[15] Ten minutes after excision of the supposed offending gland, a second blood sample is obtained for PTH; if a decrease of 50% or more from baseline is noted, the operation is terminated with no need to identify the remaining parathyroid glands. Frozen-section analysis is rarely performed. Strap muscles are closed with interrupted absorbable sutures and the skin with a subcuticular absorbable suture (Fig. 5).

Personal Experience

Patients.

From September 1998 to October 1999, 30 patients (27 women and 3 men), with a mean age of 63 ±12 (range: 38 to 89) years, underwent RGP for primary HPT at The Mount Sinai Medical Center. Three patients had undergone previous neck surgery. The mean preoperative serum calcium level was 11 +0.95 mg/dL (range: 9 to 14.3 mg/dL); the mean preoperative PTH level was 180 +167 ng/L (range: 70 to 945 ng/L).

Preoperative Localization.

All patients in the series underwent both cervical ultrasonography and technectium-99m-sestamibi scanning.

Anesthesia.

Local anesthesia was used in 26 patients, whereas two refused local anesthesia and received general anesthesia. Two patients with a history of previous conventional parathyroidectomy underwent superficial cervical block.

RESULTS

Preoperative ultrasound examination successfully disclosed a parathyroid adenoma in 28 patients, but was negative in two. Preoperative sestamibi scanning successfully localized a parathyroid adenoma in 100% of patients. Mean operative time was 46 +14 (range: 22 to 85) minutes. Two patients required conversion to general anesthesia due to technical difficulty (deep location and intrathymic location); however, a targeted approach was completed in both of these patients. The post-excision PTH level decreased by more than 50% in all patients. In 23 (77%) patients, the gamma probe was helpful in directing the surgical dissection; however, it provided confusing information or was not helpful in seven, all of whom underwent a unilateral neck exploration under local anesthesia. Pathologic findings confirmed the presence of a benign parathyroid adenoma in all patients. No complications were noted. Twenty-eight patients were discharged from the hospital the same day of surgery, but the two converted to general anesthesia were admitted for 23 hours of observation.

CONCLUSIONS

RGP is a valuable, minimally invasive technique for treatment of primary sporadic HPT, including first-time operations and reoperations for persistent or recurrent disease. It can be performed safely under local anesthesia as an outpatient procedure. A successful preoperative localization with sestamibi scanning is mandatory. Selection criteria include: absence of concomitant thyroid disease and no history of multiple endocrine neoplasia (MEN) or familial HPT. By minimizing the extent of exploration, RGP allows an excellent cosmetic result while potentially decreasing the risk of complications associated with conventional parathyroidectomy. Despite the availability of radioguidance and intraoperative PTH monitoring, the most important factor in surgical management of HPT is the experience of the operating surgeon.

ACKNOWLEDGMENT

The authors thank Gae O. Decker-Garrad for editorial assistance.

REFERENCES

1. Clark OH. Surgical treatment of primary hyperparathyroidism. Adv Endocrin Metab 1995; 6:1-16.
2. Malhotra A, Silver CE, Deshpande V, et al. Preoperative parathyroid localization with sestamibi. Am J Surg 1996;172:637-40.
3. Inabnet WB, Fulla Y, Richard B, et al. Unilateral neck exploration under local anesthesia: the approach of choice for asymptomatic primary hyperparathyroidism. Surgery 1999;126:1004-10.
4. Irvin GL III, Deriso GT. A new, practical intraoperative parathyroid hormone assay. Am J Surg 1994;219:574-81.
5. Gordon LL, Snyder WH III, Wians F, et al. The validity of quick intraoperative parathyroid hormone assay: an evaluation in seventy-two patients based on gross morphologic criteria. Surgery 1999;126(6):1030-5.
6. Norman J, Chheda H. Minimally invasive parathyroidectomy facilitated by intraoperative nuclear mapping. Surgery 1997;122:998-1004.
7. Norman JG, Jaffray CJ, Chheda H. The false-positive parathyroid sestamibi. A real or perceived problem and a case for radioguided parathyroidectomy. Ann Surg 2000;231(1):31-7.
8. Norman J, Denham D. Minimally invasive radioguided parathyroidectomy in the reoperative neck. Surgery 1998;124:1088-93.
9. Coackley AJ, Kettle AG, Wells CP, et al. Technetium-99m sestamibi: a new agent for parathyroid imaging. Nucl Med Commun 1989;10:791-4.
10. Pattou F, Huglo D, Proye C. Radionuclide scanning in parathyroid diseases. Br J Surg 1998;85:1605-16.
11. Denham DW, Norman J. Cost-effectiveness of preoperative sestamibi scan for primary hyperparathyroidism is dependent solely upon the surgeon's choice of operative procedure. Am J Coll Surg 1998;186:293-305.
12. Brown RC, Aston JP, Weeks I, et al. Circulation intact parathyroid hormone measured by a two-site immunochemiluminometric assay. J Clin Endocrinol Metab 1987;65:407-14.
13. Irvin GL, Prudhomme DL, Deriso GT, et al. A new approach to parathyroidectomy. Ann Surg 1994;219:574-81.
14. Irvin GL III, Sfakianakis G, Yeung L, et al. Ambulatory parathyroidectomy for primary hyperparathyroidism. Arch Surg 1996;131:1074-8.
15. Murphy C, Norman J. The 20% rule: a simple, instantaneous radioactivity measurement defines cure and allows elimination of frozen sections and hormone assays during parathyroidectomy. Surgery 1999;126:1023-9.

Minimally Invasive Repair of Groin and Ventral Hernias Using A Self-Expanding Mesh Patch

ROBERT D. KUGEL, M.D., F.A.C.S.
DIRECTOR, HERNIA TREATMENT CENTER NORTHWEST
OLYMPIA, WASHINGTON

The high risk of hernia recurrence as reported in the literature[1,2] has prompted a significant increase in use of prosthetic materials for repair of groin hernias.[3,4,5] The speed of recovery after surgery, as well as cost and simplicity, has become a much more important consideration than in the past, now that the risk of recurrence has been lowered with modern techniques.[6,7]

Development of a self-expanding mesh, the "Kugel Patch™" (Davol, Inc., Cranston, RI) occurred over a period of about two years. It began as a simple, single piece of mesh material, which ultimately developed into the current patch. The patch was developed to facilitate performance of a sutureless groin hernia repair performed in a completely tension-free fashion. The goal was to achieve the fastest recovery possible within acceptable limits of cost, difficulty, risk, and recurrence. The patch was then used in repair of ventral hernias as well. The result is a uniform system of repair that can be applied in a similar manner to both groin and ventral hernias.

In both groin and ventral hernia repairs, the patch is placed in a totally preperitoneal position. By placing the patch deep to the hernia defect, without rigid suture fixation in groin hernias (or minimal suture fixation with ventral hernias), the repair takes advantage of intra-abdominal pressure and hydrostatic tissue forces to help secure the patch in position.[8,9]

BACKGROUND

For many years, the only way to surgically repair a hernia was to actually close the defect, which involved and depended on use of the patient's own tissue. These techniques have been collectively referred to as the "traditional" repairs. The primary concern with traditional repairs has been the risk of recurrence.[10] Tension on the suture line was recognized as a potential problem and modifications were introduced to reduce tension.[11,12]

The pioneering contributions of surgeons such as Usher, Gannon,[13] Rives,[14] Stoppa, Lichtenstein, and colleagues[15] have resulted in widespread acceptance of the concept of "tension-free" hernia surgery. All the newer repairs for hernia are considered "tension-free" and use a prosthetic piece of mesh to bridge, plug, and/or patch the hernia defect. This procedure has decreased the importance of, and dependence on, the patient's sometimes marginal tissue.

Prevention and treatment of femoral hernias has attracted new attention in recent years as well.[16] Laparoscopic and other preperitoneal approaches have demonstrated that both occult femoral hernias and wide femoral canals are present more frequently than believed previously. Protecting the entire groin, including the femoral canal, at the time of herniorrhaphy is a prudent practice.

Before the advent of laparoscopic hernia surgery, many surgeons advocated the advantage of the preperitoneal approach.[17,18,19] Advocates have claimed advantages for repair of recurrent hernias, sliding hernias, large incarcerated hernias, and femoral hernias and more recently, for ventral hernias.[20] The preperitoneal approach allows for a more complete evaluation of the defects and potential defects. In addition, the preperitoneal approach

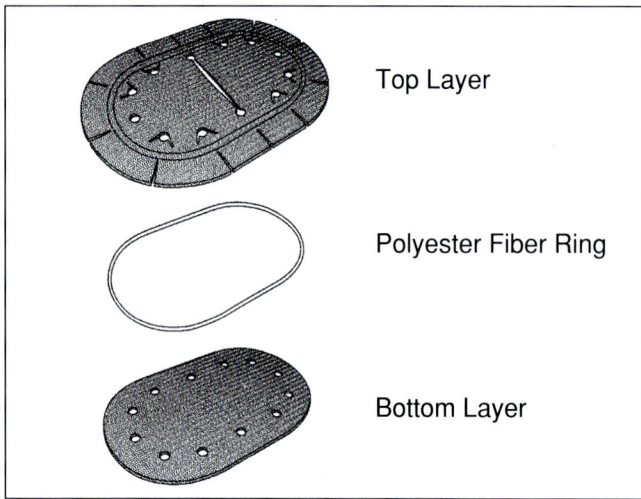

Figure 1. Mesh patch.

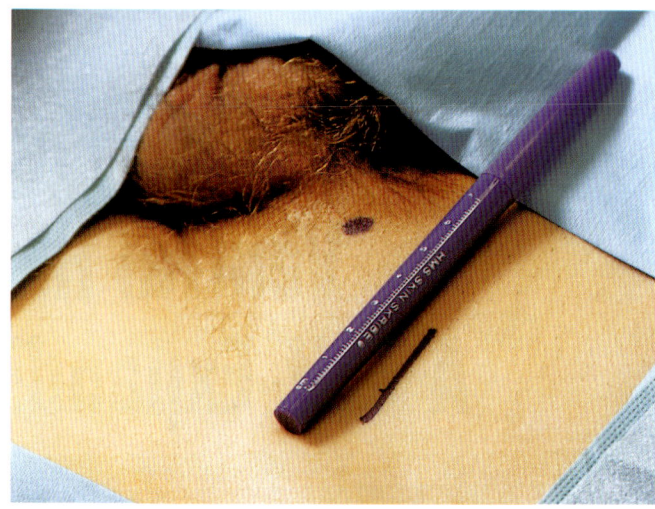

Figure 2. Incision location for a left inguinal hernia with pen marks showing the pubic tubercle, incision, and anterior superior iliac spine.

uses intra-abdominal pressure to its advantage.

The term "minimally invasive" has been applied largely to endoscopic surgery.

The concept conveys the notion that the smaller the incision and the less the dissection, the less trauma inflicted on the patient. The benefit to the patient is a potentially faster recovery. The use of this term should be applied to whatever procedure is less invasive, regardless of whether a laparoscope is used. It should include those procedures that result in the least postoperative pain and risk to the patient.

THE PATCH

The patch is composed of two overlapping layers of a monofilament polypropylene mesh material (Fig.1). The two layers are bonded together by two narrow, concentric ultrasonic "welds" approximately 1 cm in from the outer edge, which leaves an outer "apron" approximately 1 cm wide into which are cut multiple radial slits. This outer "apron" allows greater conformity of the edge of the patch to irregular surfaces (i.e., iliac vessels) and the preperitoneal pocket into which the patch is placed.

Inserted between the two mesh layers and between the two "welds" is a single, monofilament polyester fiber spring. This fiber is stiff enough to contribute some rigidity to the outer portion of the patch and, thus, help maintain the patch in an open configuration. The polyester fiber is contained between the inner and outer welds, but is not rigidly fixed to the mesh.

Just inside the innermost weld are multiple small holes that extend through both layers of the patch. These holes allow for tissue-to-tissue contact through both layers of the patch, increasing friction and resistance to movement. Small v-shaped cuts are made at each of these holes in the upper or anterior layer of the patch only. These cuts create a v-shaped piece of mesh that angles up and serves as an anchoring mechanism that further secures the patch in place.

A single transverse slit in the upper layer of the patch allows access to the pocket between the two layers of the patch. This opening is used to insert and manipulate the patch into position.

PREOPERATIVE PREPARATION

This procedure can be performed using a variety of anesthetic approaches; however, certain advantages and disadvantages exist between the various options.[21] Local anesthesia with sedation can be effective, but it may be more difficult in patients with bilateral hernias, significant obesity, or large ventral hernias. General anesthesia has the advantage of simplicity and may be necessary in patients with a limited ability to cooperate with the surgeon, but it has the disadvantage of not allowing the surgeon to test the repair at the end of the procedure. Spinal anesthesia can be effective, but the usual muscle paralysis with spinal anesthesia also limits the surgeon's ability to "test" the repair and it does not allow for re-dosing. Epidural anesthesia may be the most useful; it can be short or long-acting, and when a catheter is left in place the patient can be re-dosed.

Prophylactic antibiotics are not given routinely except to patients at higher risk (i.e., cardiac valvular disease).[22] They are used somewhat more liberally with ventral hernias, particularly in very large hernias and very obese patients where the potential for fluid collections is greater.

The operative site is prepared with a limited shave just before surgery. A wide antiseptic scrub is performed which includes the lower abdomen and groin, including the scrotum, with groin hernias (this process will allow for testing the repair under sterile conditions), and extends well beyond the extent of any possible ventral hernias.

GROIN HERNIAS

Operative Technique
Incision

The pubic tubercle and anterior superior iliac spine are identified by palpation and marked with a marking pen. A third mark is made at a point halfway between these two points. An oblique skin incision is made about 1/3 lateral and 2/3 medial to this third mark (Fig. 2). In an average-size adult, the procedure can usually be done through a 3- to 4-cm incision. A larger incision may be necessary in obese patients and while learning the approach. The goal is to divide the transversalis fascia and enter the preperitoneal space at a point just superior to the internal ring.

Scarpa's fascia and the subcutaneous

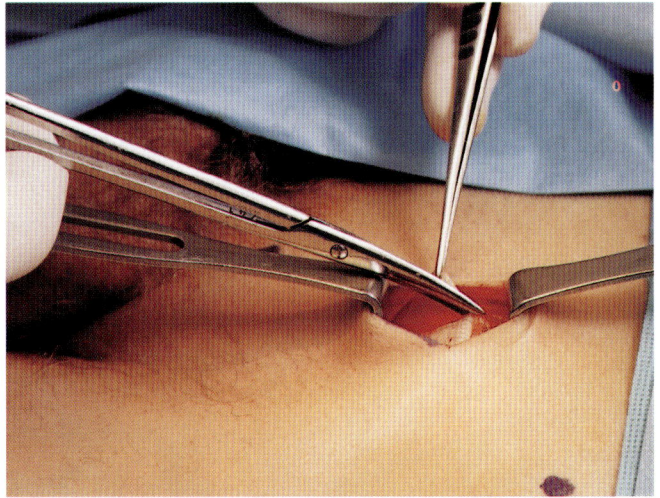 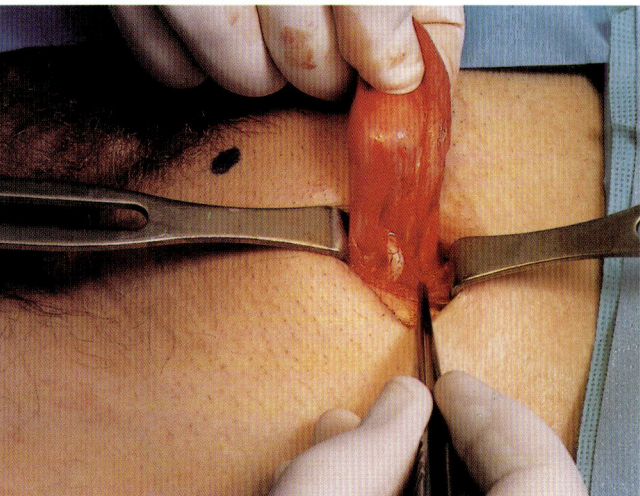

Figure 3. Cutting the external oblique fascia.

Figure 4. Indirect hernia sac with cord structures and vas exposed.

tissues are divided using electrocautery. The fascia of external oblique is opened a short distance parallel with its fibers, but not through the external ring (Fig. 3). The underlying internal oblique muscle is bluntly separated, exposing the underlying transversalis fascia (and occasionally a few fibers of transversus abdominus muscle). This procedure is similar to a "muscle-splitting" approach for an appendectomy, although a little lower. The muscle should be split about 5- to 10-mm lateral to the edge of the rectus sheath. The transversalis fascia is opened vertically (more or less parallel to the inferior epigastric vessels), but not through the internal ring.

Dissection

The preperitoneal space is entered using blunt dissection. Gentle traction is placed on the peritoneum while bluntly separating it from the preperitoneal fat and transversalis fascia. This constitutes an important difference when compared with an "anterior" approach where traction is typically placed on the cord structures. In general, traction maintained continually on the peritoneum while doing the dissection is the easiest way to identify the correct plane and develop the space. A plane of dissection is created between the peritoneum and overlying preperitoneal fat and transversalis fascia; these are retracted anterior along with the inferior epigastric vessels. With difficult dissections, particularly in obese patients, placing the patient in a Trendelenburg position improves exposure.

The cord structures are visible on the lateral and posterior aspect of the peritoneum and should be gently teased away from the peritoneum (while maintaining traction on the peritoneum) for a distance of about 3-cm posterior to the internal ring (Fig. 4). The peritoneum is dissected from the preperitoneal tissues first in a lateral and superior direction, and then continued anterior and medial. Cooper's ligament is then followed over to the symphysis, and the loose connective tissue is cleaned off the ligament using a sweeping action with the index finger. The preperitoneal pocket should be just large enough to accept the patch (Fig. 5).

Indirect Hernias

With indirect hernias, the hernia sac is visualized as traction is placed on the peritoneum (in a superior direction) while dissecting it free from the preperitoneal fat. The sac usually pulls through the internal ring and out of the inguinal canal without difficulty. Occasionally, the hernia sac will not free up easily. A safer method then is to divide the sac at the level of the internal ring and leave a portion of sac in the inguinal canal. To persist in attempts at removing all of a stubborn sac increases the risk of damage to the cord structures and hematoma formation in the scrotum. The resulting peritoneal defect is closed with a running stitch using absorbable suture. Large redundant sacs are excised and removed.

The cord structures must be completely separated from the hernia sac as it is pulled out of the inguinal canal.

Any large "lipoma" of the cord should be excised to prevent it from being mistaken later for a recurrent hernia.

Direct Hernias

Direct hernias are identified by finding a defect medial to the inferior epigastric vessels. With direct hernias, frequently a "pseudo-sac" is formed from the attenuated transversalis fascia, which usually everts as traction is placed on the peritoneum. Preperitoneal fat and peritoneum must be separated completely from this pseudo-sac. Dissection and exposure may be improved by placing a gauze sponge into the partially completed preperitoneal pocket and retracting the peritoneum out of the way with a malleable retractor.

To ensure the pseudo-sac is separated completely from the preperitoneum, Cooper's ligament must be visualized. Cooper's ligament should be clearly seen while doing the medial portion of the dissection even when no direct hernia is present. The loose connective tissue attached to the posterior edge of Cooper's ligament should be stripped off carefully, avoiding injury to aberrant obturator vessels that occur about 25% of the time. This procedure can usually be done bluntly with the index finger, but occasionally some sharp dissection, under direct visualization, may be required.

Femoral Hernias

The hernia patch will not lie correctly in the preperitoneal space unless the femoral canal, medial to the femoral vein, is cleared of any herniated material. This can usually be done with

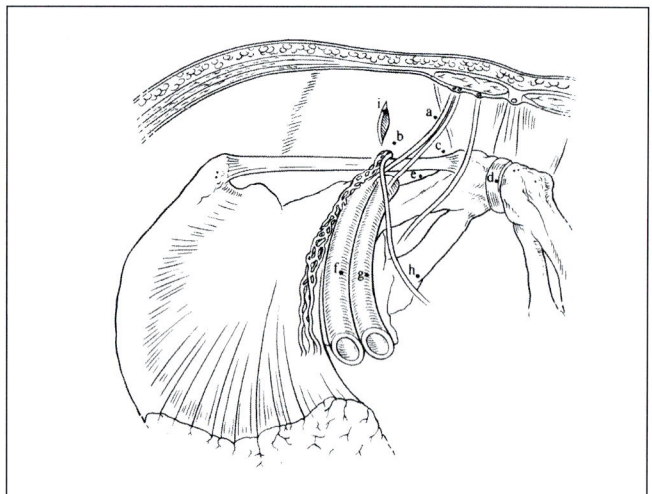

Figure 5. Preperitoneal view of left groin showing: a. inferior epigastric vessels; b. internal ring; c. direct space; d. symphysis pubis; e. femoral canal; f. iliac artery; g. iliac vein; h. vas; i. incision in transversalis fascia into preperitoneal space.

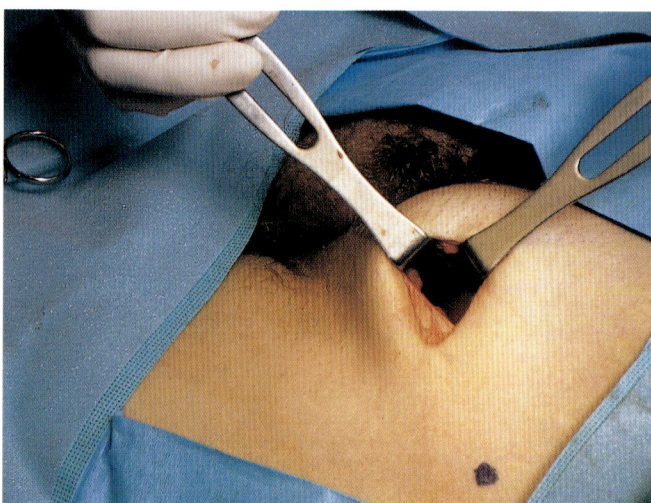

Figure 6. Finished preperitoneal pocket.

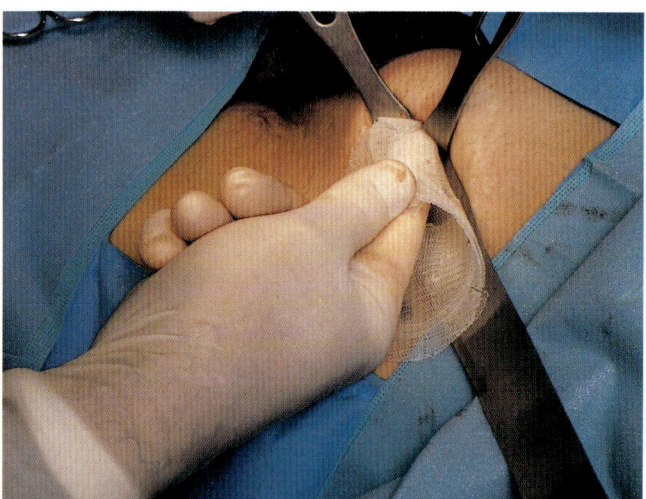

Figure 7. Patch inserted by sliding it over the malleable. Insertion of patch after folding over tip of index finger.

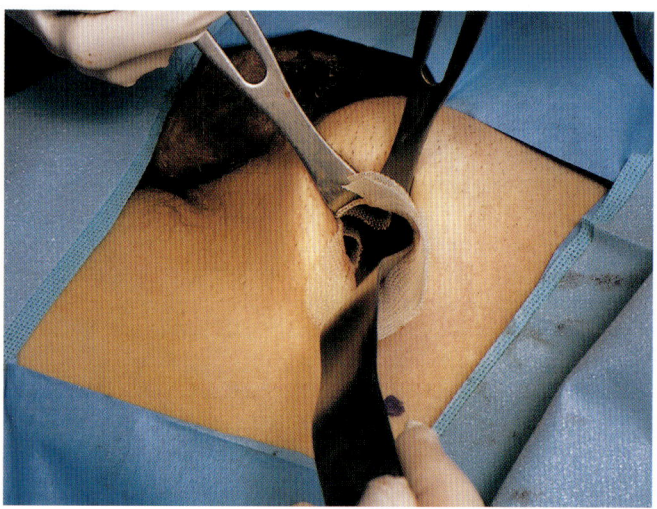

Figure 8. Using the malleable to complete insertion.

careful finger dissection and occasional limited sharp dissection under direct visualization. Care should be taken to avoid any possible injury to the iliac vein. Pressure over the femoral canal, inferior to the inguinal ligament, helps reduce an incarcerated hernia, but in rare cases a counter incision below the inguinal ligament may be necessary.

Patch Placement

The dissected preperitoneal pocket lies between the peritoneum on one side and the internal ring, cord structures, femoral canal, and Hesselbach's triangle, which are inferior and anterior, on the other. The oval-shaped pocket extends from just superior and lateral to the transversalis incision made to enter this space over to the symphysis pubis medially (Figs. 5 & 6).

An 8x12 cm mesh patch is used in most instances although many surgeons believe the 11x14 cm patch provides added insurance in larger hernias.

A dry gauze sponge is placed over the peritoneum and a narrow malleable used to retract the peritoneum out of the way. A single index finger (right-sided hernias use the left finger and left-sided hernias, use the right finger) is passed through the slit in the anterior layer of the patch, palmar surface up. The end of the patch is then folded over the tip of the finger. The patch is inserted into the preperitoneal pocket sliding on top of the malleable and along Cooper's ligament, which can be felt through the anterior layer of the patch, toward the pubic bone (Fig. 7). The finger is removed (as is the gauze sponge) and the narrow malleable inserted into the patch and used to complete insertion of the patch, if necessary (Fig. 8).

The superior edge of the patch is pushed up under the transversalis fascia into the superior portion of the preperitoneal pocket. The patch should lay completely "open" with no kinks in the outer ring. The outer "apron" is allowed to bend or fold as needed. If the patch does not open completely, the pocket is incomplete. This problem can usually be corrected by following the periphery of the patch with a single finger and breaking any fibers restraining it. While developing experience with the dissection, the patch may occasionally have to be removed to enlarge the pocket before the patch can be reinserted.

When placed properly, the medial edge of the patch lies behind (superior

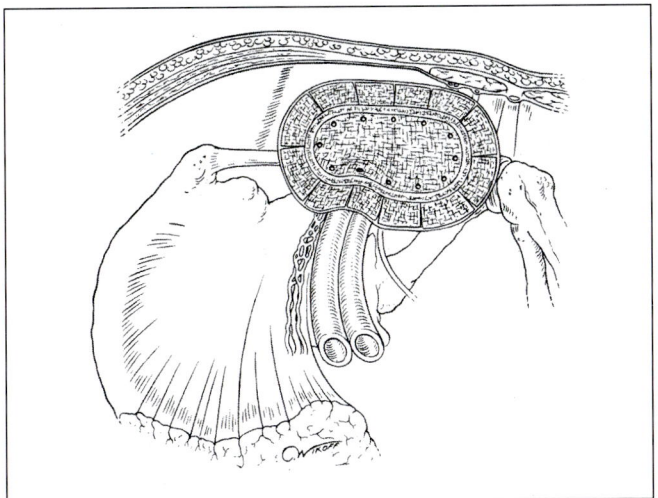

Figure 9. The 8x12 cm mesh patch positioned in the preperitoneal space.

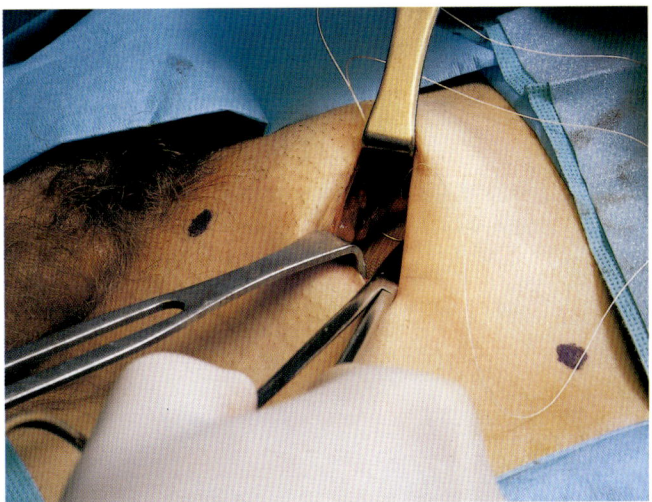

Figure 10. Single restraining stitch closing transversalis fascia and "catching" the anterior layer of the patch in the closure.

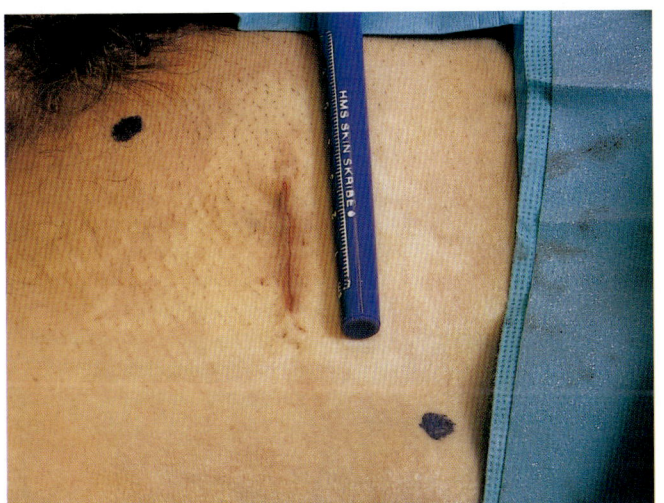

Figure 11. Closed incision.

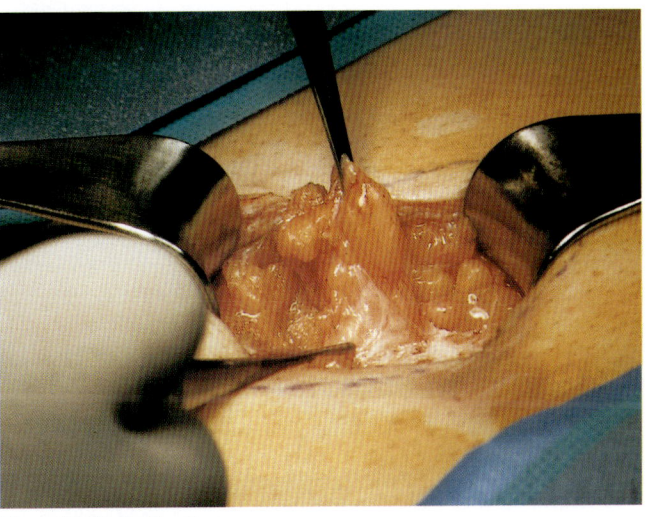

Figure 12. Ventral hernia sac.

the pubic bone and against Cooper's ligament. The posterior edge of the patch folds under the peritoneum onto the iliac vessels. The mesh lies as a barrier between the peritoneum and cord structures (round ligament) and does not encircle them (Fig. 9).

Closure

The transversalis fascia is closed with a single interrupted stitch using an absorbable suture. The anterior layer of the patch, near the medial-superior edge, is caught in this stitch to restrict the patch from moving in an anterior direction (Fig.10); this is not a rigid fixating stitch. With a very large direct hernia, placing an anchoring stitch between Cooper's ligament and the patch instead of between transversalis fascia and the patch, is occasionally of benefit. Stitches placed into the patch in two or more separate locations create two-point fixation and interfere with hydrostatic tissue forces which impair proper patch positioning and fixation and should, therefore, be avoided. A long-acting local anesthetic is then sprayed into the preperitoneal space.

The fascia of external oblique is closed using a simple running stitch with an absorbable material, avoiding injury to any underlying nerves. Local anesthetic is then infiltrated into the subfascial, subcutaneous, and deep dermal tissues. Scarpa's fascia is approximated with a single interrupted absorbable stitch, as is the deep dermis. The skin edges are reapproximated using a running, buried subcuticular stitch with absorbable suture (Fig. 11).

Postoperative Management

Patients are encouraged to cough at the end of the procedure to test the repair. A pressure dressing is applied over the wound site to minimize ecchymosis and hematoma formation. Patients are usually discharged to home within one to two hours depending on the anesthetic. Pain control is achieved after surgery using hydrocodone and acetaminophen or acetaminophen alone. No specific restrictions are placed on activities after surgery. Patients are limited only by their discomfort, but are encouraged to increase their activities gradually. Patients are usually able to resume most of their routine activities within three to seven days, including heavy lifting. The postoperative evaluation is carried out within one to two weeks.

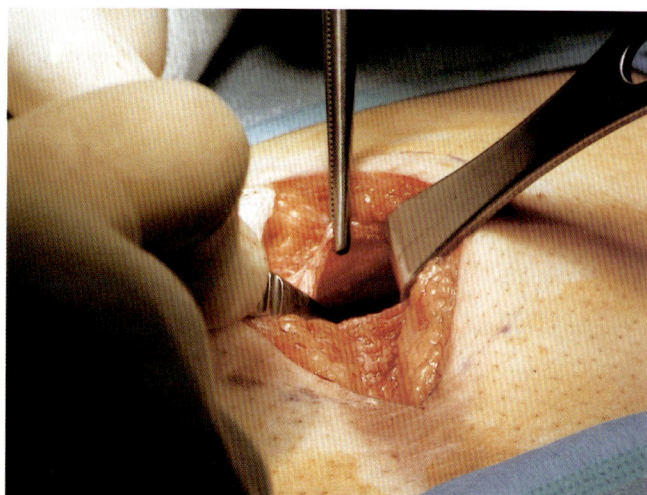

Figure 13. Edge of the defect.

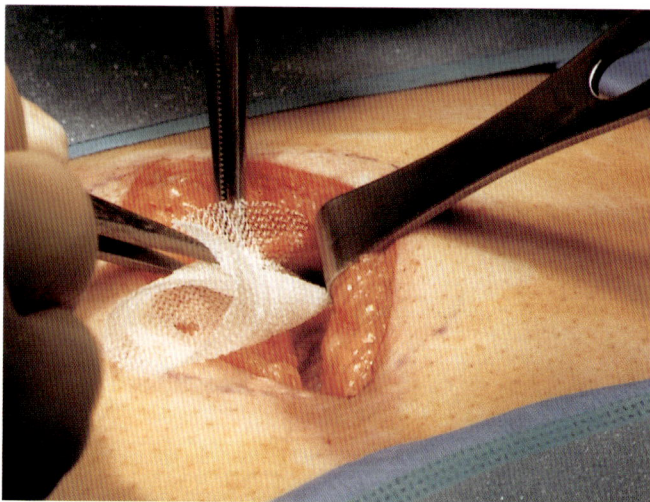

Figure 14. Inserting the patch.

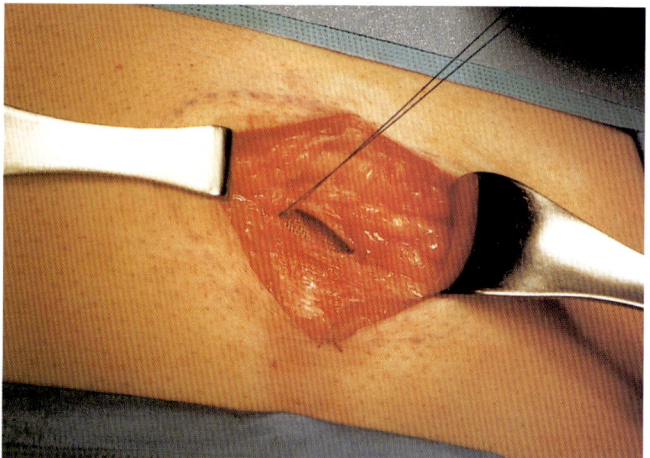

Figure 15. Anchoring the patch.

VENTRAL HERNIAS

Operative Technique

A small incision is made directly over the hernia. The hernia sac is identified and then dissected free from the surrounding subcutaneous tissue down to the fascial edge (Fig. 12). The attenuated fascia at the edge of the defect is scored with either sharp dissection or electrocautery around the circumference of the hernia defect. This maneuver allows entrance into the preperitoneal space. The hernia sac, unless very large, is inverted. Large, redundant sacs can be de-bulked taking care to then close the peritoneal opening.

The edge of the defect is elevated with clamps and the dissection is carried into the preperitoneal space (Fig. 13). When the preperitoneal space cannot be developed easily, as with multiple previous surgeries, a submuscular (retromuscular) dissection can be performed and the patch placed posterior to the rectus or oblique muscles.[23,24] This method allows use of the posterior sheath and transversalis fascia as a barrier between the patch and hollow viscera. In some instances even the posterior sheath does not provide adequate protection and it may be necessary to use omentum as a barrier.

A pocket is created in the preperitoneal space just large enough to accept the mesh patch. The patches are available in several sizes, which should allow satisfactory treatment of the majority of the ventral hernias encountered. The outer edge of the patch should extend at least 2 cm beyond the edge of the hernia defect with small hernias (2 to 4 cm) but must extend progressively farther with larger hernias. Some surgeons suggest a 3:1 ratio between size of the mesh and the size of the defect, but a certain amount of surgical judgment is required.

The mesh is inserted into the preperitoneal or submuscular pocket by loosely folding or rolling the patch (Fig. 14). It is allowed to open to its full dimension and is then anchored to the edge of the fascial defect with interrupted mattress stitches (heavy absorbable or permanent monofilament) placed between the fascia and anterior layer of the patch trying to bury the knots under the fascia (Fig. 15). The outer edge of the patch is rarely anchored except with a few stitches in large defects. Usually no attempt is made to close the fascia over the mesh unless it can be approximated without tension. Closed suction drainage is used liberally in larger ventral hernias and patients are regularly continued on oral antibiotics until the drain is removed, but the effectiveness of this regimen is unproven.[25,26]

Postoperative Management

Even large ventral hernias can usually be managed on an outpatient basis using this technique. Most of these patients are discharged to home within one to four hours after the procedure. Pain control is achieved, in most instances, using hydrocodone and acetaminophen. With more extensive procedures, pain control may require a stronger combination of oxycodone and acetaminophen with oral hydroxyzine, still allowing treatment as an outpatient.

These patients are usually discharged to resume regular activities within one to two weeks. They are seen in followup in one to two weeks; drains are removed in two to seven days.

RESULTS

Between January 1, 1994 and November 30, 1996, all the patches used were hand-made. In November 1996, the small oval patch became available commercially, followed shortly thereafter by introduction of additional sizes. The early experience with both the hand-made and commercially made patches has been reported for groin hernias.[27]

Between November 1996 and December 31, 1999, 489 total groin hernias were repaired in 401 patients using the now commercially available self-expanding mesh (Kugel Patch™). Of these, 170 were for unilateral right-sided hernias and 159 for unilateral left-sided hernias. 80 bilateral hernias were repaired; 39 of these repairs were for recurrent hernias. Only two recurrences have been identified in this group, resulting in a recurrence rate of 0.4%.

Between November 1996 and December 31, 1999, 192 total ventral hernia defects were repaired in 114 patients. These required the use of 119 commercially made patches. Of these, 48 round 8x8 cm patches were used, 25 oval 8x12 cm patches, 5 oval 11x14 cm patches, 20 round 12x12 cm patches and 22 oval 14x18 cm patches were used. Thus far, in this group only one patient has been identified as suffering a recurrence, which translates to a 0.52% recurrence rate.

DISCUSSION

Use of the preperitoneal patch allows the surgeon to approach both ventral and groin hernias using similar methods and principles. The patch and its placement is completely tension-free and uses intra-abdominal pressure and hydrostatic tissue forces to help secure it in position and reduce the need for anchoring sutures. This procedure provides easier placement (particularly in ventral hernias) and decreased pain for the patient.

The repair is less invasive than a laparoscopic groin hernia repair. It protects the entire groin, including the femoral canal, unlike most anterior approaches. If a disadvantage exists to the groin repair, it is the lack of understanding of the anatomy in this area by most surgeons. As a consequence, the repair is easy to perform but for some surgeons, a little more difficult to learn. Ventral hernia repairs are straightforward, and most surgeons do not have to learn a new approach to take advantage of the patch in these repairs.

Early results with this repair have been encouraging. Clearly, success of a hernia operation should be measured by more than just the risk of recurrence. Whereas the recurrence risk must be low, it is important that whatever repair is selected it should allow the patient to recover as rapidly as possible with the least amount of risk and in the most cost-effective manner possible. This approach to hernia repair appears to provide an ideal balance of the many factors now considered important in modern hernia surgery.

ACKNOWLEDGMENT

Figures 5 and 9 are reproduced from the American Journal of Surgery 1999 (Am J Surg, vol 178, October 1999, 298-302). Figures 2-4, 6-8, and 10-15 are reproduced by permission © Steve Vento.

REFERENCES

1. RAND Corp. Conceptualization and measurement of physiologic health of adults. Santa Monica, CA: RAND Corp Publications; 1983:15.
2. Lichtenstein IL, Shulman AG, Amid PK. The cause, prevention, and treatment of recurrent groin hernia. Surg Clin North Am 1993;73:529-44.
3. Shulman AG, Amid PK, Lichtenstein IL. The safety of mesh repair for primary inguinal hernias: results of 3,019 operations from five diverse surgical sources. Am Surg 1992;58:255-7.
4. Beets GL, van Mameren H, Go PMNYH. Long-term foreign-body reaction to preperitoneal polypropylene mesh in the pig. Hernia 1998;2:153-5.
5. Bendavid R. Prosthesis and herniorrhaphies. In: Kurzer M, Kark AE, Wantz GE, eds. Surgical management of abdominal wall hernias. London: Martin Dunitz Ltd., 1999. p 73-85.
6. Memon MA, Fitzgibbons RJ Jr. Assessing risks, costs, and benefits of laparoscopic hernia repair. Annu Rev Med 1998;49:95-109.
7. Rutkow IM, Robbins AW. 1669 mesh plug hernioplasties. Contemp Surg 1993;43:141-7.
8. Stoppa R, Petit J, Abourachid H, et al. [Original procedure of groin hernia repair: interposition without fixation of Dacron tulle prosthesis by subperitoneal median approach]. Chirurgie 1973;99:119-23.
9. Gilbert AI. Sutureless repair of inguinal hernia. Am J Surg 1992;163:331-5.
10. Rulli F, Percudani M, Muzi M, et al. From Bassini to tension-free mesh hernia repair. Review of 1409 consecutive cases. G Chir 1998;19:285-9.
11. McVay CB, Chapp JD. Inguinal and femoral hernioplasty. Ann Surg 1958;148:499.
12. Ponka JL. The relaxing incision in hernia repair. Am J Surg 1968;115:552.
13. Usher FC, Gannon JP. Marlex mesh: A new plastic mesh for replacing tissue defects. Arch Surg 1959;78:131.
14. Rives J. Surgical treatment of the inguinal hernia with Dacron patch: principles, indications, technic and results. Int Surg 1967;47:360.
15. Lichtenstein IL, Shulman AG, Amid PK, et al. The tension-free hernioplasty. Am J Surg. 1989;157:188-93.
16. Crawford DL, Hiatt JR, Phillips EH. Laparoscopy identifies unexpected groin hernias. Am Surg 1998;64:976-8.
17. Cheatle GI. An operation for the radical cure of inguinal and femoral hernia. Br Med J 1920;2:68.
18. Henry AK. Operation for femoral hernia by a midline extraperitoneal approach. Lancet 1936;1:531.
19. Nyhus LM, Condon RE, Harkins HN. Clinical experiences with preperitoneal hernial repair for all types of hernia of the groin. Am J Surg 1960;100:234.
20. Wantz GE. Incisional hernioplasty with Mersilene. Surg Gynecol Obstet 1991;172:129-37.
21. Amado WJ. Anesthesia for hernia surgery. Surg Clin North Am 1993;73:427-38.
22. Gilbert AI, Felton LL. Infection in inguinal hernia repair considering biomaterials and antibiotics. Surg Gynecol Obstet 1993; 177:126-30. [published erratum appears in Surg Gynecol Obstet 1993;177:528]
23. Flament JB, Palot JP, Avisse C, et al. In: Kurzer M, Kark AE, Wantz GE, editors. Massive multirecurrent incisional hernia prosthetic repair. London: Martin Dunitz Ltd., 1999. p 227-40.
24. Duce AM, Muguerza JM, Villeta R, et al. The Rives operation for the repair of incisional hernias. Hernia 1997;1:175-7.
25. Condon RE. In: Nyhus LM, Condon RE, editors. Hernia. Philadelphia: JB Lippincott Company, 1995. p 319-28.
26. White TJ, Santos MC, Thompson JS. Factors affecting wound complications in repair of ventral hernias. Am Surg 1998;64:276-80.
27. Kugel, RD. Minimally invasive, nonlaparoscopic, preperitoneal, and sutureless, inguinal herniorrhaphy. Am J Surg 1999;178:298-302.

LITT Outpatient TREATMENT is now a REALITY.

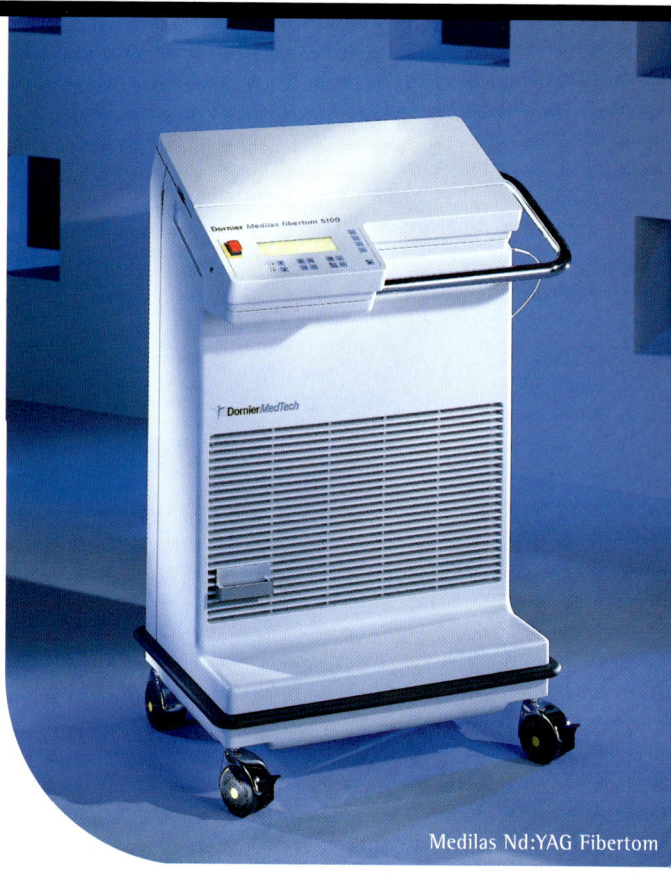

Medilas Nd:YAG Fibertom

Laser Induced Thermal Therapy (LITT) has changed the concept of modern oncological treatment. With the use of the Dornier *MedTech* Nd:YAG Fibertom or the Medilas D 940 nm Diode Laser, liver tumor treatment is now a minimally invasive, outpatient procedure. After an extensive, 5-year, European study, Dornier *MedTech*

Introducing the Dornier *MedTech* Fibertom Nd:YAG and Medilas D Lasers for LITT surgery.

is making this revolutionary procedure available to doctors everywhere. With treatment options like these, you can experience the advantage of using Dornier *MedTech's* leading edge technology.

Call Dornier *MedTech* today for more information on our LITT Laser options.

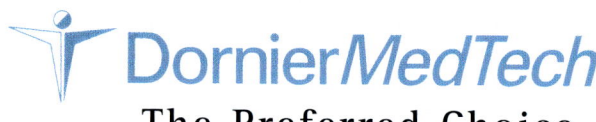

Dornier*MedTech*
The Preferred Choice.

Visit our website at www.dml-lasers.com, or read the conclusions for yourself in the adjacent article.

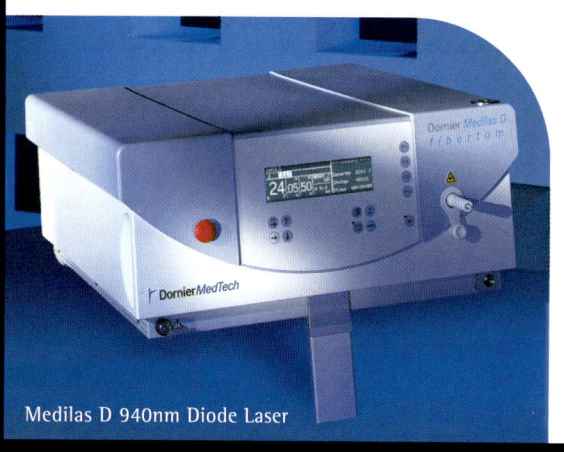

Medilas D 940nm Diode Laser

Magnetic Resonance (MR)-Guided Percutaneous Laser-Induced Interstitial Thermotherapy (LITT®) for Malignant Liver Tumors

THOMAS J. VOGL, M.D.
MARTIN G. MACK, M.D.
RALF STRAUB, M.D.
KATRIN EICHLER, M.D.
ANDRE ROGGAN, M.D.
STEPHAN ZANGOS, M.D.
DIRK WOITASCHEK, M.D.
MARIAN BÖTTGER, M.D.

INSTITUTE FOR DIAGNOSTIC AND INTERVENTIONAL RADIOLOGY
JOHANN WOLFGANG GOETHE-UNIVERSITY CLINIC
FRANKFURT AM MAIN, GERMANY

The liver has a central role in human metabolism and represents one of the organ systems most often affected, especially by tumor diseases. The group of colorectal carcinomas metastatically almost exclusively attacks this organ, which, according to studies by Weiss and colleagues, can be attributed to venous drainage of the intestines through the portal vein.[1,2] A large number of primary tumors often cause liver metastases as well as bone, lung, and brain metastases. After curative sanitation of the primary tumor, the liver infestation has a decisive influence on survival time of affected patients in many instances.

The therapeutic strategy for malignant liver lesions is based on a number of factors such as the underlying primary tumor, localization, stage the tumor has reached, and general factors, such as age or any existing concomitant illnesses. In the instance of hepatocellular carcinoma (HCC), when the tumor is at an appropriate stage, liver resection or hemihepatic resection or liver transplant is the essential curative treatment. If contraindications are present, transarterial chemoembolization combined with a local alcohol injection is used as a palliative therapeutic strategy. Interstitial procedures such as laser-induced thermotherapy (LITT®, Dornier, Germering, Germany) or radio-frequency (RF) ablation show a high rate of controlling the site of the tumor and are currently being clinically evaluated.

Strategies for liver metastases are considerably more complex. To date, liver resection of solitary lesions has been the only potential curative treatment. However, the high rate of intrahepatic relapses and a possible exponential increase of the intrahepatic growth in metastases within the framework of tumor stimulation through released growth-stimulating substances are considered problematic. For this reason, over the last few years there has been great interest in further developments in interstitial procedures such as laser coagulation or RF ablation. LITT®

is a newly developed, minimally invasive, local-regional form of treatment, whose coagulative effects lead to tumor destruction in solid organs. Due to the comparatively high penetrative depth of the photons and possibility of problem-free radiation transmission by fiber-optic waveguides, nearly infra-red (NIR) lasers are used for LITT®. The most commonly used are the ND:YAG-Laser (1064 nm)–already widely distributed clinically–or the semiconductor laser (800 to 950 nm) which has become available in the market recently.

In the instance of RF therapy, the energy generated is conducted through the guide directly into the target volume, in which mono or bipolar application systems are available. Interstitial treatment produces a circumscribed coagulation necrosis, sparing the surrounding structures as much as possible. Percutaneous access, local anesthesia, and out-patient therapy management are the considerable advantages of this minimally invasive procedure, which offers a curative or palliative treatment option to patients already under a great deal of stress.

In the following overview, we present the methods, findings, and treatment strategies for interstitial therapeutic measures for malignant liver tumors, and focus on liver metastases and the primary HCC.

LASER-INDUCED THERMOTHERAPY (LITT®)

LITT® makes available a photothermal tumor destruction technique, which permits solid tumor configurations inside parenchymatous organs to be destroyed. Expansion of the tissue-destroying effect is dependent on the choice of radiation capacity and radiation time. Therefore, the parameters must be pre-selected in such a way that all tumor cells, if possible, are exposed to the coagulative effect, and there must also be a safety margin of at least 10 mm in width. At the same time, it must be taken into account that within the immediate vicinity of a tumor there may be other sensitive structures that must not be damaged. Selecting the right laser is based on the following points: an optimal depth effect in a tissue, determined by the absorption properties of water and hemoglobin, can be achieved with a wave length between 1060 and 1200 nm. ND:YAG and semiconductor lasers of the wavelength, 1060 nm or 940 nm, fulfill these requirements. The ND:YAG laser is the solid-state laser used most often and has a wavelength of 1604 nm. The laser can be both pulsed and operated continuously and supplies output power of up to 100 W. The tissue-dependent penetration depth of the photons is an essential parameter of the absorption in different depths of tissue layers. The range of the resulting increase in temperature is not restricted to the optical penetration depth, but is extended by thermal conduction processes substantially. Normal cells are less sensitive with regard to thermal exposition; malignant cells show a significantly higher sensitivity. The altered metabolic status of malignant cells with pronounced hypoxia causes this high sensitivity.

To do justice to the coagulation of a three-dimensional tumor geometry, it must be possible to heat an approximately spherical volume of tissue at the same time. For this reason, application systems of defined spatial radiation characteristic have been developed, the distal ends of which are prepared in such a way that the result is an even circumference of radiation. With conventional applicators, almost spherical coagulation zones with a diameter of 20 to 25 mm can be achieved. Apart from the applicator geometry, the radiation capacity and radiation time are crucial parameters for the dimensions of the coagulation zone, as are the specific tissue properties such as optical parameters or perfusion rate.

The temperature-dependent effects of the laser light on the tissue are defined as enzyme induction, edema formation, and membrane relaxation in a temperature range of 40°C to 45°C. From 60°C, protein denaturation takes place; from 80°C, collagen denaturation as far as drying; and over 150°C carbonization.

Applicators

Tissue carbonization must be avoided at all costs to achieve large-volume coagulation zones and be able to guarantee a safe application. The critical value is a power density of approximately 5 W/cm². Depending on the applicator, this means laser power of 3 to 10 W. Higher power can produce carbon layers that result in a "hot spot." Photon migration into deep tissue is impeded by absorption in the carbon layer. The only heat diffusion, still active, limits the LITT® zone to a small volume (1 cm diameter). To avoid this carbonization effect, which greatly reduces the volume, a dome-shaped applicator ("scattering dome") was developed. The optimized radiation characteristic of the scattering dome applicator used was to achieve a maximum penetration depth of the photons into the tissue. Additional heat propagation results in deeper tissue layers and, hence, a virtual "expansion" of the applicator, through which the diffusion

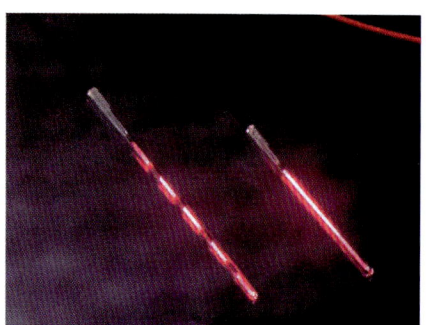

Figure 1a. Structure of the applicator system: the fiber glass light with glass dome stuck on the end as active zone, which causes a diffuse, spherical radiation characteristic of the laser light generated.

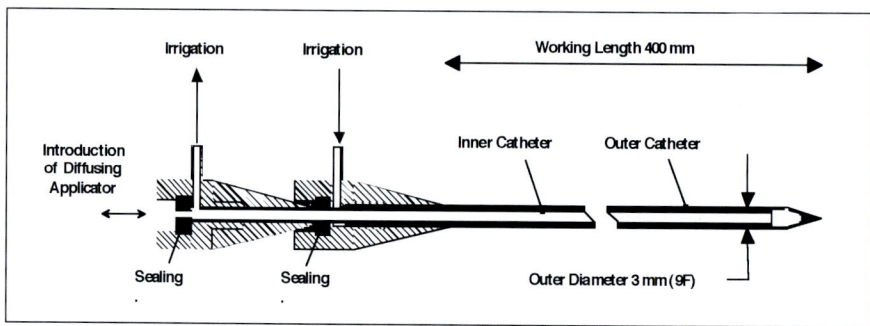

Figure 1b. Structure of the applicator system: the sluicing system with markings and thermostable translucent sheathed catheter with tip. This system enables the applicator to be repositioned along the length of its axis.

processes of the heat propagation become dominant, because of absorption and convection processes occurring there. Technically easier and more effective is to adapt the scatter applicator to the given therapeutic situation (Fig. 1). Radiation times over a period of 30 minutes do not lead to substantial additional expansion of the damaged tissue volume (diffusion equilibrium).

Application Techniques

An essential step in clinical LITT® was the development of application systems that could be applied percutaneously, and could also be used for laparoscopic or operative procedures. First, a conventional system was available that consisted of a scattering dome applicator, sluicing system, and thermostable sheathed catheter, through which the LITT® applicator could be positioned sterile and as required (Fig. 1b).

By further developing the irrigated application system,[3] additional expansion of the laser-induced necrosis was achieved and, hence, an optimization of the treatment. This system has been developed from a 9-French sluicing system with centimeter markings and a 7-French sheathed catheter with irrigated double lumina. A sterile common salt solution at room temperature is a proven irrigation medium. With a pump system integrated into the laser, irrigation rates of 30 to 60 mL per minute can be reached and, thus, a reliable cooling of the applicator zone achieved.

The following application techniques permit further treatment optimization: for the mono-application, an application system is placed in the lesion by percutaneous access and removed after an application of heat.

A method of modifying the size and morphology of the necrosis is a multi-application with unifocal access ("pull-back" technique). The applicator is withdrawn through the single percutaneous access point after the end of the first heat application by 1 to 2 cm in the puncture track, and a further heat application is carried out.

As well as mono-applicators, multi-applicators are also used (multi-applications with multi-focal access). In this study, two or up to four applicators were laid parallel and operated simultaneously. Prerequisites were the corresponding number of laser devices or beam splitters. In this way, treatment of larger malignant lesions could be speeded up substantially; however, the disadvantage was the higher number of punctures required.

Treatment Monitoring

According to findings to date, magnetic resonance tomography (MRT) and MR thermometry (MRTE) are the optimum imaging procedures for treatment monitoring, based on several factors such as multiplanar representation and the high soft-tissue contrast of MRT. In principle, sequences that emphasize these parameters can be used for noninvasive temperature measuring because numerous image-characterizing MRT parameters, such as perfusion or diffusion, are temperature-dependent. These parameters include the diffusion coefficient of the water, photon resonance frequency or chemical shift, and T1 relaxation time. Due to the relatively low sensitivity with regard to movement artifacts, their wide availability and speed of data acquisition, thermosensitive T1-weighted MRTE sequences are applied for clinical implementation of LITT® in the area of the liver. The longitudinal or spin-lattice relaxation time of a tissue is temperature-dependent, in that a local rise in temperature results in a signal drop in the MRT-image. *In vivo* examinations, and the findings of our team and others, showed a virtually linear correlation between the drop in signal in the image and temperature. Appropriately weighted gradient echo sequences (FLASH and Turbo-FLASH), with measuring times between 6 and 15 seconds in the breath-holding technique, have proved suitable to represent the laser-induced temperature changes in the range between 60°C to 110°C.

Before and after LITT®, a test certificate of T1- and T2-weighted spin-echo and gradient-echo sequences is used for treatment planning and control. In addition, contrasting agent-aided (0.1 mmol GD-DTPA per kg of body weight) T1-weighted sequences are used (Fig. 2).

Computer-aided treatment planning, which has been expanded through *in vivo* comparative tests, is available for further treatment optimization. This technique makes it possible to calculate the optimal parameters for radiation capacity and radiation time for each individual fiber before carrying out the laser treatment. Progress of the current temperature and irreversible damage distribution can be represented at the same time as progress of the treatment by means of real-time simulation, so by means of MRT, indirect "monitoring" is available as an extension of virtual on-line monitoring. Implementing and evaluating computer-aided thermoplaning for LITT® applications is costly, however, because the expected irreversible damage zone depends on various parameters in a complex way. Influencing factors are laser capacity, radiation time, applicator characteristics, and optical and thermal tissue parameters such as tissue perfusion and blood flow. Initial applications of this kind of system lead us to expect a further improvement in precision during the treatment.

Criteria Defined for Clinical LITT® in the Instance of Malignant Liver Tumors

Inclusion criteria
- Primary tumor must be resected completely
- Liver metastases smaller or equal to 5 cm in diameter
- Number of lesions less than 5
- Informed consent from the patient in writing after a verbal and written explanation at least 24 hours before the operation
- Significance of the lesion must be verified bioptically and clinically and with a morphologic image

Exclusion criteria
- Existence of extrahepatic metastatic spread
- Absolute contraindications for an MRT examination
- Coagulation parameter more than 50% below normal values

Local Tumor Control Rates

The local tumor control rate after a percutaneous hepatic tumor ablation is defined as verification the tumor has been destroyed completely with no local recurrences in the imaging and clinical follow up. Results of the local tumor control rate for primary and secondary malignant liver tumors were evaluated in different groups. Patients treated during phase 1 and 2 studies were combined in Group 1 (patients 1 to 100; period 06/93 to 10/96). In this study, LITT® was carried out using conventional applicators in mono or dual application. The patients in Group 2 (phase III study, patients 101 to 176;

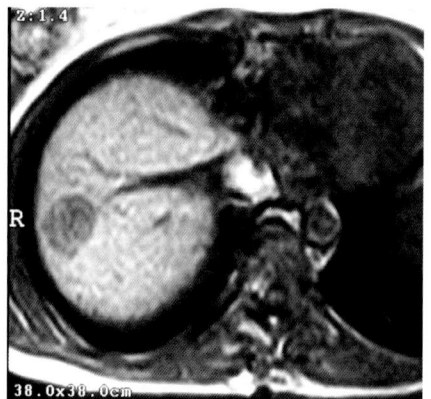

Figure 2a. 35-year old woman with liver metastasis from a colorectal carcinoma (initial tumor stage pT3, N1, M1). The T1-weighted thermosensitive gradient echo sequence in axial tomographic orientation shows the metastasis in liver segment 8 before starting the laser.

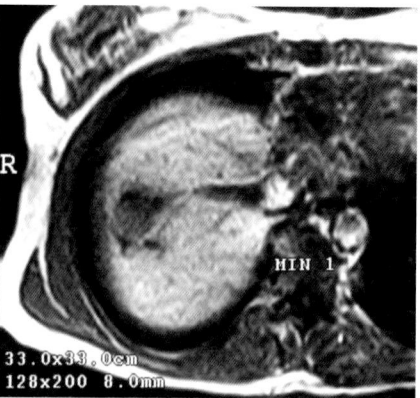

Figure 2b. T1-weighted thermosensitive gradient echo sequence in axial tomographic orientation in the 1st minute. Clear drop in signal intensity in the heated area.

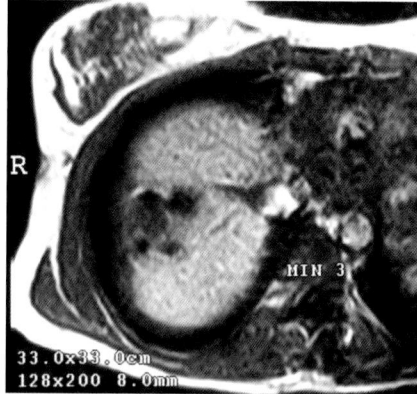

Figure 2c. T1-weighted thermosensitive gradient echo sequence in axial tomographic orientation in the 3rd minute. Clear drop in signal intensity in the heated area.

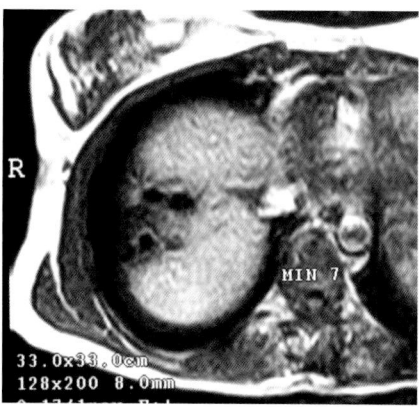

Figure 2d. T1-weighted thermosensitive gradient echo sequence in axial tomographic orientation in the 7th minute. Clear drop in signal intensity in the heated area.

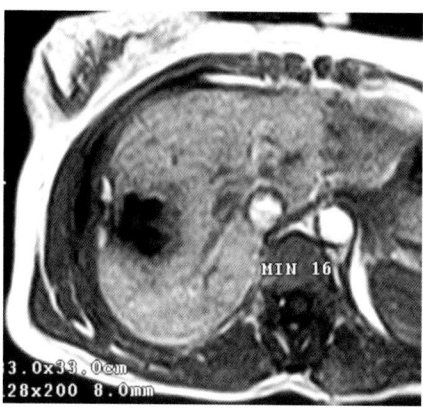

Figure 2e. T1-weighted thermosensitive gradient echo sequence in axial tomographic orientation in the 16th minute. Clear drop in signal intensity in the heated area.

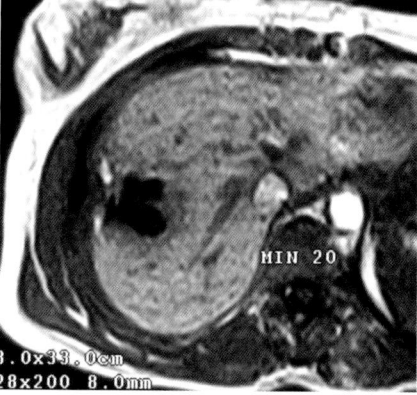

Figure 2f. T1-weighted thermosensitive gradient echo sequence in axial tomographic orientation in the 20th minute. Clear drop in signal intensity in the heated area.

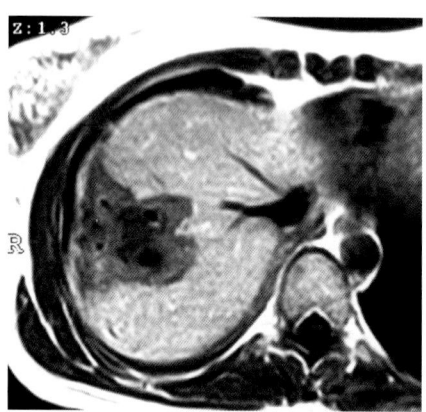

Figure 2g. T1-weighted spin echo sequence in axial tomographic orientation after the administration of gadolinium-DTPA (0.1 mL/kg body weight). Sharp demarcation of the LITT®-induced necrosis with a safety margin surrounding the lesion.

period 10/96 to 08/97) were treated using the multi-applicator technique. All patients from 08/97, treated outside studies within the framework of a clinical application observation, were combined as Group 3 (patients 177 to 729), and treated by means of irrigated power application using the multi-applicator or pullback technique. To manage large-volume laser-induced necroses, it can additionally be used cumulatively during the LITT®.

The tumor control rate in the 3-month check-up was 65% for the Phase I patients and 80% for those in Group 2. The values for the tumor control rate in the 6-month check-up was somewhat lower, with values of 29% for Group I and 67% for Group II. In the 3-month check-up, evaluation of all patients in Group 3 from 08/97 regarding local tumor control by means of unmodified and contrast-enhanced MRT showed local tumor control of 99% and in the 6-month check-up, 97%. This high rate of local tumor control in Group 3 was the result of the optimized application technique, both the findings with regard to optimum choice of the laser parameters and puncture paths, and consistent coagulation of a circular, 10-mm safety margin around the metastasis.

Evaluation showed the unenhanced and contrast-enhanced T1-weighted gradient echo sequences, carried out in the breath-holding technique, were the diagnostically important sequences. After the laser treatment, the successfully treated metastases in the unenhanced T1-weighted sequence typically appeared with a discretely increased signal intensity due to a low-grade hemorrhagic imbibition. After contrasting agent application, the induced coagulation necrosis could be portrayed hypointensive in comparison with the surrounding hepatic tissue. In addition, in the T2-weighted image, the coagulation necrosis showed a moderate increase regularly in signal intensity in the border area in the sense of a concomitant edema. Both the initial complete destruction of the tumor and coagulation of an appropriate safety margin of 10 mm around the metastasis are crucial for the success of LITT® treatment. If anatomically possible, this safety margin should be at least 10 mm. The exact control and monitoring of the LITT® necessary can only be carried out during the on-going LITT® treatment by means of MRTE; here, sonography or CT are inferior to the MRT regarding precision. The predominant aim of monitoring during LITT® must be to ensure the tumor is coagulated fully.

SURVIVAL DATA

The cumulative survival rate of patients treated with LITT® was calculated using the Kaplan-Meier method. The cumulative survival rate, both for the period from the first LITT® treatment and that of initial diagnosis of the lasered metastasis, was calculated.

Total Patient Population: 729 Patients with 2041 Lesions, 1707 LITT® Sessions with 7470 Laser Applications

The mean cumulative survival time (Fig. 3a) calculated from the time of initial diagnosis of the metastasis/metastases treated with LITT® was 48.0 (95% confidence interval: 44.4 to 52.8) months. The period between the initial diagnosis of the metastasis and first laser treatment was, on average, 3.1 months.

Colorectal Carcinoma

The mean cumulative survival rate of patients with liver metastases from a colorectal carcinoma (n=407 patients, 1243 metastases, 4818 laser applications) was 41.8 (95% confidence interval: 37.3 to 46.4) months. The period between initial diagnosis of the metastasis and the first laser treatment was, on average, 2.9 months.

Carcinoma of the Breast

Incorporating the 129 patients treated with LITT® for liver metastases (n=336) from a carcinoma of the breast, the results of the data were as follows: the cumulative survival rate was 51.6 (95% confidence interval: 43.2 to 60) months. The period between initial diagnosis of the metastasis and the first laser treatment was, on average, 4.6 months.

Hepatocellular Carcinomas (HCC)

Our series comprises of 33 patients, of whom 52 sources were treated with 231 laser applications. Mean survival

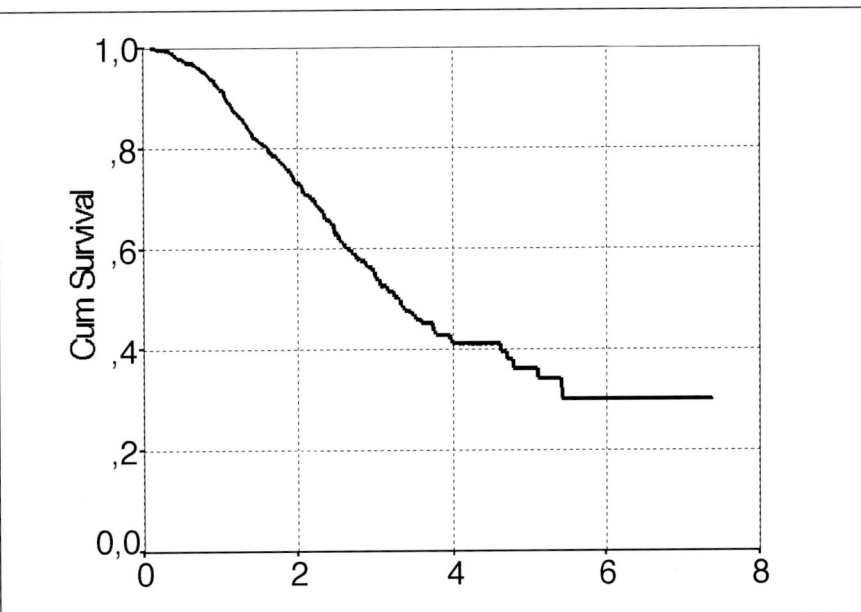

Figure 3a. Mean survival time in the total population of patients with liver metastases is 48.0 (95% confidence interval: 44.4 to 52.8) months.

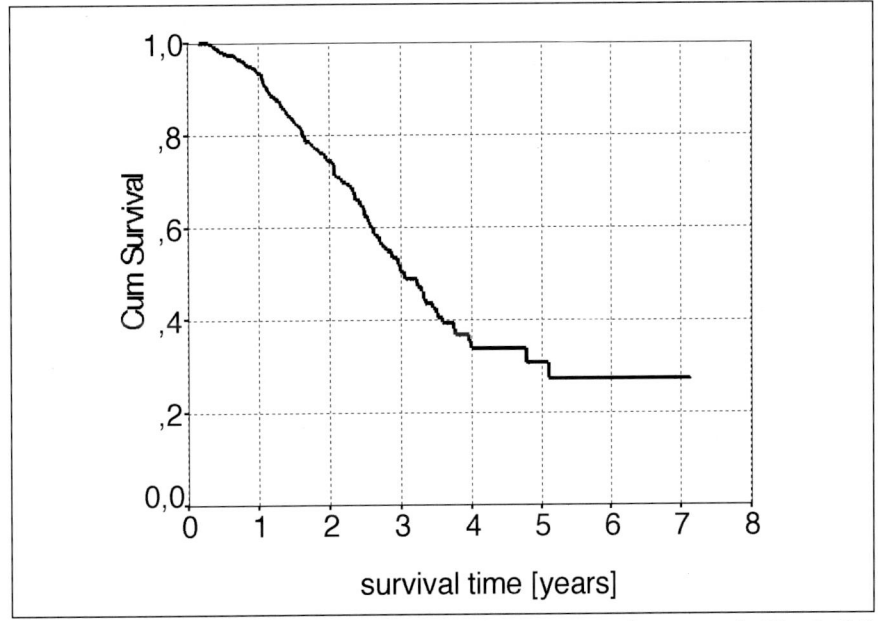

Figure 3b. For patients with liver metastases from a colorectal carcinoma the mean survival time is 41.8 (95% confidence interval 37.3 to 46.4) months.

times of 46.8 (95% confidence interval: 37.2 to 57.6) months were documented.

No statistically significant difference could be proved regarding survival rates in a comparative analysis between the various primary tumors (Log Rank, Breslow, Tarone-Ware-Test).

Complication Rate

Despite receiving out-patient treatment in between, as a rule the patients tolerated the LITT® well with a local anesthetic and systemically applied low doses of analgesics. Within the framework of clinical tests and imaging treatment check-ups, the following side effects and complication rates–referring to the number of LITT® sessions–were documented: pleural effusion (7.28%), subcapsular hematoma (2.46%), intrahepatic abscess formation (0.42%), or a local infection at the puncture site (0.31%). With the exception of the complications listed below, all side effects and complications were not clinically relevant and could only be detected as images on the check-up radiographs after 24 hours: in 0.94% of patients, pleural effusion was tapped;

four abscesses were cured by percutaneous drainage; and three infections at the puncture site were treated with local, conservative measures.

One patient with a central relapse metastasis after an extended hemi-hepatectomy was carried out, already had an infiltration of the bile ducts documented by image. An intensive explanation was then given to the patient regarding a possible treatment strategy, which consisted of removing the metastasis thermoablatively as far as the biliary passage and then treating the biliary passage with a stent by way of the percutaneous transhepatic cholangio-drainage (PTCD) access. It was possible to remove the metastasis completely using this technique.

Radio-Frequency (RF) Treatment

RF waves have been used since the 1960s for treating intracerebral tumors, controlled stereotaxically. For some years, RF treatment has also been used for treating soft tissue, focusing on the treatment of malignant liver tumors. As with LITT®, a coagulation necrosis is caused through a local temperature increase. Frequencies between 300 to 500 kHz are introduced into the tissue through mono or bipolar antennae systems, resulting in the target area heating up to temperatures of 90°C, caused by high tissue resistance.

Application Systems

In previous studies, monopolar systems were used almost exclusively. The necessity for an external second electrode on patients makes an uncontrolled energy flow outside the required target zone possible in theory, meaning burns cannot be safely ruled out. Bipolar application systems integrate both poles in one applicator. Initial clinical studies and our own attempts demonstrate the safe operation of bipolar application systems, which also can be applied irrigated with appropriately constructed sheathed catheters. Continuous insulation is stretched over the entire length of the needle, leaving only the active tip area free, approximately 2 to 3 cm, depending on the system. The RF generators are relatively small and supply information on the applied output, tissue resistance, and temperature at the tip of the applicator during treatment.

Modes of Application

Using conventional RF systems, the necroses attained have a cylindrical configuration approximately 2 cm in length and 1.6 cm in diameter. The multi-applicator also was used in these patients for increasing the necrosis using several applicators approximately 1.5 cm apart. Increases in the necrosis zone of 3 cm in diameter were noted. Cooling the tip of the applicator in RF treatment was introduced parallel to LITT®, which achieved an increase of the induced necrosis of 4 to 5 cm in diameter.

Most RF teams insert and position the RF applicators using sonography, sometimes using computer tomography (CT). Then immediately after the procedure, and in the follow ups, polyphase spiral CT and contrasting agent-guided MRT are used.

The outstanding findings using MRT as a monitoring procedure in LITT® cannot be implemented straight away in RF, because despite the different frequencies (2.5 GHz vs. 8 to 63 MHz) there has been interference and image artifacts, which indicate sufficient image evaluation is not possible. Systems for shutting down the RF application quickly during the MRT data acquisition are being tested, and whether resulting breaks in the application hinder the achievement of an optimum coagulation zone is being evaluated currently. Our findings currently indicate it has no effect on the size of necrosis.

Sonography is used as another monitoring procedure. An increase in a hyperechogenuity zone around the tip of the applicator is imposed by a morphologic image during the heating process. The operation is carried out currently both under local anesthetic, and in some centers using intubation anesthesia. In this study, neuroleptic analgesia administered with droperidol and fentanyl always required the additional presence of anesthesia personnel.

RESULTS

In 1996, Rossi and colleagues treated 11 patients with 13 metastases using mono and bipolar systems and the multi-applicator technique. Although the tumors were less than 3.5 cm in size, one year after the operation only one patient was tumor-free and a relapse rate was approximately 55%. Findings for the 39 patients with HCC were better; a relapse rate of only 10% and mean survival times of 44 months were calculated.[4]

In 1997, Solbiati and colleagues published a study of 29 patients with 44 liver metastases (size: 1.3 to 5 cm) of colorectal, stomach, breast, and pancreatic carcinomas. Among them were 20 patients with solitary lesions. The operation took place using cooled systems, and a complete tumor ablation was achieved in 91% of the patients. At the 3- and 6-month check-ups, 66% of the treated lesions remained inactive. Survival rates of 100%, 94%, and 86% after 6, 12, and 18 months, respectively, were documented.[5] Further work by Solbiati and co-workers showed over 31 metastases in 16 patients, with a tumor control rate of 66% after RF therapy. All inactive tumors were less than 3 cm. One-year and two-year survival rates of 100% and 62%, respectively, were reported.[6]

Livraghi and colleagues attempted an approach using conventional systems and simultaneous irrigation with NaCl solution in 14 patients with 24 liver metastases (1.2 to 4.5 cm in size), but only 52% of the lesions were inactive after six months.[7]

In 1999, Livraghi and colleagues presented a direct comparison of RF therapy (42 patients, 52 lesions) with percutaneous alcohol injection (PAI) (44 patients with 60 tumors) in treating HCC-the first direct comparison of these two different treatments in similarly structured patient populations. Eighty percent of tumors were removed completely using PAI and 90% using RF (no statistical significance). The main advantage of RF therapy proved to be the smaller number of treatment sessions (1.2 vs. 4.8); however, a higher complication rate (2% serious, 8% less serious complications vs. 0% for PAI) was documented.[8] Side effects with regard to punctures were relevant in this study; e.g., pneumothorax or hemothorax (2%), injury of the bile ducts and gallbladder, intraperitoneal bleeding (8%), and pleural effusions. Depending on the procedure, some cases had to be upgraded from local to general anesthesia due to severe pain during the energy application.

DISCUSSION

The most frequent primary tumor with virtually exclusively hepatic metastatic spread is by far the colorectal carcinoma. In 1995, approximately 140,000 new cases of this type of tumor occurred in the USA, with approximately 56,000 patients dying of this disease. In Germany, the proportion in total cancer mortality rate among men is 12% and among women, 14%. Current estimated figures for the annual incidence in the whole of Germany are 14,000 among men and 19,000 among women for carcinoma of the colon, and for carcinoma of the rectum, 8800 and 8700. These figures place colorectal carcinoma among the male population in second place behind bronchial carcinoma, and among women in third place as the most common cancer after breast and lung cancer. The risk of developing an intestinal cancer clearly increases after the age of 40 for both sexes.[9]

In 1986, a study was published with autopsy data on 1541 patients who died from a colorectal carcinoma or its metastases. These findings supported the "cascade model" favored by Weiss and other authors; i.e., metastatic spread of gastrointestinal tumors, where tumor cells are carried with the venous bloodstream step-by-step into the next organs and from there further through the body.[10,11] Furthermore, a dependency on its blood flow is assumed (mL/min/g tissue). According to the above assumption, the liver and then the lungs are the next focal points for metastatic spread, through the venous drainage of the portal vein of the gastrointestinal system. Results showed that the cascade model applied to 85% of the patients studied. In the instance of 73% of the patients with hepatogenic metastatic spread, secondary metastases were not noted in any other organs,[1] which appear to indicate that for many of those affected the intensity of the hepatic infestation is the first determining factor for survival time.

Stangl and colleagues observed 1099 patients in this context, those who received no treatment (n=484), those administered systemic (n=70) or regional chemotherapy (n=123), or those surgically resected (n=340). If they were not treated, the patients survived on average 7.5 months; the 1-, 2-, 3-, and 5-year survival rates were 31%, 7.9%, 2.6%, and 0.9%, respectively. For the patients who received chemotherapy, the median survival time was 12.7 and 11.1 months; however, no patients survived longer than four years (Table 1).[12]

Smaller studies by Bengmark, Palmer, and their colleagues also documented median survival rates of 7.5 months and 12 months for untreated liver metastases, regardless of patient age and position of the primary tumour.[13,14] Therefore, one could predict the survival time for patients with untreated liver metastases from a colorectal carcinoma would be between 4 and 12 months from the time of diagnosis. A wide variation is suggested that, according to bibliographic references, mostly depends on how much of the hepatic tissue is affected.[15,16]

The current "gold standard" of liver metastases is surgical resection. Current studies with large patient numbers were undertaken by Scheele, Nordinger, and their colleagues. Of a population of 1766 patients recorded from 1960 to 1993 due to hepatic metastatic spread of a colorectal carcinoma, 473 were eventually able to undergo a liver resection with the intention of a cure; i.e., less than 30%! In this group, taking into account the operation mortality rate (4%, region of 12% to 4%) survival rates of 46%, 33%, 22%, and 18% for 3, 5, 10, and 20 years, respectively, were achieved cumulatively.[17,18]

According to the judgment of many authors, because up to 60%s to 70% of the patients had intrahepatic tumor relapses after the initial treatment, consistent follow-up evaluations are of the utmost importance. Furthermore, it has been documented that, overall, the majority of patients died despite having the operation on the original hepatic tumor or an operation when they relapsed.[19,20]

A prerequisite for efficiency of the local procedure is removal of the tumor as close to 100% as possible, with a safety margin of at least 10 mm.

All the disadvantages were related to

Table 1. Overview of literature - Interventional treatment of liver metastases.

Author	Year	Technique	Primary tumor	Median SR
Rossi et. al.[4]	1996	RF	Colorectal and other	11 months
Lencioni et al.[27]	1998	RF, cooled	Colorectal, stomach, carcinoid	6.5 months
Ravikumar et al.[28]	1991	Cryotherapy	Colorectal	5 months to 5 years
Vogl et. al.[29]	1997	LITT®	Colorectal, stomach, breast, pancreas, lung, thyroid, melanoma	40.8 months
Lopez et. al.[30]	1997	Chemoembolization		10 months
Martin et. al.[31]	1995	Chemoembolization	Neuroendocrine	33 months
Sanz-Altamira et al.[32]	1997	Chemoembolization	Colorectal	10 months
Amin et. al.[33]	1993	PEI, ILP	Colorectal	ILP: 27 mon. PEI: 7 mon.

PEI: percutaneous ethanol instillation, ILP: interstitial laser photocoagulation, TAE: transarterial chemoembolization, RF: Radio-frequency therapy, TAE: transarterial chemoembolization, PAI: percutaneous alcohol injection

Table 2. Overview of literature - Interventional therapy of hepatocellular carcinomas (HCC).

Author	Year	Technique	No. of Patients	Complications	Local Tumor Control	Survival
Lau et al.[23]	1998	Intraarterial infusion of 90 ytt. Microspheres	71	Nausea	-	median 9.4 months
Rossi et al.[4]	1996	Percutaneous RF	39	Pains	Follow up period of 22 months: 5% local relapse, 36% new lesions	44 months, still alive after 22 months 28%
Hesse et al.[24]	1997	Combined TAE+PAI	17	Raised temperature and pains	8 of 17: 50% necrosis, 6 further 90% necrosis	41 months followup time with 75% alive
Livraghi et al.[25]	1995	PAI	746	Abscess, pains, pleural effusion, haematoma	17% local relapse	Child A and <5cm. 1 y. 98%, 3 y. 79%, 5.y. 47%
Kanematsu et al.[26]	1993	TAE	20	Pains	-	1. y. 90%, 3 y: 50%, 5 y. 17.5%
Livraghi et al.[8]	1999	RF versus PAI	86	RF: pains, pleural effusion, cholecystitis	RF: 90% complete PAI: 80% (immediately after intervention)	

SR: survival rate, RF: radio frequency, LITT(r) laser-induced interstitial thermotherapy, PEI: percutaneous ethanol instillation, ILP interstitial laser photocoagulation.

shortcomings of the local treatment regarding the character of the basic disease. Contraindications to the MRT examination such as metal implants and metal splinters, intense claustrophobia, or pacemakers make it difficult to monitor treatment sufficiently.

Our findings in a population of more than 381 patients with liver metastases from different primary tumors, in the main colorectal carcinomas, can only be compared with the other local ablative procedures to a limited extent, because in these studies mostly HCCs have been treated (Table 2). In our study, only comparative statements on local tumor control were possible. Due to the improved application systems that have become available in the meantime, and the completed learning curve regarding the puncture technique and choice of laser and irrigation parameters, we are seeing positive data with regard to local tumor control in LITT® (Table 3).

The survival rates achieved, which represent the most relevant success criteria for a treatment, are similar among patients with metastases from a colorectal carcinoma or carcinoma of the breast to those in surgically-resected patients. It must be considered in this study, however, that a surgical resection was not, or was no longer, an option among most of the patients being treated due to metastatic relapse after surgical resection or a bilobibular pattern of infestation. Nevertheless, it was possible to achieve survival rates comparable to surgical resection among these patients, who were in a group with a worse prognosis. Compared with the extensively publicized historic survival data after surgical metastatic resection, LITT® offers a good further treatment option. Due to the survival data and local tumor control rates achieved thus far, in our opinion randomized studies that compare LITT® with chemotherapy solely in patients who fulfill the inclusion criteria for LITT® are no longer ethically tenable.

Advantages of LITT® have proved to be:

1. good tolerance through local anesthesia and percutaneous access
2. low rate of complications
3. no perioperative mortality
4. treatment managed through out patient's department
5. low costs in comparison with hepatectomy
6. can be repeated almost at will

In the modern oncologic concept of treatment, the internationally defined terms of "clinical benefit," "performance status," and "quality of life" are of the utmost importance. These terms apply predominantly to patients suffering from local and generally advanced tumors no longer curative. Above all, however, intensive chemotherapy, systemic or regional, with marked toxic side effects severely affects the quality of life in the majority of patients. With this in mind, all the more attention must be paid to treatment concepts described in this study, because minimally invasive techniques are applied that adversely affect patients less and shorter-term.

Consequently, the prerequisites are given to integrate these new procedures into oncologic treatment programs that have been carried out up to date. In the

Table 3. Overview: Comparative representation of the ablative treatment of liver tumours (valency increasing + ++) Survival rate.							
Technique	Curative Metastases	Max. No. of	Max. Size	Expenditure	Complications	Local Tumor Control	Survival Data
LITT®	(+)	5	50 mm	+++	1-3%	96-99%	5J-SR 21-34%
RF	(+)	5	50 mm	++	2-5%	91%	2 J-SR % (HCC)
Alcohol (PEI)	(+)	5	60 mm	+	2-6%	93-99%	5 J-SR 30-50% (HCC)
Chemoembol. (TAE)	-	-	-	++	3-4%	80-91%	3 J-SR 10% (HCC)
Cryotherapy (OP)	(+)	5	70 mm	+++	20%	~80%	5 J-SR 10-30%

LITT® : laser-induced interstitial thermotherapy, RF: radio-frequency, PEI: percutaneous ethanol instillation, TAE: transarterial chemoembolization, OP: operating, HCC: hepatocellular carcinomas, SR: survival rate.

palliative approach, a laser-guided intrahepatic metastatic removal in combination with chemotherapy can be of great help, because the correlation between tumor mass and response to chemotherapy can be documented. LITT®, which has been used for the past two years within the framework of the clinical routine and can be carried out on an out-patient basis, can have a great part in modern oncologic treatment concepts.

The much-discussed problem of spreading tumor cells by manipulating the tumor tissue with needles, scalpels, or other surgical instruments affects both the surgery and radiologic intervention in the instance of resections, biopsies, or therapeutic intervention.

Current publications assume an incidence among percutaneous biopsies of 1/10 000 to 1/33 000, in which 48% of the population studied had pancreatic biopsies. Occasionally, individual cases are reported in the literature.[21,22] No figures are available on possible cell spreading in the instance of open or laparoscopic operations.

Tumor cells can spread and are implanted mainly along the puncture channel and subcutaneously in the puncture area. Over the months, the growing masses drop in the instance of CT or MRT examination, or detected through tactile findings in the course of clinical examinations. Effects of the tumor manifestations on the survival time, or on further clinical progress of the affected patients, have not been examined sufficiently, but appear to have no real influence. Overall, tumor cell spreading must be evaluated as a potential, but seldom-occurring complication during intervention. The procedure we use of installing tissue glue by way of a double lumina catheter in the puncture canal appears to have a beneficial effect. In our patient population, no spreading of tumorous cells in the puncture canal has been observed to date.

CONCLUSIONS

The percutaneous MR-guided interstitial LITT® of malignant liver tumors is a reliable treatment concept for destroying tumors palliatively and is also potentially curative. In this study, the treatment concept must be differentiated according to the underlying histology: for HCC, a local ablative procedure instead of, or in combination with, the local alcohol installation (PEI) or transarterial chemoembolization (TACE) can be used. According to the latest studies, local procedures such as RF ablation and laser therapy (LITT®) permit reliable local tumor control in the instance of HCC.[3,8,32,34]

Regarding liver metastases, the therapeutic situation must be discussed within the context of the primary tumors. Currently, using MR-guided LITT® for liver infestation restricted to a local area without extrahepatic manifestations can be justified clinically. MRT proves to be an indispensable tool for monitoring and controlling percutaneous LITT®. MRT is used both for monitoring and controlling complete tumor removal as well as for the follow-up process, and has proved to be the optimum examination procedure in assessing small tumor manifestations.

REFERENCES

1. Weiss L, Grundmann E, Torhorst J, et al. Haematogenous metastatic patterns in colonic carcinoma: an analysis of 1541 necropsies. J Pathol 1986;150:195-203.
2. Weiss L. Inefficiency of metastasis from colorectal carcinomas. Boston: Kluwer Academic Publishers; 1994. p 35-7.
3. Vogl TJ, Mack MG, Roggan A, et al. Internally cooled power laser for MR-guided interstitial laser-induced thermotherapy of liver lesions: initial clinical results. Radiology 1998;209:381-5.
4. Rossi S, Di Stasi M, Buscarini E, et al. Percutaneous RF interstitial thermal ablation in the treatment of hepatic cancer. Am J Roentgenol 1996;167:759-68.
5. Solbiati L, Goldberg SN, Ierace T, et al. Hepatic metastases: percutaneous radio-frequency ablation with cooled-tip electrodes. Radiology 1997;205:367-73.
6. Solbiati L, Ierace T, Goldberg SN, et al. Percutaneous US-guided radio-frequency tissue ablation of liver metastases: treatment and follow-up in 16 patients. Radiology 1997;202: 195-203.
7. Livraghi T, Goldberg S, Monti NF, et al. Saline-enhanced radio-frequency tissue ablation in the treatment of liver metastases. Radiology 1997;202:205-10.
8. Livraghi T, Goldberg N, Lazzaroni S, et al. Small hepatocellular carcinoma: treatment with radio-frequency ablation versus ethanol injection. Radiology 1999;210:655-61.
9. Wingo PA, Tong T, Bolden S. Cancer statistics, 1995. CA Cancer J Clin 1995;45:8-30.
10. Bross IDJ, Blumenson LE. Metastatic sites that produce generalized cancer: identification and kinetics of generalizing sites. In: Weiss L, ed. Fundamental aspects of metastasis. Amsterdam: North-Holland; 1976. p

359-75.

11. Viadana E, Bross IDJ, Pickren JW. The metastatic spread of cancers of the digestive system in man. Oncology 1978;35:114-26.

12. Stangl R, Altendorf-Hofmann A, Charnley RM, et al. Factors influencing the natural history of colorectal liver metastases. The Lancet 1994;343:1405-10.

13. Bengmark S, Hafström L. The natural history of primary and secondary malignant tumors of the liver. Cancer 1969;23:198-202.

14. Palmer M, Petrelli NJ, Herrera L. No treatment option for liver metastases from colorectal adenocarcinoma. Dis Colon Rectum 1989;32:698-701.

15. Kemeny N, Niedzwiecki D., Shurgot B, et al. Prognostic variables in patients with hepatic metastases from colorectal cancer. Cancer 1989;63:742-7.

16. Ringe B, Bechstein WO, Raab R, et al. Leberresektion bei 175 patienten mit colorektalen metastasen. Chirurg 1990;61:272-9.

17. Scheele J, Altendorf-Hofmann A, Stangl R, et al. Surgical resection of colorectal liver metastases: gold standard for solitary and completely resectable lesions. Swiss Surg Suppl 1996;4:4-17.

18. Nordlinger B, Guiguet M, Vaillant JC, et al. Surgical resection of colorectal carcinoma metastases to the liver: a prognostic scoring system to improve case selection, based on 1568 patients. Association Francaise de Chirurgie. Cancer 1996;77:1254-62.

19. Adson MA. Resection of liver metastases-when is it worthwhile? World J Surg 1987;11:511-20.

20. Mazzaferro V, Dindazans VJ, Makova L, et al. Approach to hepatic metastases from colorectal adenocarcinoma. Semin Liver Dis 1988; 8:247.

21. Chapman W C, Sharp KW, Weaver F, et al. Tumor seeding from percutaneous biliary catheters. Ann Surg 1989;6:708-15.

22. Loew R, Dueber C, Schwarting A, et al. Subcutaneous implantation metastasis of a cholangiocarcinoma of the bile duct after percutaneous transhepatic biliary drainage (PTBD). Eur Radiol 1997;7:259-61.

23. Lau W Y, Ho S, Leung TWT, et al. Selective internal radiation therapy for nonresectable hepatocellular carcinoma with intraarterial infusion of yttrium microspheres. Int J Radiat Oncol Biol Phys 1998; 40:583-92.

24. Hesse UJ, Troisi R, Defreyne L, et al. Die kombinierte transarterielle chemoembolisation (TAE) und perkutane ethanolinjektion (PEI) beim hepatozellulären karzinom vor transplantation. Langenbecks Arch Chir 1997;I(Forumband):121-5.

25. Livraghi T, Giorgio A, Marin G, et al. Hepatocellular carcinoma and cirrhosis in 746 patients: long-term results of percutaneous ethanol injection. Radiology 1995;197:101-8.

26. Kanematsu T, Matsumata T, Shirabe K. A comparative study of hepatic resection and transcatheter arterial embolization for the treatment of primary hepatocellular carcinoma. Cancer 1993;71:1281-6.

27. Lencioni R, Goletti O, Armillotta N, et al. Radio-frequency thermal ablation of liver metastases with a cooled-tip electrode needle: results of a pilot clinical trial. Eur Radiol 1998;8:1205-11.

28. Ravikumar TS, Kane R, Cady B, et al. A 5-year study of cryosurgery in the treatment of liver tumors. Arch Surg 1991;126:1520-4.

29. Vogl TJ, Mack MG, Straub R, et al. Percutaneous MRI-guided laser-induced thermotherapy for hepatic metastases for colorectal cancer. The Lancet 1997;350:29.

30. Lopez R L, Pan SH, Lois JF, et al. Transarterial chemoembolization is a safe treatment for unresectable hepatic malignancies. Am Surg 1997;63:923-6.

31. Martin M, Tarara D, Wu YM, et al. Mitros Intrahepatic arterial chemoembolization for hepatocellular carcinoma and metastatic neuroendocrine tumors in the era of liver transplantation. Am Surg 1996; 62:724-32.

32. Sanz-Altamira PM, Spence LD, Hubermann LS, et al. Selective chemoembolization in the management of hepatic metastases in refractory colorectal carcinoma: a phase II trial. Dis Colon Rectum 1997;40:770-5.

33. Amin Z, Bown SG, Lees WR. Local treatment of colorectal liver metastases: a comparison of interstitial laser photocoagulation (ILP) and percutaneous alcohol injection (PAI). Clin Radiol 1993;48:166-71.

Radiofrequency Ablation of Primary and Metastatic Liver Tumors

STEVEN A. CURLEY, M.D., F.A.C.S.
PROFESSOR OF SURGERY
CHIEF, GASTROINTESTINAL TUMOR SURGERY
THE UNIVERSITY OF TEXAS M.D. ANDERSON CANCER CENTER
HOUSTON, TEXAS

FRANCESCO IZZO, M.D.
ASSOCIATE PROFESSOR OF SURGERY
CHIEF, HEPATOBILIARY TUMOR SURGERY
THE G. PASCALE NATIONAL TUMOR INSTITUTE
NAPLES, ITALY

Worldwide, hepatocellular carcinoma (HCC) is one of the most common and deadly solid cancers. At least one million new patients are diagnosed annually with this cancer.[1] Incidence in non-Western countries is related to infections of hepatitis B virus and dietary ingestion of aflatoxins, whereas in Western countries alcohol-related cirrhosis and chronic hepatitis C virus infection are leading causes of HCC.[2] In the United States, approximately 155,000 new cases of cancer of the liver and bile duct occur annually, with the majority being colorectal metastases.[3]

Surgical resection of these tumors is considered the only treatment modality with a curative effect, as it has a five-year survival rate of 20% to 35% for patients with primary and metastatic liver tumors.[4-6] However, for a tumor to be considered appropriate for resection, there must not be any extrahepatic disease or severe hepatic dysfunction, the tumor or tumors must not be so extensive that too little functioning liver remains following the resection, at least a 1-cm tumor-free margin should be attained, and there should not be any involvement of the confluence of the portal vein.[7,8] As a result, only 10% to 30% of patients with HCC or liver metastases are eligible for surgical resection.

To provide treatment for the 70% to 90% of patients diagnosed with liver cancer who are not candidates for surgical resection, several alternative treatment methods have been developed, including systemic and regional chemotherapy;[9,10] and interstitial therapies such as chemoembolization;[11,12] or localized ablative techniques involving either freezing (cryoablation[13,14]), chemical desiccation (alcohol ablation[15,16]), or heating (laser,[17,18] microwave,[19] or radiofrequency ablation [RFA][20-22]) of hepatic tumor. Systemic toxicity due to prolonged exposure to antineoplastic agents limits their long-term efficacy, and systemic chemotherapy has response rates of less than 20% in HCC and metastatic colorectal cancer patients.[2] Among the interstitial therapies, rapid freezing of tissue with exposure to liquid nitrogen cryoprobes at $-196°C$ has a high risk of liver fracture, hemorrhage, and tumor-lysis syndromes, and alcohol injection results in non-homogeneous distribution within tumors and results in incomplete areas of necrosis. Neither of these local therapies produces extended long-term survival in most patients (Table 1).

Table 1. Clinical outcomes following treatment of primary and metastatic liver tumors with either surgical resection, cryoablation, injection of ethanol, or chemoembolization

	Percentage of patients alive 1 year after procedure	Percentage of patients alive 3 years after procedure	Percentage of patients alive 5 years after procedure
TUMORS			
Primary Liver			
Surgical resection[44,48,50,51]	46% - 90%	22% - 75%	14% - 64%
Cryoablation[43,45,56]	33% - 77%	12% - 32%	4% - 51%
Ethanol Injection[52,57,58]	83% - 95%	33% - 78%	13% - 55%
Chemoembolization[48,52,55]	24% - 90%	13% - 50%	6% - 18%
Metastatic Liver			
Surgical resection[46,47,53]	83% - 93%	50% - 60%	28% - 50%
Cryoablation[38,43,49,54]	77%	51% - 60%	36% - 44%

HEAT TREATMENT OF CANCER TUMORS

The use of heat to treat tumors has been part of medical practice since the Greek and Roman times, when superficial tumors were subjected to cautery.[18] In general, thermal injury to cells begins at 42°C, with the exposure times to low-level hyperthermia needed to achieve cell death ranging from 3 to 50 hours depending upon the tissue type and conditions.[23] As one increases the temperature above 42°C, there is an exponential decrease exists in the exposure time necessary for a lethal response. For example, only eight minutes at 46°C is needed to kill malignant cells, and 51°C can be lethal after only two minutes.[24,25] At temperatures above 60°C, intracellular proteins become denatured and cell death is inevitable.[26]

In the 1970s and early 1980s, application of heat from an external source became a focus of care when it was noted that malignant cells were more sensitive to heat than nondiseased cells.[27] Although this appeared to be a promising modality, problems existed with the equipment used and in accurately predicting the extent of target and adjacent tissue heating for any given treatment regimen.[28]

Radiofrequency (RF) energy has been the focus of increasing research and practice for the past few years.[29-33] During the application of RF energy, a high-frequency alternating current moves from the tip of an electrode into the tissue surrounding that electrode. As the ions within the tissue attempt to follow the change in direction of the alternating current, their movement results in frictional heating of the tissue. As the temperature within the tissue becomes elevated beyond 60°C, cells begin to die, resulting in a region of necrosis surrounding the electrode (Fig. 1).[34]

The use of RF energy to cause necrosis has been used in patients who did not meet the criteria for resectability of HCC and metastatic liver tumors, yet were candidates for a liver-directed procedure based upon the presence of liver-only disease. A needle electrode is advanced into the unresectable liver tumor by way of either a percutaneous, laparoscopic, or open (laparotomy) route. The needle electrode used most frequently is a 15-gauge, 12 to 15 cm long insulated cannula containing ten individual hook-shaped electrode arms or tines (Fig. 2). Upon deployment, the array of tines extends to a diameter of either 2.0, 3.0, or 3.5 cm. Using ultrasound to guide placement, the needle electrode is advanced to within 5 mm of the center of the targeted tumor, and the individual wires or tines of the electrode are deployed into the tissues (Fig. 3). After the tines have been extended or deployed into the tissue, the needle electrode is attached to a RF generator and two dispersive electrodes (return or grounding pads) are placed on the patient, one on each thigh. The RF energy is applied beginning at 50 Watts and increased in 10-Watt increments every 60 seconds until 90 Watts are being applied through the needle electrode. As the RF energy (alternating current) moves from the active needle electrode to the dispersive electrodes (return pads) ionic agitation occurs, resulting in frictional heating of the tissue. As the tissue around the tines of the electrode begin to heat, the system

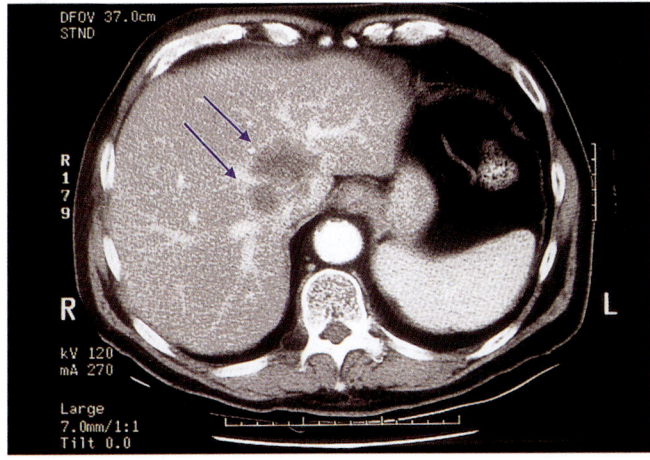

Figure 1a. CT scan of an unresectable hepatocellular cancer (arrows) near inferior vena cava, right, middle, and left hepatic veins before radiofrequency ablation.

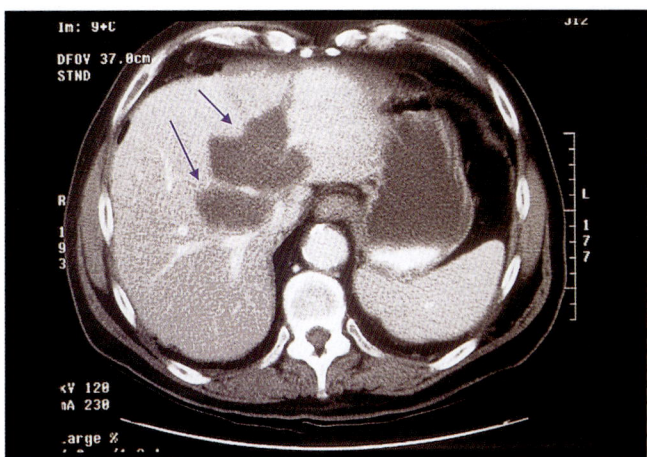

Figure 1b. CT scan three months after intraoperative radiofrequency ablation of hepatocellular carcinoma in liver. Thermal lesions (solid arrows) encompass an area larger than original tumor.

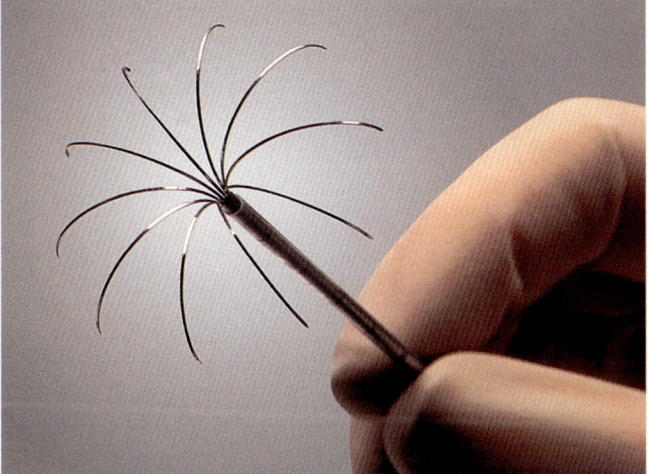

Figure 2. Multi-wire array deployed fully from tip of a 15-gauge needle cannula. Ten individual tines of the LeVeen multiple array needle electrode can be deployed to a full 3.5-cm diameter.

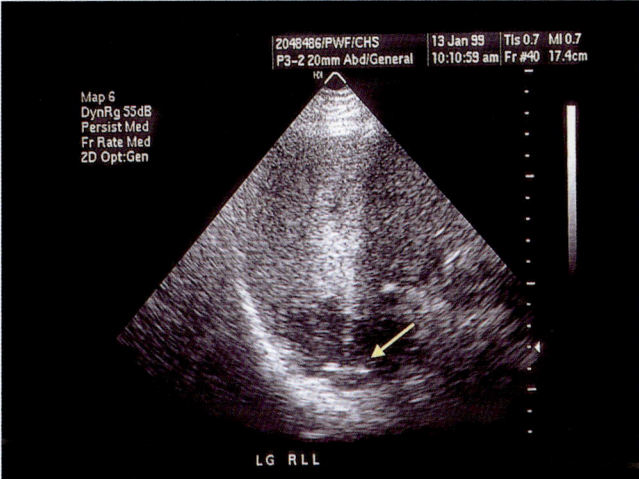

Figure 3. Tines of the multiple array LeVeen needle electrode (solid arrow) advanced into tissue surrounding metastatic liver tumor, as visualized with 7.5-MHz intraoperative ultrasound probe.

impedance begins to rise because the necrotic tissue acts as an insulating, high-resistance layer (Fig. 4). A tissue impedance measurement of over 400 ohms completely blocks the flow of RF energy to the return pads and essentially shuts off the RF system, signaling completion of the thermal lesion. Using a second-phase application of RF energy, after waiting approximately 30 seconds, results in a complete thermal lesion slightly greater than the diameter of the deployed tines.

Tumors less than 3 cm in their greatest diameter can be ablated with the placement of a needle electrode with an array diameter of 3.5 cm when the electrode is positioned in the center of the tumor. Tumors larger than 3 cm require more than one deployment of the needle electrode. Typically, we place the array first at the most posterior interface between the tumor and nondiseased liver parenchyma, and then reposition and redeploy the array anteriorly at 2.0-2.5-cm intervals within the tissue. To mimic a surgical margin in these unresectable tumors, the needle electrode is used to produce a thermal lesion that incorporates not only the tumor but also nondiseased liver parenchyma in a zone 1 cm wide surrounding the tumor (Figs 1a-b).

Radiofrequency Ablation (RFA) of Primary Liver Tumors

Use of RFA to treat primary and metastatic liver tumors in patients from the University of Texas M.D. Anderson Cancer Center and the G. Pascale National Cancer Institute has been reported recently.[22] The sizes of HCC addressed in this patient population ranged from 1 to 7 cm in their greatest dimension. As the size of the tumor increased, the number of deployments of the needle electrode and total time of applying RF energy increased (Table 2). Primary liver tumors tend to be highly vascular, so a vascular heat sink phenomenon may contribute to the extended ablation times. As with tumors metastatic to the liver, we strive to mimic a surgical margin of approximately 1 cm of nonmalignant liver tissue surrounding the tumors, which required additional deployments of the needle electrode beyond the leading edge of the tumors.

Procedure-related complications were minimal in patients with HCC. Complications immediately after the application of RF energy (i.e., symp-

Table 2. Number of deployments of a needle electrode and total elapsed time to system-wide impedance in primary liver tumors of varying diameters

Greatest diameter of liver tumor(cm)	No. of Tumors	Mean number of deployments of needle electrode taken		Mean elapsed time to system-wide impedance (minutes)	
0.1- 1.0	2	1	(1 - 2)*	13	(8 - 20)
1.1- 2.0	14	2	(2 - 4)	19	(15 - 33)
2.1 - 3.0	14	3	(2 - 5)	27	(17 - 35)
3.1 - 4.0	17	5	(4 - 8)	49	(36 - 71)
4.1 - 5.0	7	7	(5 - 9)	83	(47 - 95)
> 5.0	3	10	(6 - 12)	94	(56 - 110)

* Values in parentheses are ranges of the measurements

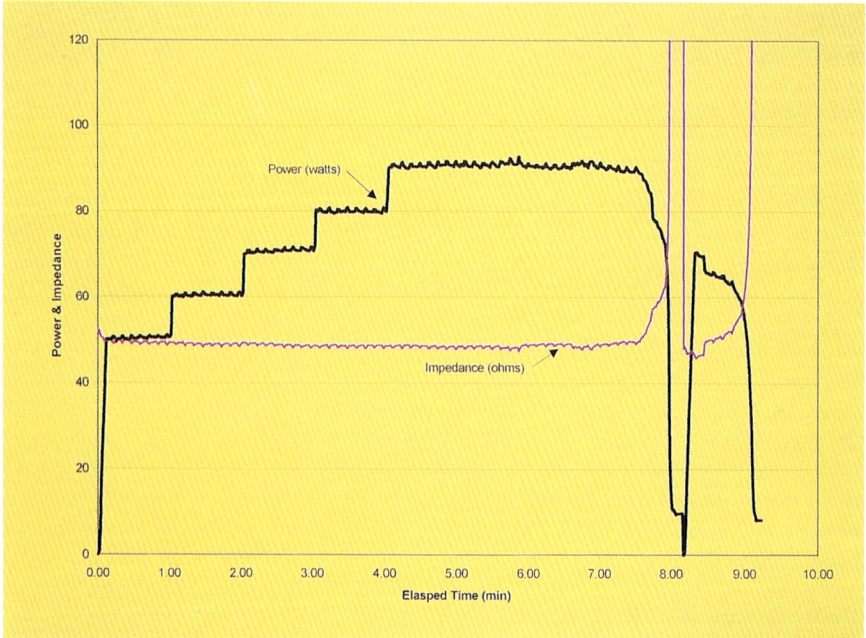

Figure 4. Graphic display of power (in watts) and tissue impedance (in ohms) during radiofrequency ablation of liver tissue. After needle electrode is placed and tines deployed fully into the tissue, radiofrequency generator is set to 50 Watts and treatment started. Every minute the power is increased by 10 Watts until a maximum power of 90 Watts is achieved. As tissue coagulation begins, impedance increases and power output decreases to less than 10 Watts. After waiting 30 seconds to allow heat to dissipate, power again is applied in a second-phase treatment, beginning at approximately 75% of maximum power achieved in first phase; this power is applied until impedance again increases and power falls off.

toms presenting within one day post-procedure) were noted in 27% of the HCC patients. These complications included asymptomatic pleural effusion, fever, pain, subcutaneous hematoma, subcapsular hematoma, and ventricular fibrillation. In addition, one patient developed ascites. All patient events resolved with appropriate clinical management within one week following the RFA procedure, with the exception of the development of ascites, which resolved with use of diuretics within three weeks of the treatment. No patient developed thermal injury to adjacent tissues, hepatic insufficiency, renal insufficiency, or coagulopathy following the application of RF energy into the target tumors.

All patients returned first at one month post-procedure and then every three months for computed tomographic (CT) scan or magnetic resonance imaging (MRI) of the liver. In all but one patient, CT scan of the zone of necrosis produced by the application of RF energy showed non-viable tumor. The patient with

Table 3. Number of deployments of a needle electrode and total elapsed time to system-wide impedance in metastatic liver tumors of varying diameters

Greatest diameter of liver tumor(cm)	No. of Tumors	Mean number of deployments of needle electrode taken		Mean elapsed time to system-wide impedance (minutes)
0.2 - 1.0	11	1	(1 - 2)*	12 (6 - 14)
1.2 - 2.0	27	2	(2 - 4)	17 (13 - 19)
2.1 - 3.0	22	3	(2 - 6)	21 (14 - 28)
3.1 - 4.0	13	6	(4 - 7)	43 (27 - 51)
4.1 - 5.0	12	6	(5 - 8)	68 (43 - 92)
> 5.0	13	11	(6 - 16)	72 (55 - 97)

* Values in parentheses are ranges of the measurements

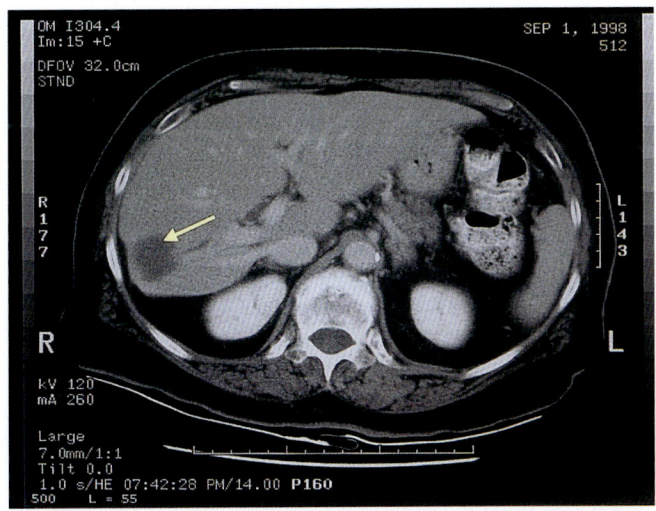

Figure 5A. CT scan in patient with metastatic colorectal cancer liver tumors. Scan was performed three months after radiofrequency ablation and shows one of the areas where tumor was ablated intraoperatively (arrow).

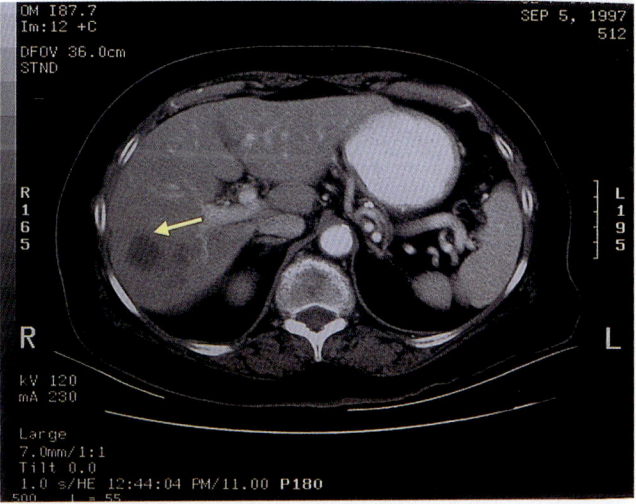

Figure 5B. CT scan approximately one year after radiofrequency ablation of tumors. Intrahepatic cystic area at site of radiofrequency ablation has involuted and does not show any persistence of viable tumor cells at point of ablation.

incompletely ablated tumor was retreated with percutaneous RFA in the area of viable tumor. At up to 12 months following the procedure, recurrence or persistence at the point of the RFA was noted in only one HCC tumor, for a recurrence rate of approximately 2%. This region of viable tissue contrast enhancement on CT scan was found at the periphery of the thermal lesion in a single tumor greater than 5 cm in diameter; no recurrence or persistence was noted within the boundary of any of the other thermal lesions produced by RFA. This represents a recurrence/persistence rate in the RF ablated tumors of less than 1% at 12 months post-procedure, based upon the total number of zones of RF lesions produced.

RF Ablation of Metastatic Liver Tumors

The sizes of the unresectable metastatic liver tumors treated with RF energy ranged from 0.5 to 12 cm in their greatest dimension (Table 3).[22] As expected, as the size of the tumor increased, the number of deployments of the needle electrode and total elapsed time of applying RF energy

Table 4. Complications reported with cryoablation and radiofrequency ablation of liver tumors

Complication	Reported with cryoablation	Noted with radiofrequency ablation
Hemorrhage	X	X
Perihepatic abscess	X	X
Intrahepatic abscess	X	X
Renal insufficiency	X	
Symptomatic pleural effusion	X	X
Pneumothorax	X	
Bile leak fistula	X	X
Coagulopathy	X	
Myoglobinuria	X	
Hepatic "cracking"	X	
Fever	X	X
"Cryoshock" (multiple organ failure, severe coagulopathy, & disseminated intravascular coagulation)	X	
Pain	X	X
Hematoma	X	X
Ventricular fibrillation	X	X
Ascites	X	X

increased. For tumors whose largest dimension was less than 1 cm, typically only one deployment was necessary, whereas those lesions greater than 1 cm in diameter were treated with two or more separate deployments (Table 3). CT scans performed after RFA of primary or metastatic liver tumors initially demonstrate a cystic-density lesion larger than the original tumor; the size of this cystic area decreases slightly over time (Fig. 5).

Procedure-related complications were minimal in patients with metastatic liver tumors. A few (10%) of the sites of intraoperative RFA expressed bleeding when the needle was withdrawn from the needle electrode track, but in all cases this was minimal (<5 cc of blood lost) and controlled easily with electrocauterization of the puncture site at the surface of the liver. Complications immediately after the procedure (i.e., symptoms presenting within one day post-procedure) were noted in 33% of the patients. The complications included asymptomatic pleural effusion, fever, and pain. All events resolved with appropriate clinical management within one week following the procedure.

No patient developed thermal injury to adjacent tissues, hepatic insufficiency, renal insufficiency, or coagulopathy following application of RF energy into the target tumors. No hepatic abscesses were noted in the regions of RF-induced necrosis in primary or metastatic tumors.

New occurrences of additional metastatic liver tumors were found in 28% of the patients within 12 months post-procedure. New occurrences of metastatic tumors are a result of the growth of subclinical or microscopic deposits of malignant cells into clinically detectable tumors. Most of the patients with new occurrences of metastatic tumors were scheduled for systemic infusion of an antineoplastic agent; the others either received another RFA of the new tumors or no further treatment at the time of diagnosis.

Recurrence or persistence of metastatic tumors at the point of the RFA was rare. At a point up to 12 months following the procedure, follow-up imaging with CT scans or MRI disclosed a recurrence rate of approximately 7%. All regions of recurrence or persistence were at the periphery of the necrotic tissue of the ablated tumors; one was near the inferior vena cava, between the right and middle hepatic veins. No recurrence or persistence was noted within the center of the thermal lesions produced by RFA.

For both HCC and metastatic liver tumor patients, serum liver function tests (e.g., alanine aminotransferase, aspartate aminotransferase, and gamma glutamyl transferase) were slightly elevated immediately following the procedure, but for most patients these values returned to baseline levels within seven days, and for all patients the values were normal within one month after the procedure. The serum tumor markers, alpha fetoprotein (AFP) or carcinoembryonic antigen (CEA), were elevated in 85% of the patients before the application of RF energy, but one month later were noted to have returned to normal levels in 72% of the patients. Those patients in whom these markers did not decrease after the procedure eventually developed clinically detectable new metastases in other regions of the liver or at distant organ sites.

Radiofrequency Ablation (RFA) in Contrast to Cryoablation of Liver Tumors

Complications associated with cryoablation include up to a 4% mortality rate, significant intraoperative hemorrhage, injury to adjacent organs, biliary fistulas, coagulopathies, acute renal failure, intrahepatic abscess, and symptomatic pleural effusions (Table 4).[35-38] Procedure-related complications from cryoablation have been reported to range from between 8% and 25% in treatment of primary liver tumors and between 8% and 58% in treatment of metastatic liver tumors (Table 1).

More important to the management of these patients is the success rate of the procedure, as represented by recurrence or persistence of the tumor at the point of the ablative procedure. The recurrence/persistence rates with the use of RF energy in a recent study was less than 2% at a median follow-up period of 15 months,[22] with none of the recurrences within the boundaries of the original thermal lesions. In contrast, incidence of recurrence or persistence of tumor cells at the site of cryoablation has been reported at rates from 10% to 22%,[39-41] especially with metastatic tumors larger than 5 cm in diameter. Local recurrence of tumors after surgical resection can only occur at the margin/edge of the resection, and it has been reported at low levels of incidence.[42]

Summary

The use of RF energy to treat unresectable liver tumors does not have a curative intent for most patients; however, a subset of patients treated with RFA may achieve long-term disease-free survival. New metastatic tumors developed in several of these patients, and at a rate comparable with those treated with surgical resection or cryoablation. Surgical resection remains the "gold" standard for treating metastatic and primary liver tumors; however, few patients are candidates for hepatic resection because of tumor size, number, location, or the presence of cirrhosis too severe to permit liver resection. Cryoablation of unresectable tumors has been an option for several years, but complications associated with freezing tissue can be problematic. Coagulation necrosis, induced by RF energy, of unresectable liver tumors has been shown to provide a relatively safe, highly effective method to achieve local disease control in liver cancer patients. Continuing research and refinements in RFA techniques and equipment may permit effective treatment of larger liver tumors and malignant tumors at other body sites.

REFERENCES

1. Di Bisceglie A, Rustgi V, Hoffnagle J, et al. NIH conference on hepatocellular carcinoma. Ann Intern Med 1988; 108: 390-401.
2. Spitz FR, Bouvet M, Yahanda AM. Hepatobiliary cancers. Pages 223-55. Feig BW, Berger DH, Fuhrman GM eds. The M.D. Anderson surgical oncology handbook. Philadelphia, PA: Lippincott Williams & Wilkins; 1999. p 551
3. Landis SH, Murray T, Bolden S, et al. Cancer statistics 1998. Can J Clin 1998; 48(1): 6-23.
4. Fong Y, Cohen AM, Fortner JG, et al. Liver resection for colorectal metastases. J Clin Oncol 1997; 15: 938-46.
5. Blumgart LH, Fong Y. Surgical options in the treatment of hepatic metastases from colorectal cancer. Curr Probl Surg 1995; 32: 333-421.
6. Tuttle T. Hepatectomy for noncolorectal liver metastases. Curley SA ed. Liver Cancer. New York; Springer-Verlag Publishers; 1998. P 201-1.
7. Adson MA, VanHeerden JA, Adson MH, et al. Resection of hepatic metastases from colorectal cancer. Arch Surg 1984; 119: 647-51.
8. Steele G, Ravikumar TS. Resection of hepatic metastases from colorectal cancer. Ann Surg 1989; 210: 127-38.
9. Ohya T, Kikuchi S, Kato K, et al. Clinical studies of chemotherapy for primary hepatocellular carcinoma. Jpn J Cancer Chemother 1982; 9: 1623-7.
10. Falkson G, MacIntyre JM, Moertel CF, et al. Primary liver cancer: an Eastern Cooperative Oncology Group trial. Cancer 1984; 54: 970-7.
11. Nakamura H, Mitani T, Murakami T, et al. Five-year survival after transcatheter chemoembolization for hepatic carcinoma. Cancer Chemother Pharmacol 1994; 33(Suppl): S89-S92.
12. Hashimoto T, Nakamura H, Tomoda K, et al. Hepatocellular carcinoma patients showing long-term complete responses to chemoembolization. Sem Oncol 1997; 24(Suppl): S6-26-S6-28.
13. Zuro LM, Staren ED. Cryosurgical ablation of unresectable hepatic tumors. AORN-J 1996; 64(2): 231-44.
14. Tandam VR, Harmantas A, Gallinger S. Long-term survival after hepatic cryosurgery versus surgical resection for metastatic colorectal carincoma: a critical review of the literature. Can J Surg 1997; 40(3): 175-81.
15. Ishii H, Okada S, Nose H, et al. Local recurrence of hepatocelluar carcinoma after percutaneous ethanol injection. Cancer 1996; 77: 1792-6.
16. Liviraghi T, Bolondi L, Lazzaroni S, et al. Percutaneous ethanol injection in the treatment of hepatocellular carcinoma in cirrhosis. Cancer 1992; 69: 925-9.
17. Bremer E, Allkemper T, Menzel J, et al. Preliminary clinical experience with laser-induced interstitial thermotherapy in patients with hepatocellular carcinoma. JMRI 1998; 8: 235-9.
18. LeVeen RF. Laser hyperthermia and radiofrequency ablation of hepatic lesions. Sem Interven Radiol 1997; 14(3): 313-24.
19. Mitsuzaki K, et al. CT appearance of hepatic tumors after microwave coagulation therapy. Am J Roentgenol 1998; 171(5): 1397-403.
20. MaGahan JP, Schneider P, Brock JM, et al. Treatment of liver tumors by percutaneous radiofrequency electrocautery. Sem Interven Radiol 1993; 10(2): 143-9.
21. Rossi S, Di Stasi M, Buscarini E, et al. Percutaneous radiofrequency interstitial thermal ablation in the treatment of small hepatocellular carcinoma. Cancer J Sci Am 1995; 1: 73-81.
22. Curley SA, Izzo F, Delrio P, et al. Radiofrequency ablation of uresectable primary and metastatic hepatic malignancies: results in 123 patients. Ann Surg 1999; 230(1): 1-8.
23. Dickson JA, Calderwood SK. Temperature range and selective sensitivity of tumors to hyperthermia: a critical review. Ann NY Acad Sci 1980; 335: 180-205.
24. Hill RP, Hunt JW. Hyperthermia: Tannock IF, Hill RP eds. The basic science of oncology. New York: Pergamon Press; 1987. P 416.
25. Haines DE, Watson DD, Halperin C. Characteristics of heat transfer and determination of temperature gradient and viability threshold during radiofrequency fulguration of isolated perfused canine right ventricle. Circulation 1987; 76: 278.
26. Grundfest WS, Litvack FI, Doyle DL, et al. Laser-tissue interactions: considerations for cardiovascular applications.: White RA, Grundfest WS eds. Lasers in cardiovascular disease. Chicago: Yearbook Medical Publishers;1987. p 32-43.
27. Coley WB. The treatment of malignant tumors by repeated innoculations of erysipelas with a report of ten original cases. Ann J Med Sci 1893; 105: 487.
28. LeVeen HH, Ahmed N, Piccone VA, et al. Radiofrequency therapy: clinical experience. Ann NY Acad Sci 1980; 335: 362-71.
29. Siperstein AE, Rogers SJ, Hansen PD, et al. Laparoscopic thermal ablation of hepatic neuroendocrine tumor metastases. Surgery 1997; 122: 1147-55.
30. Goldburg SN, Gazelle GS, Solbiati L, et al. Ablation of liver tumors using percutaneous RF therapy. Am J Res 1998; 170: 1023-8.
31. Lencioni R, Goletti O, Armillotta N, et al. Radio-frequency thermal ablation of liver metastases with a cooled-tip electrode needle: results of a pilot clinical trial. Eur Radiol 1998; 8(7): 1205-11.
32. Nagata Y, Hiraoka M, Nishimura Y, et al.

Clinical results of radiofrequency hyperthermia for malignant liver tumors. Int J Radiat Oncol Biol Phys 1997; 38(2): 359-65.
33. Curley SA, Vecchio R. New trends in the surgical treatment of colorectal cancer liver metastases. Tumori 1998; 84: 281-8.
34. MaGahan JP, Brock JM, Tesluk H, et al. Hepatic ablation with use of radio-frequency electrocautery in the animal model. JVIR 1992; 3: 291-7.
35. Seifert JK, Morris DL. World survey on the complication of hepatic and prostate cryotherapy. World J Surg 1999; 23(2): 109-13.
36. Sarantou T, Bilchik A, Ramming KP. Complications of hepatic cryosurgery. Semin Surg Oncol 1998; 14(2): 156-62.
37. McCarty TM, Kuhn JA. Cryotherapy for liver tumors. Oncology 1998; 12(7): 979-87.
38. Riley DK, et al. Infection complications of hepatic cryosurgery. Clin Infect Dis 1997; 24: 1001-3.
39. Seifert JK, Morris DL. Repeat hepatic cryotherapy for recurrent metastases from colorectal cancer. Surgery 1999; 125(2): 233-5.
40. Nagao T, et al. Postoperative recurrence of hepatocellular carcinoma. Ann Surg 1990; 211: 28-33.
41. Sasaki Y, et al. Regional therapy in the management of intrahepatic recurrence after surgery for hepatoma. Ann Surg 1987; 206: 40-7.
42. Seifert JK, Morris DL. Cryotherapy of the resection edge after liver resection from colorectal cancer metastases. Aust N Z J Surg 1998; 68(10): 725-8.
43. Adam R, et al. Place of cryosurgery in the treatment of malignant liver tumors. Ann Surg 1997; 225: 38-9.
44. Al-Hadeedi S, Choi TK, Wong J. Extended hepatectomy for hepatocellular carcinoma. Br J Surg 1990; 77: 1247-50.
45. Bilchik AJ, et al. Cryosurgery causes a profound reduction in tumor markers in hepatoma and noncolorectal hepatic metastases. Ann Surg 1997; 63: 796-800.
46. Cady B, Stone MD, McDermott WV JR, et al. Technical and biological factors in disease-free survival after hepatic resection for colorectal cancer metastases. Arch Surg 1992; 127: 561-9.
47. Hughes KS, et al. Resection of the liver for colorectal carcinoma metastases: a multi-institutional study of indications for resection. Surgery 1988; 103: 278-88.
48. Kanematsu T, et al. A comparative study of hepatic resection and transcatheter arterial embolization for the treatment of primary hepatocellular carcinoma. Cancer 1993; 71: 2181-86.
49. Korpan NN. Hepatic cryosurgery for liver metastases. Long-term follow-up. Ann Surg 1997; 225: 193-201.
50. Nagorney DM, et al. Primary hepatic malignancy: surgical management and determinants of survival. Surgery 1989; 106: 740-9.
51. Patt YZ, et al. Hepatocellular carcinoma: a retrospective analysis of treatments to manage disease confined to the liver. Cancer 1988; 61: 1884-8.
52. Ryu M, et al. Therapeutic results of resection, transcatheter arterial embolization and percutaneous transhepatic ethanol injection in 3225 patients with hepatocellular carcinoma: a retrospective multicenter study. Jpn J Clin Oncol 1997; 27: 251-7.
53. Scheele J, Stangl R, Altendorf-Hafmann A. Hepatic metastases from colorectal carcinoma: impact of surgical resection on the natural history. Br J Surg 1990; 77: 1241-6.
54. Yeh KA, et al. Cryosurgical ablation of hepatic metastases from colorectal carcinomas. Ann Surg 1997; 63: 63-8.
55. Yamada R, et al. Transcatheter arterial embolization in unresectable hepatocellular carcinoma. J Cardiovasc Intervent Radiol 1990; 13: 135-9.
56. Zhou XD, et al. An 18-year study of cryosurgery in the treatment of primary liver cancer. Asian J Surg 1992; 15: 43-47.
57. Ebra M, et al. Percutaneous ethanol injection for the treatment of hepatocellular carcinoma: study of 95 patients. Gastroenterol Hepatol 1990; 15: 615-26.
58. Lencioni R, et al. Long-term results of percutaneous ethanol injection therapy for hepatocellular in cirrhosis: a European experience. Eur Radiol 1997; 7: 514-9.

Laparoscopic Cholecystectomy in Situs Inversus Totalis: A Case Report

DR. KULDIP SINGH, MS
CONSULTANT LAPAROSCOPIC SURGEON
DEPARTMENT OF SURGERY
DAYANAND MEDICAL COLLEGE & HOSPITAL
LUDHIANA, INDIA

DR. ARUN DHIR, MS, DNB(SURG), FRCS(ED)
SENIOR RESIDENT
DEPARTMENT OF SURGERY
DAYANAND MEDICAL COLLEGE & HOSPITAL
LUDHIANA, INDIA

Some of the numerous anomalies of the biliary tract and its vasculature are incompatible with life, whereas others are only medical curiosities.[1] Many, however, are the cause of symptoms, and all are of particular concern to the surgeon who must operate in this area. An example is situs inversus totalis, an anomaly of the biliary tract that can present difficulties in management of abdominal disorders. We present a case of transposition of the viscera (situs inversus) with cholelithiasis, treated successfully with laparoscopy cholecystectomy. This article further affirms the safety and efficacy of laparoscopy in the setting of situs inversus totalis after giving due attention to the details of left-right reversal.

CASE REPORT

A 42-year-old woman was referred with epigastric pain, flatulence, and dyspepsia. Her liver functions were normal. An abdominal ultrasound disclosed a "left-sided" liver with the gallbladder fundus to the left of midline. The walls of the gallbladder were thickened and filled with multiple stones. Situs inversus totalis was confirmed on preoperative chest X-ray – displaying the reversed cardiac outline. Laparoscopy showed reversed positions of major abdominal viscera with the gallbladder located to the left of the falciform ligament. Additional ports were inserted to define the course of the cystic duct and any associated structural or vascular anomaly (Fig. 1). The cystic duct-hepatic duct junction was a mirror image of the normal; i.e., the cystic duct joining the hepatic duct from the left. The cystic artery and duct were clipped individually after meticulous dissection and prior identification. The gallbladder was deeply buried in the liver, requiring careful haemostasis. The postoperative course was uneventful. The patient remains symptom free six months later.

DISCUSSION

Anomalies of the extrahepatic biliary apparatus are infrequent radiographic and surgical findings. These may occur either in isolation or may be a part of associated anomalies. Situs inversus totalis is one such condition wherein totally reversed position of the major abdominal viscera is present. This auto-

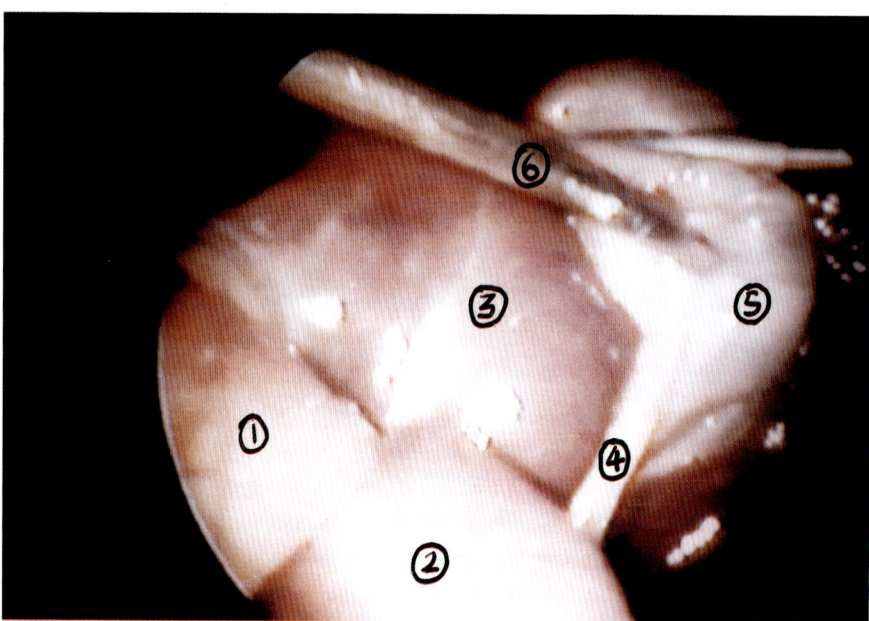

Figure 1. Laparoscopic cholecystectomy in a patient with situs inversus totalis — (1) Falciform ligament, (2) Rt. lobe of liver, (3) Lf. Lobe of Liver, (4) Cystic duct, (5) Gallbladder, (6) Grasper.

somal recessive condition occurs with a frequency of one in 35,000 births and is more common in males. Situs inversus totalis is associated with various other developmental anomalies including dextrocardia, asplenia, polysplenia, right-sided spleen, and immotile cilia Katageners syndrome (sinusitis, brochieactasis, and dextrocardia). If only some organs are reversed, the condition is known as partial situs inversus.

Gallbladders in patients with situs inversus may occasionally be the seat of disease. This situation then presents as a diagnostic and therapeutic challenge to the treating surgeon.

With the development of new radiologic modalities such as spiral computed tomography (CT), magnetic resonance (MR) cholangiography, and biliary scintigraphy, congenital anomalies of the biliary system are being increasingly diagnosed preoperatively.

The growing popularity of laparoscopy as a diagnostic and therapeutic option of choice in biliary disease deserves special mention in this context.[2] Laparoscopic cholecystectomy in situs inversus gallbladders depends primarily upon good exposure,[3] and needs careful placement of additional ports with reference to the anomalous gallbladder and falciform ligament. Suspicion of such a possibility may arise during a routine diagnostic evaluation; however, it is not unusual for such anomalies to surprise the surgeon in the theatre.

As in our situation where the operating surgeon was right-hand dominant, standing between the legs of the patient (French) – or better still on the right side of the patient—might not only facilitate dissection but also safeguard the common bile duct (CBD) with the dissection conducted away from it. Surgeons possessed with an equally dexterous left hand are able to perform better in such a clinical situation.

A successful laparoscopic cholecystectomy in situs inversus is based on the prime aim of a good exposure facilitating careful dissection. Additional port placement is as for a normal cholecystectomy—for retracting the fundus and the Hartmann's pouch, with adjustments made for the left-right reversal.

A review of the literature disclosed the role of laparoscopy as a preferred option in managing anomalous gallbladders.[1,5] Lipschutz et al.,[6] and more recently, Crosher et al in 1998,[2] all highlight the need for a meticulous dissection and clear definition of structures before cutting them. In the presence of a high incidence of associated structural, anomalies, emphasis is placed on intraoperative cholangiography not only to prevent damage to the CBD but also rule out accessory bile connections at any level.

The laparoscopic surgeon should be aware of this rare congenital anomaly, with particular attention to the preoperative confirmation of diagnosis and intraoperative left-right reversal of viscera. This case report further reaffirms the role of laparoscopy as an attractive approach for treatment of anomalous gallbladders.

ACKNOWLEDGMENT

The authors thank Mr. Tara Singh and Dr. Ravinder Malhotra for their editorial assistance.

REFERENCE

1. Gross RE. Congenital anomalies of the gall bladder. A review of 148 cases, with report of double gallbladder. Arch Surg 1936; 32: 131-62.
2. Crosher RF, Harnarayan P, Bremmer DN. Laparoscopic cholecystectomy in situs inversus totalis. J R Coll Surg Edinb 1996; 41(3): 183-4
3. D'Agata A, Boncompagni G. Video laparoscopic cholecystectomy in situ vicerum inversus totalis. Minerva Chir 1997; 52: 271-5.
4. Takei HT, Maxwell JG, Clancy TV, et al. Lap. chole. in situs inversus totalis. J Lap Surg 1992; 2: 171-6
5. Goh P, Tekant Y, Shims NS, et al. Lap. chole. in a patient with empyema and situs inversus. Endoscopy 1992; 24: 799-800.
6. Lipschutz JH, Canial DF, Hawes RH, et al. Lap. chole. and ERCP with stenting in an elderly patient with situs inversus totalis. Am J Gastro 1992; 87 : 218-220.

An Adjustable Silicone Gastric Band for Laparoscopic Treatment of Morbid Obesity— Techniques and Results

FRANCO FAVRETTI, M.D.
GIANNI SEGATO, M.D.
FRANCESCO DE MARCHI, M.D.
MAURIZIO DE LUCA, M.D.
MARIO LISE, M.D.

OBESITY CENTER
UNIVERSITY OF PADOVA, ITALY

GUY-BERNARD CADIERE, M.D.
JACQUES HIMPENS, M.D.
ELIE CAPELLUTO, M.D.
QUENTIN GAUDISSART, M.D.

SURGICAL DEPARTMENT
FREE UNIVERSITY OF BRUXELLES, BELGIUM

The laparoscopic application[1,2] of an adjustable silicone gastric band (Lap-Band™ System, Bioenterics, Carpinteria, CA) (Fig. 1), based on a similar device introduced by Kuzmak in 1986,[3] is gaining widespread acceptance as a gastric restrictive procedure in treatment of morbid obesity. The advantage of an operation that does not open the gastrointestinal tract and can be performed laparoscopically is obvious. This procedure, using the laparoscopic approach, has been performed in our institutions since 1992.[4] The goals of this article are to describe both our standardized surgical technique that minimized the morbidity rate[5,6] and its results.

SURGICAL TREATMENT

1. Positioning of the patient (Fig. 2). The patient lies supine, with thighs full abducted and slightly bent. The operating table has a 30° reversed Trendelenburg tilt. The surgeon stands between the patient's legs, the first assistant on the patient's left side and second assistant on the right.

2. Insufflation. A long Verres needle is introduced, usually above the umbilicus. Intraperitoneal insufflation is carried out. Intra-abdominal pressure is monitored at 15 mm Hg.

3. Placement of the trocars and instrumentation (Fig. 3). Five trocars are placed in the following sequence:
a) a 10-mm trocar for a 30° optical system, 6 finger breadths below the xyphoid.;
b) a 10-mm trocar for the liver retractor (sub-xyphoid);

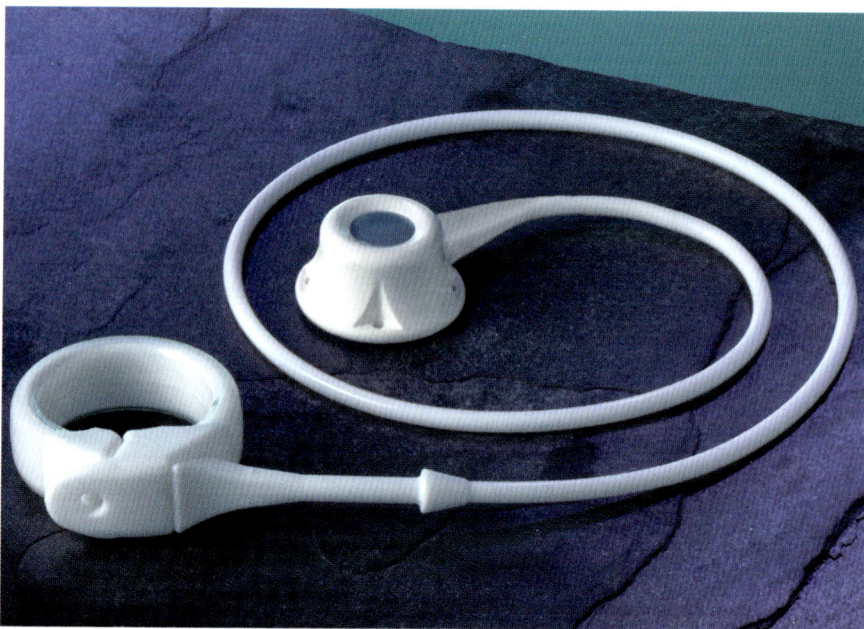

Figure 1. Lap Band™ System (Bioenterics Corporation, Carpinteria, CA).

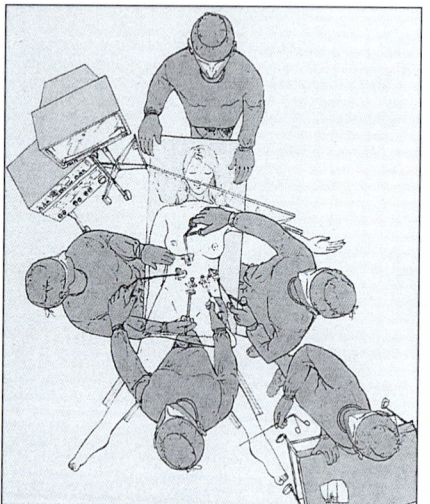

Figure 2. Patient positioning

Figure 3. Placement of trocars and instruments

c) a 10-mm trocar for the grasping forceps, articulating dissector, and Lap-Band™ closure tool (in the right upper quadrant);

d) a 10-mm trocar for the cautery hook, Endostitch (USSC-Tyco Healthcare, Norwalk, CT), grasping forceps, and reservoir placement (in L upper quadrant); and

e) a 10-mm trocar for the endo-babcock and band introduction (on the left anterior axillary line below the costal margin).

To minimize damage to the parietal vessels and abdominal organs, we routinely use an optical trocar (Visiport System, USSC-Tyco Healthcare, Norwalk, CT).

4. Initial dissection (Fig. 4). The anesthetist introduces a balloon-tipped nasogastric tube to the stomach, and insufflates 25 mL of air in the intragastric balloon, blocked at the gastroesophageal (GE) junction. The bulge seen on the stomach allows the surgeon to decide on the level of the initial dissection. The dissection on the lesser curvature begins at the equator of the calibration balloon. When decided, this level is marked by scoring the peritoneum on the lesser curvature with the coagulating hook. Therefore, the reference point on the lesser curvature is the equator of the balloon, which on the phrenogastric ligament (greater curvature), correlates to the left crus.

5. Dissection of the lesser curvature (Fig. 5). The lesser curvature is then dissected with the coagulating hook approximately 2 cm caudal from the

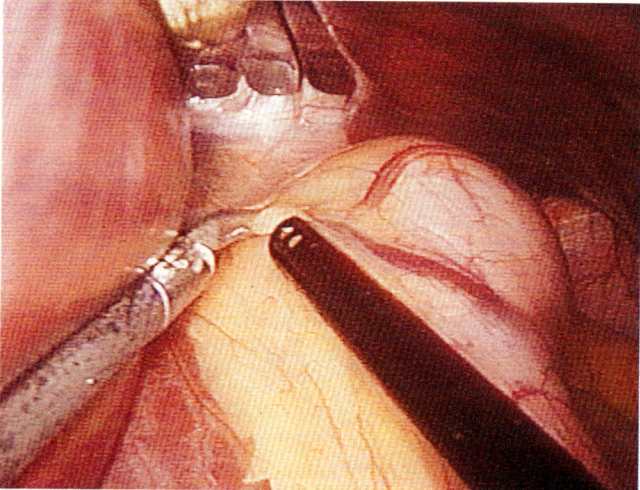

Figure 4. Initial dissection of the lower curvature begins at the equator of the calibration balloon.

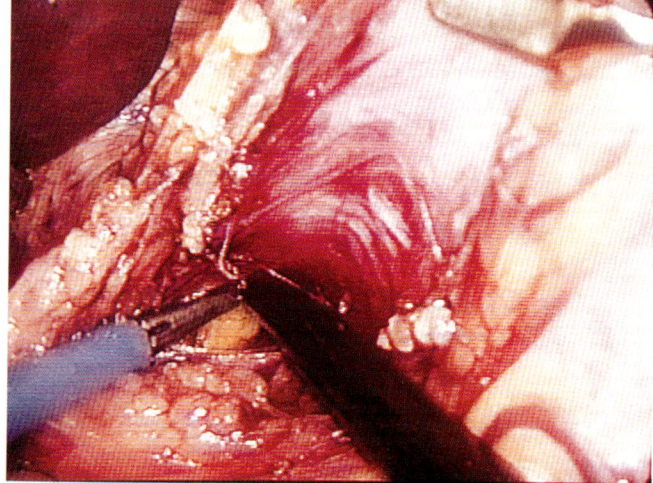

Figure 5. Dissection of Lower Curvature.

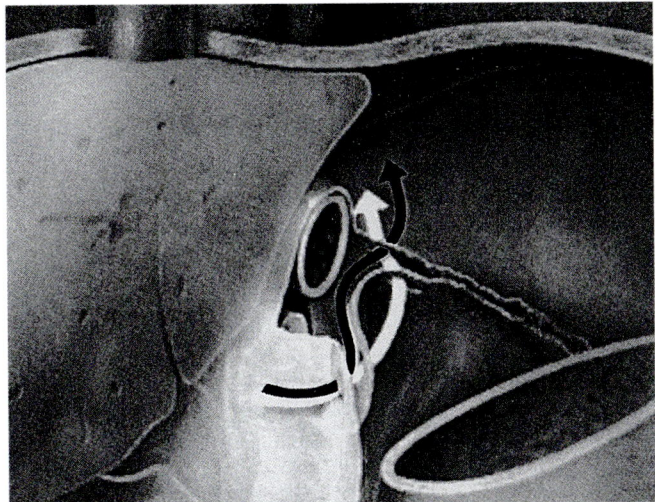
Figure 6. Retrogastric Dissection: above or below the peritoneal reflection of the bursa omentalis.

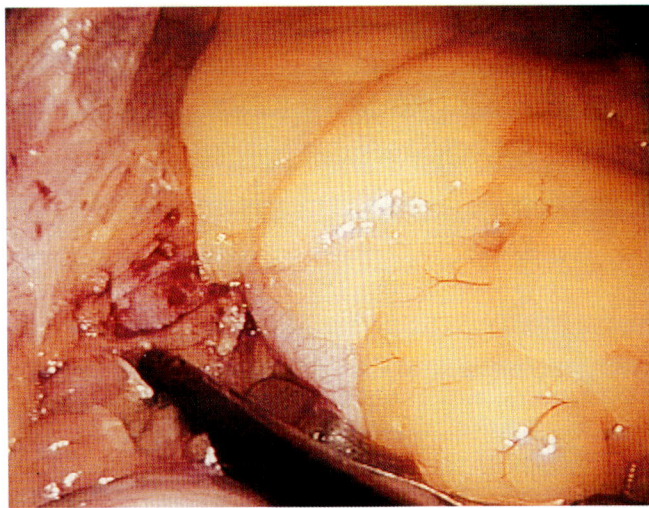
Figure 7. Dissection of phrenogastric ligament.

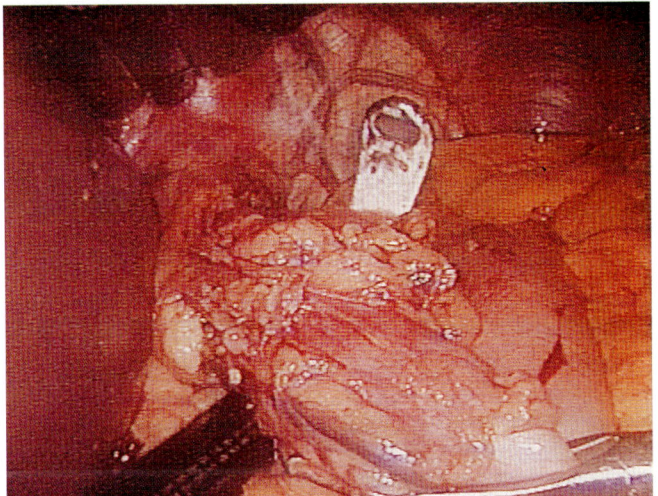
Figure 8. Articulating grasper is introduced into the retrogastric tunnel.

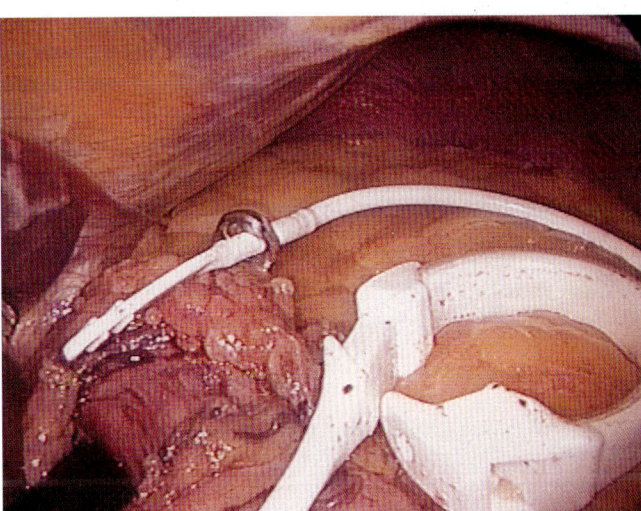
Figure 9. The adjustable silicone gastric band (Lap Band™) is grasped by the articulating dissector and looped around the stomach at the level of dissection.

cardia. From the right upper quadrant the grasping forceps holds the gastrohepatic ligament, the endo-babcock grasps the gastric wall from the left-most lateral trocar. This technique puts the peritoneum on the lesser curvature under tension. Dissection should be undertaken as close as possible to the gastric wall, care being taken not to damage it, and should preserve the nerve of Latarjet. Under direct vision, the full thickness of the gastrohepatic ligament is dissected from the gastric wall so as to make a narrow and limited opening. The posterior gastric wall is clearly recognizable. The dissection has to be of the same size as the band, or even less, to prevent the band from slipping.

To avoid stomach wall injuries, the calibration tube must be withdrawn during dissection, and should be carried out perpendicularly so as not to enter the inferior mediastinum along the esophagus.

6. Retrogastric dissection (Fig. 6). Two methods are possible:
   a) above the peritoneal reflection of the bursa omentalis, or
   b) below the peritoneal reflection of the bursa omentalis.

The authors prefer route a).

7. Dissection of the phrenogastric ligament (Fig. 7). The gastric fundus is pulled caudally by the grasper within the most lateral trocar, thereby putting the phrenogastric ligament under tension. A small window is then created in this ligament by using the coagulation hook. The location of this second window usually corresponds to the most prominent part of the left crus.

8. Retrogastric tunnel (Fig. 8). An articulating dissector (Endograsp Roticulator, USSC-Tyco Healthcare, Norwalk, CT), is introduced into the right upper quadrant trocar and advanced into the retrogastric tunnel under direct vision. The instrument is then curved and its extremity becomes visible in the dissection area of the phrenogastric ligament in front of the left crus. The coagulation hook can deal with the remaining fibrous strings and the articulating dissector is advanced until it emerges.

9. Introduction and placement of the adjustable silicone gastric band: Lap-Band™ (Fig. 9). In the path of the left most lateral 10-mm trocar, a Lap-Band

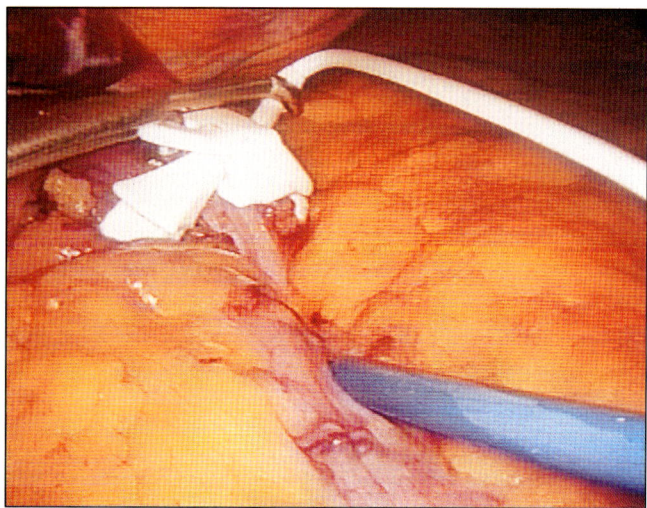

Figure 10. The band closing device is introduced and the band is tightened and locked

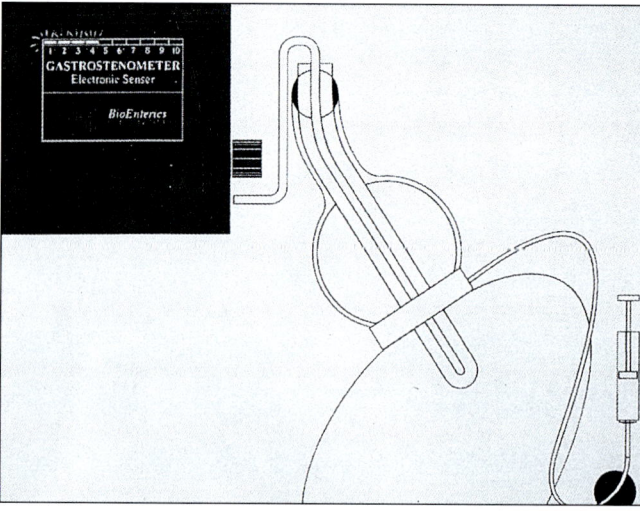

Figure 11. Calibration of the Lap Band™

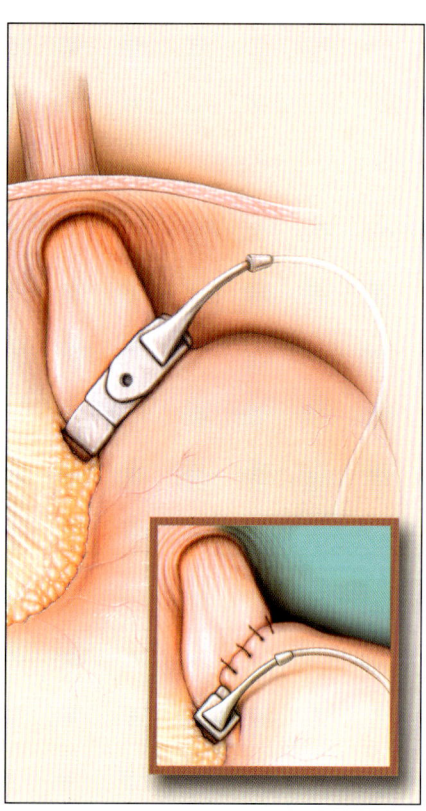

Figure 12. The Lap Band™ before and after completion of the gastrogastric suture stabilization.

with its tubing is introduced intraperitoneally. To introduce the Lap-Band™ no need exists for ports wider than 10 mm. The port is removed and its path used. The Lap-Band™ is subsequently grasped by the articulating dissector and looped around the stomach at the level of dissection. The tip of the tubing is introduced into the locking area of the band. The silicone band is tightened around the stomach.

10. Tightening (Fig. 10). The anesthetist reinsufflates 25 mL in the balloon-tipped nasogastric tube and again pulls it back until it hits the GE junction. The surgeon can now be assured of the correct positioning of the band. A specific tool for tightening of the band is introduced through the right upper quadrant trocar and the band is tightened and locked.

11. Calibration of the band (Fig. 11). The tip of the nasogastric tube contains pressure sensors. Saline solution is injected into the inflatable balloon of the silicone band with a syringe connected to the end of the non-kinking tube outside the abdominal cavity. This technique displaces the sequential lights on a gastrotenometer electronic sensor to the right until the fourth light is reached. The fourth light corresponds to the 12-mm stoma. This calibration is usually achieved with 2-4 mL of saline. The tube is double clamped with rubber-shod clamps and the redundant part cut and removed.

12. Suture stabilization of the silicone band (Fig. 12). The anesthetist withdraws the calibration tube. Three to five stitches are placed between the serosa of the stomach just proximal and distal to the band to avoid slipping.

Finally, a posterior fixation is performed, after opening the parts flaccida of the gastrohepatic ligament, only if the band has been placed below the peritoneal reflection of the bursa omentalis. These retention sutures prevent band and/or stomach slippage, and are placed between the seromuscular layer of the stomach just proximal and distal to the band. These anti-slippage sutures should start as close as possible to the greater curvature, achieving an "embedment" of the band.

If a gap is present on the lesser curvature it has to be closed by applying one or two stitches distal to the band between the lesser curvature and gastrohepatic ligament, taking care not to damage the vagus nerve.

Finally, a "virtual" pouch, based on a 25-mL measurement, is achieved.

13. Placement of the injection reservoir. The non-kinking tube is withdrawn through the port in the left hypochondrium. The port is subsequently removed and non-kinking tube cut to an appropriate length and connected to the injection reservoir. The reservoir is fixed with four stitches to the abdominal fascia in the left hypochondrium.

Thanks to this reservoir, the size of the gastric stoma can be adjusted by inflating the gastric band.

14. Silicone band (Lap-Band™) adjustment. The adjustment is performed in the radiology department postoperatively. Stoma size is adjusted depending on the patient's needs, weight loss curve, and x-ray.

PATIENTS

In 1992, Cadiere first showed the feasibility of using the laparoscopic approach for the Kuzmak adjustable gastric banding technique in five patients. A few modifications had to be introduced to make the band suitable for laparoscopy.

After these changes, from September 1993 to November 2000, a total of 830 patients (F: 78%; M: 22%) (Table 1) selected on the basis of the criteria of the American Society of Bariatric Surgery, underwent the laparoscopic adjustable gastric banding procedure (with Lap-Band™) at the Obesity Center of Padova University. Median age was 38 (15-65) years. The average body weight (BW) was 128 ± 23 (83-255) kg, and the body mass index (BMI) 46.5 ± 7 (33-76). Thirty-one percent of the patients had had previous abdominal surgery.

RESULTS

In our series, the mean operative time was 80 (49-240) minutes. In twenty-two (2.7%) patients, laparoscopy was abandoned because of (1) risky perigastric dissection (seven patients), (2) giant left liver lobe hypertrophy (six patients), (3) gastric perforation (four patients), (4) bleeding from a retrogastric vessel (two patients), (5) inadequate instrumentation (two patients, 0.3%), and (6) band malpositioning (one patient) (Table 2).

The mean hospital stay was 2-3 days. Gastrographin swallow was performed on the first postoperative day to check for leakage.

Morbidity and Mortality

The mortality rate was zero. Thirty-three patients (3.9%) experienced major complications (Table 3) and required reoperation. In the early postoperative course (<30 days) the Lap-Band™ had to be removed due to gastric perforation in one patient on the first postoperative day. The device had to be repositioned due to stomach slippage in another patient on day 14 postoperatively.

In the late postoperative course, seventeen (2%) patients experienced stomach slippage; in twelve patients the band was repositioned, and in five removed. In six (0.7%) patients a malpositioning of the band required repositioning. In four (0.5%) other patients band erosion occurred, requiring removal of the prosthesis. In three (0.4%) the prosthesis was removed for psychological intolerance and in one patient, for AIDS.

Eighty-two (9.8%) patients showed minor complications related to the reservoir. In two (0.2%) patients the reservoir was twisted, necessitating fixation. In three (0.4%) patients an

Table 1. LAP-BAND PATIENT CHARACTERISTICS

Period	September 1993-November 2000
Number of Patients	830 (female 78%, male 22%)
Age (years)	38 (range 15-76)
Weight (kg)	128 ± 23 (range 83-255)
Body Mass Index (BMI)	46.5 ± 7 (range 33-76)
Previous abdominal surgery	31%

Table 2. Lap-Band
Padova Series: 830 patients/September 1993-November 2000

Conversions

Risky perigastric dissection	7	(0.8%)
L. liver lobe hyeperthrophy	6	(0.7%)
Gastric perforation	4	(0.5%)
Bleeding (retrogastric vessel)	2	(0.2%)
Inadequate instruments	2	(0.2%)
Band malpositioning	1	(0.1%)
Total	22	(2.7%)

Table 3. LAP-BAND: MAJOR COMPLICATIONS REQUIRING REOPERATION
Padova Series: 830 patients, September 1993-November 2000

Early	Gastric Perforation (removal)	1 (0.1%)
	Stomach Slippage (repositioning)	1 (0.1%)
Late	Stomach Slippage: (12 repositioning, 5 removal)	17 (1.9%)
	Malpositioning (6 repositioning)	6 (0.8%)
	Erosions (4 removal)	4 (0.5%)
	Psychological Intolerance (3 removal)	3 (0.3%)
	AIDS (1 removal)	1 (0.1%)
Total		33 (3.9%)

Table 4. LAP-BAND: WEIGHT LOSS IN THE MORBIDLY OBESE GROUP
Padova Series: September 1993-November 2000

Years	0	1	2	3	4	5	6
Body weight (kg)	118.6	95.9	94.3	94.7	94.7	92.8	96.9
Body Mass Index	42.7	34.6	34.0	34.6	34.6	34.7	37.6
Patients	595	476	347	223	141	56	21

Table 5. LAP-BAND: WEIGHT LOSS IN THE SUPER OBESE GROUP

Padova Series: September 1993-November 2000

Years	0	1	2	3	4	5	6
Body weight (kg)	151.6	119.4	116.0	119.0	119.0	113.0	145.0
Body Mass Index	55.7	44.1	42.7	43.3	43.0	41.5	56.0
Patients	235	183	132	82	44	18	3

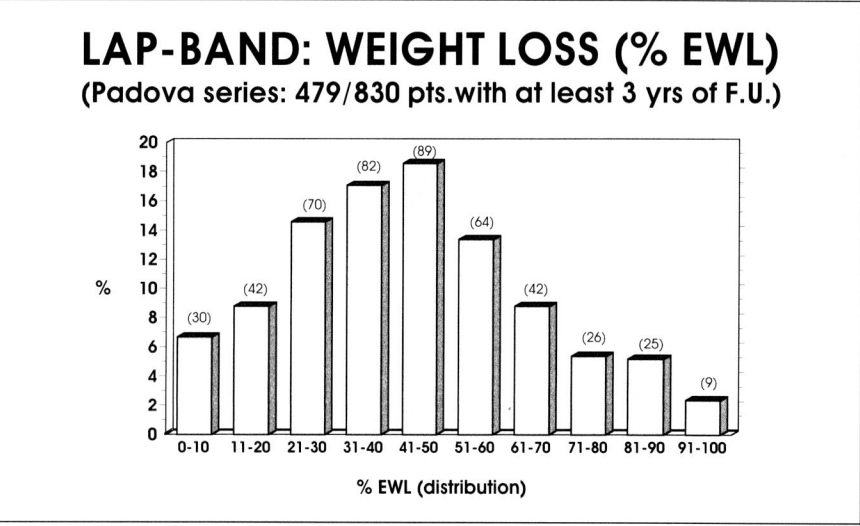

Figure 13. Three-year Lap Band™ patient weight loss follow-up: percentage excess weight loss (% EWL).

infection required removal of the reservoir. In 77 (9.2%) patients, the connecting tube had broken down and the reservoir was substituted.

Considering the weight loss (% EWL) in 479 of 830 patients with at least 3 years of follow up (Fig. 13), there is a total failure (≤20% EWL) in seventy-two (8.7%) patients. This group of patients did not lose enough weight, in most instances due to lack of compliance (59 patients), or to defective surgical technique (13 patients).

The weight loss in the morbidly obese group and in the super obese group is shown in Fig. 14 (BW), and in Fig. 15 (BMI). Weight loss (BW, BMI) in the (1) morbidly obese group is shown in Table 4 and (2) super obese group in Table 5.

CONCLUSION

The laparoscopic application [7,8] of a new adjustable silicone gastric band (Lap-Band™) belongs in the category of advanced laparoscopic procedures, and technical details of the procedure are of importance in reducing morbidity rates.

In an era of widespread acceptance of laparoscopic functional procedures, in which the role of the consequential quality of life is becoming of paramount importance, the Lap-Band™ can be considered a first procedure of choice for most morbidly obese patients.

REFERENCES

1. Cadiere GB, Bruyns J, Himpens J, et al. Laparoscopic gastroplasty for morbid obesity. Br J Surg 1994;81;1524-5.
2. Cadiere GB, Favretti F, Bruyns J, et al. Gastroplastic par coelio-videoscopie: Technique. Le Journal de Coelio-Chirurgie 1994;10:27-41.
3. Kuzmak L. Gastric Banding in Deitel M, ed.: Surgery for the morbidly obese patient. Philadelphia: Lea & Febbiger; 198.; p. 225-59.
4. Favretti F, Cadiere GB, Segato G, et al. Laparoscopic adjustable silicone gastric Banding (Lap Band): how to avoid complications. Obes Surg 1995:364-71.
5. Favretti F, Cadiere GB, Segato G, et al. Laparoscopic adjustable silicone gastric band (Lap-Band): how to avoid complications. Obes Surg 1997; 7:352-8.
6. Favretti F, Cadiere GB, Segato G, et al. Bariatric analysis and reporting outcome system (BAROS) applied to laparoscopic gastric banding patients. Obes Surg 1998;8:500-04.
7. Cadiere GB, Bruyns J, Himpens J, et al. Laparoscopic gastroplasty for morbid obesity. Br J Surg 1994;81;1524-5.
8. Cadiere GB, Favrett F, Bruyns J, et al. Gastroplastic par coelio-videoscopie: Technique. Le Journal de Coelio-Chirurgie 1994;10:27-41.

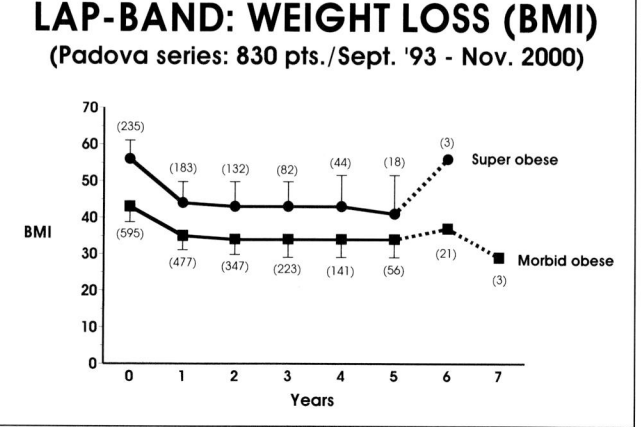

Figure 14. Three-year Lap Band™ patient weight loss follow-up: body weight (BW).

Figure 15. Three-year Lap Band™ patient weight loss follow-up: body mass index (BMI).

A New Technique for Laparoscopic Left Adrenalectomy

ANDRAS PAPP, M.D.
ANDRAS VERECZKEI, M.D.
ÖRS PETER HORVÁTH, M.D., D.SC.
DEPARTMENT OF SURGERY, MEDICAL UNIVERSITY OF PÉCS
PÉCS, HUNGARY

ZOLTÁN SZÁBO, PH.D., F.I.C.S.
MICROSURGERY & OPERATIVE ENDOSCOPY TRAINING INSTITUTE
SAN FRANCISCO, CA

After the first description of laparoscopic adrenalectomy was published in 1992,[1] this method rapidly attracted widespread interest.[2,3] Similar to conventional open techniques two main approaches have been established for the minimally invasive adrenalectomy: the transabdominal and the retroperitoneal.[4] With the transabdominal technique several different routes for exploration of the glands are possible as the patient can be operated on in a lateral, semi-lateral, or even in a supine position for both glands. Determining the best approach for the left side is further complicated because of the many possible techniques for exploration: through the gastrolienal, gastrocolic, or splenophrenic ligaments.[5,6,7,8] The authors have developed a new method for the left laparoscopic adrenalectomy using the splenophrenic approach.

METHOD

The patient is positioned in a semi-lateral, reverse-Trendelenburg position with the left side elevated. A Veress needle is used to establish a pneumoperitoneum through an incision cranial to and left of the umbilicus. After insufflation is established a 10-mm trocar is introduced through the initial opening for the camera. A 5-mm trocar caudal to the xyphoid process, and a 10-mm trocar in the midline between the two previously positioned trocars, are also introduced. The fourth trocar is placed in the anterior axillary line caudal to the costal margin to provide access for the fan retractor to hold the spleen in lateral and caudal directions. In significantly obese patients a fifth port can be placed between the camera and retractor ports to enhance exposure. Hemostatic dissection is accomplished with the use of an ultrasonic dissector.

Exploration is begun with an incision in the splenophrenic ligament, proceeding left from the left crus of the diaphragm. The upper pole of the left adrenal gland immediately comes into view and dissection is continued along the medial margin of the adrenal, until the upper pole of the kidney is visualized (Fig.1). In some cases dissection of the short gastric vessels may be necessary, and is performed in the same manner as in a fundoplication. Careful preparation along the lower margin is needed to isolate the main inferior vein of the gland. Once accomplished, two central and one peripheral clips are applied, and the vein is transected. Afterwards, further dissection of the lateral and posterior attachments with the ultrasonic dissector is performed.

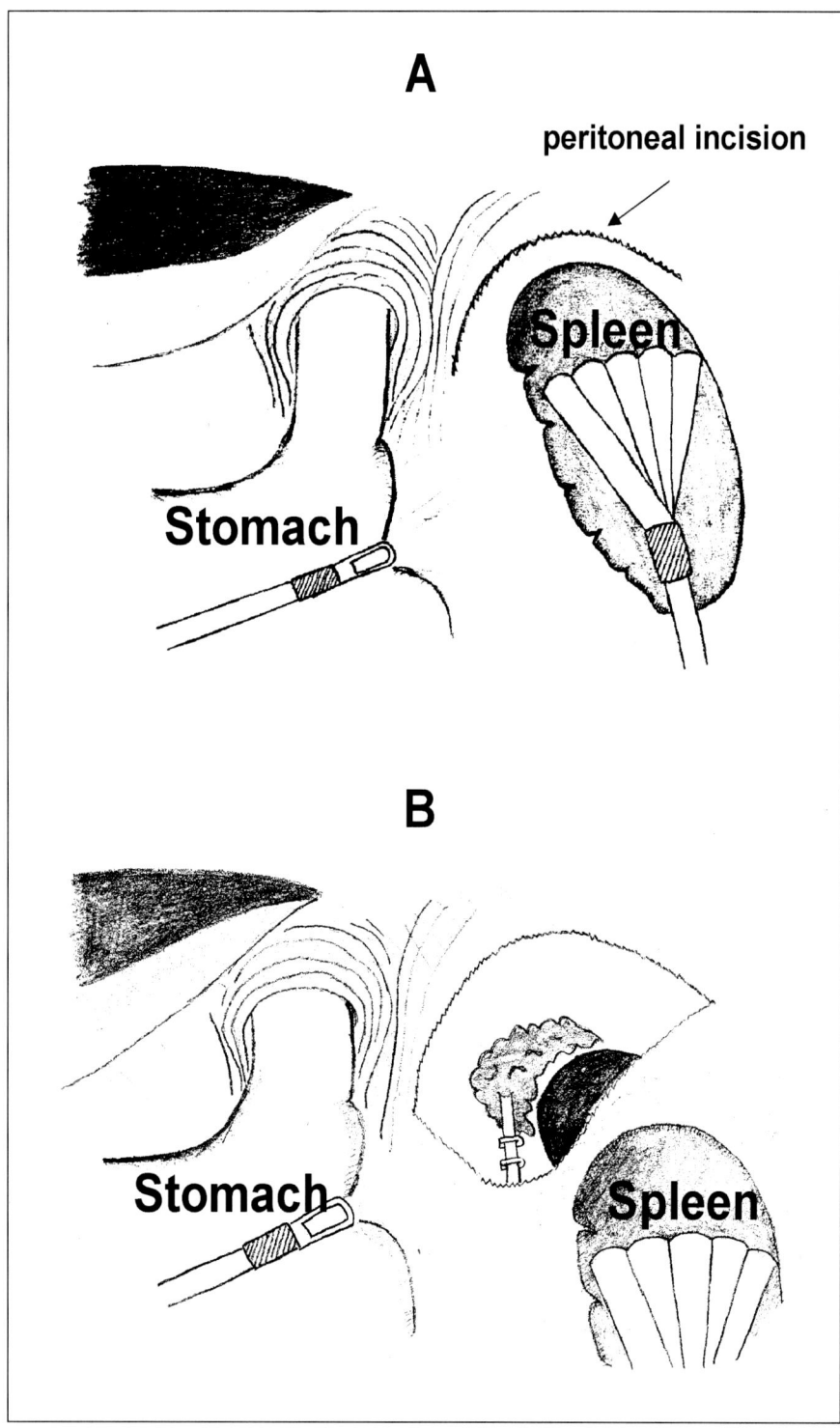

Figure 1. Left-sided supragastric approach to the adrenal gland, with (A) the peritoneal incision site and (B) retraction of the spleen.

Bleeding can occur from the inferior diaphragmatic vessels and from the short gastric vessels if dissection is not performed with sufficient care.

At the end of the operation the gland is removed in a laparobag, the operative field is irrigated, and after hemostasis is carefully established, a drain is placed under the left diaphragm.

RESULTS

Between June 1997 and April 2001, 32 cases of left laparoscopic adrenalectomies were attempted with this new method. The surgical indications, complications, operative times, transfusion requirements and mean hospital stays are presented in Table 1. In four cases conversion was necessary due to excessive bleeding: in one case the main polar vein at the inferior side was effected, and in the other three the short gastric vessels were involved. Two units of red blood cell transfusions were necessary in each of these converted cases.

In another case an intraoperative hypertensive episode occurred in a pheochromocytoma patient but was successfully controlled by the anesthetist. There were no trocar wound site infections and the postoperative course was uneventful in all 32 cases. The longer hospital stay (total of 8.5- 9.5 days: 2-3 days pre-operative and 6.5 days postoperative) were characteristic of our national custom rather than of actual patient need.

DISCUSSION

A new technique for left laparoscopic adrenalectomy, adapted from the conventional open method by the authors, was safely introduced and performed in 28 out of 32 cases (87.5%). The 4 converted cases could be attributed to the early learning curve associated with a new approach. The 80-minute average operative time is significantly lower than those of techniques previously reported in the literature (123-240 minutes),[2,3,9] and results from the improved accessibility of the left adrenal gland.

With all previously described approaches, considerable time is needed to first expose the adrenal gland, prior to beginning the essential aspects of the procedure. With the new technique, visualization of the left adrenal gland is accomplished early in the procedure, immediately following dissection of the splenophrenic ligament. In most cases the main inferior suprarenal vein at the inferior pole can also be completely visualized, together with the left renal vein, thereby obviating the need for mobilization of the tail of the pancreas, the colon, or the stomach, and consequentially avoiding a primary morbidity factor associated with laparoscopic adrenalectomy. Preparation around the gland could be further expedited with the use of an ultrasonic dissector.

CONCLUSION

Elimination of the significant wound site infection rate (approximately 10% in

Table 1. Patient clinical and operative data

Patients	Male	7	
	Female	25	
	Mean age in years (and range of age)	48.43	(21-75)
Indications	Elevated aldosterone level with hypertension	10	
	Elevated cortisol level with hypertension and obesity	16	
	Elevated cathecolamine level with hypertension	2	
	Elevated DHEA level with virilization, and allopecia or hypertension	4	
Histology	Cortical adenoma	21	
	Phaeochromocytoma	2	
	Focal nodular hyperplasia	7	
	Cortical adrenal cyst	2	
Complications	Conversions due to bleeding	4	
	Intraoperative bleeding without conversion	2	
	Intraoperative hypertensive episode (220/130)	1	
Operative time	Mean operative time in minutes (and range)	80.18	(42 -125)
Hospitalization	Total hospitalization in days (and range)	6.5	(4-12)
	Postoperative hospitalization in days (and range)	3.7	(2-9)

the authors' experience) associated with the conventional approach is accomplished with all laparoscopic approaches. However, with reduced complication rates and zero mortality experienced to date, it can be concluded that this procedure is be a viable alternative to the existing approaches to the left transabdominal laparoscopic adrenalectomy.

REFERENCES

1. Gagner M., Lacroix A., Bolte E.: Laparoscopic adrenalectomy in Cushing's syndrome and pheochromocytoma. New Engl. J. Med. 327, 1003-1006, 1992.
2. Gagner M., Pomp A., Heniford T.B., et al.: Laparoscopic adrenalectomy. Lessons learned from 100 consecutive procedures. Ann. Surg. 226, 3, 238-247, 1997.
3. Terachi T., Matsuda T., Terai A., et al.: Transperitoneal laparoscopic adrenalectomy: experience in 100 patients. J. Endourol. 11, 361-365, 1997.
4. Brunt M.L., Soper N.J.: Laparoscopic adrenalectomy. In: Arregui M.E., Fitzgibbons, R.J.jr., Katkhouda N., et al.: Principles of laparoscopic surgery. Springer Verlag, 1995. 366-378.
5. Bonjer H.J., Lange J. F., Kazemier W.W.: Comparison of three techniques for adrenalectomy. Br. J. Surg., 84, 679-682, 1997.
6. Duh Q.Y., Siperstein A.E., Clark O. H., et al.: Laparoscopic adrenalectomy. Comparison of the lateral and posterior approaches. Arch.Surg. 131, 870-875, 1996.
7. Filiponi S., Guerrieri M., Arnaldi G., et al.: Laparoscopic adrenalectomy: a report on 50 operations. Eur. J. Endocrinol. 138, 548-553, 1998.
8. Lezoche E., Guerrieri M., Paganini A.M., et al.: Laparoscopic adrenalectomy by the anterior transperitoneal approach: results of 108 operations in unselected cases. Surg. Endosc. 14(10), 920-925, 2000.
9. Henry J.F., Defechereux T., Raffaelli M., et al.: Complications of laparoscopic adrenalectomy: results of 169 consecutive procedures. World J. Surg. 24(11), 1342-46, 2000.

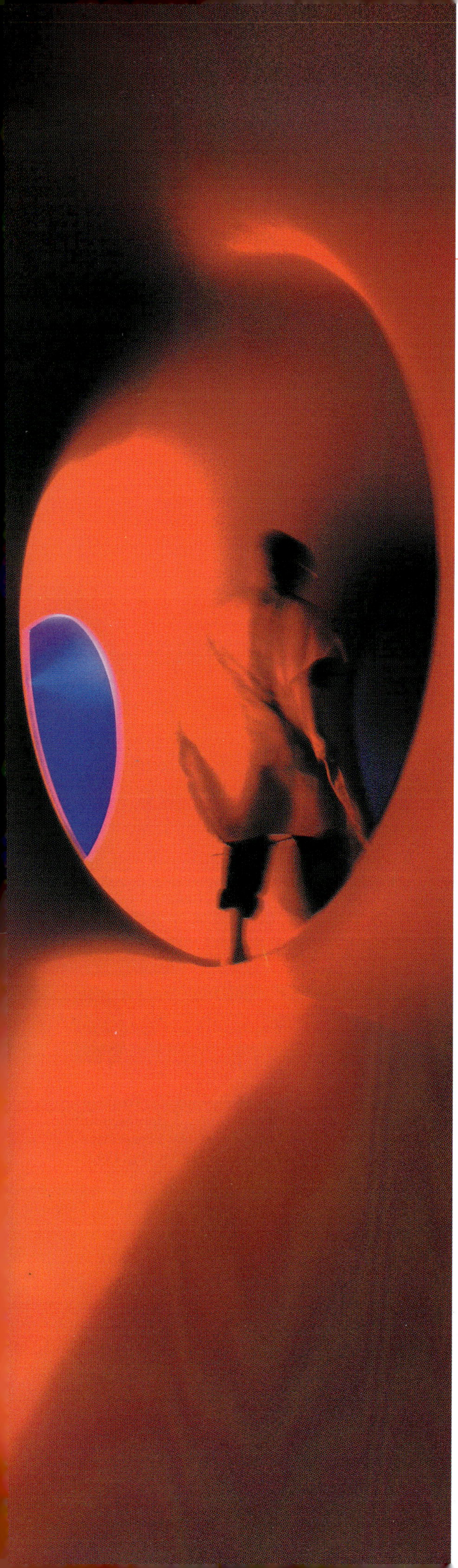

THE FUTURE TODAY

IN
CARDIOVASCULAR & THORACIC SURGERY

The surgical procedures and techniques of Cardiovascular and Thoracic Surgery demand an increasingly specialised range of products dedicated to complimenting the surgeon's skill.

CardioVations meets this need by providing a range of technically advanced products supported by superior service and a dedicated education programme.

Select CardioVations and experience 'The Future Today'.

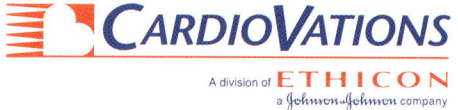

A division of ETHICON
a Johnson-Johnson company

European Marketing, Oststraße 1, 22844 Norderstedt, Germany

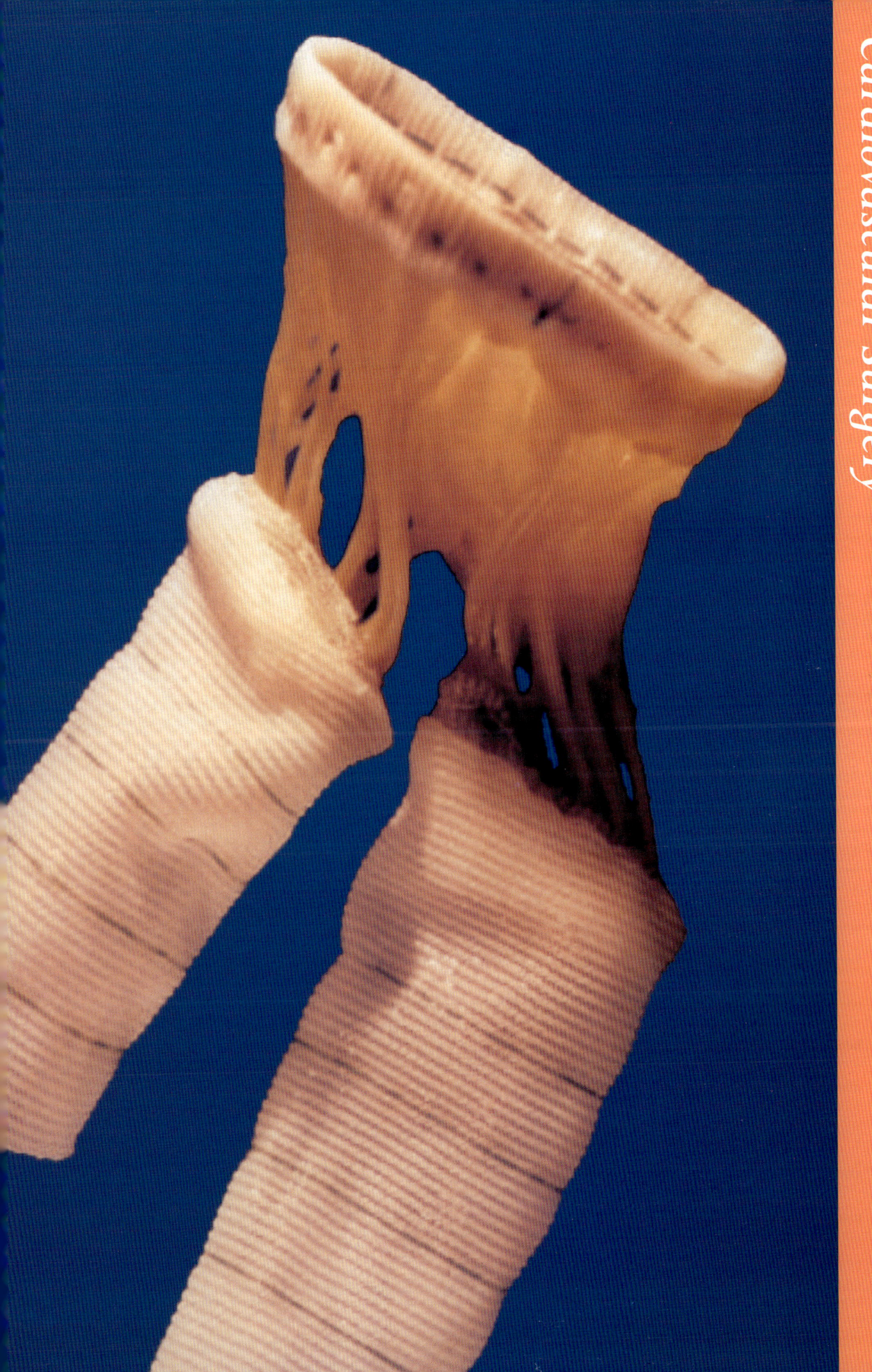
Cardiovascular Surgery

ST. JUDE MEDICAL

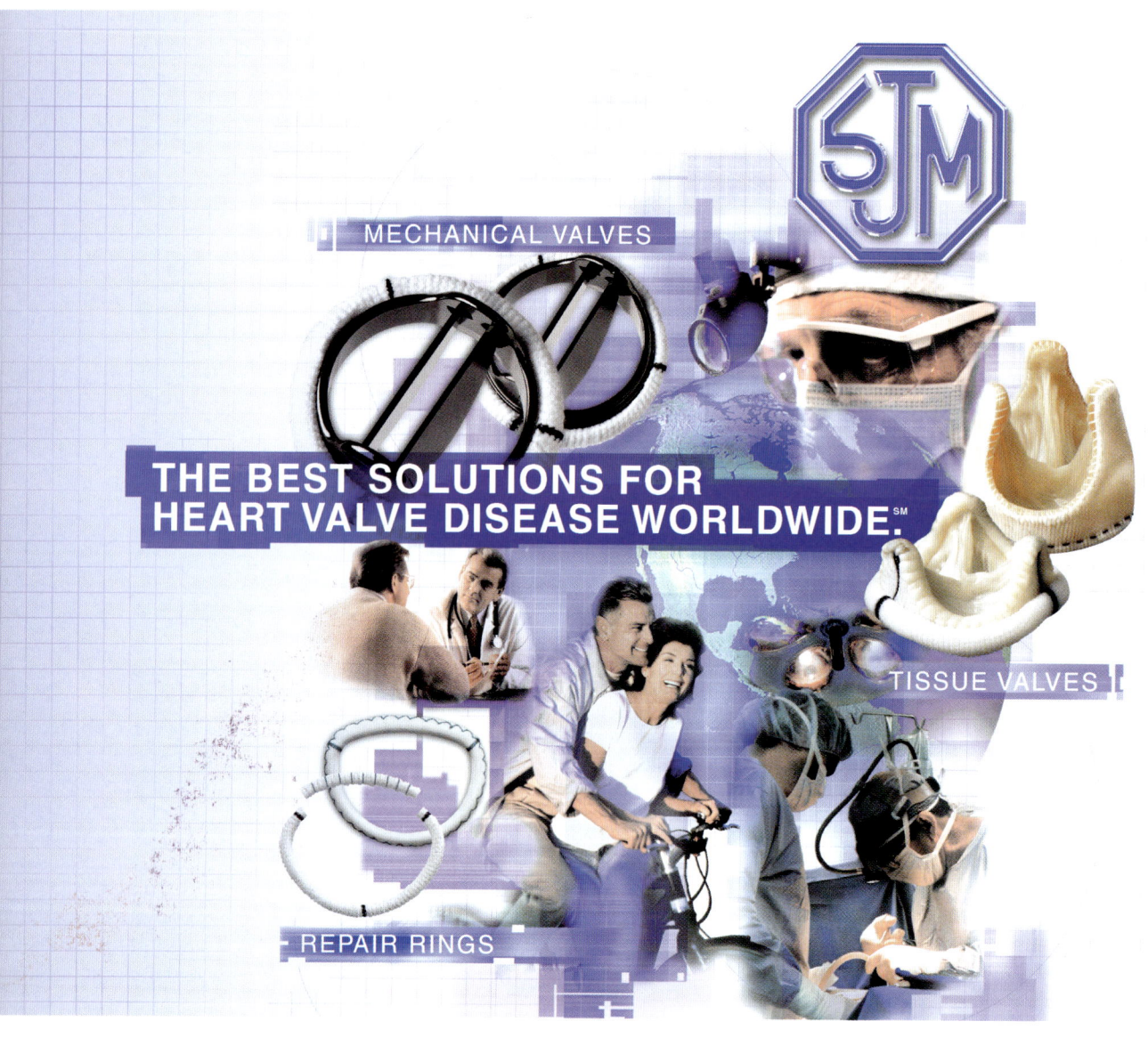

THE BEST SOLUTIONS FOR HEART VALVE DISEASE WORLDWIDE.℠

MECHANICAL VALVES

TISSUE VALVES

REPAIR RINGS

For more than 20 years, St. Jude Medical's innovative technologies and products have advanced the field of heart valve repair and replacement. Our full line of mechanical valves, tissue valves and repair rings continue to set the industry standard for performance and reliability. Yet, providing the best solutions means more than supplying the best products. It also means understanding and meeting the needs of physicians, demonstrating leadership, responsibility, and having an unwavering commitment to patient safety and well-being, every single day. St. Jude Medical. *The Best Solutions for Heart Valve Disease Worldwide.*℠ Yesterday. Today. And Tomorrow.

1 MILLION IMPLANTS 1977–2000 MECHANICAL HEART VALVES

SOME OF THESE DEVICES MAY NOT BE COMMERCIALLY AVAILABLE IN THE UNITED STATES OR IN OTHER INTERNATIONAL MARKETS PENDING REGULATORY REVIEW AND APPROVAL. The Best Solutions for Heart Valve Disease Worldwide is a service mark of St. Jude Medical, Inc. Patents pending. St. Jude Medical Heart Valve Division. ©2000 St. Jude Medical, Inc. All rights reserved. 0300200423EN **VISIT OUR WEBSITE AT** http://www.sjm.com

Current and Advanced Prostheses for Cardiac Valvular Replacement and Reconstructive Surgery

W. R. Eric Jamieson, M.D., F.R.C.S. (C)
Professor of Surgery and Director of Surgical Research-Heart Center
University of British Columbia
University Heart Centre, St. Paul's Hospital, Vancouver Hospital and Health Sciences Centre
Vancouver, Canada

The purpose of this communication is to provide an overview of modern cardiac valvular devices for replacement and reconstruction used worldwide, as well as innovative technologies and devices poised to improve clinical performance.

Advancements in cardiac valvular replacement devices over the past 25 years have left residual problems with biological and mechanical prostheses. The extensive developments were introduced to reduce or eliminate valve-related complications, namely thromboembolism, anticoagulant-related hemorrhage, and structural failure; and optimize hemodynamic performance. Residual problems persist with both biological and mechanical prostheses. Structural failure of porcine and pericardial bioprostheses persist over time, with leaflet degeneration and dystrophic calcification. Thrombus formation from blood stasis, and the resultant thromboembolic phenomena despite anticoagulant management, remain a continuing problem with mechanical prostheses. The innovative technologies under investigation will likely improve the clinical performance of both biological and mechanical prostheses significantly.

The current mechanical prostheses have been developed to eliminate structural failure, facilitate intraoperative leaflet positioning, and facilitate radioopacity for evaluation of prosthesis function. The present biological valvular prostheses have been developed with tissue preservation, together with stent designs, that contribute to preservation of anatomical characteristics and biomechanical properties of the leaflets.

The current mechanical and biological prostheses are designated in Tables 1 and 2. Current devices to support reconstructive atrioventricular valvular procedures are designated in Table 3. The experimental and developmental replacement and reconstructive devices are listed in Tables 4 and 5, respectively.

For the past 30 years, there has been a choice of bioprostheses and mechanical prostheses for cardiac valve replacement surgery.[1-3] These developments over the past two decades have been introduced to reduce or eliminate valve-related complications, namely thromboembolism and thrombosis, and anticoagulant-related hemorrhage with mechanical prostheses, and structural failure of bioprostheses. The prostheses designs have facilitated optimal hemodynamic performance. The prostheses, current and advanced generation, illustrated in this article have not significantly altered the incidence of these valve-related complications. The advanced technologies that will be incorporated in prosthesis design and formulation in the future are discussed in this overview.

Surgical management of valvular heart disease is not limited to the use of porcine and bovine pericardial bioprostheses and mechanical prostheses. Valvular reconstructive techniques, for mitral valve predominately over aortic valve, have been developed and popularized primarily by Carpentier, Cosgrove, David, Duran, Yacoub, Miller and their colleagues.[4-13] Mitral-valve reconstruction has provided superior results for degenerative disease over chronic rheumatic disease.[4] Aortic valve reconstruction has been used primarily for manifestations of congenital disease, but long-term results have yet to be reported.

Biological prostheses have not been limited to heterographic tissue. The allograft (homograft) has long been used as an aortic valve substitute either as a cryopreserved valve, or a hypothermic "homovital" valve, obtained from hearts explanted at transplantation.[14,15] The allograft is usually implanted as a subcoronary valve, or as an aortic root replacement with reconstruction of the coronary ostia.[16,17] The allograft is limited by availability and usually reserved for younger patients or management of native and prosthetic valve endocarditis.

The pulmonary autograft is another alternative for aortic valve replacement, especially in children for reconstruction of complex congenital disease. The autograft is recommended for children because it remains viable, grows in proportion to somatic growth, and the annulus and sinotubular junction is increased in size to the normal range.[18,19] The experience of the pulmonary autograft in young to middle-aged adults in the past decade is currently becoming available.

PROSTHETIC FAILURE MODES AND REMEDIES IN ADVANCEMENT

Several identified modes of failure of valvular prostheses have been attributed to the structural components of the prostheses. Structural valve deterioration has been the predominant valve-related complication of glutaraldehyde-preserved biological prostheses.[20-32] Porcine, or bovine pericardial bioprostheses, fail over extended periods of implantation—related to age at implantation—by dystrophic calcification, primary stress-related tears, or perforations or tears secondary to minimal or moderate calcification.

The prosthetic failure modes of mechanical prostheses have been structural failure, predominantly historical, and thromboembolic phenomena, including thrombosis.[23,33-38]

MECHANICAL PROSTHESES—CURRENT

The principle mechanical prostheses available primarily worldwide are listed in Table 1. The original successful mechanical prosthesis was the Starr-Edwards caged-ball valve, the gold standard prosthesis for over 20 years until the early 1980s. Mechanical prostheses subsequently were either monoleaflet or bileaflet prostheses with pyrolytic carbon leaflets, and titanium or pyrolytic carbon housing. Tungsten is used to facilitate radio-opacity of the leaflets, as well as the metallic-band reinforcement, if used. The housing is rotatable within the sewing ring in most prostheses. Retrograde washing facilitates prevention of blood stasis and thrombus formation. The monoleaflet prostheses have crossing bars or central guides to control leaflet travel, whereas bileaflet prostheses, in general, have pivot recesses in parallel flat segments of the orifice to control leaflet travel.

Table 1. Mechanical Prostheses—Current

Caged-Ball
- Starr-Edwards Mechanical Prosthesis

Monoleaflet
- Björk-Shiley Monostrut Mechanical Prosthesis
- Sorin Monoleaflet Allcarbon Mechanical Prosthesis
- Medtronic-Hall Mechanical Prosthesis
- Omnicarbon Mechanical Prosthesis
- Ultracor Mechanical Prosthesis

Bileaflet
- St. Jude Medical Mechanical Prosthesis
- Carbomedics Mechanical Prosthesis
- Edwards Tekna Mechanical Prosthesis
- Sorin Bicarbon Mechanical Prosthesis
- Edwards Mira Mechanical Prosthesis
- ATS Mechanical Prosthesis
- On-X Mechanical Prosthesis
- Medtronic Advantage Mechanical Prosthesis

MECHANICAL PROSTHESIS—CAGED-BALL

Starr-Edwards Mechanical Prosthesis

The caged-ball Starr-Edwards mechanical prosthesis (Edwards Lifeservices, Irvine, California, U.S.A.) has been marketed in current version since 1968 (Figs. 1-1 & 1-2). The Starr-Edwards silastic ball valve prosthesis is composed of a polished Stellite alloy cage with a combination of polytetrafluoroethylene (PTFE) and polypropylene cloth sewing ring. The PTFE cloth is wrapped around a porous silastic sponge insert to facilitate tissue infiltration. The ball is made of silicone rubber and contains barium sulfate for radiopacity. The Stellite cage is made from single

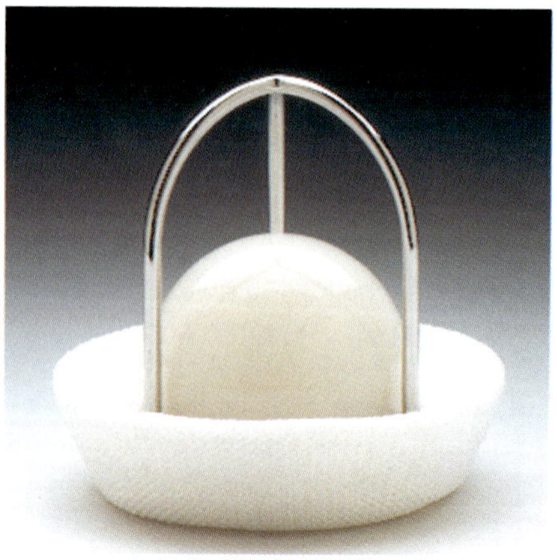

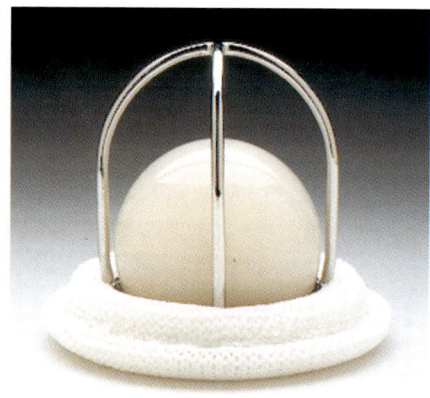

Figure 1-1. Starr-Edwards Aortic Mechanical Prosthesis.

Figure 1-2. Starr-Edwards Mitral Mechanical Prosthesis.

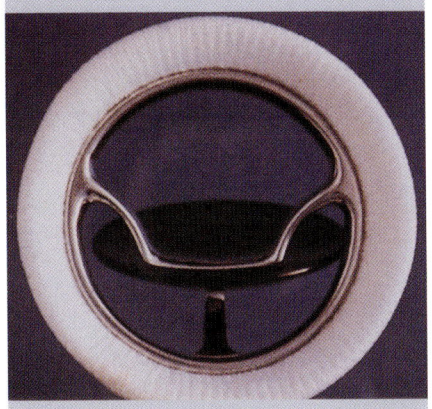
Figure 2. Björk-Shiley Monostrut Mechanical Prosthesis.

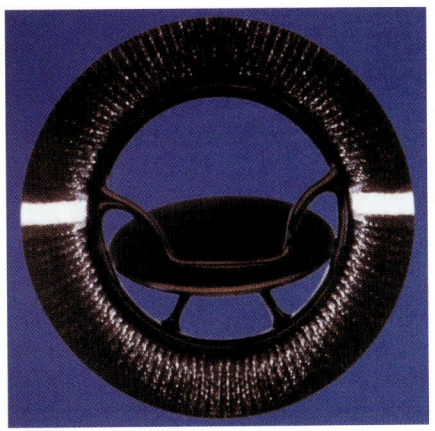
Figure 3. Sorin Monoleaflet Allcarbon Mechanical Prosthesis.

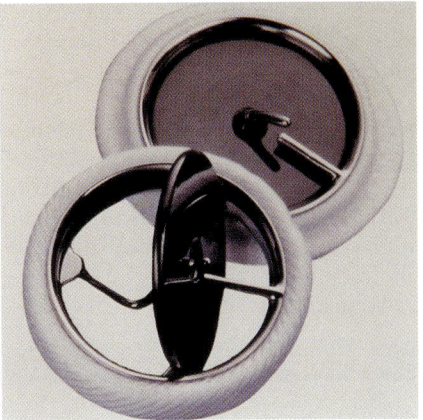
Figure 4. Medtronic-Hall Mechanical Prosthesis.

casting and is radiopaque with three struts in the aortic prosthesis and four struts in the mitral prosthesis. The ball can be removed from the aortic prosthesis (not the mitral prosthesis) for ease of implantation. The aortic prosthesis is model 1260 (Fig. 1-1) with a pediatric prosthesis model 1200. The mitral prosthesis is model 6120 (Fig. 1-2).

MECHANICAL PROSTHESES—MONOLEAFLET

Björk-Shiley Monostrut Mechanical Prosthesis

The Björk-Shiley Monostrut mechanical prosthesis is a monoleaflet prosthesis (Fig. 2). The orifice ring and integral struts are constructed from a single piece of cobalt chromium alloy. A pyrolytic carbon disc contains a radio-opaque tantalum marker. The opening angle is 70° and the valve can be rotated within the sewing ring. Leaflet motion is by rotation and translation. Retrograde washing is by relatively low-velocity blood flow through controlled backflow between the leaflet edge and orifice. This prosthesis is currently not manufactured.

Sorin Monoleaflet Allcarbon Mechanical Prosthesis

The Sorin Monoleaflet Allcarbon mechanical prosthesis (Sorin Biomedica, Saluggia, Italy) is a monoleaflet prosthesis constructed of a cobalt chromium alloy housing coated with a thin film of pyrolytic carbon (Carbofilm™), with a single monoleaflet of pyrolytic carbon (Fig. 3). The strut mechanism is integral with the housing with no welds. The sewing ring is carbon coated to reduce and stabilize surface-tissue reaction.

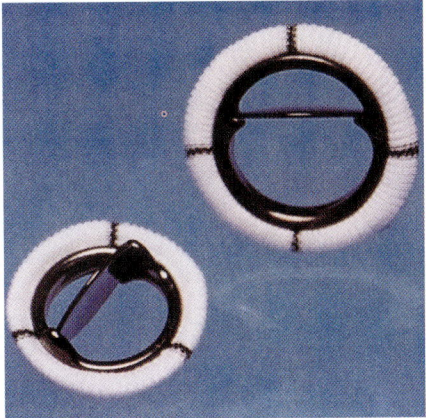
Figure 5. Omnicarbon Mechanical Prosthesis.

Medtronic-Hall Mechanical Prosthesis

The Medtronic-Hall mechanical prosthesis (Medtronic, Inc., Minneapolis, Minnesota, U.S.A.) is a monoleaflet prosthesis with a central guide for leaflet travel (Fig. 4). The housing and central guide are made of titanium and the disc of pyrolytic carbon. The prosthesis can be rotated within the sewing ring; leaflet motion is by rotation and translation. The opening angle is 70° to 75°. The disc has a tungsten-loaded substrate for radio-opacity.

Omnicarbon Mechanical Prosthesis

The Omnicarbon mechanical prosthesis (CV Medical, Inc., Inver Grove Heights, Minnesota, U.S.A.) is a monoleaflet prosthesis with a pyrolitic carbon coating over a graphite substrate orifice and a pyrolitic carbon disc (Fig. 5). The disc motion is controlled by short struts. The opening angle is 80°. The Omniscience mechanical prosthesis

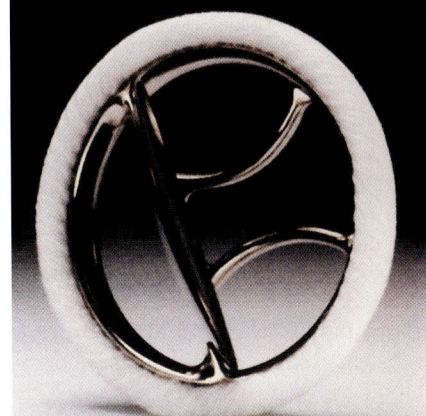

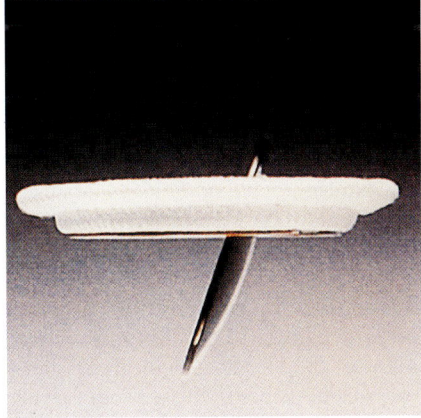
Figure 6 a & b. Ultracor Mechanical Prosthesis.

is similar except the housing is made of titanium.

Ultracor Mechanical Prosthesis

The Ultracor mechanical prosthesis (Aortech Europe, Ltd., Bellshill, Scotland, UK) is a monoleaflet prosthesis with a plano convex disc with pyrolitic carbon coating on a tungsten-impregnated graphite substrate (Fig. 6 a & b). The prosthesis design eliminates flow impedence structures in the lesser orifice by the single strut. The orifice ring is machined from solid titanium, eliminating welds. The opening angle is 73° in the aortic and 68° in the mitral. The central location of the disc pivot axis increases laminar blood flow. The sewing ring is made of knitted Teflon™ to promote rapid tissue ingrowth. The sewing ring allows *in situ* rotation of the housing. The disc is radiographic for imaging.

MECHANICAL PROSTHESES—BILEAFLET

St. Jude Medical Mechanical Prostheses

The St. Jude Medical mechanical prosthesis (St. Jude Medical, Inc., St. Paul, Minnesota, U.S.A.) is a bileaflet prosthesis with pyrolytic carbon over graphite substrate for housing and leaflets (Fig. 7-1). The leaflets are flat and impregnated with tungsten for radio-opacity. The two semicircular leaflets open to 85°, resulting in central, near laminar flow. The leaflets are orifice-orientated and closing forces are supported by the pivot system. The pivot guards are raised above the housing, and leaflet motion is by rotation. Relatively high-velocity blood and approximately 10% to 15% regurgitant flow wash the pivot recesses. In the original prosthesis, the housing could not be rotated. The prosthesis has been altered in the Masters (Fig. 7-2) series to rotate within the sewing ring and provide radio-opacity of the annular rotating mechanism.

The St. Jude Medical HP (high performance) (Fig. 7-3) and Regent™ (Fig. 7-4) prostheses have been introduced and are designed to optimize hemodynamics (Fig. 7-3). Development of the St. Jude Medical mechanical prosthesis has led to a progressively greater geometric orifice area while maintaining the same tissue annulus dimension (Fig. 7-5). In the standard cuff St. Jude Medical mechanical prosthesis, part of the cuff fabric is intra-annular, whereas in the HP Series prosthesis this fabric has shifted to an entirely supra-annular position. The St. Jude Medical Regent™ prosthesis shifts the carbon rim from intra-annular to entirely supra-annular.

Carbomedics Mechanical Prostheses

The Carbomedics mechanical pros-

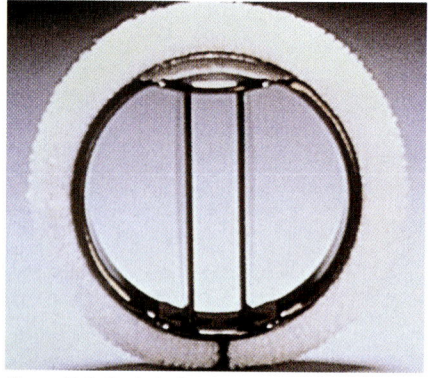

Figure 7-1. St. Jude Medical Standard Mechanical Prosthesis.

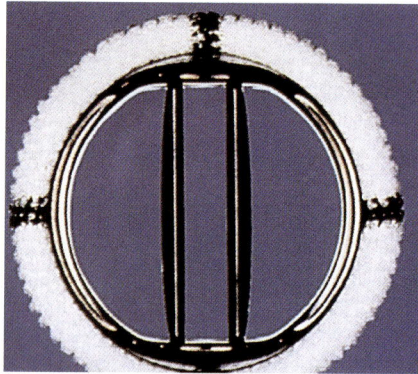

Figure 7-2. St. Jude Medical Masters Mechanical Prosthesis.

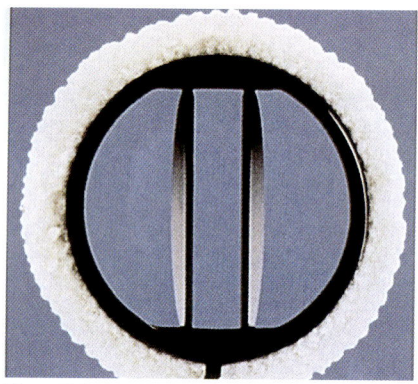

Figure 7-3. St. Jude Medical HP Mechanical Prosthesis.

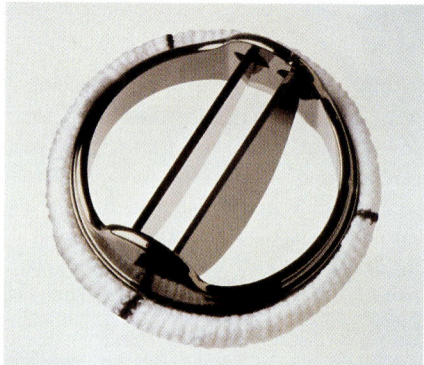

Figure 7-4. St. Jude Medical Regent™ Mechanical Prosthesis.

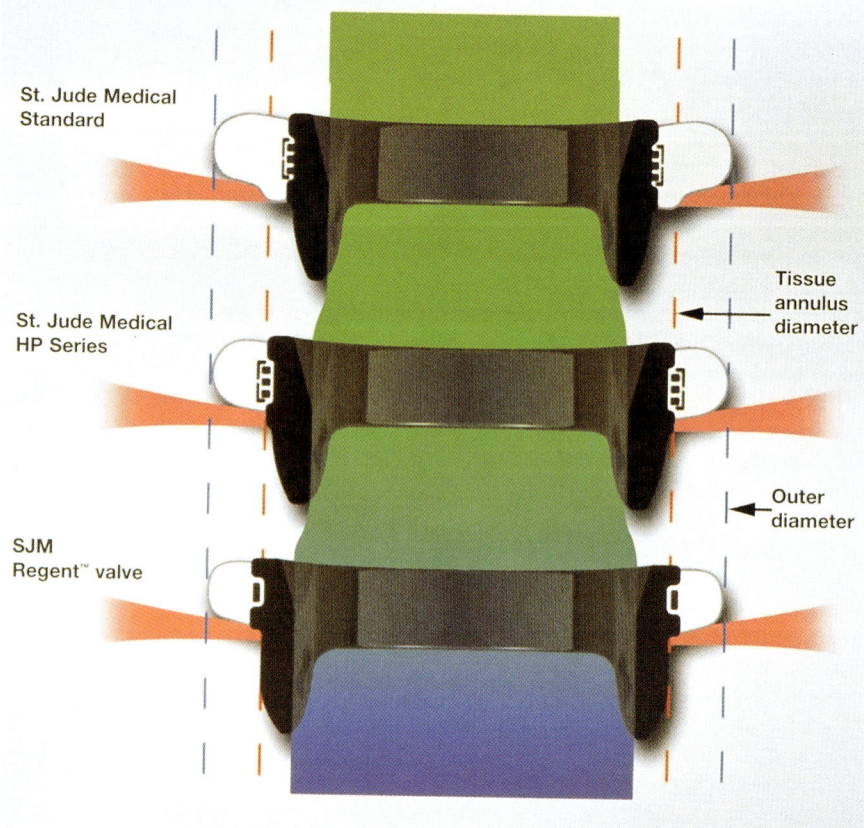

Figure 7-5. St. Jude Medical Design Modifications Mechanical Prosthesis.

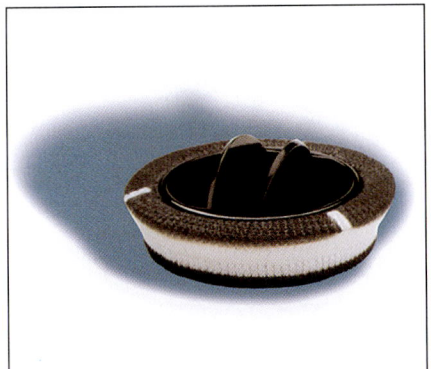

Figure 8-1. Carbomedics Standard Aortic Mechanical Prosthesis.

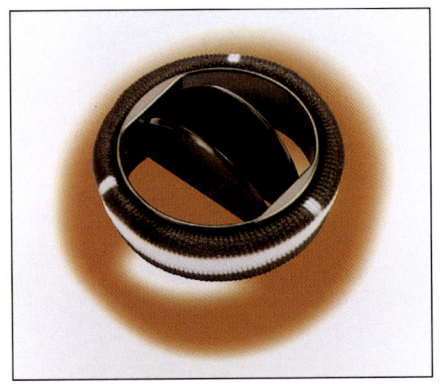

Figure 8-2. Carbomedics Aortic "R" Series Mechanical Prosthesis.

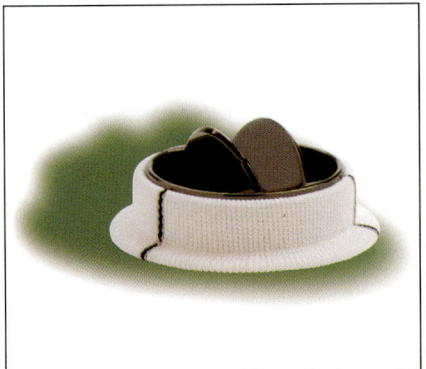

Figure 8-3. Carbomedics Aortic Top-Hat™ Mechanical Prosthesis.

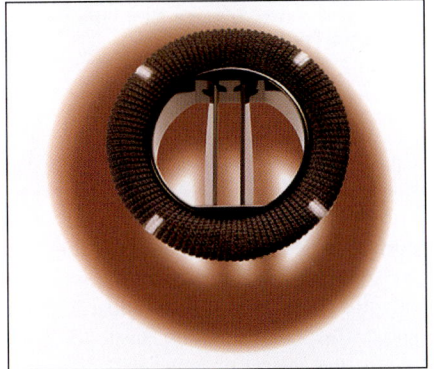

Figure 8-4. Carbomedics Mitral Mechanical Prosthesis.

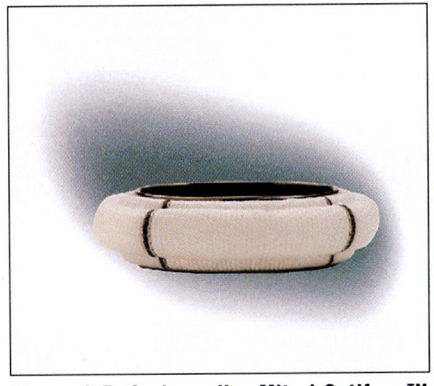

Figure 8-5. Carbomedics Mitral-Optiform™ Mechanical Prosthesis.

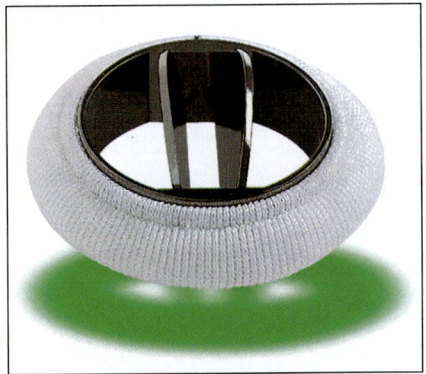

Figure 8-6. Carbomedics Orbis™ Aortic Mechanical Prosthesis.

thesis (Sulzer-Carbomedics, Inc., Austin, Texas, U.S.A.) is a bileaflet prosthesis with solid pyrolitic carbon housing and flat leaflets of pyrolytic carbon coated over tungsten-loaded graphite substrate (Figs. 8-1 & 8-2). The prosthesis has excellent radio-opacity with a radio-opaque titanium stiffening ring and increased tungsten content in the leaflet substrate. The opening angle of the leaflets is 78°, which encourages synchronous closure. The leaflet pivot retention mechanism is within the housing without pivot guards, struts, or orifice projections. Leaflet motion is by rotation. The housing can be rotated within the sewing ring. The Carbomedics Top-Hat™ prosthesis is designed for supra-annular aortic implantation and improved hemodynamic performance in small sizes (Fig. 8-3). The Carbomedics Optiform™ mitral valve is a reconfiguration of the mitral prosthesis (Figs. 8-4 & 8-5) with a generous, symmetrical polyester sewing cuff to allow either intra-annular or supra-annular implantation (Fig. 8-5). The Optiform™ prosthesis is useful in small, hypertrophied, or both, left ventricles; double-valve replacement; and reoperative mitral surgery. The Carbomedics Orbis™ prosthesis configuration has a multipurpose cuff design for aortic implantation in the scarred and calcified annulus (Fig. 8-6).

Edwards Tekna Mechanical Prosthesis

The Edwards Tekna mechanical prosthesis is a bileaflet prosthesis (Edwards Lifesciences, Irvine, California, U.S.A.) with a solid pyrolytic carbon housing and curved leaflets of pyrolytic carbon coated over tungsten-loaded graphite substrate (Fig. 9). Housing stability is increased by a stellite stiffener ring over a solid pyrolytic-valve housing. The pivot hinge mechanism is located within the housing, and leaflet motion is by rotation and translation. The opening angle of the aortic prosthesis is 77° and the mitral prosthesis is 73°. The curved leaflets enhance central flow and rapid closure. Aortic and mitral housing, which has a low profile, and leaflets can be rotated within the sewing ring. The pivot ball and pivot-slot mechanism facilitate retrograde washing by relatively high-velocity jets. Leaflets close on a

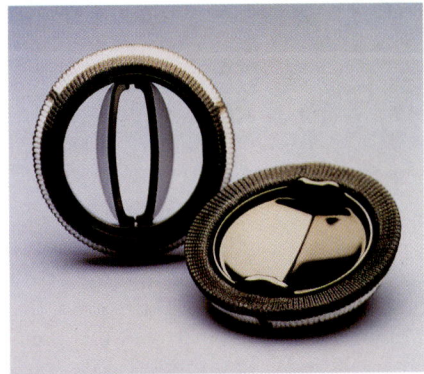

Figure 9. Edwards Tekna Mechanical Prosthesis.

circular ledge within the housing to reduce regurgitation and avoid stress on the hinge mechanism. The pivot ball hinge closes by rotation and translation. This prosthesis is currently not manufactured.

Sorin Bicarbon Mechanical Prosthesis

The Sorin Bicarbon mechanical prosthesis (Sorin Biomedica, Saluggia, Italy) is a bileaflet prosthesis with a titanium alloy housing coated with a thin film of pyrolytic carbon (Carbofilm™)

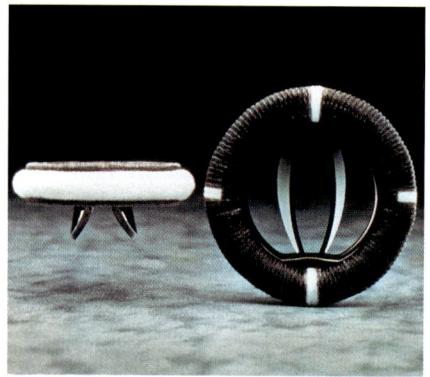

Figure 10. Sorin Bicarbon Mechanical Prosthesis.

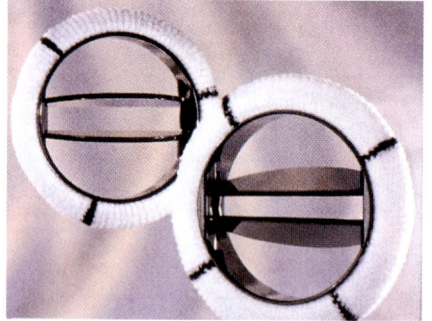

Figure 12a. ATS Mechanical Prosthesis.

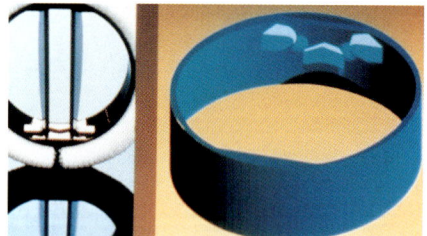

Figure 12b. ATS Mechanical Prosthesis.

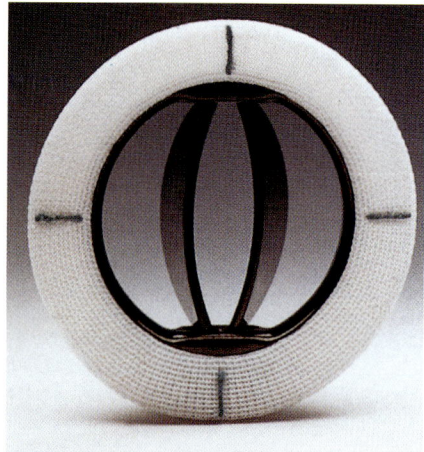

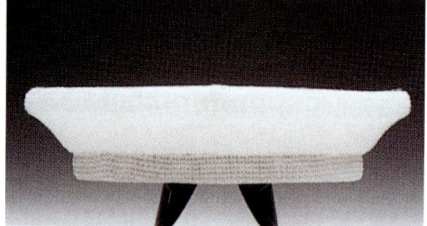

Figure 11-1 a & b. Edwards Mira Mechanical Prosthesis.

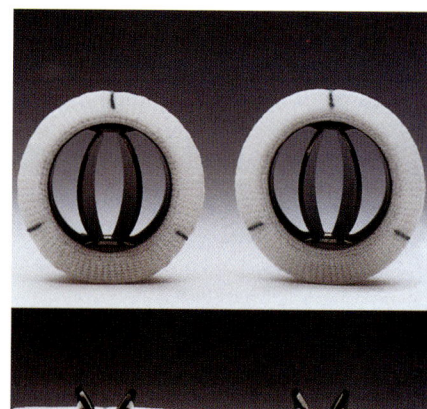

Figure 11-2 a & b. Edwards Mira Ultra Finesse Mechanical Prosthesis.

(Fig. 10). A titanium housing strengthens the prosthesis and the minimal thickness increases the effective orifice. The hinge cavity supports a constantly varying, single point of contact between pivot and housing, and two effluent passages provide continuous washing even in the closed position. The curved leaflets, made of pyrolytic carbon coated over a graphite and tungsten substrate, separate the orifice into three sections with similar resistance to flow, low-pressure gradients, and minimal turbulence. The hinge mechanism supports a rolling motion. The opening angle of both the aortic and mitral prosthesis is 80°, and both prostheses can be rotated within the sewing ring. The sewing ring is made with polyethylene terephthalate (PET) and carbon-coated PTFE.

Edwards Mira Mechanical Prosthesis

The Edwards Mira mechanical prosthesis (Edwards Lifesciences, Irvine, California, U.S.A.) is the Sorin Bicarbon mechanical prosthesis with the unique StarRing sewing cuff (Fig. 11-1 a & b). The prosthesis features a curved-leaflet profile as well as a slim, Carbofilm™-coated titanium-alloy housing. The rolling hinge provides a constantly varying point of contact in the hinge area between the leaflet and housing. An open channel in the hinge cavity allows continuous hinge washing during the entire cardiac cycle. The prosthesis has unique sewing rings designed specifically for mitral and aortic applications, as well as a special aortic version for small annuli (Fig.11-2 a & b Mira Ultra Finesse). Each sewing ring design enhances the function of the prosthesis in its position and size, including the unique hyperbolic shape of the mitral valve and downstream extension of the aortic prosthesis. The hyperbolic shape of the mitral sewing ring enhances non-everting supra-annular placement, as well as everting intra-annular placement. Downstream extension of the aortic sewing ring is customized with smaller extension in smaller sizes. The sewing rings are formulated of seamless knitted polyester cloth surface with a silicone sponge insert to provide enhanced compliance to the status of all annular irregularities. The prosthesis is radio-opaque with the graphite and tungsten substrate. The opening angle of both aortic and mitral prostheses is 80°, and both prostheses are rotatable within the sewing ring.

ATS Mechanical Prosthesis

The ATS mechanical prosthesis (ATS Medical, Inc., Minneapolis, Minnesota, U.S.A.) is a bileaflet prosthesis with pyrolytic carbon housing and pyrolytic carbon leaflets, with the housing and leaflets containing graphite substrate (Figs.12a & 12b). The prosthesis has a convex hinge mechanism with protrusions on the inner aspect of the housing supporting the leaflets. The prosthesis has no protruding struts with this hinge mechanism. The convex hinge mechanism is designed to facilitate retrograde washing. The opening angle is 85°. The aortic and mitral prostheses can be rotated within the sewing ring.

On-X Mechanical Prosthesis

The On-X mechanical prosthesis (Medical Carbon Research Institute, Austin, Texas, U.S.A.) is a bileaflet prosthesis with a pure, non-silicon carbide alloyed pyrolytic-carbon housing and flat leaflets of pyrolytic carbon-coated over tungsten-loaded graphite substrate (Fig. 13). The prosthesis design provides a curved housing in-

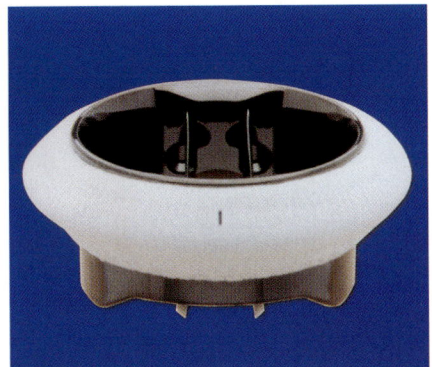
Figure 13. On-X Mechanical Prosthesis.

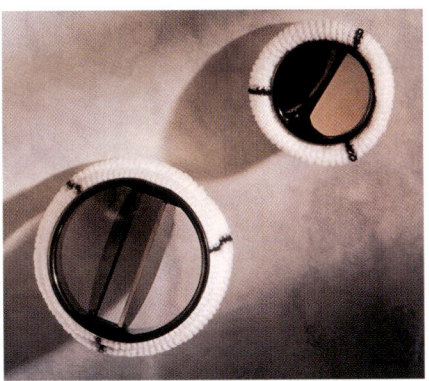
Figure 14. Medtronic Advantage Mechanical Prosthesis.

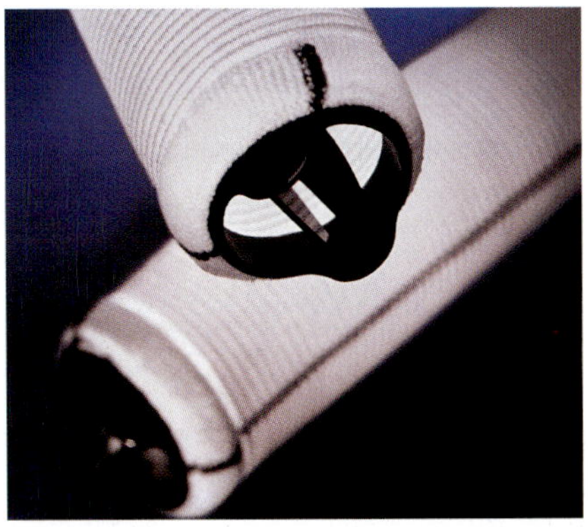

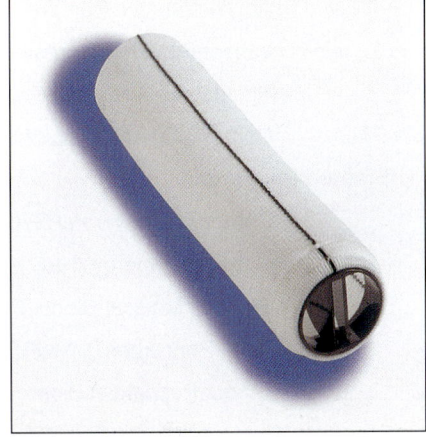
Figure 15. St. Jude Medical Masters Aortic Valved Prosthesis.

flow geometry and an orifice diameter-to-housing height ratio to minimize the vena contracta phenomenon and facilitate laminar blood flow. The leaflets of the mitral prosthesis are protected within the housing. The leaflet motion is by translation and rotation. The opening angle is no greater than 90° to the housing, but usually opens to an unstopped position of 85°. The leaflets travel an arc of 50°, closing at an angle of 40°. The regurgitant volume washes the pivot mechanism. The sewing ring is made of PTFE, the housing is rotatable within the sewing ring. Small titanium rings provide radio-opaque markers for location of the valve. The internal diameter of all mitral prosthesis sizes is 25 mm.

Medtronic Advantage Mechanical Prosthesis

The Medtronic Advantage mechanical prosthesis (Medtronic Inc., Minneapolis, Minnesota, U.S.A.) is an investigational bileaflet prosthesis consisting of a pyrolytic carbon housing with two pyrolytic carbon leaflets and a rotatable PET sewing ring (Fig. 14). The leaflets are widely spaced to increase the central-flow volume, reduce central-flow-velocity, and diminish the tendency of turbulence formation. The leaflets are radio-opaque and open to 86°. Washing of the hinge areas is facilitated by the enlarged central orifice and butterfly-hinge socket. The butterfly-hinge socket was designed to reduce flow stasis and thrombus. This design was facilitated by the engineering techniques incorporating laser Doppler velocimetry, computational fluid dynamics, and microscopic-flow visualization.

MECHANICAL PROSTHESES — AORTIC VALVED GRAFTS

The majority of mechanical prostheses, bileaflet and monoleaflet, are provided as a valved-conduit for aortic root reconstruction. Porcine aortic valve-conduits were previously available, whereas porcine stentless aortic root bioprostheses are now used, together with homografts and autografts, for aortic root reconstruction.

St. Jude Medical Masters Aortic Valved Graft Prosthesis

The St. Jude Medical Masters aortic valved graft (St. Jude Medical, Inc., St. Paul, Minnesota, U.S.A.) incorporates the St. Jude Medical valve and the Hemashield™ woven double velour graft (Meadox Medicals, Inc.) (Fig. 15). The woven graft is collagen impregnated to control homeostasis and reduce hemorrhagic complications. The gradual resorption rate of the collagen impregnation prolongs graft seal during the critical postoperative period. The collagen from bovine source promotes host tissue integration. The graft has no pleats to facilitate coronary anastomoses and ease stress on the coronary buttons. The double velour cuff enhances implantability and conformation of the graft to the annulus. The valve is rotatable and supports reduction of interference between the leaflets and subvalvular structures. The graft length is of increased length from previous generations to provide greater versatility.

Carbomedics Carbo-Seal™ Aortic Valved Graft Prosthesis

Sulzer-Carbomedics Carbo-Seal™ Aortic Valved Graft Prosthesis (Sulzer-Carbomedics, Inc., Austin Texas,

Figure 16. Carbomedics Carbo-Seal™ Aortic Valved Prosthesis.

U.S.A.) incorporates the Carbomedics mechanical prosthesis and low porosity, zero-preclot twill woven graft (Fig. 16). The woven graft is impregnated with gelatin and hydrolysis occurs over 14 days. The graft configuration minimizes interference and suture stress of coronary ostia implantation. Orientation markers provide easy suture positioning. The prosthesis has a pliable, cork-shaped sewing cuff, which conforms to the annulus. The prosthesis incorporates a titanium stiffening ring that allows rotatability in-situ and minimizes the possibility of leaflet lock-up or escape. The prosthesis has a full-sized orifice for improved hemodynamics. The woven graft enhances tissue ingrowth.

Sorin Carbon Art™ Aortic Valved Graft Prosthesis

The Sorin Carbon Art™ Aortic Valved Graft Prosthesis (Sorin Biomedica, Saluggia, Italy) incorporates the Bicarbon™ bileaflet valve and a vascular conduit of seamless, knitted poly-

Table 2. Bioprostheses—Current

Stented Porcine
- Hancock Standard Porcine Bioprosthesis
- Carpentier-Edwards Standard Porcine Bioprosthesis
- Carpentier-Edwards Supra-Annular Porcine Bioprosthesis
- Hancock II Porcine Bioprosthesis
- Hancock Modified Orifice Porcine Bioprosthesis
- St. Jude Medical-Biocor Porcine Bioprosthesis
- St. Jude Medical-Bioimplant Porcine Bioprosthesis
- Medtronic Mosaic Porcine Bioprosthesis
- AorTech Aspire Porcine Bioprosthesis
- Labcor Porcine Bioprosthesis
- St. Jude Medical Epic Porcine Bioprosthesis
- Carbomedics Synergy™ ST Porcine Bioprosthesis

Stented Pericardial
- Carpentier-Edwards PERIMOUNT Pericardial Bioprosthesis
- Mitroflow Synergy™ PC Pericardial Bioprosthesis
- St. Jude Medical-Biocor Pericardial Bioprosthesis
- Sorin Pericarbon™ MØRE Pericardial Bioprosthesis
- Labcor Pericardial Bioprosthesis

Stentless Porcine and Pericardial
- St. Jude Medical-Toronto SPV Stentless Porcine Bioprosthesis
- Medtronic Freestyle™ Stentless Porcine Bioprosthesis
- Cryolife-O'Brien Stentless Porcine Bioprosthesis
- Cryolife-Ross Stentless Porcine Pulmonary Bioprosthesis
- Edwards Prima™ Plus Stentless Porcine Bioprosthesis
- Sorin Pericarbon™ Freedom Stentless Pericardial Bioprosthesis
- AorTech Aspire Stentless Porcine Bioprosthesis
- St. Jude Medical Biocor Stentless Porcine Bioprosthesis
- Labcor Stentless Porcine Bioprosthesis
- St. Jude Medical Quattro™ Stentless Mitral Bioprosthesis
- Shelhigh Skeletorized Super-Stentless Aortic Porcine Bioprosthesis
- Shelhigh Porcine Pulmonic Valve Conduit
- Medtronic-Venpro Contegra Pulmonary Valved Conduit

Allografts
- Cryo Valve Aortic Valve With/Without Conduit
- Cryo Valve Mitral Valve
- Cryo Syner Graft Valve

Autografts
- Pulmonary Autografts for Aortic Root
- Autologous Pericardial Aortic Valve

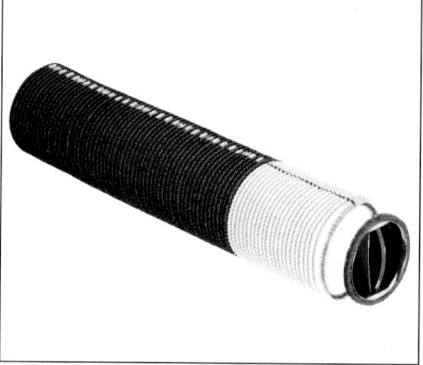

Figure 17. Sorin Carbon Art™ Aortic Valved Graft Prosthesis.

ester (Fig. 17). The Bicarbon™ heart valve and vascular conduit are both coated with Carbofilm™. The device, which features a modified Bicarbon™ aortic serving ring, is intended for use as a replacement for the aortic valve and ascending aorta. The valve section of the prosthesis is coated with Carbofilm™ on the inflow surface side and surrounded by a soft, seamless, knitted polyester cuff. The sewing ring is securely attached to a woven polyester graft coated, both internally and externally, with Carbofilm™.

BIOPROSTHESES—CURRENT

Biological valvular prostheses are formulated from porcine aortic valves or bovine pericardium (Table 2). The natural aortic valve possesses unique architectural and material characteristics consistent with functional requirements. Porcine bioprostheses have had tissue preservation at high pressure, at low pressure, or pressure free with glutaraldehyde to preserve bioprosthetic function and provide durability. The tissue preservation, together with stent designs, contribute to the anatomical characteristics and biomechanical properties of the leaflets. The first-generation porcine bioprostheses—Hancock standard and Carpentier-Edwards standard—had the porcine tissue fixed with glutaraldehyde at high pressure, 60 to 80 mm Hg. These prostheses are still marketed. The current-generation porcine prostheses are either low (<2 mm Hg) pressure or zero pressure glutaraldehyde-fixed prostheses. The bovine pericardial prostheses have used pressure-free fixation with glutaraldehyde; the current generation has used advanced engineering to formulate the tissue-

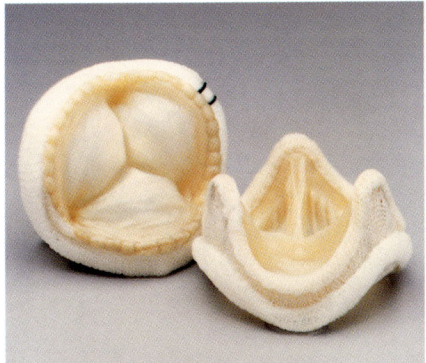

Figure 18. Carpentier-Edwards Supra-Annular Porcine Bioprosthesis.

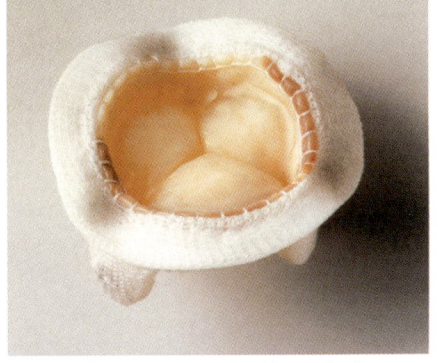

Figure 19. Hancock II Porcine Bioprosthesis.

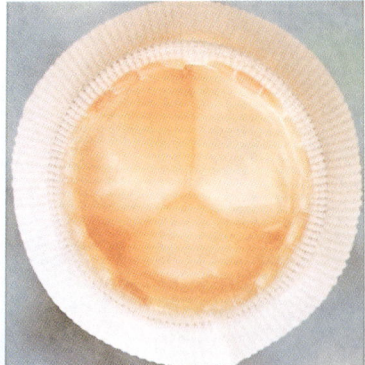

Figure 20. Hancock Modified Orifice Porcine Bioprosthesis.

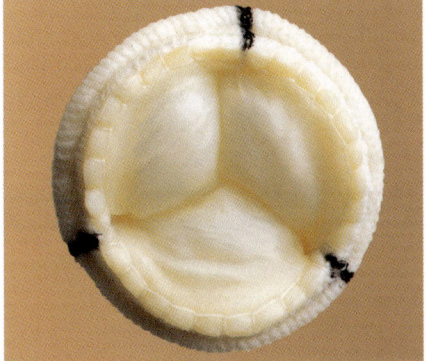

Figure 21. St. Jude Medical-Biocor Porcine Bioprosthesis.

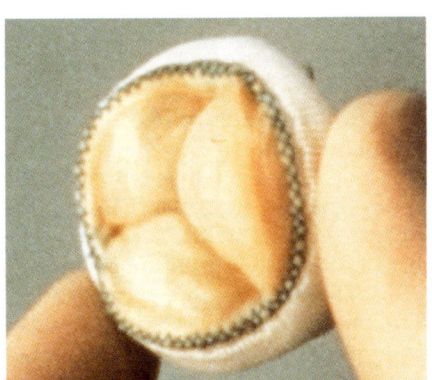

Figure 22 a & b. St. Jude Medical-Bioimplant Porcine Bioprosthesis.

stent relationship.

BIOPROSTHESES — STENTED

Carpentier-Edwards Supra-Annular Porcine Bioprosthesis

The Carpentier-Edwards supra-annular porcine bioprosthesis (Edwards Lifesciences, Irvine, California, U.S.A.) has a supra-annular configuration, mounted on a flexible Elgiloy™ wire frame for stress reduction (Fig. 18). The prosthesis has a reduced stent profile and the tissue is preserved with glutaraldehyde at low pressure fixed at less than 4 mm Hg. The tissue is treated with the calcium mitigation agents, polysorbate 80 and ethanol (XenoLogiX). The original Carpentier-Edwards standard porcine bioprosthesis remains in use in the United States, but with low-pressure fixation substituted for high-pressure fixation.

Hancock II Porcine Bioprosthesis

The Hancock II porcine bioprosthesis (Medtronic, Inc., Minneapolis, Minnesota, U.S.A.) is a supra-annular prosthesis (Fig. 19). The prosthesis has a Delrin™ stent, scalloped aortic sewing ring, reduced stent profile, and is fixed with glutaraldehyde at low pressure, subsequently, for a prolonged period at high pressure. The prosthesis is treated with sodium dodecyl sulfate to retard calcification.

Hancock Modified Orifice Porcine Bioprosthesis

The Hancock modified orifice porcine bioprosthesis (Medtronic, Inc., Minneapolis, Minnesota, U.S.A.) is similar in configuration to the Hancock standard porcine bioprosthesis except for the composite leaflet placement (Fig. 20). In this composite configuration, the non-coronary leaflet from another porcine root is used to replace the right coronary leaflet that contains a muscle shelf. The prosthesis was designed to optimize hemodynamics in small aortic roots. The prosthesis is also provided with a supra-annular configuration.

St. Jude Medical-Biocor Porcine Bioprosthesis

The St. Jude Medical-Biocor porcine bioprosthesis (St. Jude Medical, Inc., Belo Horizonte, MG, Brazil) is a zero-pressure, glutaraldehyde-fixed porcine bioprosthesis (Fig. 21). The prosthesis is formulated as a triple-composite design, with the leaflets devoid of a muscle bar. The stent posts and rails are covered with a rim of bovine glutaraldehyde-preserved pericardium. The design of the prosthesis includes a polyacetal stent and polyester sewing ring.

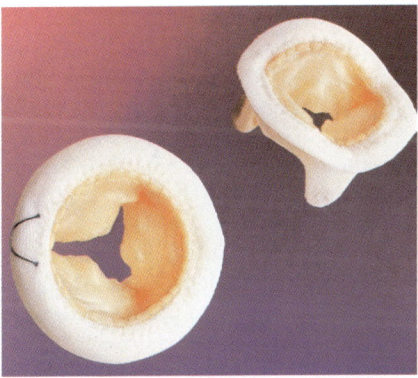

Figure 23. Medtronic Mosaic™ Porcine Bioprosthesis.

St. Jude Medical-Bioimplant Porcine Bioprosthesis

The St. Jude Medical-Bioimplant (formerly Liotta) porcine bioprosthesis (St. Jude Medical, Inc., St. Paul, Minnesota, U.S.A.) is an early-generation valve (Fig. 22 a & b). The prosthesis has a low-profile supra-annular configuration with low-pressure, glutaraldehyde-fixed tissue.

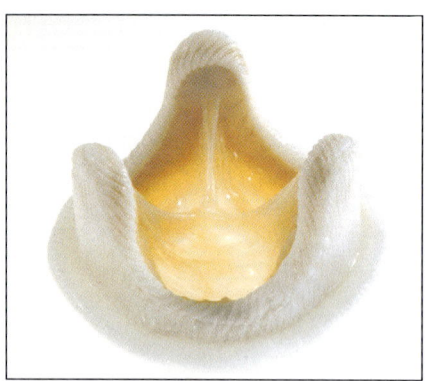

Figure 24. AorTech Aspire Porcine Bioprosthesis.

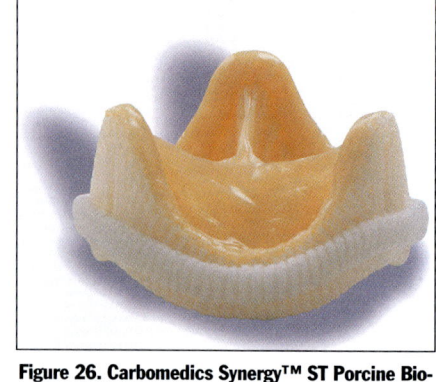

Figure 26. Carbomedics Synergy™ ST Porcine Bioprosthesis.

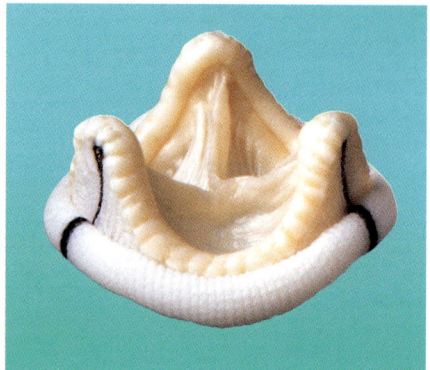

Figure 27. St. Jude Medical Epic Porcine Bioprosthesis.

![Figure 25]

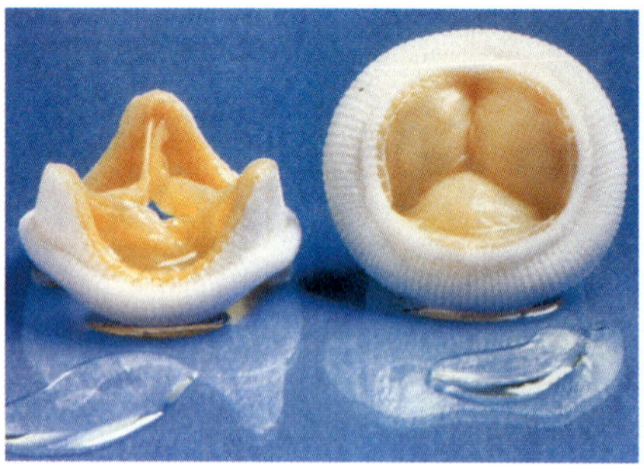

Figure 25. Labcor Stented Porcine Bioprosthesis.

Medtronic Mosaic™ Porcine Bioprosthesis

The Medtronic Mosaic™ porcine bioprosthesis (Medtronic, Inc., Minneapolis, Minnesota, U.S.A.) is a third-generation prosthesis (Fig. 23). The prosthesis has a supra-annular configuration with a Delrin™ stent, scalloped aortic sewing ring, and reduced stent profile. The tissue is pressure-free fixed with glutaraldehyde, and the aortic wall predilated to reduce deformation of the commissures. The prosthesis is treated with alpha oleic acid to retard calcification.

AorTech Aspire Porcine Bioprosthesis

The AorTech Aspire porcine bioprosthesis (AorTech, Bellshill, Scotland) is a low-pressure (<2 mm Hg) glutaraldehyde-fixed stented porcine bioprosthesis (Fig. 24). The bioprosthesis is formulated by a process of "fresh mounting" to allow correct alignment of the commissures. Dilation of the valve during preparation allows correct functional sizing. Dilation in conjunction with low-pressure fixation increases the angle of inclination of the leaflet and produces a reduction in open leaflet bending deformation. The valve tissue is selected to ensure minimal size of the muscle shelf.

Labcor Stented Porcine Bioprosthesis

The Labcor stented porcine bioprosthesis (Labcor, Inc., Belo Horizonte, MG, Brazil) is a stented, tri-composite prosthesis of low-profile design (Fig. 25). The tri-composite prosthesis has three non-coronary leaflets glutaraldehyde-preserved at zero-pressure fixation. The three non-coronary leaflets with no muscle shelf provide a large, effective blood-flow area.

Carbomedics Synergy™ ST Porcine Bioprosthesis

The Carbomedics Synergy™ ST porcine bioprosthesis (Sulzer Carbomedics, Inc., Austin, Texas, U.S.A.) is a stented, tri-composite supra-annular prosthesis of low-profile design (Fig. 26). The tri-composite prosthesis has three non-coronary leaflets glutaraldehyde-preserved at zero-pressure fixation. The three non-coronary leaflets with no muscle shelf provide a large, effective blood-flow area. The stent posts and stent rails are covered with glutaraldehyde-preserved pericardium. The porcine and pericardial tissue is treated with an advanced calcium mitigation therapy.

St. Jude Medical Epic Porcine Bioprosthesis

The St. Jude Medical Epic porcine bioprosthesis (St. Jude Medical, Inc., St. Paul, Minnesota, U.S.A.) is a minimal-pressure, glutaraldehyde-fixed porcine bioprosthesis (Fig. 27). The prosthesis is formulated as a triple-composite design devoid of muscle bar, and is a low-profile design in both aortic and mitral positions. The stent-posts and rails are covered with a rim of glutaraldehyde-preserved bovine pericardium. The prosthesis has a polyacetal stent and polyester sewing ring. In the Linx™ technology, ethanol is used to prevent calcification.

BIOPROSTHESES—STENTED PERICARDIAL

Carpentier-Edwards PERIMOUNT Pericardial Bioprosthesis

The Carpentier-Edwards PERIMOUNT pericardial bioprosthesis (Edwards Lifesciences, Irvine, California, U.S.A.) is constructed with an Elgiloy™ stent at the orifice and commissures for flexibility and pericardium fixed without pressure in glutaraldehyde. Leaflets are produced by computer-aided design for optimal leaflet to stent matching (Fig. 28). Leaflets achieve satisfactory coaptation without stent-post sutures. The tissue is treated with the calcium mitigation agents, polysorbate 80 and ethanol (XenoLogiX).

Mitroflow Synergy™ PC Pericardial Bioprosthesis

The Mitroflow Synergy™ PC pericardial bioprosthesis (Sulzer Mitroflow, Richmond, British Columbia, Canada) is formulated with a acetyl homopolymer stent for flexibility and pericardium pressure-free fixed with glutaraldehyde (Fig. 29). Pericardium is used as a single component without critical stent-post sutures. The Dacron™ cloth of the prosthesis (current version) has the smooth, rather than ribbed, PET in contact with the pericardium.

St. Jude Medical-Biocor Pericardial Bioprosthesis

The St. Jude Medical-Biocor pericardial bioprosthesis (St. Jude Medical, Inc., Belo Horizonte, MG, Brazil) is a zero-pressure, glutaraldehyde-fixed pericardial bioprosthesis with the stent-posts and rails covered with pericardium (Fig. 30). The design incorporates a polyacetal stent and polyester ring.

Sorin Pericarbon™ MØRE Pericardial Bioprosthesis

The Sorin Pericarbon™ MØRE pericardial bioprosthesis (Sorin Biomedica, Saluggia, Italy) is made with two sheets of pressure-free fixed pericardium over a semiflexible polymeric stent covered with polyester fabric (Fig. 31). One sheet forms the three cusps with reduced stress on the commissures and a cylindrical shape in the open position. The other sheet coats the inner surface of the stent. The prosthesis is low profile, has a radio-opaque metal wire marker and carbofilm-coated polyester fabric sewing ring (to control pannus overgrowth). The sewing ring in the aortic position is designed for supra-annular positioning. The tissue is submitted to detoxification post-glutaraldehyde aimed at neutralizing residues of unbound aldehyde groups. The valve is stored in a solution free from aldehyde.

Labcor Stented Pericardial Bioprosthesis

The Labcor stented pericardial bioprosthesis (Labcor, Inc. Belo Horizonte, MG, Brazil) is a tri-composite prosthesis with precisely determined individual cusp shape with the tissue selected for mounting of uniformity and thickness (Fig. 32). The prosthesis is formulated with a copolymer scalloped flexible stent to reduce stress on the tissue. The fabrication technique produces uniformity and consistency in valve function. The attachment of the pericardium at the stent post facilitates stress reduction and reinforces apposition of the leaflets. The prosthesis is also constructed to avoid contact of the pericardial membrane with the polyester and reduction of abrasion by means of pericardial padding of the inner surface of the valve at the post.

BIOPROSTHESES—STENTLESS PORCINE AND PERICARDIAL

St. Jude Medical-Toronto SPV Stentless Porcine Bioprosthesis

The St. Jude Medical-Toronto SPV stentless porcine bioprosthesis (St. Jude Medical, Inc., St. Paul, Minnesota,

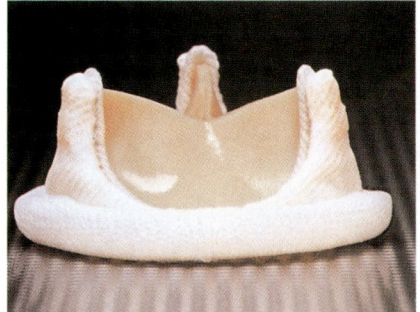
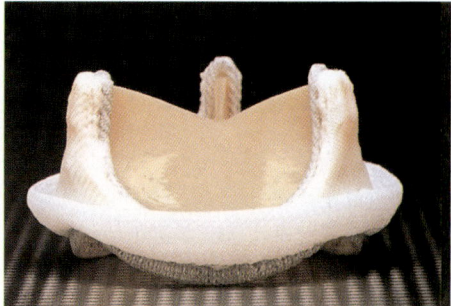

Figure 28(a-mitral, b-aortic). Carpentier-Edwards PERIMOUNT Pericardial Bioprosthesis.

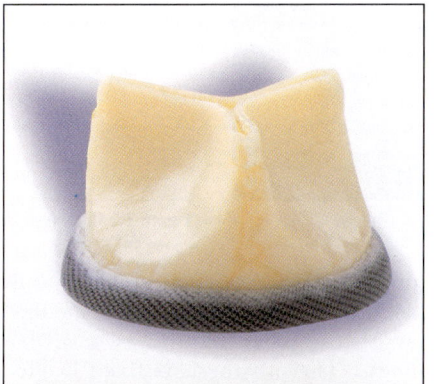

Figure 29. Mitroflow Synergy™ PC Pericardial Bioprosthesis.

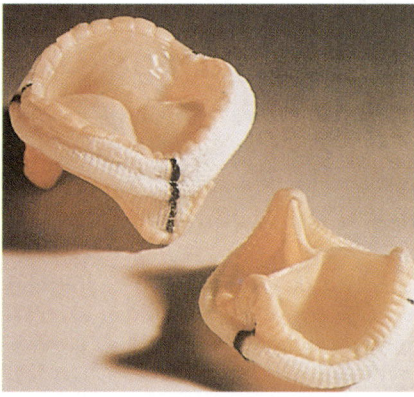

Figure 30. St. Jude Medical-Biocor Pericardial Bioprosthesis.

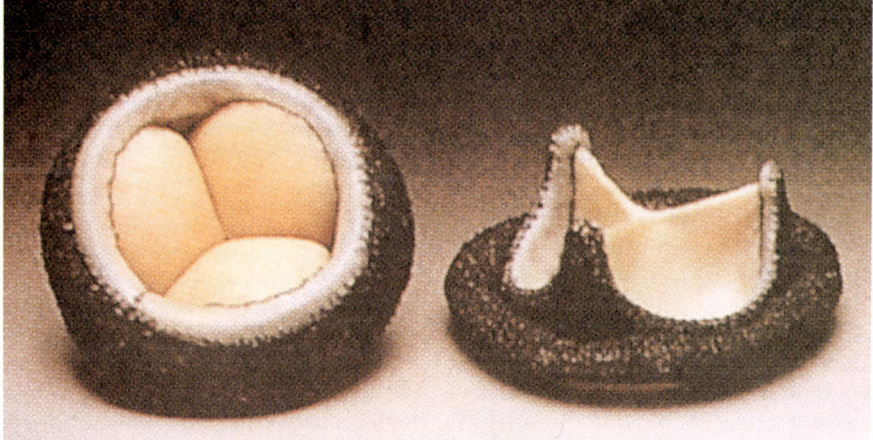

Figure 31. Sorin Pericarbon™ MØRE Pericardical Bioprosthesis.

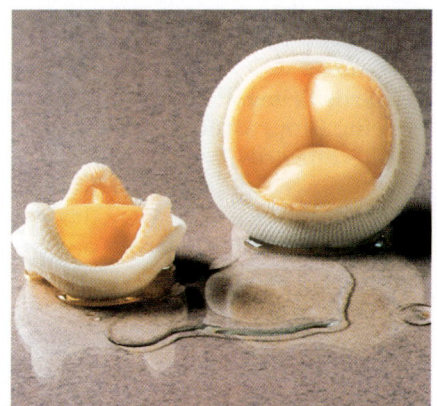

Figure 32. Labcor Pericardial Bioprosthesis.

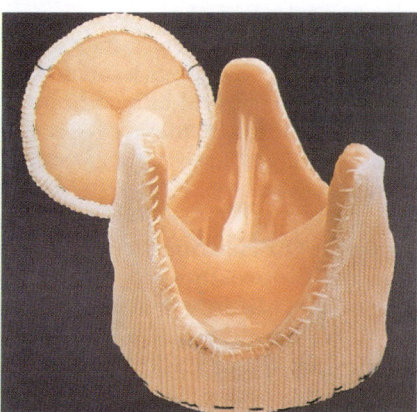

Figure 33. St. Jude Medical-Toronto SPV Stentless Porcine Bioprosthesis.

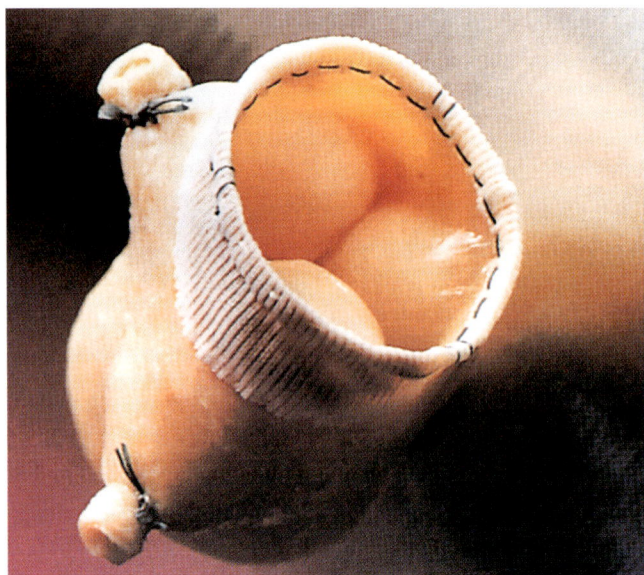

Figure 34. Medtronic Freestyle™ Stentless Porcine Bioprosthesis.

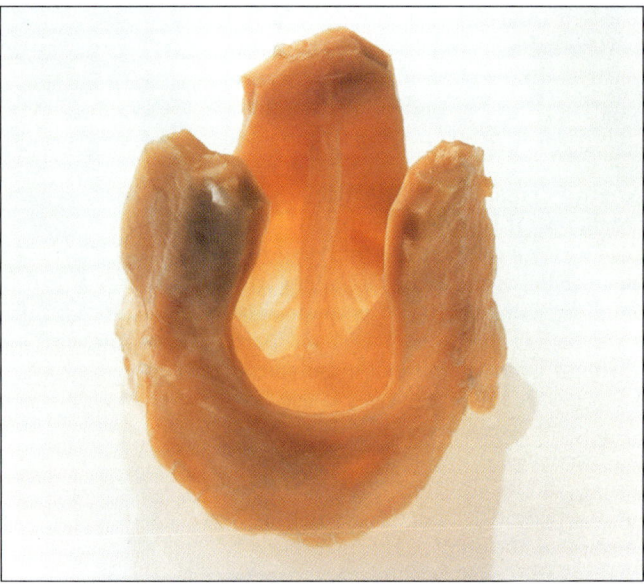

Figure 35. Cryolife-O'Brien Stentless Porcine Bioprosthesis.

U.S.A.) is a subcoronary stentless porcine bioprosthesis with an external surface, including muscle shelf covered with fine Dacron™ mesh (Fig. 33). The proximal sewing ridge is covered with fine Dacron™. The porcine tissue is preserved with low-pressure glutaraldehyde fixation. The future generation of the Toronto SPV bioprosthesis will be the Toronto SPV-Duo™ incorporating the Linx™ technology with ethanol for calcium mitigation.

Medtronic Freestyle™ Stentless Porcine Bioprosthesis

The Medtronic Freestyle™ stentless porcine bioprosthesis (Medtronic, Inc., Minneapolis, Minnesota, U.S.A.) is fashioned as a porcine aortic root for implantation using the subcoronary (allograft freehand-like), miniroot cylinder or aortic root technique (Fig. 34). Tissue is pressure-free fixed with glutaraldehyde and the aortic wall predilated to reduce deformation of the commissures. Tissue is treated with alpha amino oleic acid to retard calcification. Dacron™ mesh covers the muscle shelf and forms a fine proximal sewing cuff.

Cryolife-O'Brien Stentless Porcine Bioprosthesis

The Cryolife-O'Brien stentless porcine bioprosthesis (Cryolife, Inc., Kennesaw, Georgia, U.S.A.) is a stentless prosthesis with composite leaflets (Fig. 35). The prosthesis is designed only for distal suture-line implantation, above the annulus, in contrast to other stentless porcine bioprostheses that require two suture lines. The prosthesis is fixed in glutaraldehyde. The Cryolife-O'Brien stentless porcine bioprosthesis also is fashioned as an aortic root for implantation using the subcoronary, miniroot cylinder or aortic-root technique.

Cryolife-Ross Stentless Porcine Pulmonary Bioprosthesis

The Cryolife-Ross stentless porcine pulmonary bioprosthesis (Cryolife International Inc., Kennesaw, Georgia, U.S.A.) is available in pediatric sizes (11 to 13 mm) and adult sizes (19 to 29 mm) (Fig. 36). The porcine tissue is glutaraldehyde-fixed at low pressure (<2 mm Hg). The stentless design with the symmetrical muscle bar yields optional hemodynamics. The prosthesis has the potential increase in durability due to lower calcium content in pulmonary leaflets and wall compared to aortic counterparts.

Edwards Prima™ Plus Stentless Porcine Bioprosthesis

The Edwards Prima™ Plus is a stentless porcine bioprosthesis (Edwards Lifesciences, Inc., Irvine, California, U.S.A.) designed as a versatile cylinder without prefashioned coronary openings (Fig. 37). The prosthesis has a Dacron™ mesh that covers the muscle shelf and forms a thin proximal cuff. The porcine tissue is glutaraldehyde-fixed at low pressure with sinus-area dilitation. The prosthesis can be

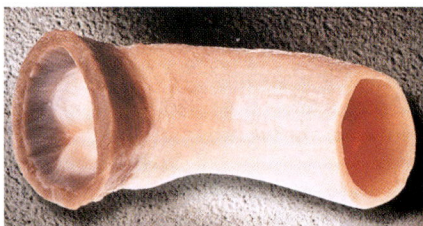

Figure 36. Cryolife-Ross Stentless Porcine Pulmonary Bioprosthesis.

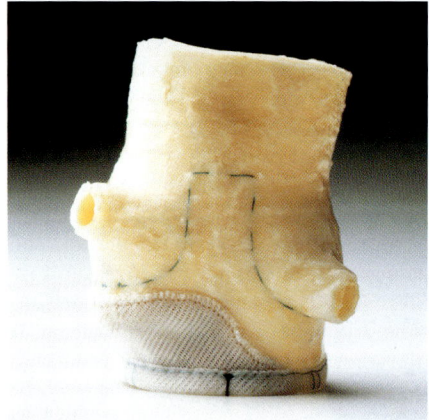

Figure 37. Edwards Prima™ Plus Stentless Porcine Bioprosthesis.

implanted as freehand subcoronary, miniroot cylinder, or aortic-root replacement technique.

Sorin Pericarbon™ Freedom Stentless Pericardial Bioprosthesis

The Sorin Pericarbon™ Freedom stentless pericardial bioprosthesis (Sorin Biomedica, Saluggia, Italy) is a stentless pericardial valve made of two separate

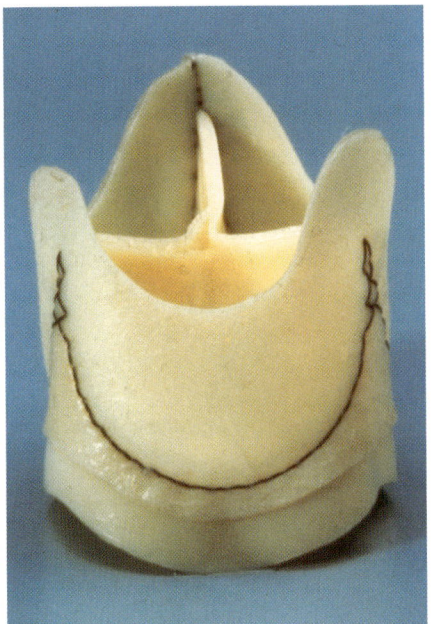

Figure 38. Sorin Pericarbon™ Freedom Stentless Pericardial Bioprosthesis.

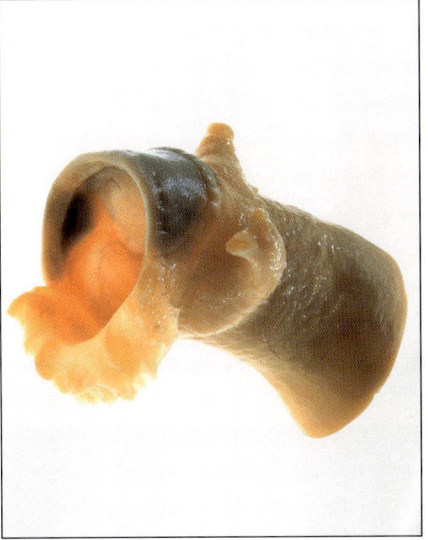

Figure 39-1. AorTech Aspire Stentless Porcine Bioprosthesis (Aortic).

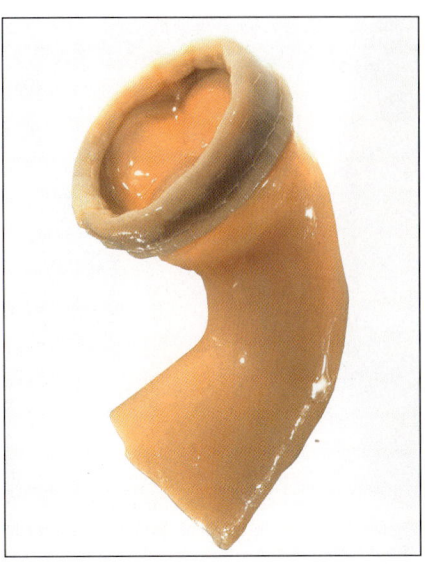

Figure 39-2. AorTech Aspire Stentless Porcine Bioprosthesis (Pulmonary).

sheets of low-pressure, glutaraldehyde-treated bovine pericardium (Fig. 38). The first sheet is shaped to form the three leaflets by means of a process of atraumatic tissue fixation without the use of molds, and then sutured to the second sheet using a carbofilm-coated suture. The suture line is designed especially to minimize the mechanical stress at the level of the commissures. The tissue is submitted to detoxification post-glutaraldehyde aimed at neutralizing residues of unbound aldehyde groups. The valve is stored in a solution free from aldehyde.

AorTech Aspire Stentless Porcine Bioprostheses

The AorTech Aspire stentless porcine bioprosthesis (AorTech, Bellshill, Scotland) is low-pressure (<2 mm Hg) glutaraldehyde-fixed with aortic and pulmonary root formulations (Figs. 39-1 & 39-2). The aortic roots are supplied with the anterior leaflet of the mitral valve intact. The inflow of both aortic and pulmonary roots are reinforced using porcine pericardium. The distal root is dilated, which facilitates the physiological connection between the porcine implant and the patient aorta. The pulmonary root is also provided in a bifurcated fashion. The aortic root, pulmonary root, and pulmonary root bifurcated are provided in both adult and pediatric root configurations. The aortic prosthetic root can be implanted as subcoronary, cylinder, or root techniques.

St. Jude Medical-Biocor Stentless Porcine Bioprosthesis

The St. Jude Medical-Biocor stentless porcine bioprosthesis (St. Jude Medical, Belo Horizonte, MG, Brazil) is a stentless prosthesis with individual porcine cusps to mount a composite bioprosthesis, avoiding leaflets with muscular bands (Fig. 40). The leaflets are treated under no pressure and tanned with different glutaraldehyde solutions for three months. The leaflets are sutured to a conduit of glutaraldehyde-treated bovine pericardium. The conduit is then shaped in a scalloped manner to mimic the natural aortic valve.

Labcor Stentless Porcine Bioprosthesis

The Labcor stentless porcine bioprosthesis (Labcor, Inc., Belo Horizonte, MG, Brazil) is a stentless prosthesis of tri-composite design with three non-coronary leaflets (Fig. 41). The leaflets are preserved in glutaraldehyde at no pressure. The tri-composite design provides a large, effective blood-flow area.

St. Jude Medical Quattro™ Stentless Mitral Bioprosthesis

The St. Jude Medical Quattro™ mitral bioprosthesis (St. Jude Medical, Inc., St. Paul, Minnesota, U.S.A.) is a stentless bovine pericardial mitral prosthesis (Fig. 42). The pericardium is preserved with glutaraldehyde and treated with polyol technology to reduce calcification. The prosthesis is

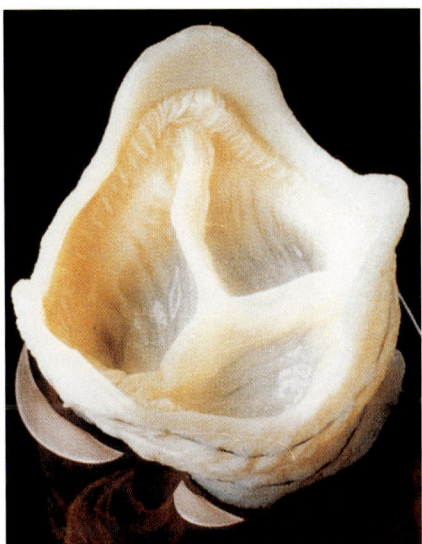

Figure 40. St. Jude Medical-Biocor Stentless Porcine Bioprosthesis.

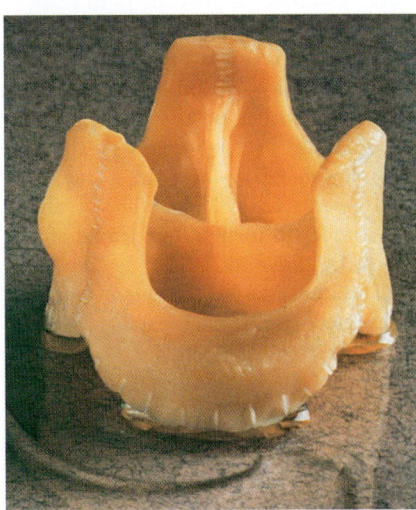

Figure 41. Labcor Stentless Porcine Bioprosthesis.

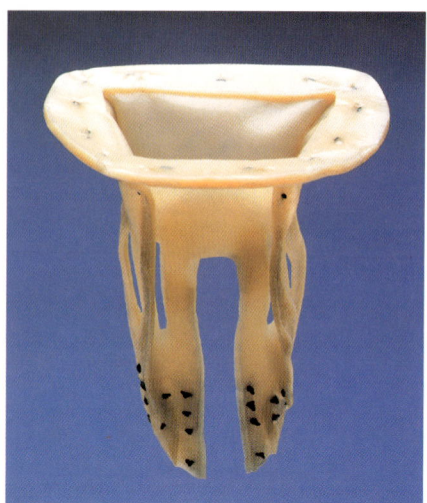

Figure 42. St. Jude Medical Quattro™ Stentless Mitral Bioprosthesis.

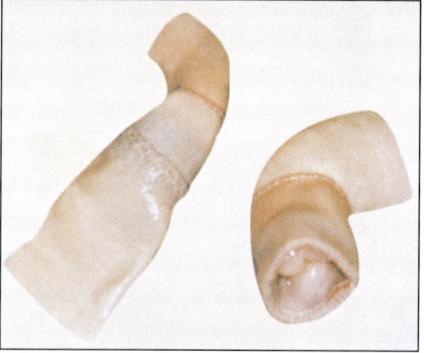

Figure 44. Shelhigh Porcine Pulmonic Valve Conduit.

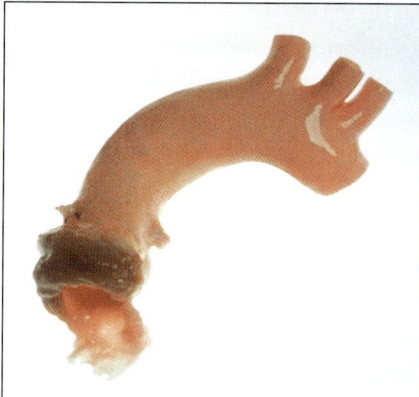

Figure 46-1. CryoValve with/without Conduit (Aortic).

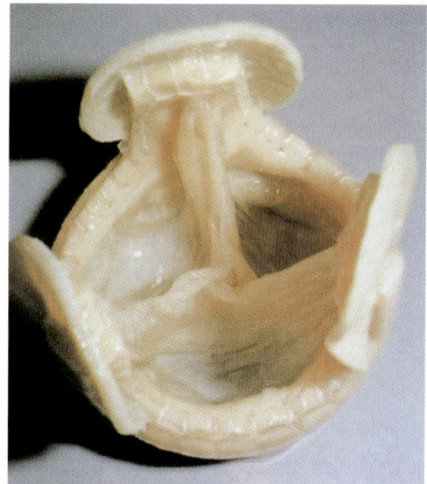

Figure 43. Shelhigh Skeletonized Super-Stentless™ Aortic Porcine Bioprosthesis.

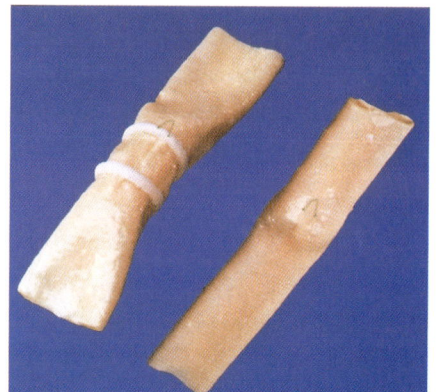

Figure 45. Medtronic-Venpro Contegra Pulmonary Valved Conduit.

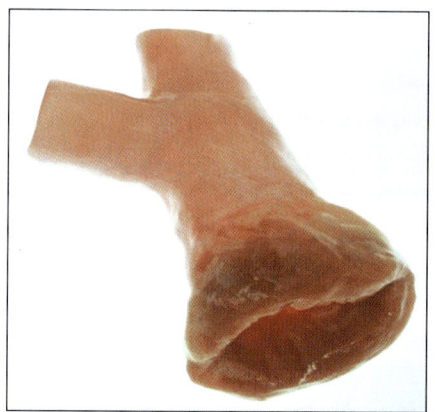

Figure 46-2. CryoValve with/without Conduit (Pulmonary).

composed of a "D-shaped" sewing cuff with one large anterior leaflet and one posterior leaflet containing three scallops. Chordal support for both leaflets on the anterolateral (left) side of the prosthesis is brought together, forming one anterolateral papillary flap. Similarly, the chordae on the posteromedial (right) side are brought together to form another papillary flap. The valve components are held together by aligning stitches to form a four-leaflet stentless mitral prosthesis.

The implantation technique incorporates anchoring of each papillary flap to the corresponding papillary muscle with two horizontal or longitudinal pledgetted mattress sutures. The aligning sutures in the prosthesis sewing ring and papillary flaps guide the placement of sutures during implantation. The Quattro™ prosthesis is available in mitral sizes 26 mm, 28 mm, and 30 mm.

Shelhigh Skeletonized Super-Stentless™ Aortic Porcine Bioprosthesis

The Shelhigh Skeletonized Super-Stentless™ (Shelhigh, Inc., Milburn, New Jersey, U.S.A.) aortic porcine bioprosthesis is a composite porcine bioprosthesis (Fig. 43). The valve is mounted on a super-flexible ring (skeleton), preserved with glutaraldehyde, detoxified, and heparin-treated with the No-React™ anticalcification treatment. The No-React™ treatment is a tissue-detoxification and stabilization process that makes cross-linking permanent and prevents the toxic glutaraldehyde molecules from leaching out of the tissue. The Shelhigh Super-Stentless™ valve has stentless hemodynamics and the implantation is as easy as that of a stented valve. The valve has a "volume-less" annulus that facilitates upsizing by one size.

Shelhigh Porcine Pulmonic Valve Conduit

The Shelhigh porcine pulmonic valve conduit (Shelhigh, Inc., Milburn, New Jersey, U.S.A.) is a glutaraldehyde-fixed porcine pulmonic valve and pulmonary artery extension to formulate the conduit (Fig. 44). The conduit is treated with the No-React™ tissue-detoxification process to reduce or delay the onset of calcification. The porcine pulmonic valve conduit has segments of bovine pericardial tissue to allow trimming to fit. The valve conduit is available in sizes 9 to 27 mm, and in the U.S.A. up to 18 mm.

Medtronic-Venpro Contegra Pulmonary Valved Conduit

The Medtronic-Venpro Contegra™ pulmonary valved conduit (Venpro, Minneapolis, Minnesota, U.S.A.) is a bioprosthesis consisting of a heterologous bovine jugular vein having a trileaflet venous valve and possessing a natural sinus slightly larger in diameter than its lumen (Fig. 45). The conduit is preserved in buffered glutaraldehyde in low concentration to preserve the flexibility of the leaflet material. The conduit is available in both unsupported and supported models. In the support-

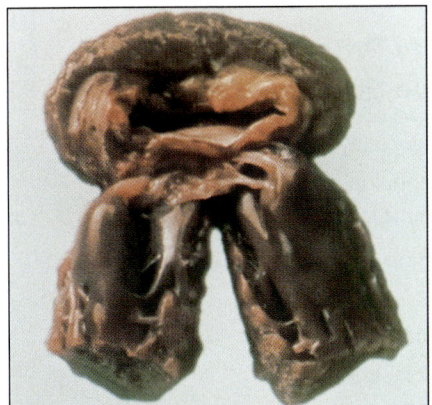
Figure 47. CryoValve Mitral Valve.

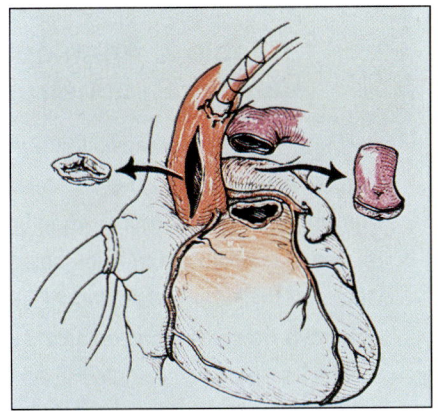
Figure 49. Pulmonary Autograft for Aortic Root.

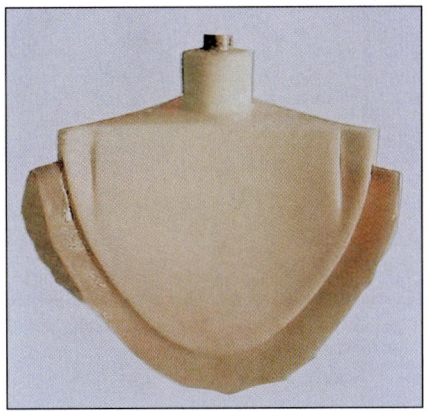
Figure 50. Autologous Pericardial Aortic Valve.

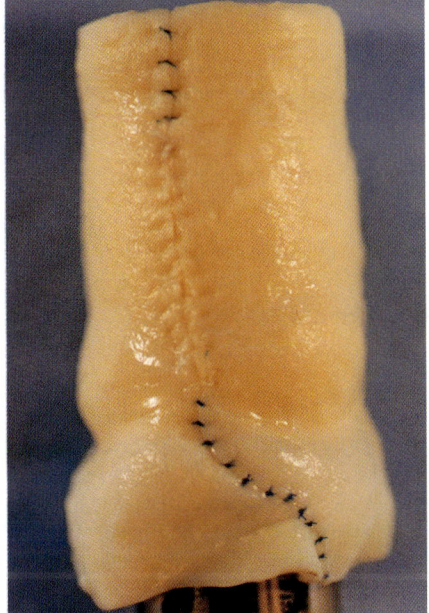
Figure 48. CryoSyner Graft Valve.

ed model, two external cloth-covered polypropylene rings provide additional support on either side of the valve. The available sizes are 12 to 22 mm.

BIOPROSTHESES—ALLOGRAFTS

CryoValve Aortic and Pulmonary Valve With/Without Conduit

CryoValve Aortic valve with or without conduit (Cryolife International, Inc., Kennesaw, Georgia, U.S.A.) is a cryopreserved human cadaveric aortic allograft for aortic-root replacement or freehand aortic valve (Fig. 46-1). The aortic valve is transected from the left ventricle containing the muscle band with or without the anterior mitral leaflet. The aortic allograft (homograft) also is available from institutional or regional tissue banks. The allograft aortic valve is acceptable for pediatric and adult valve replacement, small aortic root, women of childbearing age, and infective endocarditis. CryoValve pulmonary valve with conduit is a cryopreserved human cadaveric pulmonary allograft for pulmonary-root replacement (Fig. 46-2).

CryoValve Mitral Valve

CryoValve Mitral valve (Cryolife International, Inc., Kennesaw, Georgia, U.S.A.) is a cryopreserved mitral valve (Fig. 47). The mitral valve is transected from the left ventricle containing the muscle band and anterolateral and posteromedial papillary muscles, with the chordae tendineae attached. The mitral-valve prosthesis is used for both mitral- and tricuspid-valve replacements. The allograft valve is accepted for adult- and pediatric-valve replacement, women of childbearing age, infective endocarditis, and contraindication for anticoagulation therapy.

CryoSyner Graft Valve

The CryoSyner graft valve (CryoLife International, Inc., Kennesaw, Georgia, U.S.A.) is an acellular composite porcine-valve bioprosthesis (Fig. 48). The valve contains three sized and symmetry-matched decellularized porcine non-coronary cusp units, each with aortic leaflet, anterior mitral leaflet, and aortic conduit. This construct contains no myocardium. Its inflow is created from pendant anterior mitral leaflets, and outflow is formed from the three segments of the aortic wall. The bioprosthesis is designed for right ventricular outflow tract reconstruction, but also may be used for left ventricular-outflow tract, aortic-root reconstruction. The acellular, non-glutaraldehyde-prepared tissue facilitates repopulation with host fibroblastoid cells.

BIOPROSTHESES—AUTOGRAFTS

Pulmonary Autograft for Aortic Root

The pulmonary autograft is used to replace and/or reconstruct the aortic root. Pulmonary allograft is usually used to replace the pulmonary root; stentless porcine root is another alternative (Fig. 49).

Autologous Percardial Aortic Valve

Autologous pericardial aortic valve (CardioMed, Santa Barbara, California, U.S.A.) can be achieved by special instrumentation to formulate the stentless semilunar valve reconstruction with the autologous tissue (Fig. 50). The autologous tissue is treated initially with a brief immersion in 0.625% buffered glutaraldehyde solution. The chemical treatment stiffens the tissue, makes it easier to handle, and prevents thickening and shrinkage. The instruments include a sizer to assess leaflet height and commissural symmetry in addition to annular diameter, an intraoperative tissue tester to assess the mechanical properties of the tissue before it is used, a tool to cut a precisely sized novel geometric pattern, and formers to hold the tissue in anatomical orientation during valve reconstruction. The concept of autologous pericardial aortic valve has been used on an institutional, not commercial, basis without advanced instrumentation.

ANNULOPLASTY PROSTHESES FOR VALVULAR RECONSTRUCTIVE SURGERY—CURRENT

The techniques of mitral-valve reconstruction have been well established, but there remains controversy regarding the types of annuloplasty

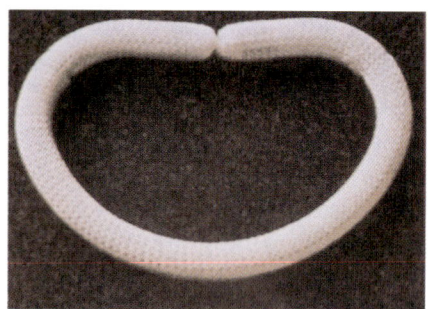

Figure 51. Carpentier-Edwards Classic Mitral Annuloplasty Ring.

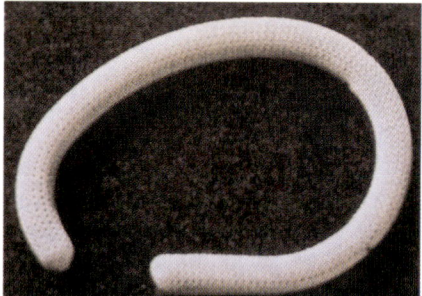

Figure 52. Carpentier-Edwards Classic Tricuspid Annuloplasty Ring.

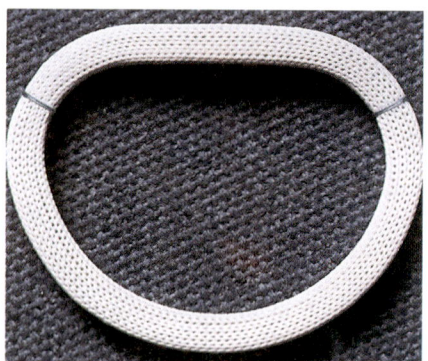

Figure 53. Carpentier-Edwards Physio Annuloplasty Ring.

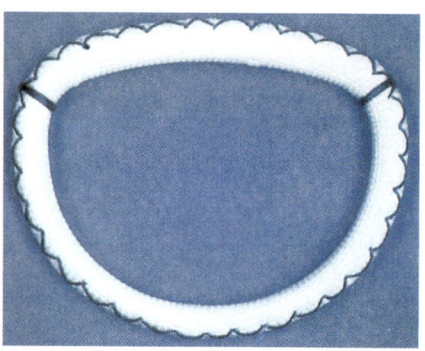

Figure 54. St. Jude Medical Seguin Annuloplasty Ring.

Table 3. Annuloplasty Prostheses for Valvular Reconstructive Surgery – Current

Carpentier-Edwards Classic Mitral Annuloplasty Ring
Carpentier-Edwards Classic Tricuspid Annuloplasty Ring
Carpentier-Edwards Physio Annuloplasty Ring
St. Jude Medical Seguin Annuloplasty Ring
Genesee Sculptor Annuloplasty Ring
Cosgrove-Edwards Annuloplasty System
Sulzer-CarboMedics Annulo Flo Annuloplasty Ring
Sulzer-CarboMedics Annulo Flex Annuloplasty Ring
St. Jude Medical Tailor Annuloplasty Ring
Medtronic Duran Flexible Annuloplasty Ring
Medtronic Duran Flexible Annuloplasty Band
Jostra Fully Flexible Annuloplasty Ring
Jostra Rigid Mitral Annuloplasty Ring
Jostra Rigid Tricuspid Annuloplasty Ring
Jostra Rigid La Pitié Annuloplasty Ring
AorTech MRS (Mitral Repair System)
Labcor Mitral Annuloplasty Ring
Medtronic Colvin-Galloway Annuloplasty System

rings. The available annuloplasty rings are rigid, flexible, complete, partial, and semi-rigid/flexible. Several objectives exist to annuloplasty, namely remodeling of the length and shape of the dilated annulus, prevention of dilitation of the annulus, and support for the potentially fragile area after partial-leaflet resection. Annuloplasty rings may have the potential for maintaining the anatomical and physiological characteristics of the mitral annulus.

Carpentier-Edwards Classic Annuloplasty Rings

The Carpentier-Edwards Classic annuloplasty rings (Edwards Lifesciences, Irvine, Inc., California, U.S.A.) are remodeling rigid rings designed specifically for mitral and tricuspid annular reconstructive surgery (Figs. 51 & 52). The rings are formulated from titanium alloy, with the sewing-ring margin composed of a layer of silicone rubber covered with a polyester knit fabric.

Carpentier-Edwards Physio Annuloplasty Ring

The Carpentier-Edwards Physio annuloplasty ring (Edwards Lifesciences, Irvine, California, U.S.A.) is a remodeling, semi-flexible annuloplasty ring (Fig. 53). The ring is fabricated with layers of Elgiloy™ and plastic strips, with sewing-line margin that consists of a layer of silicone rubber covered by a polyester knit fabric.

St. Jude Medical Seguin Annuloplasty Ring

The St. Jude Medical Seguin annuloplasty ring (St. Jude Medical, Inc., St. Paul, Minnesota, U.S.A.) is made of a solid, one-piece core consisting of ultra-high-weight polyethylene thicker in the anterior portion and thinner in the posterior portion to enhance flexibility (Fig. 54).

Genesee Sculptor Annuloplasty Ring

The Genesee Sculptor annuloplasty ring (Genesee Biomedical, Inc., Denver, Colorado, U.S.A.) is a semi-flexible, adjustable annular ring for mitral-valve reconstruction (Fig. 55). The anterior portion of the ring contains a curved, metal stiffener, which conforms to the shape of the anterior portion of the annulus to maintain the intertrigonal distance during implantation and long term. The posterior portion of the ring is flexible to conform to the changes in annular shape and size during the cardiac cycle. Color-coded drawstrings allow any, or all, of the four adjustable segments of the

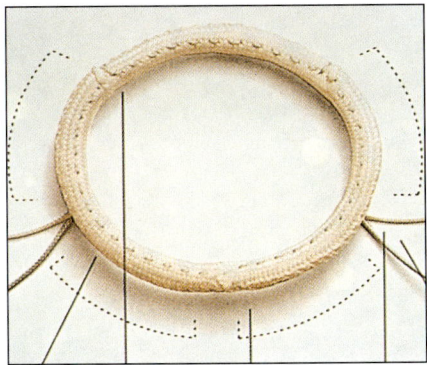

Figure 55. Genesee Sculptor Annuloplasty Ring.

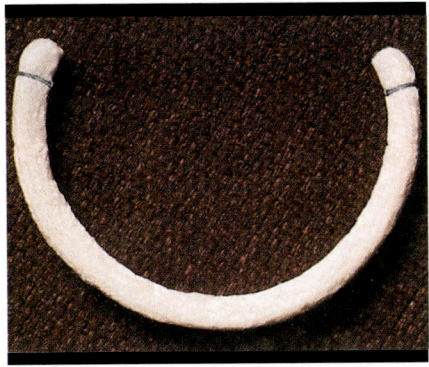

Figure 56. Cosgrove-Edwards Annuloplasty System.

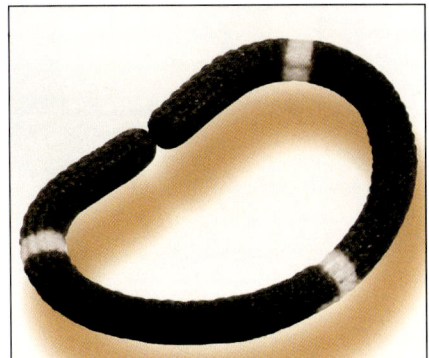

Figure 57. Sulzer-Carbomedics Annulo Flo Annuloplasty Ring.

posterior portion of the ring to be shortened, which allows for "fine-tuning" of the repair in the case of mild commissural leaks.

Cosgrove-Edwards Annuloplasty System

The Cosgrove-Edwards annuloplasty system (Edwards Lifesciences, Irvine, California, U.S.A.) is a non-remodeling, open flexible ring (Fig. 56). The ring incorporates barium sulfate-impregnated silicone rubber covered by a polyester velour cloth.

Sulzer-Carbomedics Annulo Flo Annuloplasty Ring

The Sulzer-Carbomedics Annulo Flo annuloplasty ring (Sulzer Cabomedics, Austin, Texas, U.S.A.) is a rigid remodeling annuloplasty ring (Fig. 57). The titanium-stiffening ring ensures annulus remodeling and allows radiographic analysis. Orientation markers are provided for implant placement.

Sulzer-Carbomedics Annulo Flex Annuloplasty Ring

The Sulzer-Carbomedics Annulo Flex annuloplasty ring (Sulzer-Carbomedics, Austin, Texas, U.S.A.) provides the opportunity for a partial or complete annuloplasty system (Fig. 58). Removal of the anterior portion converts the prosthesis from a complete to partial ring; two suture cut points optimize conversion to a partial ring. The full flexibility provides three-dimensional compliance that mirrors natural valve dynamics. The barium-impregnated silicon provides radiographic visualization.

St. Jude Medical Tailor Annuloplasty Ring

The St. Jude Medical Tailor annuloplasty ring (St. Jude Medical, Inc., St. Paul, Minnesota, U.S.A.) is a unique annuloplasty ring that supports multiple repair options (Fig. 59). The ring is fully flexible to accommodate the natural movement of the annulus, and can be cut anywhere within the intertrigonal area to create a customized C-ring. The ring is suitable for both mitral and tricuspid valve repair, and provides the opportunity for a complete or partial annuloplasty.

Medtronic-Duran Flexible Annuloplasty Ring

The Medtronic-Duran flexible annuloplasty ring (Medtronic, Minneapolis, Minnesota, U.S.A.), has been available for 25 years; it is a radioopaque ring (Fig. 60). The ring provides the opportunity for the annulus to decrease during systole. This flexible ring is an option to a rigid ring in

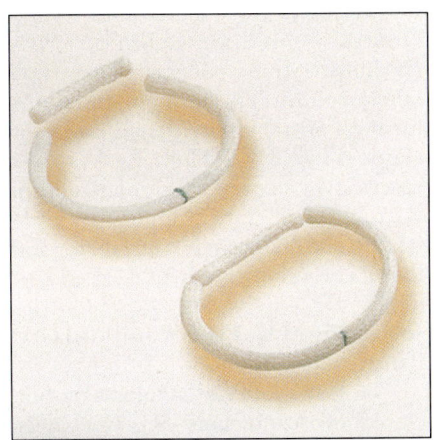

Figure 58. Sulzer-Carbomedics Annulo Flex Annuloplasty Ring.

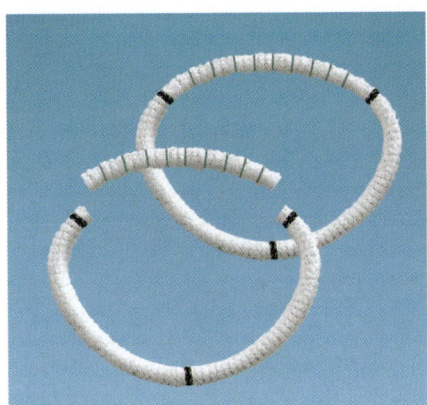

Figure 59. St. Jude Medical Tailor Annuloplasty Ring.

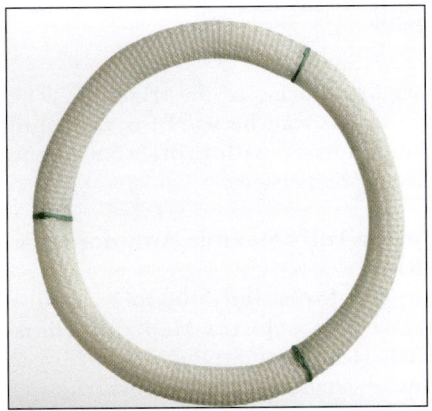

Figure 60. Medtronic-Duran Flexible Annuloplasty Ring.

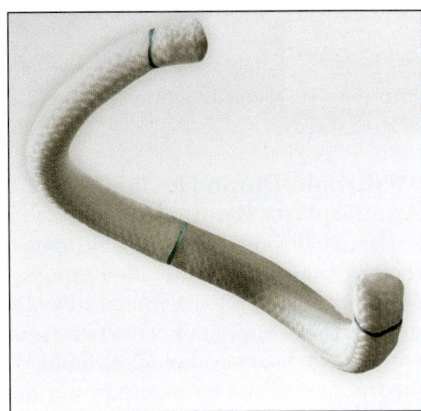

Figure 61. Medtronic-Duran Flexible Annuloplasty Band.

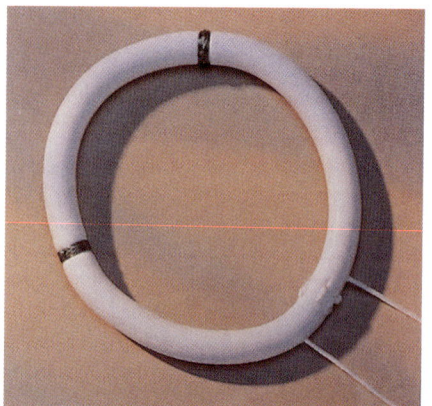

Figure 62. Jostra Fully Flexible Annuloplasty Ring.

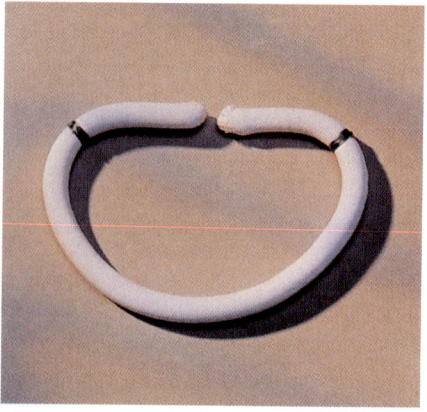

Figure 63. Jostra Rigid Mitral Annuloplasty Ring.

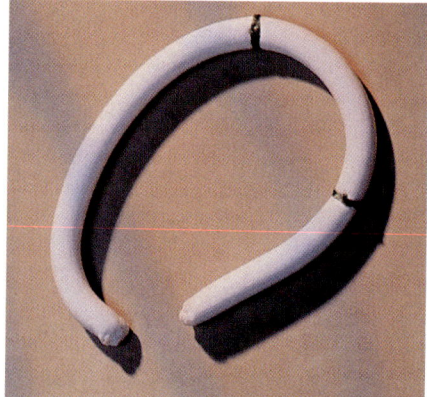

Figure 64. Jostra Rigid Tricuspid Annuloplasty Ring.

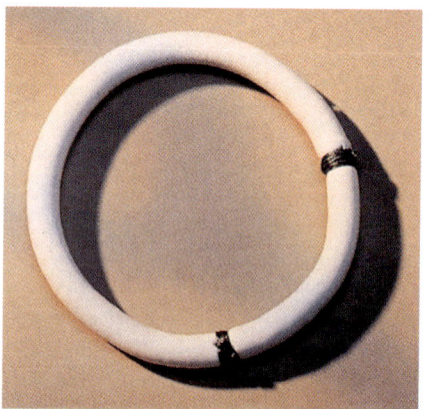

Figure 65. Jostra Rigid La Pitié Annuloplasty Ring.

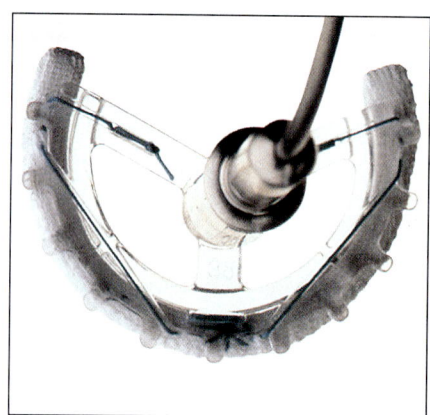

Figure 66. AorTech MRS (Mitral Repair System).

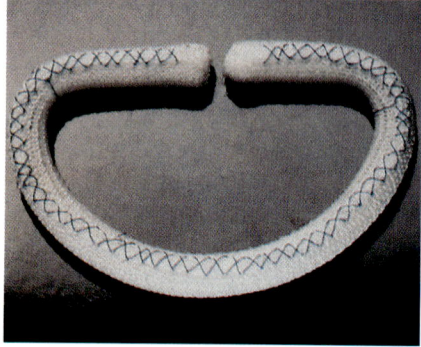

Figure 67. Labcor Mitral Annuloplasty Ring.

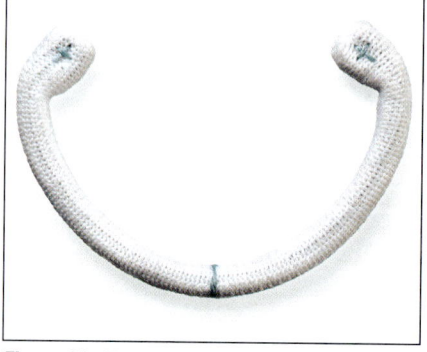

Figure 68. Medtronic Colvin-Galloway Future™ Band.

mitral-valve reconstruction for degenerative disease.

Medtronic-Duran Flexible Annuloplasty Band

The Medtronic-Duran flexible annuloplasty band (Medtronic, Minneapolis, Minnesota, U.S.A.) is a partial flexible device that supports reconstruction when the primary pathological findings incorporate dilatation of the posterior annulus (Fig. 61). The Duran band extends beyond the trigones to provide secure suturing to the trigones. The band also can be used for tricuspid annuloplasty with protection of the conduction system.

Jostra Fully Flexible Annuloplasty Ring

The Jostra fully flexible annuloplasty ring (Jostra Medizintechnik AG, Hechinger Strabe, Germany) is an adjustable ring for reconstruction of insufficient or dilated mitral or tricuspid valves (Fig. 62). The fully flexible ring allows the valve annulus to maintain both annular shape and motion. The ring is composed solely of PTFE and a polyester suture. The intertrigonal segment of the ring is unadjustable. Each side of the ring can be adjusted individually; the ring can be adjusted after implantation.

Jostra Rigid Annuloplasty Rings

The Jostra Rigid annuloplasty rings (Jostra Medizintechnik AG, Hechinger Strabe, Germany) are rigid fabric-reinforced ring, formulations for both mitral and tricuspid positions (Figs. 63 & 64). The ring has four layers over a core of rigid titanium wire covered with a highly flexible PTFE tube, polyester knit fabric, and thin PTFE tubing.

Jostra Rigid La Pitié Annuloplasty Ring

The Jostra La Pitié annuloplasty ring (Jostra Medizintechnik AG, Hechinger Strabe, Germany) is a completely flexible, fabric-reinforced annuloplasty ring for reconstruction of insufficient or dilated mitral or tricuspid valves (Fig. 65). The ring affords the opportunity for annular shape and motion. The core of the ring is a highly flexible PTFE round-shaped material covered with a polyester knit fabric and thin PTFE tubing.

AorTech MRS (Mitral Repair System)

The AorTech mitral repair system (Aortech, Bellshill, Scotland) is an open flexible annuloplasty ring made of knitted PTFE containing a radio-opaque barium-impregnated silicon marker (Fig. 66).

Labcor Mitral Annuloplasty Ring

The Labcor mitral annuloplasty ring (Labcor, Inc., Belo Horizonte, MG, Brazil) is a rigid remodeling annuloplasty ring (Fig. 67). The ring is formulated from a Celcon foundation with a silastic membrane covered with Dacron™. The prosthesis supports normal function of the mitral annulus with a rigid anterior segment and a flexible posterior segment originating at the anterior and posterior commissures.

Medtronic Colvin-Galloway Future™ Band

The Medtronic Colvin-Galloway Future™ Band (Medtronic Inc., Minneapolis, Minnesota, U.S.A.) is a low-profile, semi-rigid partial band composed of an inner core of a proprietary metal alloy possessing a combination of high strength and durability (Fig. 68). Because of this core, the band offers stiffness to provide remodeling yet flexibility to allow movement of the mitral annulus during the cardiac cycle. The band also has anchoring eyelets that align with the annular trigones for ease of attachment.

MECHANICAL PROSTHESES — DEVELOPMENTAL AND EXPERIMENTAL

Carbomedics Kinetic Mechanical Prosthesis

The Carbomedics Kinetic mechanical prosthesis (Sulzer-Carbomedics Inc., Austin, Texas, U.S.A.) is a prosthesis designed but not evaluated (Fig. 69). This investigational bileaflet design incorporates all the features of the current Carbomedics mechanical prosthesis including a solid carbon orifice, in situ rotatability, enhanced radioopacity, Biolite™ carbon-coated sewing rings, and pivots contained within the orifice protected by a solid metal ring. The prosthesis offers a new pivot design modeled with advanced computer technology to improve pivot washing. The prosthesis leaflet opening angles vary as a function of valve size. The opening angle design minimizes energy losses associated with high gradients in small sizes and reduces energy loss resulting from excessive reflux volumes with larger sizes. The increased orifice area has been achieved without increasing the exterior size of the prosthesis. The sewing ring of the mitral prosthesis has a compliant silicon filler, and a Pyrolite™ rim that serves as barrier to tissue growth.

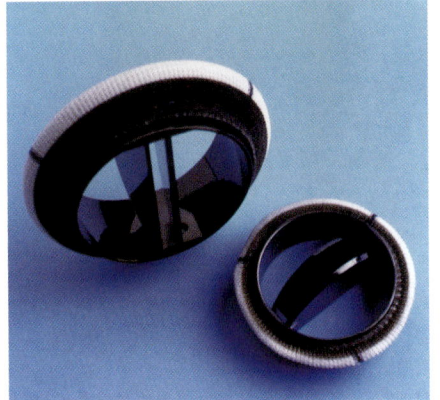

Figure 69. Carbomedics Kinetic Mechanical Prosthesis.

Triflo Medical Mechanical Heart Valve

The Triflo medical mechanical heart valve (Triflo Medical, Inc., Irvine, California, U.S.A.) is an experimental trileaflet prosthesis (Fig. 70). The leaflets are three-dimensionally shaped and the valve orifice has a nozzle-shaped, streamlined configuration. The leaflet configuration provides a soft and early-closure mechanism, similar to the natural aortic valve, with minimal regurgitation and a low tendency for cavitation and HITS generation. The streamlined design minimizes flow separation and is associated with a low gradient. The prosthesis is scheduled for clinical trials following completion of animal studies.

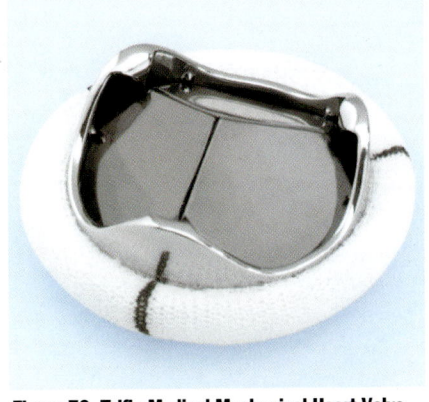

Figure 70. Triflo Medical Mechanical Heart Valve.

BIOPROSTHESES — DEVELOPMENTAL AND EXPERIMENTAL

Carbomedics Oxford Stentless Porcine Bioprosthesis

The Oxford stentless porcine bioprosthesis (Sulzer-Carbomedics, Inc.,

---

Table 4. Mechanical Prostheses – Developmental and Experimental

Carbomedics Kinetic Mechanical Prosthesis

Triflo Medical Mechanical Heart Valve

Table 5. Bioprostheses and Biomechanical Prostheses – Developmental and Experimental

3F Therapeutics™ Stentless Equine Pericardial Aortic Bioprosthesis

Carbomedics Oxford Stentless Porcine Bioprosthesis

St. Jude Medical-Toronto SPV Duo Stentless Root™ Porcine Bioprosthesis

AorTech Elan Stentless Porcine Bioprosthesis

Edwards Flexible Pericardial Aortic Bioprosthesis

Medtronic Physiologic Mitral Valve (PMV)

Robicsek-Thubrikar Graft

AorTech Aspire Polymer Prosthesis

Adiam Polyurethane Prosthesis

Sulzer-Carbomedics Polymer Prosthesis

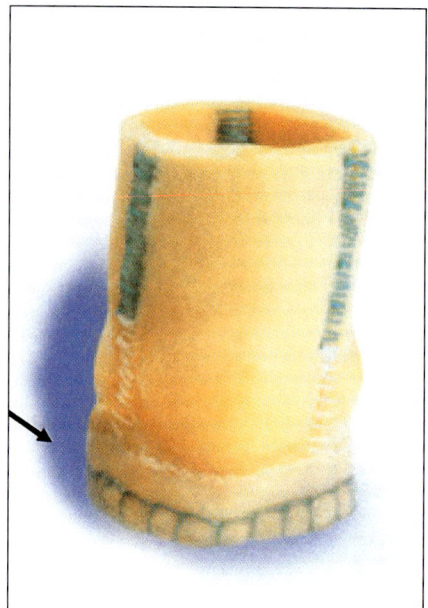

Figure 71. Carbomedics Oxford Stentless Porcine Bioprosthesis.

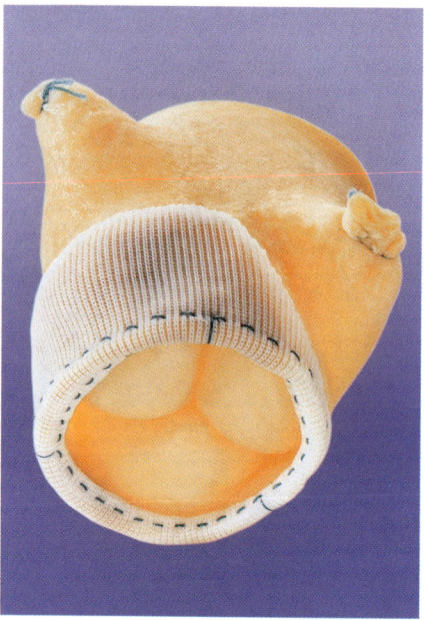

Figure 72. St. Jude Medical-Toronto SPV Duo Stentless Root™ Porcine Bioprosthesis.

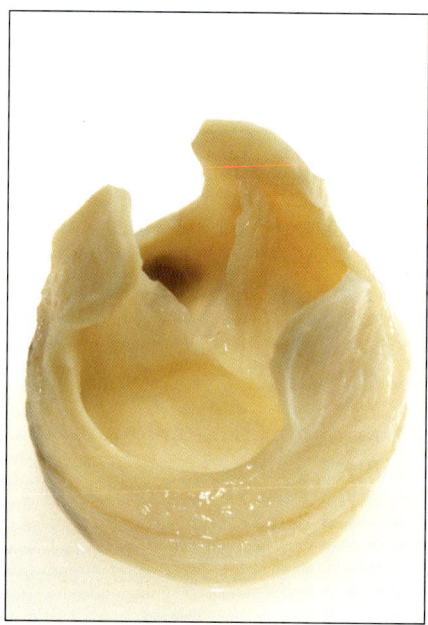

Figure 73. AorTech Elan Stentless Aortic Porcine Bioprosthesis.

Austin, Texas, U.S.A.) is a composite bioprosthesis formulated from three non-coronary porcine aortic cusps and adjacent aortic sinuses and aortic wall (Fig. 71). Fabrication of the porcine root is formulated with the suturing of the three components to facilitate use as a subcoronary or aortic-root implantation. The bioprosthesis may be introduced with glutaraldehyde-preservation and advanced calcium mitigation therapy. The bioprosthesis will be reintroduced in the future with preservation of the porcine tissue conducted by collagen cross-linking by the dye-mediated photo-oxidation technique. Proximal suturing is to be formulated in a horizontal plane at the annular level and trimming of the root tissue for distal suturing in the subcoronary and commisural placement. The total root replacement is to be implanted with the same proximal suturing technique and coronary ostial aortic buttons for the coronary artery implantation.

St. Jude Medical-Toronto SPV Duo Stentless Root™ Porcine Bioprosthesis

The St. Jude Medical-Toronto SPV Duo Stentless Root™ porcine bioprosthesis (St. Jude Medical, Inc., Minneapolis, Minnesota, U.S.A.) is a new-generation porcine aortic root for implantation as a subcoronary, freehand valve insertion or an aortic root replacement (Fig. 72). The proximal sewing ridge is covered with fine Dacron™, and the muscle shelf is also covered with fine Dacron™ mesh. The porcine tissue is preserved with low-pressure glutaraldehyde fixation. The tissue is treated with the BiLinx™ anticalcification technology, which has been identified to reduce calcification on the aortic wall tissue, as well as the aortic leaflet. The Toronto SPV Root™ is used in procedures where aortic root disease accompanies valve disease.

AorTech Elan Stentless Aortic Porcine Bioprosthesis

The AorTech Elan stentless aortic porcine bioprosthesis (AorTech, Bellshill, Scotland) is a new-generation prosthesis in early stages of clinical evaluation (Fig. 73).

Medtronic Physiologic Mitral Valve (PMV)

The Medtronic physiologic mitral valve (Medtronic, Minneapolis, Minnesota, U.S.A.) is a prosthesis-in-development based on the platform of a stentless porcine mitral xenograft (Fig. 74). The prosthesis is based on the concept that restoration of the native mitral valvular mechanics, due to non-repairable valvular disease, requires a complete functioning unit that includes both left ventricular and annular mechanics to ensure optimum valvular function. The valve is modified to facilitate implantation through addition of sewing tubes attached along the three-dimensional axial direction of the strut chordae. Annular reinforcement is provided by either cloth or porcine pericardium. Markers are provided on the sewing tube in 5-mm increments to enable trimming. Annular markers delineate the commissures as well as short axis of the valve annulus. Valve size is based on the linear intra-trigonal distance. The valvular tissue is preserved with glutaraldehyde or another non-glutaraldehyde collagen cross-linking agent, such as carbodiimide. Zero-pressure fixation is used *in situ* within a portion of the porcine left ventricle to ensure maintenance of proper valvular geometry and leaflet biomechanics. Alpha oleic acid (AOA) antimineralization treatment is provided to mitigate bioprosthetic calcification when the valve is processed using glutaraldehyde.

3F Therapeutics™ Stentless Equine Pericardial Aortic Bioprosthesis

The 3F Therapeutics™ bioprosthesis (3F Therapeutics Inc., Lake Forest, California, U.S.A.) is composed of three equal sections of equine pericardium that have been processed by fixation with a buffered formulation of glutaraldehyde, and are assembled together to form a tubular structure (Fig. 75). The glutaraldehyde formulation is of concentration low enough to preserve much of the flexibility of the raw material, and fully crosslink the collagenous structure to preserve its strength, mini-

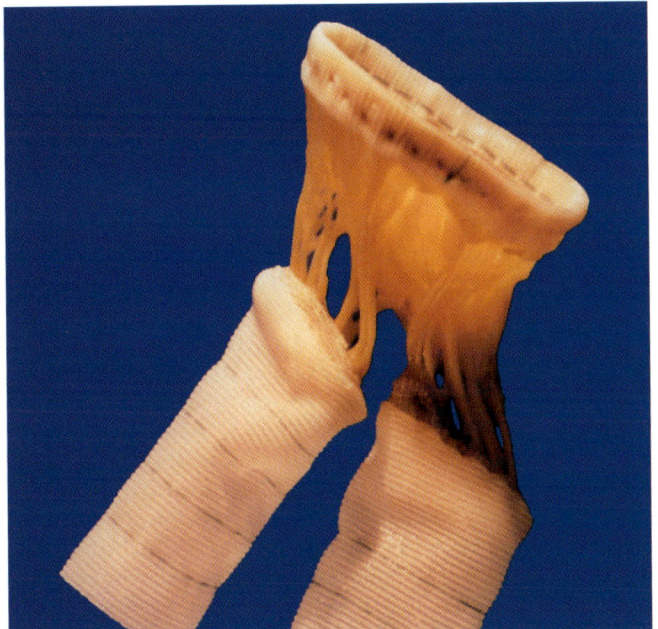

Figure 74. Medtronic Physiologic Mitral Valve.

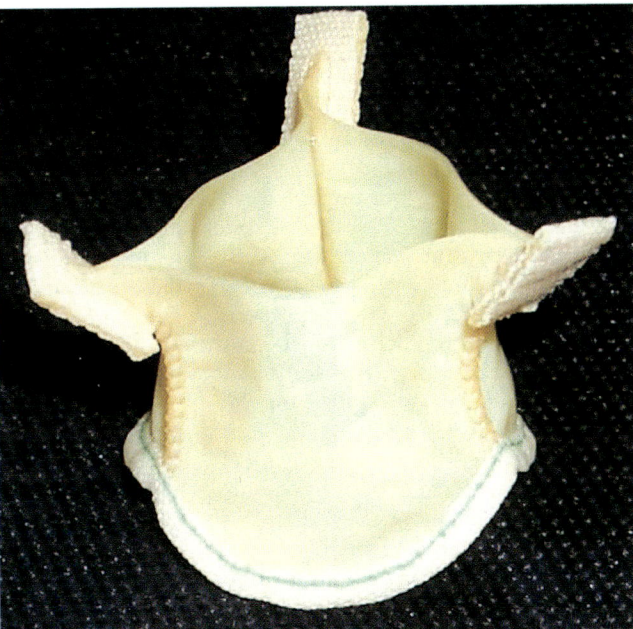

Figure 75. 3F Therapeutics™ Stentless Equine Pericardial Aortic Bioprosthesis.

mize its immunogenic and thrombogenic potentials and provide lengthened durability when implanted in the heart of the patient. In contrast with bovine pericardium, equine pericardium comes from a source that has not been implicated in transmissible spongiform encephalopathies. The inflow aspect of the bioprosthesis is fitted with a woven polyester cuff to facilitate suturing of the device to the orifice created by removal of the diseased heart valve, and allow fibrous ingrowth to help in prevention of perivalvular leakage. The junctions of the three pericardial sections that form the leaflets become the three commissures of the bioprosthetic valve. These commissural attachment sites are integral tabs of pericardium backed by woven polyester material. The polyester material serves to reinforce the tissue and firmly affix the commissural attachment sites near the sino-tubular junction of the native aorta during surgical implantation of the bioprosthesis. The 3F Therapeutics™ mitral bioprosthesis is composed of two leaflets of equine pericardium with integral tabs of pericardium for papillary muscle attachment.

Edwards Flexible Pericardial Aortic Bioprosthesis

The Edwards flexible pericardial aortic bioprosthesis (Edwards Lifesciences, Irvine, California, U.S.A.) is a prosthesis-in-development. The design integrates the proven pericardial technology of the Carpentier-Edwards Perimount pericardial tissue valve into a flexible frame that conforms to the anatomy of the native aortic valve. The flexible frame allows contraction and expansion of the valve prosthesis at the aortic root and the commissures in concert with native aortic wall motion.

The structural stent is highly flexible in a generally cylindrical configuration, with cusps and commissures permitted to move radially. The stent commissures are constructed so that the cusps are pivotably or flexibly coupled together at the commissures to permit relative movement. The stent is cloth covered and may be a single element or may be made in three separate elements for a three-cusp valve, each element having a cusp portion for each pair of adjacent stent elements combining to form the stent commissures. The cloth covering may incorporate an outward projecting flap or connecting band that follows the cusps and commissures. The valve is connected to the natural tissue along the undulating connecting band. The connecting band may be cloth-covered silicon to provide support to the stent and outer side of the valve at the commissures.

The implantation is expected to be supra-annular into the aortic wall above the native annulus, providing optimal coronary artery space in the coronary sinuses. The prosthesis incorporates a multi-legged holder used to implant the prosthesis and maintain its implant

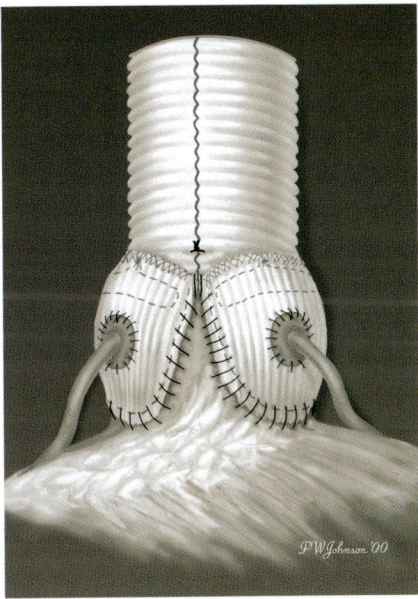

Figure 76. Robicsek-Thubrikar Graft (Aortic Root Prosthesis with Compliant Sinuses).

shape.

Robicsek-Thubrikar Graft Aortic Root Prosthesis with Compliant Sinuses

The aortic root prosthesis with compliant sinuses (Robicsek-Thubrikar Graft) is designed for use in the aortic valve-sparing operation (Fig. 76). The prosthesis has been formulated to address the concerns of the current techniques of aortic valve-sparing operations, namely–contact of the leaflets with the Dacron™ fabric wall in the tubular application and maintenance of normal dynamics of the valve leaflets in the remodeling application. The graft design is based on the design of the natural aortic root. The normal dynamics of the valve leaflets are achieved by maintenance of compliance of the graft by the re-orientation of the Z-fold in the Dacron™ tube. Presence of the sinuses prevents the leaflets from contact with the Dacron™ fabric wall by creating a space between the open leaflets and sinus wall. The leaflet-sinus assembly has a circular cross-section in the circumferential direction of the leaflet. This circularity allows the sharing of the stress between the leaflets and the sinuses, and thereby avoids stress concentration on the leaflets. It is believed that absence of stress concentration in the sinus graft-valve assembly is necessary for longevity of the leaflets. Both the sinus geometry and orientation of the Z-fold in the direction of the blood flow allow smooth formation of vortices in the spaces behind the leaflets, which has the potential to reduce the formation of thrombus and embolism. Suturing of the two coronary ostia is also made easy in the sinus graft because the graft wall comes closer to the coronary buttons and attachment of the left and right coronary arteries appears natural and dynamics of the graft are maintained. The sinus graft offers benefit by the potential for reduction of thromboembolic phenomena and enhancement of the functional life of the leaflets. The prosthesis is formulated in the operating room from a Meadox (Meadox Medical Ltd.) graft to the specifications of the patient.

AorTech Aspire Stentless Mechanical Flexible Prosthesis

The AorTech Elast Eon™ synthetic bioprosthesis (AorTech, Bellshill, Scotland) is an experimental prosthesis-in-development. The new tri-leaflet prosthesis is composed of a unique soft segment that combines the best properties of silicone and polyurethane. The material has exhibited biostability, biocompatibility, and durability *in vitro* and *in vivo*.

Adiam Polyurethane Prosthesis

The Adiam polyurethane mechanical (flexible) prosthesis (Adiam Life Science, Bernhard-Hahn, Germany) is an experimental prosthesis-in-development. The prosthesis is formulated by a specific polyurethane composition. The prosthesis-type is formulated as a trileaflet aortic prosthesis and bileaflet mitral prosthesis. The prostheses are totally formulated, inclusive of the sewing cuff, of polyurethane. The chemical composition of the polyurethane is formulated to support mitigation of calcium and prevent prosthesis degeneration.

Sulzer-Carbomedics Polymer Prosthesis

The Sulzer-Carbomedics polymer mechanical (flexible) prosthesis (Sulzer-Carbomedics, Austin, Texas, U.S.A.) is an experimental prosthesis-in-development. Sulzer-Carbomedics has developed a proprietary tear-resistant polymer similar to polyetherurethane urea (PEU) alternatives, including polycarbonateurethane (PCU) and polysiliconeurethane (PSU).[39,40]

Nearly 30 years ago, a trileaflet PEU valve proved too prone to thrombosis and mineralization in a juvenile sheep model.[41] Sulzer-Carbomedics' experience with a prototype polymer valve design suggested that valve mineralization is associated primarily with adherent thrombus rather than leaflet material.[42-44] Surface modification of the prototype PEU valve with either of two different non-thrombogenic ligands virtually eliminated leaflet thrombus accumulation and mineralization, which implied that any material or material treatment that reduces accumulation of thrombus upon polymer valve leaflets should inhibit leaflet mineralization.[45] Development efforts at Sulzer-Carbomedics have been driven by the belief that a prosthetic polymer valve, fabricated of a durable polymeric material and surface treated with a non-thrombogenic reagent, provides durability greater than that offered by current clinical tissue valves, yet may not require chronic patient anticoagulation as do mechanical valves.

The durability of fatigue/degradation resistance of available polymers have proved unacceptable in heart-valve application. Despite a reported 20-year lifetime in accelerated durability testing *in vitro* of at least one polymer valve, no valve or material has proved adequately durable and hemocompatible in pre-clinical animal studies, much less human clinical studies.[46] Polyetherurethanes used commonly in the medical device industry have excellent initial mechanical properties, but appear susceptible to biodegradation in both *in vitro* and animal models.

The polymer developed by Sulzer-Carbomedics has demonstrated that constitutive modeling and finite element analysis predicts polymer will have durability beyond 20-year clinical valve lifetime in an appropriate design.[47] An acceptable design must minimize leaflet stresses and incorporate appropriate hemodynamics, while maintaining fatigue resistance and exploiting material surface chemistry. Design features that minimize leaflet stresses must not result in valve thrombosis. The ultimate design of the valve is a formidable challenge but must perform adequately in all aspects (fatigue resistance, durability, thrombosis resistance, and hemodynamics).

TECHNOLOGICAL ADVANCES

Technology has been striving to bring forward advances that improve the durability of bioprostheses and reduce the thrombogenicity of mechanical prostheses. The current status of technological progress is showing promise at meeting these objectives.

BIOPROSTHESES

Glutaraldehyde has been used effectively to stabilize connective tissue for porcine and bovine pericardial heart valve substitutes over the past 25 years. Glutaraldehyde cross-linking of collagen reduces biodegradation significantly. Of the aldehydes, glutaraldehyde produces the most chemically, biologically, and thermally stable collagen cross-links. Long-term durability of glutaraldehyde-preserved bioprostheses has remained the most significant concern.[48-51] Dystrophic calcification was identified initially in children and young adults.[52,53] Glutaraldehyde has been implicated in the calcification process.[54-59] Mechanical stress also has been implicated as a causative factor of calcification.[60-62] In porcine bioprostheses, stresses were lowest at the base of the leaflet, whereas highest near the commissures where calcification is found most frequently. The highest stresses of heterograft prostheses are in the areas of greatest flexion.[63] These observations have identified that both glutaraldehyde and mechanical stresses are of the utmost importance.

Glutaraldehyde is both a biomaterial-stabilizing agent and a sterilizing agent, but does provide a significant element of toxicity.[64-66] The stabilization or tanning effect of glutaraldehyde is dependent on concentration, exposure time, temperature, pH, and concentration. The toxicity of glutaraldehyde contributes to lack of endothelial cell coverage in human implants due to aldehydes released from the treated tissue.[54] It also is believed that the toxicity from leaching of the unbound glutaraldehyde, or its polymers from the treated tissue or aldehyde storage solutions, cause the tissue propensity to develop calcification.[50,55,58,67-69]

The appropriate management of this problem has been reviewed by Myers and colleagues,[68] emphasizing the need to ameliorate the toxicity of glutaraldehyde or identify effective means of preserving tissue not involving aldehydes. Measures have been taken over the past 10 to 15 years to control this glutaraldehyde toxicity. Surfactants, particularly sodium dodecyl sulfate and polysorbate-80, have been incorporated in the preservation process of the current-generation bioprostheses.[57,70] Jones and colleagues,[70] reporting in 1989, disclosed that only surfactants reduced calcification substantially in experimental models, but only in porcine and not pericardial bioprostheses.

Control of residual aldehydes, following glutaraldehyde fixation, with amino-oleic acid (AOA) has been evaluated extensively and used currently in the Medtronic prostheses, stented Mosaic porcine, and stentless Freestyle™ porcine.[55,71-75] In 1992, Gott and co-authors[75] reported that AOA reduced mineralization of porcine prostheses dramatically in a juvenile sheep model. It was noted subsequently that, whereas the aortic cusps remained free of calcification, the aortic wall developed calcification. The investigators reported that with increasing AOA concentration during treatment, increasing penetration was present into the wall. Chen and co-authors[71] indicated that the aortic wall had less AOA binding and differences in calcium-diffusion kinetics. These characteristics are important, especially if the Medtronic Freestyle™ is used as a root replacement.

Alternatives to glutaraldehyde cross-linking of collagen are being pursued actively. The agents being studied either are incorporated into the tissue (e.g., glutaraldehyde or epoxide), or act as promoters of the cross-linking process (e.g., acyl azide or dye-mediated photo-oxidation). The epoxide compounds, such as Denacol, form strong cross-links with the carboxyl and amino protein groups.[76,77] The compound, acyl azide, facilitates cross-linking without incorporating the agent into the fixed tissue.[78,79] The agent, carbodiimide, also leaves no residual cross-linking chemical as part of the bridge between polypeptide chains.[68] The carbodiimide cross-linked tissue is completely non-toxic, and both shrink temperature and collagenase digestion are similar to glutaraldehyde. This process reduces calcification only in the valve cusps and not the aortic wall.

An additional method of preventing calcification of glutaraldehyde- preserved porcine tissue is preincubation with a combination of aluminum chloride and ethanol.[80-82] The combination inhibited calcification in both the cusps and aortic wall. The hypothesis of calcification inhibition is the interaction of membrane-lipid removal and ethanol-induced collagen structural changes. Ethanol-treated cusps were free of calcification in rat subdermal implants and sheep mitral replacements but aortic wall had focal calcification. In tissue treated only with glutaraldehyde, there was marked cuspal and aortic wall mineralization. The extracellular calcification of aortic wall elastin is inhibited by aluminum chloride.[83]

Dye-mediated photo-oxidation also is a promoting process of collagen cross-linking.[84-86] The porcine tissue is treated with an aqueous solution, including the photo-oxidative dye and light irradiated. Several amino acids of the collagen polypeptide chains are modified. Moore and co-authors[86] reported that enzymatic digestion, chemical digestion, and shrink temperature are similar to tissue treated with glutaraldehyde. In the juvenile sheep model, there was minimal cusp mineralization at one year.[86]

The concept of acellular matrix has received more consideration because cellular components may be the focus of calcification.[87] Novel tissue-engineering approaches are being investigated to improve replacement heart-valve durability.[88-90] These tissue-engineering techniques are focused on fabricating the intricate architecture of the valve leaflets. Scaffolds have been developed from synthetic and naturally occurring polymers and then cellularized from host endothelial cells in tissue culture. Besides synthetic scaffolds, both heterograft and allograft valvular tissue can be decellularized and repopulated *in vitro* with the predetermined host cells. O'Brien and colleagues[91] have developed stentless allograft bioprosthetic valves that have been fabricated from acellular tissues, cryopreserved, and implanted as pulmonary root replacements in juvenile sheep. After 150 days, the grafts showed intact leaflets with in-growth of host fibroblastoid cells in all explanted porcine valves and no evidence of calcification. The decellularization process with heterografts replaces the use of glutaraldehyde for collagen cross-linking to limit xenograft antigenicity. The predominant issues with this modality of tissue engineering is the maintenance of balancing scaffold disappearance and interstitial cell reseeding, and support a desirable host cellular response not susceptible to antigenic recognition and immunologic rejection. Elkins and collaborators[92] have implanted porcine decellularized conduits in both the pulmonary and aortic outflow tracts in humans.

The future bioprostheses will be treated with glutaraldehyde and various agents to control active aldehyde residues, or with collagen cross-linking promoters that facilitate amino acid residues on adjacent chains to cross-link.

MECHANICAL PROSTHESES

The demonstrated new standards for *in vitro* analysis of mechanical prostheses will likely contribute to prosthesis designs to reduce incidence of thromboembolic phenomena, including thrombosis. The flow fields within the hinge pockets of prostheses are believed to contribute to thrombus formation. Microstructural flow visualization, computational fluid dynamics modeling, laser Doppler velocimetry measurements, and laser Doppler anemometry measurements have all contributed to prostheses hinge-pocket performance and design.[93-96]

These investigative technologies should be used in development of all

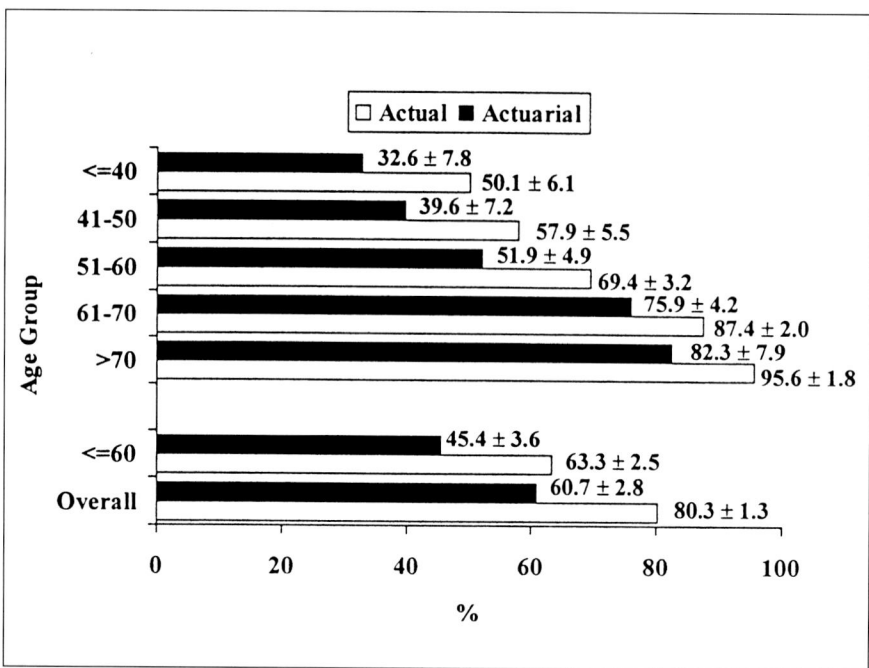

Figure 77. Freedom from structural valve deterioration (actuarial and actual) for aortic valve replacement. Published with Permission From: Jamieson WRE, Burr LH, Miyagishima RT, et al. Actuarial versus actual freedom from structural valve deterioration with the Carpentier-Edwards porcine bioprostheses. Can J Cardiol 1999;15(9):973-8.

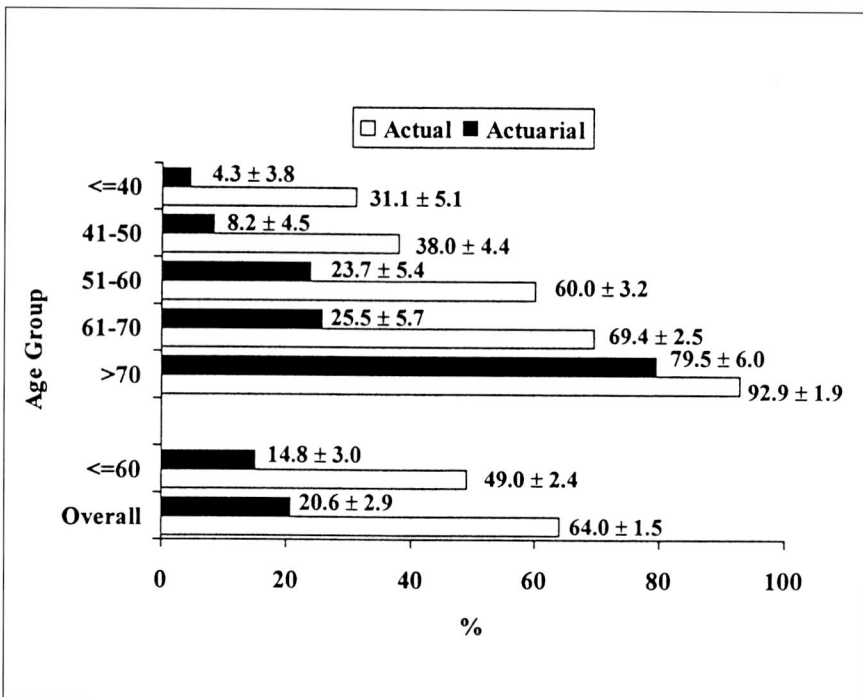

Figure 78. Freedom from structural valve deterioration (actuarial and actual) for mitral valve replacement. Published with Permission From: Jamieson WRE, Burr LH, Miyagishima RT, et al. Actuarial versus actual freedom from structural valve deterioration with the Carpentier-Edwards porcine bioprostheses. Can J Cardiol 1999;15(9):973-8.

the wide array of current developmental and experimental bioprostheses and mechanical prostheses is beyond the scope of this monograph article. Sections on implantation considerations were part of "Cardiac Valve Replacement Surgery: Prostheses and Technological Considerations" in Surgical Technology International III and "Cardiac Valvular Replacement Devices: Residual Problems and Innovative Investigative Technologies" in Surgical Technology International VII.

CLINICAL PERFORMANCE—INDICATIONS FOR PROSTHESIS TYPE

Cardiac valvular prostheses are evaluated by clinical and hemodynamic performance. The current-generation stented and stentless porcine and pericardial bioprostheses have, generally, satisfactory hemodynamic performance. The clinical performance is judged according to the "Guidelines for Reporting Morbidity and Mortality After Cardiac Valvular Operations."[97] The complications of cardiac valvular prostheses are structural-valve deterioration, non-structural dysfunction, thromboembolism (including thrombosis), hemorrhage, and prosthetic-valve endocarditis. Structural-valve deterioration is the predominant complication of bioprostheses, whereas thromboembolism and hemorrhage is of mechanical prostheses.

The University of British Columbia and its affiliated teaching hospitals have an extensive experience with bioprostheses, currently totalling over 6,000 patients. The experience has not identified appreciable differences between prostheses. The prostheses are the Carpentier-Edwards standard, Carpentier-Edwards supra-annular, Carpentier-Edwards PERIMOUNT, and Medtronic Intact and Mosaic porcine bioprostheses. Structural-valve deterioration is the predominant valve-related complication of bioprostheses, more in mitral over aortic prostheses, and younger than elderly patients. The freedom from structural-valve deterioration, actuarial and actual, is demonstrated in Figures 77 and 78 for aortic- and mitral-valve replacements.[25] The actual freedom is the most realistic evaluation because it determines the percentage of patients who would experience the valve-related complication (i.e., structural-valve deterioration) before they die from

future prosthetic designs. The likelihood exists of reduced thromboembolism and thrombosis with future prostheses and the potential for reduction of levels of anticoagulation. The only investigational prostheses that have been evaluated, formulated, or both, by these evaluative modalities are the Medtronic Advantage, the Carbomedics Kinetic, and On-X mechanical prostheses.

IMPLANTATION CONSIDERATIONS

The implantation considerations for

unrelated causes; actuarial analysis means describing patient-risk, provided that patients were experiencing immortality. The actuarial and actual composites of valve-related complications, namely valve-related mortality and valve-related reoperation, are illustrated in Tables 6 and 7 and for aortic and mitral valve replacements.[24]

The data indicate bioprostheses are often recommended for aortic-valve replacements in the elderly (≥65 years of age), with either stented porcine or bovine pericardial prostheses. The stentless porcine bioprostheses are used more currently in the elderly, but the potential for improved durability due to the lack of rigid stents may not be apparent until long-term experience with 50- to 65-year age groups is available. The hemodynamic benefit of stentless porcine bioprostheses may contribute to optimal regression of left ventricular hypertrophy and potentially improved patient survival.[98-107] Bioprostheses, as demonstrated, have a limited role in mitral-valve replacement, primarily in patients over 70 years of age and women of child-bearing age.

The incidence of thromboembolism with bioprostheses in aortic-valve replacement is 1.5% to 2.0%/patient-year, whereas for mitral-valve replacement is 2%/patient-year, but 30% to 40% of patients require anticoagulation for risk factors of thromboembolism.

Thromboembolism remains the major complication of mechanical prostheses. The University of British Columbia experience with bileaflet mechanical prostheses in aortic-valve replacement in patients less than 65 years of age is 3.5%/patient-year overall and 1.5%/patient-year for major events.[36] Mechanical prostheses, bileaflet and monoleaflet, are recommended for the age group 40 to 65 years, along with allografts. Mechanical prostheses, allografts, and autografts are the alternatives for the 16- to 40-year age group.

Mechanical prostheses are generally recommended for mitral replacement surgery when reconstructive surgery is not feasible or indicated. Thromboembolism remains the major valve-related complication of mechanical prostheses (bileaflet); 5.0%/patient-year overall, major 2.5%/patient-year, and thrombosis 0.6%/patient-year.[37,38,108] The incidence of bleeding from anticoagulant management is 1.5%/patient-

Table 6. Patient Survival and Freedom From Valve-Related Mortality and Valve-Related Reoperation at 15 Years After Aortic Valve Replacement

Data* are presented by age group

Age (Years)	Patient Survival	Valve-Related Mortality		Valve-Related Reoperation	
		Actuarial	Actual	Actuarial	Actual
21-40	74.2 ± 7.4	94.1 ± 2.6	94.5 ± 2.4	28.8 ± 6.9	38.2 ± 6.3
41-50	57.3 ± 7.4	82.8 ± 7.0	86.5 ± 5.3	37.3 ± 7.0	52.5 ± 5.6
51-60	51.8 ± 4.0	84.4 ± 3.4	87.9 ± 2.5	46.8 ± 4.8	62.5 ± 3.4
61-70	30.9 ± 3.1	79.3 ± 3.8	86.9 ± 2.0	79.0 ± 3.7	88.1 ± 1.8
>70	18.1 ± 3.2	72.8 ± 4.8	84.9 ± 2.1	86.3 ± 7.2	96.1 ± 1.6

* Values are percentages

Published with Permission From:
Jamieson WRE, Miyagishima RT, Burr LH, et al. Carpentier-Edwards Porcine Bioprostheses: clinical performance assessed by actual analysis. J Heart Valve Dis 2000;9(4):530-5.

Table 7. Patient Survival, and Freedom from Valve-Related Mortality and Valve-Related Reoperation at 15 Years After Mitral Valve Replacement

Data* are presented by age group

Age (Years)	Patient Survival	Valve-Related Mortality		Valve-Related Reoperation	
		Actuarial	Actual	Actuarial	Actual
21-40	63.2 ± 8.2	78.1 ± 9.2	81.8 ± 7.6	6.1 ± 3.7	25.7 ± 4.8
41-50	46.7 ± 8.0	68.3 ± 12.4	77.7 ± 6.8	8.0 ± 4.3	32.3 ± 4.4
51-60	35.6 ± 4.4	69.0 ± 6.1	79.6 ± 3.6	22.3 ± 4.7	53.7 ± 3.2
61-70	16.1 ± 2.9	59.5 ± 5.8	79.5 ± 2.6	32.6 ± 6.1	71.0 ± 2.5
>70	2.8 ± 1.9	26.1 ± 15.0	82.0 ± 3.2	83.4 ± 5.4	93.3 ± 1.8

* Values are percentages

Published with Permission From:
Jamieson WRE, Miyagishima RT, Burr LH, et al. Carpentier-Edwards Porcine Bioprostheses: clinical performance assessed by actual analysis. J Heart Valve Dis 2000;9(4):530-5.

year.[37,38,108]

Several reports have been published on optimal anticoagulant management and establishment of guidelines.[109-119] The recommended International Normalization Ratio (INR) for aortic mechanical prostheses is 2.5 to 3.0; the recommended INR for mitral mechanical prostheses is 3.0 to 3.5.[109]

The cryopreserved mitral allograft is an experimental prosthesis and requires special sizing and measurement evaluated by preoperative echocardiography.[120] The cryopreserved mitral allograft can be used for tricuspid valve replacement, as well as mitral valve replacement.[121]

Biological prostheses also are indicated in special circumstances, such as contraindications for anticoagulation, women of child-bearing age (noted above), and patients with reduced life expectancy from compromised ventricular function, coronary artery disease, or other systemic disease. Mechanical prostheses, however, are considered indicated in hypercalcemic syndromes and chronic renal failure.

The implantation of both mechanical prostheses and bioprostheses in the mitral position should incorporate preservation of the subvalvular papillary muscle-chordal apparatus to support ventricular function.[12,122-139]

The clinical performance of biological and mechanical prostheses at the University of British Columbia was analyzed for predictors of survival, valve-related complications, and composites of valve-related complications.[140] The significant predictors for both aortic- and mitral-valve replacement were age, valve type, and concomitant coronary artery bypass surgery. The evaluation disclosed a considerable preference for bioprostheses for aortic-valve replacement and mechanical prostheses for mitral-valve replacement.

REFERENCES

1. Jamieson WRE. Valvular surgery-mechanical and bioprosthetic aortic valve replacement. In: Edmunds LH Jr, ed. Cardiac surgery in the adult. New York: McGraw-Hill Publishers; 1996. p 859-909.
2. Cohn LH, Reul RM. Mechanical and bioprosthetic mitral valve replacement. In: Edmunds LH, ed. Cardiac surgery in the adult. New York: McGraw Hill-Health Profession Division; 1997. p 1025-150.
3. Jamieson WRE. Modern cardiac valve devices-bioprostheses and mechanical prostheses: state of the art. J Card Surg 1993;8(1): 89-98.
4. Carpentier A. Cardiac valve surgery-the French correction? J Thorac Cardiovasc Surg 1983;86(3):323-37.
5. Carpentier A, Chauvaud S, Fabiani JN, et al. Reconstructive surgery of mitral incompetence. Ten-year appraisal. J Thorac Cardiovasc Surg 1980;79(3):338-48.
6. Cosgrove DM III. Aortic valve repair. Ann Thorac Surg 1992; 54(5):1014-5.
7. Cosgrove DM III, Rosenkranz ER, Hendren WG, et al. Valvuloplasty for aortic insufficiency. J Thorac Cardiovasc Surg 1991; 102(4):571-6.
8. David TE, Uden DE, Strauss HD. The importance of the mitral apparatus in left ventricular function after correction of mitral regurgitation. Circulation 1983;68(3 Pt 2):II76-82.
9. Duran CG. Repair of anterior mitral leaflet chordal rupture or elongation (the flip-over technique). J Cardvasc Surg 1986;1(2):161-6.
10. Duran CG, Pomar JL, Cucchiara G. A flexible ring for atrioventricular heart valve reconstruction. J Thorac Cardiovasc Surg 1974;19(4):417-20.
11. Yacoub M, Halim M, Radley-Smith R, et al. Surgical treatment of mitral regurgitation caused by floppy valves. Repair versus replacement. Circulation 1981;64(2 Pt 2):II210-6.
12. Yun KL, Miller DC. Mitral valve repair versus replacement. Cardiol Clin 1991;9(2): 315-27.
13. Fraser CD Jr, Cosgrove DM III. Aortic valve reparative procedures. Adv Cardiac Surg 1996;7:65-86.
14. O'Brien MF, Stafford EG, Gardner MAH, et al. Allograft aortic valve replacement: long-term follow-up. Ann Thorac Surg 1995; 60(2 Suppl):S253-70.
15. Yacoub M, Rasmi NR, Sundt TM, et al. Fourteen-year experience with homovital homografts for aortic valve replacement. J Thorac Cardiovasc Surg 1995;110(1):186-93.
16. O'Brien MF. Allograft aortic root replacement: standardization and simplification of technique. Ann Thorac Surg 1995;60(2 Suppl):S92-4.
17. O'Brien MF, Finney RS, Stafford EG, et al. Root replacement for all allograft aortic valves: preferred technique or too radical? Ann Thorac Surg 1995;60(2 Suppl):S87-91.
18. Elkins RC, Knott-Craig CJ, Ward KE, et al. Pulmonary autograft in children: realized growth potential. Ann Thorac Surg 1994; 57(6):1387-93.
19. Doty DB. Replacement of the aortic valve with cryopreserved aortic allograft: the procedure of choice for young patients. J Cardiovasc Surg 1994;9(2 Suppl):192-5.
20. Burdon TA, Miller DC, Oyer PE, et al. Durability of porcine valves at fifteen years in a representative North American patient population. J Thorac Cardiovasc Surg 1992; 103(2):238-51.
21. Jamieson WRE, Burr LH, Tyers GFO, et al. Carpentier-Edwards supraannular porcine bioprosthesis: clinical performance to twelve years. Ann Thorac Surg 1995;60(2 Suppl): S235-40.
22. Klepetko W, Moritz A. Leaflet fracture in Edwards-Duromedics bileaflet valves. J Thorac Cardiovasc Surg 1989;97(1):90-4.
23. Jamieson WRE, Rosado LJ, Munro AI, et al. Carpentier-Edwards standard porcine bioprosthesis: primary tissue failure (structural valve deterioration) by age groups. Ann Thorac Surg 1988;46(2):155-62.
24. Jamieson WRE, Miyagishima RT, Burr LH, et al. Carpentier-Edwards Porcine Bioprostheses: clinical performance assessed by actual analysis. J Heart Valve Dis 2000;9(4): 530-5.
25. Jamieson WRE, Burr LH, Miyagishima RT, et al. Actuarial versus actual freedom from structural valve deterioration with the Carpentier-Edwards porcine bioprostheses. Can J Cardiol 1999;15(9):973-8.
26. Jamieson WRE, Janusz MT, Burr LH, et al. Carpentier-Edwards supra-annular porcine bioprosthesis: second generation prosthesis in aortic valve replacement. Ann Thorac Surg 2001;71:S224-7.
27. Jamieson WRE, Lemieux MD, Sullivan JA, et al. Medtronic Intact porcine bioprosthesis: experience to twelve years. Ann Thorac Surg 2001;71:S278-81.
28. Lemieux MD, Jamieson WRE, Landymore RW, et al. Medtronic Intact porcine bioprosthesis: clinical performance to seven years. Ann Thorac Surg 1995;60(2 Suppl): S258-63.
29. Pomar JL, Jamieson WRE, Pelletier LC, et al. Mitroflow pericardial bioprosthesis: clinical performance to ten years. Ann Thorac Surg 1995;60(2 Suppl):S305-9.
30. Burr LH, Jamieson WRE, Munro AI, et al. Porcine bioprostheses in the elderly: clinical performance by age groups and valve positions. Ann Thorac Surg 1995;60(2 Suppl):S264-9.
31. Thomson DJ, Jamieson WRE, Dumesnil JG, et al. Medtronic Mosaic porcine bioprosthesis: midterm investigational trial results. Ann Thorac Surg 2001;71:S269-720.
32. Pelletier LC, Carrier M, Leclerc Y, et al. The Carpentier-Edwards pericardial bioprosthesis: clinical experience with 600 patients. Ann Thorac Surg 1995;60(2 Suppl):S297-302.
33. Chandran KB, Lee CS, Aluri S, et al. Pressure distribution near the occluders and impact forces on the outlet struts of Björk-Shiley convexo-concave valves during closing. J Heart Valve Dis 1996;5(2):199-206.
34. Graf T, Reul H, Detlefs C, et al. Causes and formation of cavitation in mechanical heart valves. J Heart Valve Dis 1994;3 Suppl 1:S49-64.
35. Horstkotte D, Burckhardt D. Prosthetic valve thrombosis. J Heart Valve Dis 1995; 4(2):141-53.
36. Jamieson WRE, Miyagishima RT, Grunkemeier GL, et al. Bileaflet mechanical prostheses for aortic valve replacement in patients younger than 65 years and 65 years of age or older: major thromboembolic and hemorrhagic complications. Can J Surg 1999;42(1): 27-36.
37. Jamieson WRE, Miyagishima RT, Grunkemeier GL, et al. Bileaflet mechanical prostheses performance in mitral position. Euro J Cardio-thoracic Surg 1999;15(6): 786-94.

38. Jamieson WRE, Munro AI, Miyagishima RT, et al. Multiple mechanical valve replacement surgery comparison of St. Jude Medical and CarboMedics prostheses. Euro J Cardio-thoracic Surg 1998;13(2):151-9.
39. Tanzi MC, Mantovani D, Petrini P. Chemical stability of polyether urethanes versus polycarbonate urethanes. J Biomed Mater Res 1997;36(4):550-9.
40. O'Conner BO, Bernacca GM, Straub I, et al. Mechanical testing of flexible polyurethanes: candidate selection for a prosthetic heart valve. In: Sixth World Biomaterials Congress Transactions, Society for Biomaterials, Minneapolis, MN; 2000. p 294.
41. Hilbert SL Ferrans VJ, Yomita Y, et al. Evaluation of explanted polyurethane trileaflet cardiac valve prostheses. J Thorac Cardiovasc Surg 1987;94(3):419-29.
42. Wisman CB, Pierce WS, Donachy JH, et al. A polyurethane trileaflet cardiac valve prosthesis: in vitro and in vivo studies. Trans ASAIO 1982;28:164-8.
43. Chinn JA, Frautschi JR, Phillips RE Jr. In vitro and in vivo mineralization of polymers: further comparison with device performance. In: Surfaces in Biomaterials '93 Symposium, Surfaces in Biomaterials Foundation, Minneapolis, MN, 1993.
44. Chinn JA, Frautschi JR, Phillips RE Jr. In vitro and in vivo mineralization of polymers: a comparison with device performance. In: Surfaces in Biomaterials Symposium, Surfaces in Biomaterials Foundation, Minneapolis, MN, 1992.
45. Chinn J, Phillips R Jr, Moore M. A new generation of heart valves. Sulz Tech Rev 1996; 4(96):34-5.
46. Bernacca GM, MacKay TG, Gulbransen MJ, et al. Polyurethane heart valve durability: effects of leaflet thickness and material. Int J Artif Organs 1997;20(6), 327-31.
47. Sarnowski E. Characterization of a silicone elastomer for use in a medical device. J Appl Med Poly 2001 (In Press).
48. Ishihara T, Ferrans VJ, Boyce SW, et al. Structure and classification of cuspal tears and perforations in porcine bioprosthetic cardiac valves implanted in patients. Am J Cardiol 1981;48(4):665-78.
49. Schoen F. Pathologic considerations in the surgery of adult heart disease. In: Edmunds LH, ed. Cardiac surgery in the adult. New York: McGraw Hill; 1997. p 85-144.
50. Schoen FJ, Levy RJ. Pathology of substitute heart valves: new concepts and developments. J Card Surg 1994;9(2 Suppl): 222-7.
51. Schoen FJ, Levy RJ. Pathophysiology of bioprosthetic heart valve calcification. In: Bodnar E, Yacoub M, eds. Biologic and bioprosthethic valves. New York: Yorke Medical Books; 1986. p 418-32.
52. Silver MM, Pollock J, Silver MD. Calcification in porcine xenograft valves in children. Am J Cardiol 1980;45(3):685-9.
53. Thandroyen FT, Whitton IN, Pirie D, et al. Severe calcification of glutaraldehyde-preserved porcine xenografts in children. Am J Cardiol 1980;45(3):690-6.
54. Eybl E, Griesmacher A, Grimm M, et al. Toxic effects of aldehydes released from fixed pericardium on bovine aortic endothelial cells. J Biomed Mater Res 1989;23(11): 1355-65.
55. Girardot MN, Torrianni M, Dillehay D, et al. Role of glutaraldehyde in calcification of porcine heart valves: comparing cusp and wall. J Biomed Mater Res 1995;29(7):793-801.
56. Gong G, Ling Z, Seifter E, et al. Aldehyde tanning: the villain in bioprosthetic calcification. Eur J Cardiothorac Surg 1991;5(6):288-93.
57. Hirsch D, Drader J, Thomas TJ, et al. Inhibition of calcification of glutaraldehyde pretreated porcine aortic valve cusps with sodium dodecyl sulfate: pre-incubation studies and controlled release studies. J Biomed Mater Res 1993;27(12):1477-84.
58. Levy RJ. Glutaraldehyde and the calcification mechanism of bioprosthetic heart valves. J Heart Valve Dis 1994;3(1):101-4.
59. Speer DP, Chvapil M, Eskelson CD, et al. Biological effects of residual glutaraldehyde in glutaraldehyde-tanned collagen biomaterials. J Biomed Mat Res 1980;14(6): 753-64.
60. Sabbah HN, Hamid MS, Stein PD. Mechanical stresses on closed cusps of porcine bioprosthetic valves: correlation with sites of calcification. Ann Thorac Surg 1986;42(1): 93-6.
61. Butterfield M, Fisher J, Davies GA, et al. Leaflet geometry and function in porcine bioprostheses. Eur J Cardiothorac Surg 1991;5(1):27-32.
62. Thubrikar MJ, Deck JD, Aouad J, et al. Role of mechanical stress in calcification of aortic bioprosthetic valves. J Thorac Cardiovasc Surg 1988;86(1):115-25.
63. Christie GW. Anatomy of aortic heart valve leaflets: the influence of glutaraldehyde fixation on function. Eur J Cardiothorac Surg 1992;6(Suppl 1):S25-32.
64. Flomenbaum MA, Schoen FJ. Effects of fixation back pressure and antimineralization treatment on the morphology of porcine aortic bioprosthetic valves. J Thorac Cardiovasc Surg 1993;105(1):154-64.
65. Hey KB, Lachs CM, Raxworthy MJ, et al. Crosslinked fibrous collagen for use as a dermal implant: control of the cytotoxic effects of glutaraldehyde and dimethylsuberimidate. Biotech Appl Biochem 1990;12(1): 85-93.
66. Huang-Lee LL, Cheung DT, Nimni ME. Biochemical changes and cytotoxicity associated with the degradation of polymeric glutaraldehyde derived crosslinks. J Biomed Mater Res 1990;24(9):1885-201.
67. Myers D. New tissue-processing techniques. In: Piwnica A, Westaby S, eds. Stentless bioprostheses. Oxford: Isis Medical Media; 1997. p 448-59.
68. Myers DJ, Gross J, Nakaya G. Stentless heart valves: biocompatibility issues associated with new antimeralization and fixation agents. In: Piwnica A, Westaby S, eds. Stentless bioprostheses. Oxford: Isis Medical Media; 1995. p 100-17.
69. Myers DJ, Nakaya G, Girardot MN, et al. A comparison between glutaraldehyde and diepoxide-fixed stentless porcine aortic valves: biochemical and mechanical characterization and resistance to mineralization. J Heart Valve Dis 1995;4 (Suppl 1):S98-101.
70. Jones M, Eidbo EE, Hilber SL, et al. Anticalcification treatments of bioprosthetic heart valves: in vivo studies in sheep. J Card Surg 1989;4(1):69-73.
71. Chen W, Kim JD, Schoen FJ, et al. Effect of 2-amino oleic acid exposure conditions on the inhibition of calcification of glutaraldehyde cross-linked porcine aortic valves. J Biomed Mater Res 1994;28(12): 1485-95.
72. Girardot MN, Girardot JM, Schoen FJ. Development of the AOA process as antimineralization treatment for bioprosthetic heart valves. Trans Soc Biomat 1993;19: 266.
73. Girardot MN, Girardot JM, Torrianni M. Alpha-aminooleic acid (AOA) anticalcification effect on glutaraldehyde-fixed heart valves: shelf life studies. In: Gabby S, Frater RWM, eds. New horizons and the future of heart valve bioprostheses, 1st ed. Austin, Texas: Silent Partners, Inc.; 1994. p 41-52.
74. Girardot MN, Torrianni M, Girardot JM. Effect of AOA on glutaraldehyde-fixed bioprosthetic heart valve cusps and walls: binding and calcification studies. Int J Artif Organs 1994;17(2):76-82.
75. Gott JP, Pan-Chih, Dorsey L, et al. Calcification of porcine valves: a successful new method of antimineralization. Ann Thorac Surg 1992;53(2):207-15.
76. Imamura E, Sawatani O, Koyanagi H, et al. Epoxy compounds as a new cross-linking agent for porcine aortic leaflets: subcutaneous implant studies in rats. J Card Surg 1989;4(1):50-7.
77. Sung HW, Shen Sh, Tu R, et al. Comparison of the cross-linking characteristics of porcine heart valves fixed with glutaraldehyde or epoxy compounds. ASAIO Journal 1993;39(3):M532-6.
78. Petite H, Frei V, Huc A, et al. Use of diphenylphorphorylazide for cross-linking collagen-based biomaterials. J Biomed Mat Res 1994;28(2):159-65.
79. Petite H, Rault I, Huc A, et al. Use of the acyl azide method for cross-linking collagen-rich tissues such as pericardium. J Biomed Mat Res 1990;24(2):179-87.
80. Lee CH, Vyavahare N, Zand R, et al. Inhibition of aortic wall calcification in bioprosthetic heart valves by ethanol pretreatment: biochemical and biophysical mechanisms. J Biomed Mater Res 1998; 42(1):30-7.
81. Vyavahare NR, Hirsch D, Lerner E, et al. Prevention of calcification of glutaraldehyde-crosslinked porcine aortic cusps by ethanol preincubation: mechanistic studies of protein structure and water-biomaterial relationships. J Biomed Mater Res 1998; 40(4): 577-85.
82. Vyavahare N, Hirsch D, Lerner E, et al. Prevention of bioprosthetic heart valve calcification by ethanol preincubation. Efficacy and mechanisms. Circulation 1997;95(2):

479-88.
83. Vyavahare N, Ogle M, Schoen FJ, et al. Elastin calcification and its prevention with aluminum chloride pretreatment. Am J Pathol 1999;155(3):973-82.
84. Bengtsson LA, Phillips R, Haegerstrand AN. In vitro endothelialization of photooxidatively stabilized xenogeneic pericardium. Ann Thorac Surg 1995;60(2 Suppl):S365-8.
85. Bianco RW, Philips R, Mrachek J, et al. Preclinical evaluation of a new pericardial bioprosthetic with dye mediated photooxidized bovine pericardial tissue. ASAIO 1995;42(1) Suppl 39 (Abstr).
86. Moore MA, Bohachevsky IK, Cheung DT, et al. Stabilization of pericardial tissue by dye-mediated photooxidation. J Biomed Mater Res 1994;28(5):611-8.
87. Wilson GJ, Courtman DW, Klement P, et al. Acellular matrix: a biomaterials approach for coronary artery bypass and heart valve replacement. Ann Thorac Surg 1995;60(2 Suppl):S353-8.
88. Sodian R, Hoerstrup SP, Sperling JS, et al. Tissue engineering of heart valves: in vitro experiences. Ann Thorac Surg 2000; 70(1):140-4.
89. Hoerstrup SP, Zund G, Lachat M, et al. Tissue engineering: a new approach in cardiovascular surgery-seeding of human fibroblasts on resorbable mesh. Swiss Surg 1998; Suppl 2:23-5.
90. Shinoka T, Breuer CK, Tanel RE, et al. Tissue engineering heart valves: valve leaflet replacement study in a lamb model. Ann Thorac Surg 1995;60(6 Suppl):S513-6.
91. O'Brien M, Goldstein S, Walsh S, et al. The SynerGraft Valve: a new acellular (nonglutaraldehyde-fixed) tissue heart valve for autologous recellularization: first experimental studies before clinical implantation. Semin Thorac Cardiovasc Surg 1999;11(4 Suppl 1):194-200.
92. Elkins RC, Dawson PE, Goldstein S, et al. Decellularized human valve allografts. Ann Thorac Surg 2001;71:S428-32.
93. Gross JM, Shu MCS, Dai FF, et al. A microstructural flow analysis within a bileaflet mechanical heart valve hinge. J Heart Valve Dis 1996;5(6):581-90.
94. Ellis JT, Healy TM, Fontaine AA, et al. An in vitro investigation of the retrograde flow fields of two bileaflet mechanical heart valves. J Heart Valve Dis 1996;5(6):600-6.
95. Ellis JT, Healy TM, Fontaine AA, et al. Velocity measurements and flow patterns within the hinge region of a Medtronic Parallel bileaflet mechanical valve with clear housing. J Heart Valve Dis 1996;5(6):591-9.
96. Hasenkam JM, Nygaard H, Terp K, et al. Hemodynamic evaluation of a new bileaflet valve prosthesis: an acute animal experimental study. J Heart Valve Dis 1996;5(6):574-80.
97. Edmunds LH, Clark RE, Cohn LH, et al. Guidelines for reporting morbidity and mortality after cardiac valvular operations. Ann Thorac Surg 1996;62(3):932-5.
98. Yun KL, Jamieson WRE, Khonsari S, et al. Prosthesis-patient mismatch: hemodynamic comparison of stented and stentless aortic valves. Semin Thorac Cardiovasc Surg 1999; 11(4 Suppl 1):98-102.
99. David TE, Bos J, Rakowski H. Aortic valve replacement with the Toronto SPV bioprosthesis. J Heart Valve Dis 1992; 1(2):244-8.
100. Mohr FW, Walther T, Baryalei M, et al. The Toronto SPV bioprosthesis: one-year results in 100 patients. Ann Thorac Surg 1995;60(1):171-5.
101. Rao V, Jamieson WRE, Ivanov J, et al. Patient-prosthesis mismatch affects survival following aortic valve replacement. Circulation-Cardiovascular Surgery Supplement 2000;102(Suppl III):III 5-9.
102. Westaby S, Amarasena N, Ormerod O, et al. Aortic valve replacement with the freestyle stentless xenograft. Ann Thorac Surg 1995;60(2 Suppl):S422-7.
103. Sintek CF, Fletcher AD, Khonsari S. Stentless porcine aortic root: valve of choice for the elderly patient with small aortic root? J Thorac Cardiovasc Surg 1995;109(5): 871-6.
104. Del Rizzo DF, Abdoh A, Cartier P, et al. The effect of prosthetic valve type on survival after aortic valve surgery. Semin Thorac Cardiovasc Surg 1999;11(4), Suppl 1:1-8.
105. Doty DB, Cafferty A, Cartier P, et al. Aortic valve replacement with Medtronic Freestyle Bioprosthesis: 5-year results. Semin Thorac Cardiovasc Surg 1999;11(4), Suppl 1:35-41.
106. Goldman B, Christakis G, David T, et al. Will stentless valves be durable? The Toronto valve (TSPV) at 5 to 6 years. Semin Thorac Cardiovasc Surg 1999;11(4), Suppl 1:42-9.
107. Del Rizzo DF, Abdoh A, Cartier P, et al. Factors affecting left ventricular mass regression after aortic valve replacement with stentless valves. Semin Thorac Cardiovasc Surg 1999;11(4), Suppl 1:114-20.
108. Jamieson WRE, Fradet GJ, Miyagishima RT, et al. CarboMedics Mechanical Prosthesis: performance at eight years. J Heart Valve Dis 2000;9(5):678-87.
109. Ad Hoc Committee of the Working Group on Valvular Heart Disease, European Society of Cardiology: guidelines for prevention of thromboembolic events in valvular heart valve disease. J Heart Valve Dis 1993;2(4):398-410.
110. Albertal J, Sutton M, Pereyra D, et al. Experience with moderate intensity anticoagulation and aspirin after mechanical valve replacement. A retrospective, non-randomized study. J Heart Valve Dis 1993;2(3): 302-7.
111. Butchart EG. Prosthesis-specific and patient-specific anticoagulation. In: Butchart EG, Bodnar E, eds. Current issues in heart valve disease, thrombosis, embolism and bleeding, London: ICR Publishers; 1992. p 293.
112. Cannegieter SC, Rosendaal FR, Wintzen AR, et al. Optimal oral anticoagulant therapy in patients with mechanical heart valves. N Engl J Med 1995;333(1):11-7.
113. Cappelleri JC, Fiore LD, Brophy MT, et al. Efficacy and safety of combined anticoagulant and antiplatelet therapy versus anticoagulant monotherapy after mechanical heart-valve replacement: a meta-analysis. Am Heart J 1995;130(3 Pt 1):547-52.
114. Horstkotte D, Schulte HD, Bircks W, et al. Lower intensity anticoagulation therapy results in lower complication rates with the St. Jude Medical prosthesis. J Thorac Cardiovasc Surg 1994;107(4):1136-45.
115. Horstkotte D, Bergemann R, Althaus U, et al. German experience with low intensity anticoagulation (GELIA): protocol of a multi-center randomized prospective study with the St. Jude Medical valve. J Heart Valve Dis 1993;2(4):411-9.
116. Stein PD, Alpert JS, Copeland J, et al. Antithrombotic therapy in patients with mechanical and biological prosthetic heart valves. Chest 1996;108(4 Suppl):371S-95S.
117. Turpie AG, Gent M, Laupacis A, et al. A comparison of aspirin with placebo in patients treated with warfarin after heart-valve replacement. N Engl J Med 1993; 329(8):524-9.
118. Hirsh J, Fuster V. Guide to anticoagulant therapy. Part 2: oral anticoagulants. Circulation 1994;89(3):1469-80.
119. Butchart EG, Lewis PA, Grunkemeier GL, et al. Low risk of thrombosis and serious emboli events despite low-intensity anticoagulation: experience with 1,004 Medtronic Hall valves. Circulation 1988; 78(3 Pt 2):166-77.
120. Acar J, Gaer J, Chauvaud S, et al. Technique of homograft replacement of the mitral valve. J Heart Valve Dis 1995;4(1): 31-4.
121. Miyagishima RT, Brumwell ML, Jamieson WRE, et al. Tricuspid valve replacement using a cryopreserved mitral homograft-surgical technique and initial results. J Heart Valve Dis 2000;9:805-9.
122. Asano K, Furuse A. Techniques of modified mitral valve replacement with preservation of the posterior leaflet and chordae tendineae. Thorac Cardiovasc Surg 1987;35(4):206-8.
123. David TE. Mitral valve replacement with preservation of chordae tendineae: rational and technical considerations. Ann Thorac Surg 1986;41(6):680-2.
124. David TE. Papillary muscle-annular continuity: is it important? J Cardiac Surg 1994;9(2 Suppl 2):252-4.
125. Feikes HL, Daugharthy JB, Perry JE, et al. Preservation of all chordae tendineae and papillary muscle during mitral valve replacement with a tilting disc valve. J Cardiovasc Surg 1990;5(2):81-5.
126. Hansen DE, Cahill PD, DeCampli WM, et al. Valvular-ventricular interaction: importance of the mitral apparatus in canine left ventricular systolic performance. Circulation 1986;73(6):1310-20.
127. Hansen DE, Sarris GE, Niczyporuk MA, et al. Physiologic role of the mitral apparatus in left ventricular regional mechanics, contraction synergy, and global systolic performance. J Thorac Cardiovasc Surg 1989;97(4):521-33.
128. Hennein HA, Swain JA, McIntosh CL, et al. Comparative assessment of chordal preservation versus chordal resection during mitral valve replacement. J Thorac Cardiovasc Surg 1990;99(5):828-36.

129. Hetzer R, Bougioukas G, Franz M, et al. Mitral valve replacement with preservation of papillary muscles and chordae tendineae: revival of a seemingly forgotten concept. I. Preliminary clinical report. Thorac Cardiovasc Surg 1983;31(5):291-6.

130. Lillehei CW, Levy MJ, Bonnabeau RC. Mitral valve replacement with preservation of papillary muscles and chordae tendinae. J Thorac Cardiovasc Surg 1964;47:532.

131. Okita Y, Miki S, Kusuhara K, et al. Analysis of left ventricular motion after mitral valve replacement with a technique of preservation of all chordae tendineae: comparison with conventional mitral valve replacement or mitral valve repair. J Thorac Cardiovasc Surg 1992;104(3):786-95.

132. Okita Y, Miki S, Ueda Y, et al. Comparative evaluation of left ventricular performance after mitral valve repair or valve replacement with or without chordal preservation. J Heart Valve Dis 1993;2(2):159-66.

133. Pitarys CJ, Forman MB, Panayiotou H, et al. Long-term effects of excision of the mitral apparatus on global and regional ventricular function in humans. J Am Coll Cardiol 1990;15(3):557-63.

134. Rose EA, Oz MC. Preservation of anterior leaflet chordae tendineae during mitral valve replacement. Ann Thorac Surg 1994;57(3):768-9.

135. Rozich HD, Carabello BA, Usher BW, et al. Mitral valve replacement with and without chordal preservation in patients with chronic mitral regurgitation. Mechanisms for differences in postoperative ejection performance. Circulation 1992;86(6): 1718-26.

136. Sarris GE, Fann JI, Niczyporuk MA, et al. Global and regional left ventricular systolic performance in the in situ ejecting canine heart. Importance of the mitral apparatus. Circulation 1989;80(3 Pt 1):I24-42.

137. David TE, Burns RJ, Bacchus CM, et al. Mitral valve replacement for mitral regurgitation with and without preservation of chordae tendineae. J Thorac Cardiovasc Surg 1984;88(5 Pt 1):718-25.

138. Yagyu K, Matsumoto H, Asano K, et al. Importance of the mitral complex in left ventricular contraction–an analysis of the results of mitral valve replacement with preservation of the posterior mitral complex. Thorac Cardiovasc Surg 1987; 35(3):166-71.

139. Yun KL, Rayhill SC, Niczyporuk MA, et al. Mitral valve replacement in dilated canine hearts with chronic mitral regurgitation. Importance of the mitral subvalvular apparatus. Circulation 1991;84(5 Suppl): III112-24.

140. Jamieson WRE, Germann E, Fradet GJ, et al. Bioprostheses and mechanical prostheses predictors of performance. Asian Cardiovasc-Thorac Ann 2000;8:121-6.

For a future of...

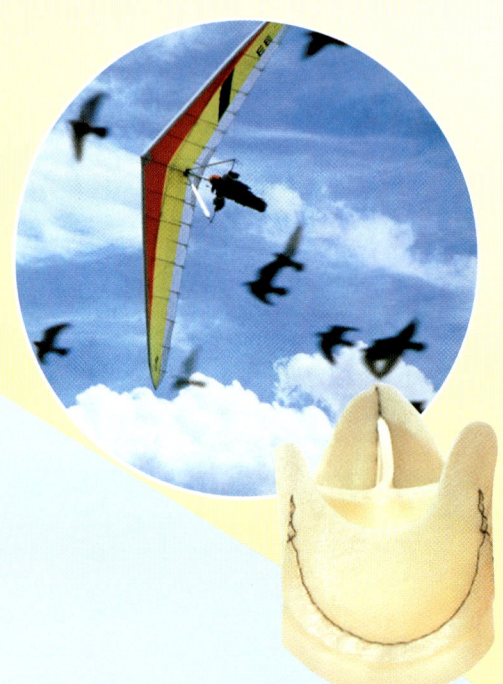

PERICARBON™ FREEDOM STENTLESS

NOT FOR SALE IN U.S.A.

The Pericarbon™ Freedom Stentless biological heart valve is proof of Sorin Biomedica's ceaseless commitment to achieving superior levels of quality and reliability in medical technology.

Pericarbon Freedom's exclusive detoxification post-treatment is the latest development after 15 years of experience with bovine pericardium biological valves.

Pericarbon™ Freedom Stentless bioprosthesis is the true stentless valve, soft and pliable. Its excellent haemodynamic performance meets the challenge of restoring the quality of life for patients.

WE TAKE RESEARCH TO HEART

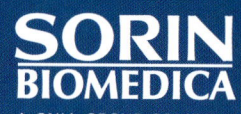

SORIN BIOMEDICA
A SNIA GROUP COMPANY

The Incomplete Ring with Modulated Flexibility: A New Concept of Mitral Annuloplasty

Wajih Maazouzi, M.D.
Younes Cheikhaoui, M.D.
Rhizlene Drissi Kacemi, M.D.
Mohammed Messouak, M.D.
Souad Bouaichi, M.D.

CARDIOVASCULAR SURGERY UNIT, IBN SINA HOSPITAL
RABAT, MOROCCO

Among the different techniques of mitral valve repair (involving chordea, commissures, papillary muscles, leaflets, or annulus), the annuloplasty remains a difficult problem-solving step. Since invention of the first ring, which was rigid and closed,[1,2] the concept of annuloplasty has taken into consideration the following objectives: to make the available leaflet tissue well fitted to the systolic mitral orifice by repairing the length and shape of the dilated annulus, prevent its further dilatation, and provide a support to the fragile area after a partial leaflet resection.[3-5]

The first implanted rings were complete and totally rigid to allow them to reach these objectives, but they did not address the natural flexibility of the annulus. As the mitral annulus is a flexible and moving component of the mitral apparatus, a second generation of annuloplasty rings, the flexible closed rings,[6] appeared to conform better to the physiological function of the mitral valve. However, they were not always successful in restoring the shape of the annulus and coaptation of the valves, whereas they could be bunched with multiple plications.

The aim of the incomplete ring with modulated flexibility (IRMF) is to incorporate, in a single device, the advantages of both rigid and flexible rings, and address the recently discovered anatomical and physiological characters of the mitral annulus at the same time. Also, the special holder and sizer match this prosthesis and allow easy measurement and implantation.

MATERIAL AND METHODS

Between May 1999 and May 2000, 50 patients (13 male, 37 female) with mitral regurgitation underwent mitral valve annuloplasty using the new incomplete and flexible ring after an enlightened consent. The mean age of the patients was 23 (range: 13 to 55) years, and the etiology was rheumatic in 45 (90%) patients. Five (10/%) patients were in functional Class II of the New York Heart Association (NYHA), and 45 (90%) in Class III.

Analysis of the valve injury was performed by echocardiography and Doppler. This exploration was completed by visual inspection during the operation. The mitral regurgitation was Grade III in 30 patients and Grade IV in 20. The left ventricular end diastolic diameter varied from 39 mm to 74 mm (average: 52 mm), and the ejection fraction varied from 33% to 78% (mean: 61%). Absence of important

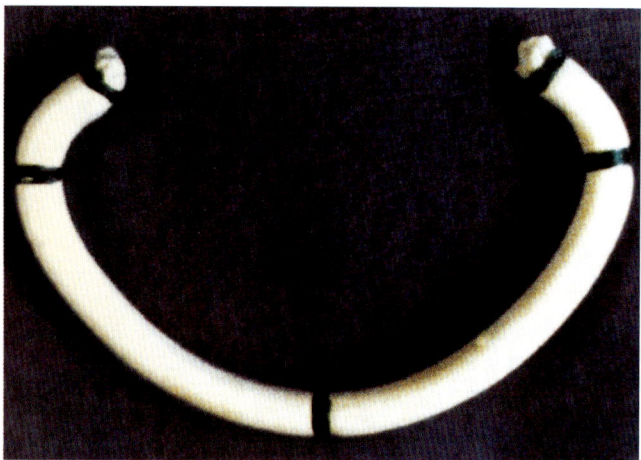

Figure 1. Shape of the incomplete ring with modulated flexibility: two thirds of a circumference.

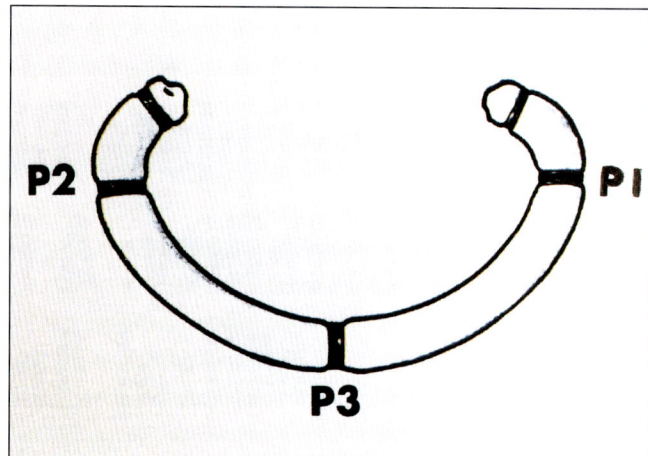

Figure 2. Ring is made of three parts: P1 and P2 are laterals, P3 is middle.

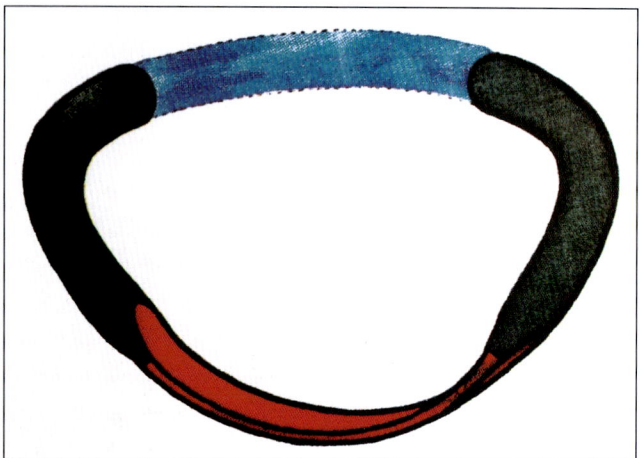

Figure 3. In the IRMF, the lateral parts of the wire are cylindrical and have a high moment of inertia (Iz0 = .1mm^r), whereas in the middle part the wire is flat and has a low moment of inertia (Iz0 = 0.058 mm^r).

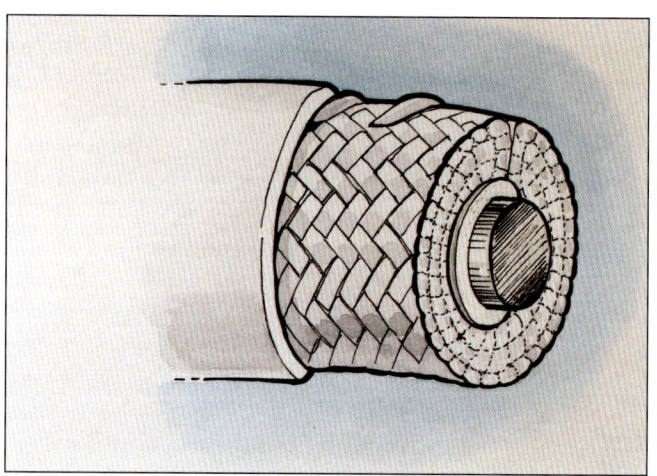

Figure 4. Three layers of synthetic tissues covering the titanium wire; the deepest is made of ePTFE, middle layer is made of polyester, and superficial area is made of an ePTFE cloth.

leaflet retraction and calcifications was the main criterion for conservative surgery.

The configuration of IRMF is two thirds of a circumference (Fig. 1). This ring is made of three parts, two laterals (P1, P2) and one in the middle (P3) (Fig. 2). The flexibility of the lateral parts (P1, P2) is lower than that of the middle part (P3). This modulated flexibility was obtained using a pure titanium wire whose thickness and shape vary according to its different parts. In the lateral parts, the metal is cylindrical and has a high moment of inertia ($Iz0 = 0.1$ mm^4), whereas in the middle part this wire is flat and has a low moment of inertia ($Izo = 0.058$ mm^4) (Fig. 3). Three layers of synthetic tissues cover the titanium wire: the deepest is made of expanded polytetrafluoroethylene (ePTFE), the middle layer is made of polyester, and the superficial area is made of an ePTFE cloth (Fig. 4).

The prosthesis is placed in a plastic holder, which adapts itself to the configuration of the mitral annulus, particularly in its aortic neighborhood, and whose upper edge is more prominent than the lower edge. This design allows passage of the suture needle into the ring without shifting it from its holder (Fig. 5). The prosthesis is set precisely in the groove of the holder so as to expose only the part subjected to suture, guiding the surgeon's needle, which has only to slide along the rear edge of the plastic base to meet the precise point of transit through the width of the ring. Finally, the device is fitted with two multigraduated, single-gesture testers (unlike the models currently in existence): an adult sizer and a child sizer. These sizers allow the appropriate prosthesis number to be selected simultaneously with a single gesture according to the intertrigonal distance and height of the anterior leaflet (Fig. 6).

In all instances, the operation was performed using moderate hypothermic bypass with blood cardioplegia. The mean bypass time was 66.6 (40 to 123) minutes. The technique of implantation of the IRMF differs from the classical one in that the sutures do not affect the anterior portion of the annulus (the aortic segment) (Fig.7). A fundamental point is that each mark at the extremities of the device has to be sutured to the trigones that act as the strong points on which fixation of the prosthesis is based, to shorten or prevent ulterior dilatation of the annulus. The incomplete character of this device allows for further repair after stitches and trials, if it appears necessary (Fig. 8).

Also, the annuloplasty was associated with other corrective procedures such as commissurotomy (n=10), leaflet resection (n=3), chordae shortening (n=10), chordae resection (n=15), chordae fenestration (n=5),

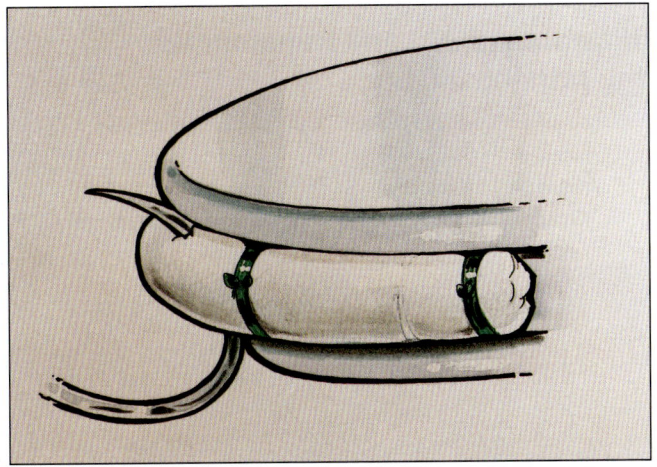

Figure 5. Prosthesis is set in the groove of the holder to expose only the part subjected to suture, guiding the surgeon's needle, which has only to slide along the rear edge of the plastic base to meet the precise point of transit through the width of the ring.

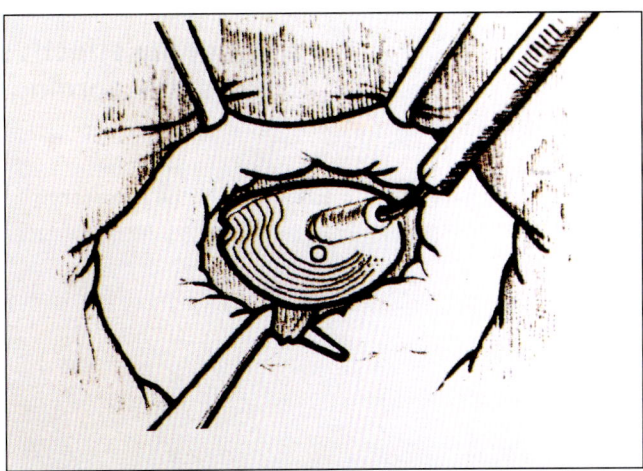

Figure 6. Sizers allow the appropriate prosthesis number to be selected simultaneously with a single gesture according to the intertrigonal distance and height of the anterior leaflet.

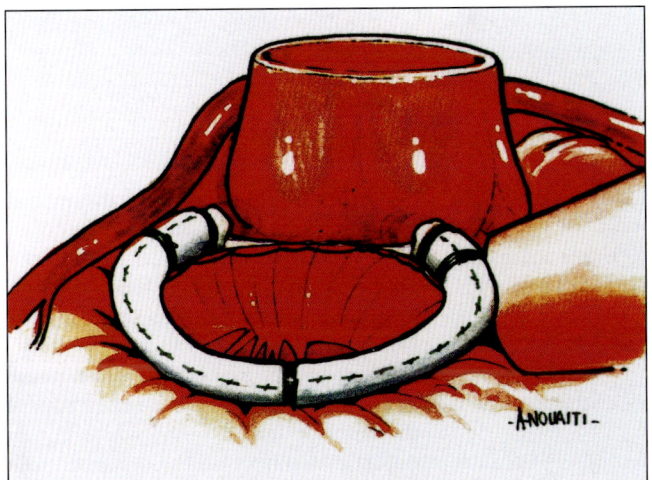

Figure 7. Technique of implantation of the IRMF differs from the classical one because the sutures do not affect the anterior portion of the annulus (the aortic segment).

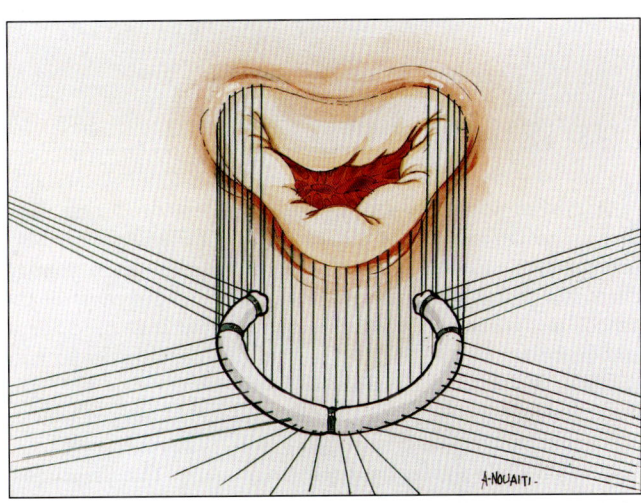

Figure 8. Incomplete character of the IRMF allows further repair after stitches and trials.

and papillotomy (n=7). Twenty-two patients have had an associated procedure (tricuspid annuloplasty, 15; aortic valve replacement, 3; and left atrium reduction.

RESULTS

Intraoperative assessment of the mitral repair was performed by using the left ventricular filling test, which showed a perfect competence in 42 patients. In eight patients, additional repair procedures were necessary after annuloplasty: chordae shortening (two patients), chordae resection (four patients), and papillotomy (two patients). These procedures were facilitated by the incomplete character of the annuloplasty ring, which allows for performing those additional repairs just by lifting up the device without withdrawing it.

The intraoperative transesophageal echocardiography was performed in three patients (persistent systolic thrill or hemodynamic instability). Minimal regurgitation was noted in two patients and no regurgitation in one.

The immediate postoperative course was smooth in 47 patients, with an average Intensive Care Unit stay of 48 hours. In three patients, the postoperative course was difficult (important doses of inotropic support, prolonged mechanical ventilation) because of pulmonary hypertension (two patients) or left ventricular dysfunction (one patient).

The patients in this study were examined after one month, six months, and one-year follow-up periods. The authors used the classification of the NYHA to determine the functional class: 47 patients were in Class I, two in Class II, and one in Class III. Among the 50 patients, ten have received antiarrhythmics and anticoagulants during three months.

Echocardiography and Doppler exploration were used in all patients: 30 (60%) patients had no regurgitation, minimal regurgitation was noted in 18 (36%), and two (4%) had regurgitation Grade III. The effective orifice area (EOA) varied from 1.8 cm^2 to 4.2 cm^2 (average: 2.71), and the average transmitral diastolic gradient was 2.4 mm Hg (Table 1). The left ventricular end diastolic diameter decreased in 37 (74%) patients, and the average was 50.3 mm. The ejection fraction varied from 50% to 80% (average: 65 %), with the exception of the patient who had left ventricular dysfunction and whose ejection fraction remained less than 50%.

Table 1. Variation of the effective orifice area (EOA) and transmitral gradient according to the prosthesis size

Prosthesis Size	Effective Orifice Area (cm²)	Average Transmitral Gradient (mm Hg)	Number of Patients (and Percentage)
26	2.3	3.7	2 (4)
28	2.5	3.0	7 (14)
30	2.6	2.7	24 (48)
32	2.6	2.3	15 (30)
34	2.6	2.0	1 (2)
36	3.2	2.0	1 (2)

A cineangiography study was performed to determine the cinesis of the prosthesis. This study confirmed the changing of the size (intertrigonal distance) in accordance with the systole and diastole.

The results were considered excellent (normal mitral valve or minimal regurgitation without transmitral gradient) in 38 (76%) patients, good (minimal regurgitation + with moderate gradient) in ten (20%), and moderate (regurgitation++) in two.

DISCUSSION

The observations the authors have made during the numerous annuloplasties performed in our unit—in a population often young, sometimes infantile, and in most of the time associated with at least mild aortic disease—have incited us to consider another design of annuloplasty device: an incomplete and flexible ring whose basis is anatomical and physiological.

This prosthesis is incomplete because the suture and fixation of the aortic portion of the mitral annulus is not useful, as the two fibrous trigones are interconnected with a curtain of fibrous tissue between the aortic valve and anterior leaflet of the mitral valve.[7] This curtain prevents dilatation of the corresponding segment of the mitral annulus,[8,9] especially in rheumatic disease. Furthermore, for fear of touching aortic cusps the surgeon tends to position some sutures in the valvular area rather than the anterior annulus itself. This procedure makes less mitral tissue available and may cause a restriction of the anterior mitral valve, which has an unfortunate effect on the dominant role of this element in closure of the valve. However, the advantages of not suturing the anterior annulus are multiple: the aortic cusps and bundle of His are not liable to injury, nor the aortic annulus to deformation, which can aggravate a potential aortic regurgitation; the ante-

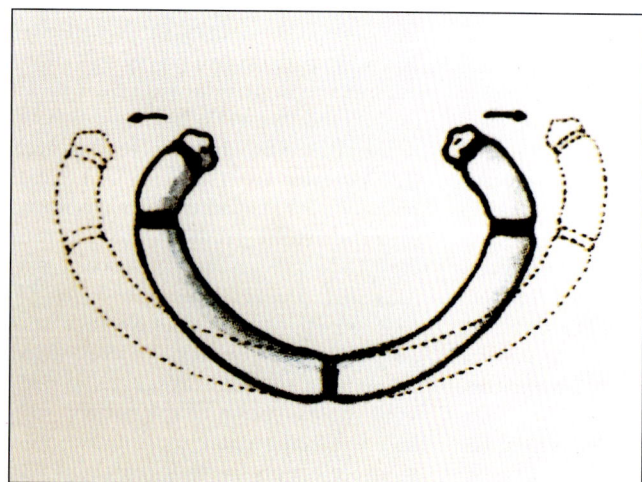

Figure 9. The IRMF is flexible in the frontal plane.

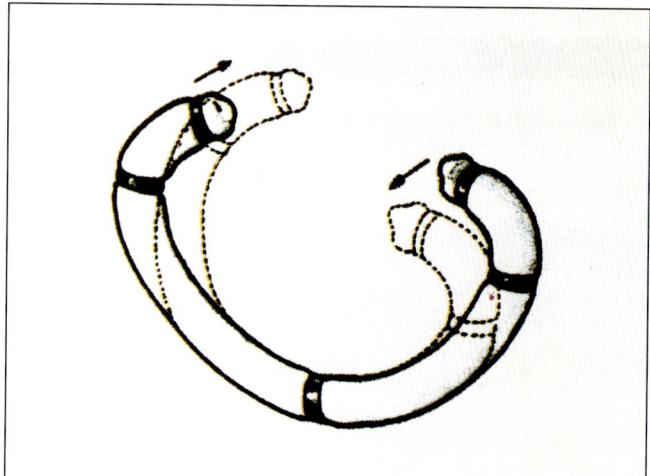

Figure 10. The IRMF is flexible in the perpendicular plane.

rior annulus (never dilated) is not shortened; it allows optimal exploitation of the anterior leaflet and provides a larger orifice area. This procedure should yield a low transmitral gradient, as we noted in most of the patients in this study. Also, we anticipate the annulus will continue to grow in the event this device is used in children.

This incomplete ring also is flexible, in the frontal plane (Fig. 9) as well as the perpendicular one (Fig. 10), because it is well documented that the mitral annulus is a dynamic structure with a sphincter-like function, which reduces its area (the difference between diastolic and systolic annulus size rises to 20%) and changes its shape (the mitral annulus is circular during diastole and becomes more elliptical in systole) as a result of shortening of the baso-constrictor muscles (bulbo and sino-spiral muscle bundle).[10-12] Furthermore, the anterior portion of the mitral annulus is probably a much more dynamic component of the mitral apparatus than previously thought. These changes in size and shape of the annulus throughout the cardiac cycle seem to have an essential role in the left ventricular systolic function and performance.[13] Use of a flexible ring for mitral regurgitation repair seems to provide better results for the left ventricular function,[14,15] whereas it decreases the risk of disinsection at the same time.

The new ring design can better assess the dynamic property of the annulus, because a flexible ring allows an expansion by approximately 10% during diastole, and more if the prosthesis also is incomplete. Another point that should be mentioned is the advantage of being able to shape the ring in any way, before definitive implantation according to the annulus one. Moreover, we have even observed a ring to take a saddle shape spontaneously when implanted in instances in which the anterior valve was long enough but its annulus too short. With another type of ring, the size implanted would have been necessarily smaller and, therefore, restrictive.

The comparison between this device and other rings is necessary to justify its interest. The IRMF allows the approximating effect of the anterior and posterior leaflets even though incomplete, by acting mainly in the commissural zones where the prosthesis has the lowest flexibility, which is not the case for totally flexible rings.[6] At the same time, the anterior and posterior annulus retain their flexibility with total respect to the anterior annulus, unlike rigid closed rings,[2] and semi-flexible closed rings.[16] Finally, unlike other open rings,[17] anchorage of the prosthesis to the trigones avoids further dilatation of the juxtacommissural annulus. Usually, the quest for adequate flexibility has led to complex devices. The new ring is monolithic and determines the precise compromise between flexibility and rigidity.

The ePTFE has been chosen as a component of this device because it is one of the most chemically inert polymers known, causing little tissue reaction with a high biocompatibility. Furthermore, the porosity of the ePTFE allows complete incorporation by the host tissue with free ingrowths of connective cells (phenomenon of rehabilitation).[18]

Investigation of all the patients in this study was satisfactory, as 47 (94%) were in functional Class I of the NYHA and echocardiography, and Doppler results were excellent (no regurgitation or minimal regurgitation without gradient) in 38 (76%). The left ventricular end diastolic and end systolic diameters decreased with improvement of the ejection fraction in most of the patients, which demonstrated an improved left ventricular function.

Results of this ring preliminary study showed the efficiency of the new concept, which can be proved by a randomized study.

CONCLUSION

If the rigid closed ring remodels the annulus to a correct size and shape, and the flexible ring allows an appropriate size without impairing the annulus dynamism, the new incomplete and flexible ring (with its support and single-gesture sizer) demonstrates the advantages of those two concepts without their disadvantages. It also allows a technique easy to perform and teach, thanks to elimination of a delicate step that also saves time. Finally, it better allows for an ultimate assessment of the repair in instances in which the surgeon is unsure of the subvalvular situation.

REFERENCES

1. Carpentier A, Deloche A, Dauptain J, et al. A new reconstructive operation for correction of mitral and tricuspid insufficiency. J Thorac Cardiovasc Surg 1971;61:1-13.
2. Carpentier A. Cardiac valve surgery-The "french correction." J Thorac Cardiovasc Surg 1983;86:323.
3. Antunes MJ, Kinsley RH. Mitral valve annuloplasty: results in an underdeveloped population. Thorax 1983;38(10):730-6.
4. Burr HB, Krayenbuhl C, Sutton MS, et al. The mitral plication suture. J Thorac Cardiovasc Surg 1977;73 (4):589-95.
5. Shore DF, Wong P, Paneth M, et al. Results of mitral valvuloplasty with a suture plication technique. J Thorac Cardiovasc Surg 1980;79(3):349-57.
6. Duran CG, UBago JL. Clinical and hemodynamic performance of a totally flexible prosthetic ring for atrioventricular valve reconstruction. Ann Thorac Surg 1976;22(5):458-63.
7. Antunes MJ. Functional anatomy of the mitral valve. In: Schulz RS. Mitral valve repair. 1989;15:28.
8. Levine RA, Triuli MO, Harrigan P, et al. The relationship of mitral annular shape to the diagnosis of mitral valve prolapse. Circulation 1987;75(4):756-67.
9. Van Rijk-Zwikker GL, Delemarre BJ, Huysmans HA. Mitral valve anatomy and morphology: relevance to mitral valve replacement and valve reconstruction. J Cardiovasc Surg 1994;9(2 Suppl):255-61.
10. Ranganathan N, Lam JHC, Wigle ED, et al. Morphology of the human mitral valve. II. The valve leaflets. Circulation 1970;41(3):459-67.
11. Tsakiris AG, Von Bernuth G, Rastelli GC, et al. Size and motion of the mitral valve annulus in anesthetized intact dogs. J Appl Physiol 1971;30(5):611-8.
12. Ormiston JA, Shah PM, Tei C, et al. Size and motion of the mitral annulus in man: a two-dimensional echocardiographic method and findings in normal subjects. Circulation 1981;64(1):113-20.
13. Glasson JR, Komeda M, Daughters GT, et al. Three dimensional regional dynamics of the normal mitral anulus during left ventricular ejection. J Thorac Cardiovasc Surg 1996;111:574-85.
14. Sarris GE, Cahill PD, Hausen DE, et al. Restoration of left ventricular systolic performance after reattachment of the mitral chordae tendinae. The importance of valvular-ventricular interaction. J Thorac Cardiovasc Surg 1988;95(6):969-79.
15. David TE, Komeda M, Pollick C, et al. Mitral valve annuloplasty: the effect of the type on left ventricular function. Ann Thorac Surg 1989;47:524-8.
16. Kurosawa H, Nakano M, Kawase M, et al. Mitral valve repair by Carpentier-Edwards physio annuloplasty ring. Jpn J Thorac Cardiovasc Surg 1999;47(8):355-60.
17. Gillinov AM, Cosgrove DM, Shiota T, et al. Cosgrove-Edwards Annuloplasty System: midterm results. Ann Thorac Surg 2000;69(3):717-21.
18. Hanel KC, Mccabe C, Abbott WM, et al. Current PTFE grafts: a biomechanical, scanning electron, and light microscopic evaluation. Ann Surg 1982;195(4):456-63.

Surgical Advances for the New Millenium

- **Updates on Recent Innovations in Surgery**

- **Peer Reviewed by Expert Specialty Surgeons**

- **Indexed on MEDLINE**

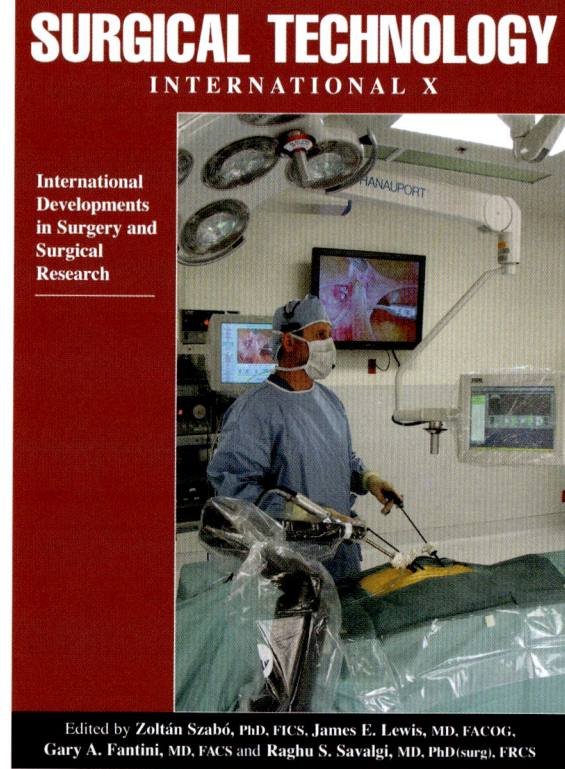

"*Surgical Technology International* does a splendid job of showcasing the many aspects of recent surgical achievement and innovation that have been possible as we hurtle forward into the new millenium."
—M. David Tilson, M.D.
Professor of Surgery
Columbia University, New York

"The authors are to be congratulated on the latest edition of what is essential reading for surgeons in every discipline."
—Tom Bates, F.R.C.S.
Consultant Surgeon
The William Harvey Hospital
Ashford, Kent, England, UK

ISBN No. 1-890131-06-7

Order a 3-year subscription now and get 50% off the bookstore price!

Yes, please enter my subscription to Surgical Techonology International for:

☐ 3 years (6 Issues) $285 ☐ 2 years (4 Issues) $215 ☐ 1 year (2 Issues) $145 ☐ Individual Copy ($95)

Please add 10% per year for shipping & handling on U.S. orders.

Please add $46 per year for shipping & handling for international orders.   ISBN No.: 1-890131-06-7

☐ Special Back Issue Set STI III - STI X - $685 US, $755 overseas - (Includes shipping)
☐ AMEX   ☐ MasterCard   ☐ VISA   ☐ Check enclosed*   ☐ Bill me

Card Number: ☐☐☐☐☐☐☐☐☐☐☐☐☐☐☐☐

Signature: _____   Expiration Date: _____
Name: _____   Institution: _____
Address: _____
City: _____   State: _____   Zip: _____
Country: _____   Phone/Fax: _____
                                      Email: _____

Please send to: Universal Medical Press, Inc., 2443 Fillmore Street, #229, San Francisco, CA 94115, USA,
or FAX YOUR ORDER TO: 1-415-436-9791. / Telephone: 1-415-436-9790 / E-mail: info@ump.com / Website: www.ump.com

*Make checks payable to **Universal Medical. Press, Inc.** California residents, please add applicable state sales tax.*

Off-Pump Coronary Artery Bypass (OPCAB) Surgery

CHRISTOPH SCHMITZ, M.D.
ARMIN WELZ, M.D.
DEPARTMENT OF CARDIAC SURGERY
UNIVERSITY OF BONN, GERMANY

During recent years, a rapid progress in the area of minimally invasive heart surgery has been seen. In addition to operations through smaller incisions and those without a complete median sternotomy, minimally invasive in cardiac surgery also means—and this might be even more important—performing the operation without cardiopulmonary bypass (CPB). Documented evidence indicates that CPB is an independent risk factor for end-organ injury after heart surgery. However, discussion continues regarding whether off-pump coronary artery bypass (OPCAB) techniques allow the same (or better) outcomes in long-term graft patency, myocardial damage, and associated morbidity compared with the classic operation done on CPB. That is one of the reasons the German insurance companies still do not accept OPCAB techniques as a viable alternative for surgical coronary revascularization, although the avoidance of CPB appears to have the greatest potential to minimize procedural costs and, consequently, provide economic benefit.

HISTORY

Coronary artery bypass grafting (CABG) was first performed without extracorporeal circulation in the early 1960s.[1] However, in the presence of evolving experience with extracorporeal circulation and development of myocardial protection methods, this technique was soon abandoned. The delicate cardiac anastomoses could be performed much more precisely when the operation was done on the arrested cardioplegic heart and in a bloodless operative field.

Almost more than three decades later, the interest in coronary revascularization without CPB was revived due to new technological developments, and the documented evidence that CPB is an independent risk factor for end-organ injury after heart surgery. Furthermore, limited availability of the heart-lung machine in some regions of the world encouraged its increasing use.

TECHNIQUES

Numerous techniques have been described for coronary revascularization without CPB during the last several years. Currently, the most important and frequently used techniques are OPCAB and minimally invasive coronary artery bypass (MIDCAB).

OPCAB is an operation performed through a complete median sternotomy, but without CPB, without cardioplegia, and under direct vision of the beating heart. MIDCAB is an operation performed without complete median sternotomy (usually through a left lateral thoracotomy), also without CPB, without cardioplegia, and under direct vision of the beating heart. Furthermore, less-popular techniques include a limited posterior left-sided approach for revascularization of the lateral wall, as described by Fonger and colleagues,[2] and a transabdominal approach for the use of multiple arterial conduits (e.g., left internal thoracic artery [LITA], right internal thoracic artery [RITA], and gastroepiploic artery [GEA]), as described by Subramanian and Patel.[3] These latter-mentioned techniques may particularly be an advantage in re-oper-

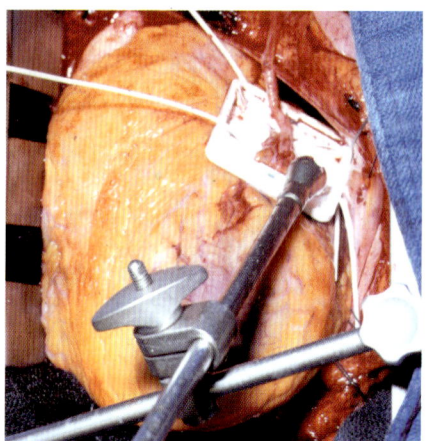

Figure 1. Stabilization of an obtuse marginal branch with the Genzyme OPCAB™ procedure system.

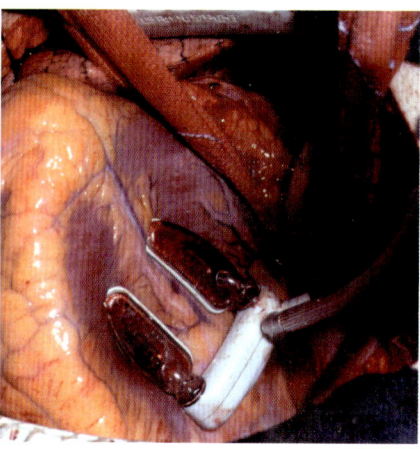

Figure 2. Rotation of the heart using deep pericardial stitches and a swap. Stabilization of the posterior descending artery with the Guidant Vortex™ stabilizer.

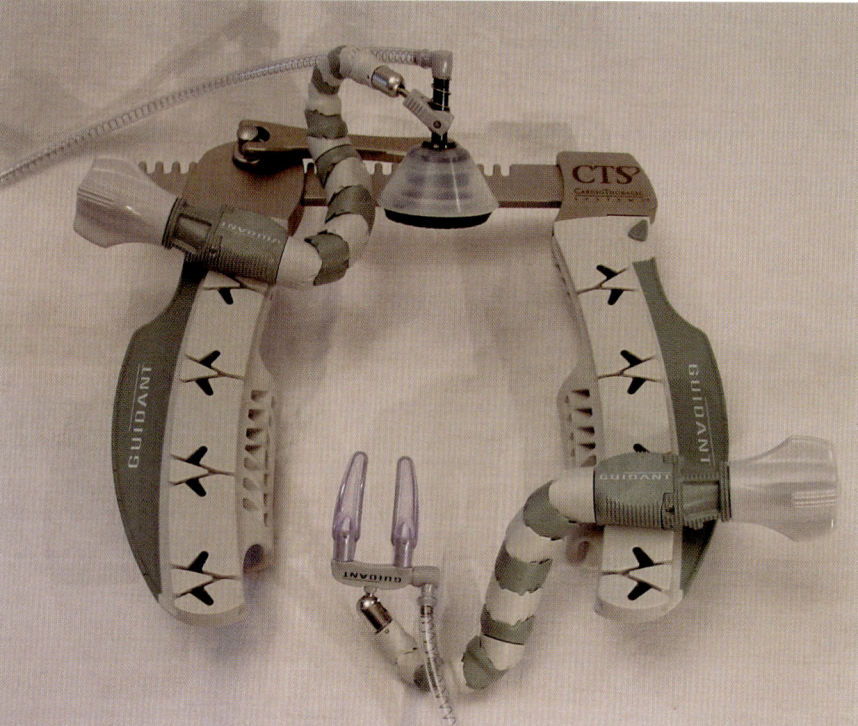

Figure 3. Guidant Axius™ Vacuum Assist Stabilizer and Guidant Xpose™ Access Device.

Table 1. Currently Commercially Available Stabilizers

Device	Type of Stystem
Estech Universal Stabilizer System™	Pressure stabilizer
Estech OPVAC™	Suction stabilizer
Genzyme-OPCAB Elite™	"Capture" stabilizer
Genyzme Immobilizer™	"Capture" stabilizer
Guidant Axius™ Mechanical Stabilizer	Pressure stabilizer
Guidant Axius™ Vacuum Assist Stabilizer	Suction stabilizer
Guidant Xpose™ Access Device	Access device
Medtronic Octopus™ 3 Flexible System Stabilization System	Suction stabilizer

ations with a patent LITA to the left anterior descending (LAD) artery.[4] All the above-described techniques can even be used in emergency cases.[5]

Several problems have to be solved to ensure a precision comparable to the standard coronary revascularization with CPB: exposure and stabilization of the operative field while providing a sufficient hemodynamic situation. This can be achieved easily when approaching branches of the anterior and posterior wall (LAD, diagonal branches, and right posterior descending), but exposure and stabilization of marginal branches, particularly in cardiomegaly, remain a challenge for the surgeon doing OPCAG procedures.

Mechanical stabilizer help to ensure an immobilized operative field. Additional medical support can be helpful, but pharmacologic agents alone (e.g., beta-antagonists) have been shown to be unacceptable in most situations. One of the most important factors in OPCAB techniques was introduction of the Octopus™-stabilizer (Medtronic, Inc., Minneapolis, MN, USA), developed by the Utrecht group by Jansen, Grundeman, and their colleagues.[6, 7] Current mechanical stabilizers use either pressure or suction for exposure of the coronary vessel and immobilization of the operative field (Fig. 1, Table 1).

Deep pericardial sutures, as first described by Ricardo Lima from Brazil, allow luxation and rotation of the heart (Fig. 2).[8] The hemodynamic impairment subsequent to the luxation or rotation of the heart is mainly due to compression of the right atrium and can, at least partially, be reversed by positioning the operative table in the Trendelenburg position.[9] Extensive right pleurotomy and deep vertical right pericardiotomy also may help enable this position. Furthermore, elevating the right hemisternum allows the apex to move behind the sternum, rotating the left lateral wall just into the center of the operative filed.

A newly developed apical suction cap, the Xpose™ Access Device (Guidant Corporation, Cupertino, CA, USA), facilitates rotation of the heart and thereby eliminates the need for periods of extreme hypotension required by the deep pericardial suture placement (Fig. 3).[10]

A further, also important feature of beating-heart surgery, is the creation of a bloodless operative field to ensure an optimal view for the surgeon. This can be accomplished by means of external occluding sutures, blowing devices, intravascular occluders, deep-bite pledgeted snares, or a combination of these different techniques.[11] Blowing devices can provide a localized wash-out of the remaining blood in the anastomotic site by using either filtered gas (e.g., CO_2) or a mixture of gas and a sterile fluid (e.g., saline).

Sometimes ECG changes or rhythm disturbances may occur when snaring a coronary vessel, particularly when occluding the proximal right coronary artery (RCA), or in patients with non-occlusive disease. In these instances, introduction of intraluminal shunts might be helpful.[12] These shunts provide the continuity of coronary flow in the distal part of the coronary, while ensuring a bloodless field.

Possible contraindications for the safe use of OPCAB techniques may be anatomic factors, including cardiomegaly and small, intramyocardial, or heavily calcified coronary vessels.[13]

The surgical strategy of coronary revascularization differs a bit from the strategy of standard techniques with CPB. In OPCABs, the LAD is usually bypassed first, which ensures the best function of the anterior and septal wall, and can be crucial before extensive manipulation of the heart. The next area, which usually is revascularized, is the RCA or its branches. The operation ends with revascularization of the obtuse marginal branches, which need the most extensive rotation of the heart. Whether the central anastomoses have to be done first or after the peripheral anastomoses remains a matter of ongoing discussion, and for that reason, varies depending on the surgeon's preference.

GRAFT PATENCY

The most important issue in coronary artery revascularization is long-term graft patency, which has been well documented for the standard operation with the use of extracorporeal circulation. OPCAB techniques have to compete with these published data. Patency rates have to be at least as good, or preferably, better.

Jansen and colleagues described angiographic findings of 100 consecutive OPCAB cases, and reported similar short-term results compared with CABG surgery with extracorporeal circulation.[14] Mack and coworkers demonstrated similar short-term patency rates in 100 patients operated off-pump by way of a left-sided mini-thoracotomy.[15] Furthermore, Omeroglu and coworkers demonstrated mid-term patency rates, comparable to the conventional techniques with CPB.[16]

MYOCARDIAL DAMAGE

The findings that postoperative markers for myocardial damage are lower in OPCAB surgery than with standard techniques with extracorporeal circulation were surprising, as the coronary vessel has to be occluded during construction of the anastomosis. Therefore, during the procedure, the surgeon produces something similar to a myocardial infarction.

Bouchard and Cartier reported a significantly lower infarction rate (creatine kinase [CK] >50 IU) and lower maximum CK-rate in patients operated off-pump as compared to those operated on-pump.[17] Wildhirt and coworkers reported similar data when they compared patients after OPCAB or CABG procedures.[18] Although the groups were relatively small–13 patients in each group–they observed a significant reduction of the cardiac specific cell damage (as measured with levels of CK-MB and Troponin-I) in the OPCAB group as compared with the on-pump group over time in the absence of acute myocardial ischemia or infarction. In addition, systemic and myocardial lipid peroxidation, as measured by the malondialdehyde levels, were lower in the OPCAB group when compared to the on-pump group. Finally, plasma levels of big-endothelin (big-ET) rose significantly in the on-pump patients but not in the off-pump patients.

These findings indicate coronary revascularization without the use of CPB and cardioplegic arrest reduces myocardial cell damage and lipid peroxidation. OPCAB procedures also are associated with a reduced activation of the potent vasoconstrictor peptide endothelin.

SYSTEMIC INFLAMMATORY RESPONSE SYNDROME (SIRS)

One of the perceived advantages of OPCAB surgery is the elimination of inflammatory reactions associated with the heart-lung machine and reperfusion injury due to cardioplegic arrest and the non-physiological flow pattern. These adverse effects of CPB have been well known for a long time; they include complement activation and neutrophil activation as well as microembolism.[19]

In a broad review of the literature, Vallely and coworkers noted that the SIRS resulting from OPCAB surgery differs markedly from that seen in conventional on-pump cardiac surgery.[20] However, they concluded one should be cautious when choosing to use OPCAB surgery on the basis of a theoretical reduction in the SIRS and ensuing end-organ injury.

In 1998, Kilger and coworkers reported a reduced procalcitonin concentration in patients after MIDCAB operation compared with those after standard CABG with CPB.[21] Also, complement activation and the release of pro-inflammatory interleukin (IL)-8 seem to be dependent on the extracorporeal circuit. In a prospective randomized study, Ascione and coworkers demonstrated that both complements C3a and C5a were elevated significantly one hour after on-pump surgery relative to OPCAB surgery.[22]

Likewise, the release of products of endothelial and leukocyte activation in the plasma is more prominent in on-pump surgery. Brasil and colleagues demonstrated a significantly greater leukocytosis after on-pump CABG surgery than that seen after OPCABG surgery.[23] However, the scarcity of cell-surfaces studies means that any interpretation of these data should be made with caution.

IL-10 is a potent anti-inflammatory cytokine that has a significant role in amelioration of ischemia and reperfusion injury.[24] IL-10 release is protective in many inflammatory syndromes such as sepsis, reducing neutrophil adhesion to activated endothelial cells, and decreasing endothelial adhesion molecule expression.[25] Wan and Yim demonstrated that IL-10 levels are increased early after CABG procedures with CPB, but are not altered in patients who undergo OPCAB surgery.[26] The absence of a rise in anti-inflammatory IL-10 after OPCAB surgery also may be deleterious, with IL-10 potentially being protective against ischemia and reperfusion injury after CPB.

The procoagulant state seen after OPCAB surgery also may be deleterious.[27] In view of the apparent clinical significance of OPCAB thrombosis, a specific perioperative prophylactic pharmacologic regimen might be advisable.

BRAIN INJURY

The finding that CPB is associated with some sort of brain damage was reported more than 30 years ago.[28] But despite various improvements in technique and technologies, use of CPB for coronary revascularization continues to be associated with some risk for stroke.

From a database of 3200 patients, Gardner and coworkers reported a 7% stroke rate for septuagenarians operated in 1983.[29] More than one decade later, Roach and coworkers noted an almost unchanged stroke rate of 6% in a series of more than 2100 patients operated with extracorporeal circulation.[30] Obviously, no improvement regarding this special problem has been achieved during this time frame. Furthermore, the mortality rate of major neurological complications is approximately 20% to 30%, and of those who die after CABG surgery 30% to 50% have had a neurological complication.[31]

Striking is the emerging evidence of the role of aortic atheroma in the genesis of perioperative stroke.[32] In this study, 23% of those with severe aortic atheroma suffered an operation-related stroke, compared to 0% of those with no detectable aortic source for embolism. Lynn and coworkers reviewed the records of 1000 patients and reported that preoperative evidence of aortic calcification was predictive of perioperative stroke.[33] Patients with diabetes who smoked and had aortic calcification and mural thrombus had a calculated probability of stroke of 93%.

CONCLUSIONS

During the last ten years, OPCAB surgery has been demonstrated to be safe and effective. Early patency rates seem to be equal to or, perhaps, better than those compared to CABG operations using CPB. Longitudinal studies are important to evaluate the real benefit for the patient who requires CABG surgery.

REFERENCES

1. Conolly E. The history of coronary artery surgery. J Thorac Cardiovasc Surg 1978; 76(6):733-44.
2. Fonger JD, Doty JR, Sussman MS, et al. Lateral MIDCAB grafting via limited posterior thoracotomy. Eur J Cardiothorac Surg 1997; 12(3):399-404.
3. Subramanian VA, Patel NU. Transabdominal mimially invasive direct coronary artery bypass grafting (MIDCAB). Eur J Cardiothorac Surg 2000;17(4):485-7.
4. Baumgartner FJ, Gheissari A, Panagiotides GP, et al. Off-pump obtuse marginal grafting with local stabilization: thoracotomy approach in reoperations. Ann Thorac Surg 1999; 68(3):946-8.
5. Hirose H, Amano A, Yoshida S, et al. Emergency off-pump coronary artery bypass grafting under a beating-heart. Ann Thorac Cardiovasc Surg 1999;5(5):304-9.
6. Jansen EW, Grundeman PF, Borst C, et al. Less invasive off-pump CABG using a suction device for immobilization: the 'Octopus' method. Eur J Cardiothorac Surg 1997; 12(3):406-12.
7. Jansen EW, Lahpor JR, Borst C, et al. Off-pump coronary artery bypass grafting: how to use the Octopus Tissue Stabilizer. Ann Thorac Surg 1998;66(2):576-9.
8. Bergsland J, Karamanoukian HL, Soltoski PR, et al. "Single suture" for circumflex exposure in off-pump coronary artery bypass grafting. Ann Thorac Surg 1999;68(4):1428-30.
9. Grundeman PF, Borst C, van Hervaarden JA, et al. Hemodynamic changes during displacement of the beating heart by the Utrecht Octopus method. Ann Thorac Surg 1997; 63(Suppl. 6):S88-92.
10. Dullum MK, Resano FG. XposeTM: A new device that provides reproducible and easy access for multivessel beating heart bypass grafting. Heart Surg Forum 2000; 3(2):113-8.
11. Benetti FJ, Mariani MA. Off-pump coronary artery bypass surgery. Surg Tech Int 1998;VII:219-26.
12. van Aarnhem EE, Nierich AP, Jansen EW. When and how to shunt the coronary circulation in off-pump coronary artery bypass grafting. Eur J Cardiothorac Surg 1999; 16(Suppl 2):S2-6.
13. Baumgartner FJ, Gheissari A, Capouya ER, et al. Technical aspects of total revascularization in off-pump coronary bypass via sternotomy approach. Ann Thorac Surg 1999; 67(6):1653-8.
14. Jansen EW, Borst C, Lahpor JR, et al. Coronary artery bypass grafting without cardiopulmonary bypass using the octopus method: results in the first one hundred patients. J Thorac Cardiovasc Surg 1998; 116(1):60-7.
15. Mack MJ, Magovern JA, Acuff TA, et al. Results of graft patency by immediate angiography in minimally invasive coronary artery surgery. Ann Thorac Surg 1999;68(2):383-9.
16. Omeroglu SN, Kirali K, Guler M, et al. Midterm angiographic assessment of coronary artery bypass grafting without cardiopulmonary bypass. Ann Thorac Surg 2000; 70(3):844-9.
17. Bouchard D, Cartier R. Off-pump revascularization of multivessel coronary artery disease has a decreased myocardial infarction rate. Eur J Cardiothorac Surg 1998;14(Suppl 1):S20-4.
18. Wildhirt SM, Schulze C, Conrad N, et al. Reduced myocardial cellular damage and lipid peroxidation in off-pump versus conventional coronary artery bypass grafting. Eur J Med Res 2000;5(5):222-8.
19. Kirklin JK, Westaby S, Blackstone EH, et al. Complement and the damage effects of cardiopulmonary bypass. J Thorac Cardiovasc Surg 1983;86(6):845-57.
20. Vallely MP, Bannon PG, Kritharides L. The systemic inflammatory response syndrome and off-pump cardiac surgery. Heart Surg Forum 2000;4(Suppl. 1):S7-13.
21. Kilger E, Pichler B, Goetz AE, et al. Procalcitonin as a marker of systemic inflammation after conventional or minimally invasive coronary artery bypass grafting. Thorac Cardiovasc Surg 1998;46(3):130-3.
22. Ascione R, Lloyd CT, Underwood MJ, et al. Inflammatory response after coronary revascularization with or without cardiopulmonary bypass. Ann Thorac Surg 2000; 69(4):1198-204.
23. Brasil LA, Gomes WJ, Salomao R, et al. Inflammatory response after myocardial revascularization with or without cardiopulmonary bypass. Ann Thorac Surg 1998;66(1):56-9.
24. Yang Z, Zingarelli B, Szabo C. Crucial role of endogenous interleukin-10 production in myocardial ischemia/reperfusion injury. Circulation 2000;101(9):1019-26.
25. Lane JS, Todd KE, Lewis MP. Interleukin-10 reduces the systemic inflammatory response in a murine model of intestinal ischemia/reperfusion. Surgery 1997;122(2): 288-94.
26. Wan S, Yim AP. Cytokines in myocardial injury: impact on cardiac surgical approach. Eur J Cardiothorac Surg 1999;16 Suppl 1: S107-11.
27. Mariani MA, Gu YJ, Boonstra PW, et al. Procoagulant activity after off-pump coronary operation: is the current anticoagulation adequate? Ann Thorac Surg 1999;67(5):1370-5.
28. Gilman S. Cerebral disorders after open heart operations. N Engl J Med 1965; 272:489-98.
29. Gardner TJ, Horneffer PJ, Gott VL, et al. Coronary artery bypass grafting in women. A ten-year perspective. Ann Surg 1985;201(6): 780-4.
30. Roach GW, Kanchuger M, Mangano CM, et al. Adverse cerebral outcome after coronary bypass surgery. N Engl J Med 1996;335: 1857-63.
31. Coffey CE, Massey EW, Roberts KB, et al. Natural history of cerebral complications of coronary artery bypass surgery. Neurology 1983;33:1416-21.
32. Hosoda Y, Watanabe G, Hirooka Y, et al. Significance of atherosclerotic changes of the ascending aorta during coronary artery bypass surgery with intraoperative detection by echocardiography. J Thorac Cardiovasc Surg 1991;32:301-6.
33. Lynn GM, Stefanko K, Reed JF, et al. Risk factors for stroke after coronary artery bypass. J Thorac Cardiovasc Surg 1992;104: 1518-23.

Endovascular Procedures Under Near-Real-Time MRI Guidance: Present Status and Future Perspectives

Yves-Marie Dion, M.D., M.Sc., F.A.C.S., F.R.C.S.C.
Associate Professor of Surgery
Laval University
Quebec City, Canada
and
Clinical Researcher
Quebec Biomaterials Institute

Geoffroy Warnier de Wailly, M.D.
Departement of Surgery
Laval University
Quebec City, Canada

Christian Moisan, Ph.D.
Director, iMRI unit
St François d'Assise Hospital
Centre Hospitalier Universitaire de Quebec
Canada

Indications for endoluminal treatment of occlusive aorto-iliac disease are well known. Endovascular grafting is a technique currently being evaluated for its efficacy for treatment of aneurysmal disease. The success of those techniques is due to their favorable results and non-invasive characteristics. X-ray contrast angiography (CA) is the most currently used imaging modality for endovascular procedures; however, the iodinated contrast agent is directly responsible for systemic and renal adverse effects in 3% to 12% of patients.[1]

X-ray irradiation could also be a problem for patients and the interventionist; consequently, other imaging modalities have been explored. The two main alternatives, computerized tomography (CT) scan and magnetic resonance angiography (MRA), are presently under evaluation.[2-4] Another technique, intravascular ultrasound (IVUS), has been used intra-operatively to assist placement of aortic endografts.[5] Martin and colleagues have demonstrated a high correlation between IVUS, MR images, and histologic findings.[6] However, MRI provides a most comprehensive anatomic picture with axial, coronal, and sagittal views. It also allows for three-dimensional (3-D) reconstruction and preoperative exploration of occlusive and aneurysmal diseases.

In 1995, Schenck and colleagues proposed a superconducting open-configuration MR imaging system to guide therapy.[7] This system allows acquisition of high-quality, near-real-time MR images under direct control of the interventionist, who can perform certain procedures while standing within the magnet itself.

We investigated the potential of such a near-real-time MRI system to guide endovascular procedures. First, the precision of this technology was tested in an *in vitro* model with a vascular anthropomorphic phantom, used to simulate insertion of aortic endoprostheses.[8] Then, the feasibility of insertion of endovascular stents and precision of the open-field interventional magnetic resonance imaging (iMRI) technology was tested in an *in vivo* model.[9]

The iMRI system used a 0.5T open configuration MRI unit (SIGNA SP*i* system, General Electric Medical Systems, Milwaukee, WI, USA, Fig. 1). To obtain high-resolution near-real-time images, a fast two-dimensional (2-D) Gradient Recalled Echo sequence with a 30° flip angle, a TE/TR of 13.2/44.9 msec along with a field of view of 34x34 cm^2, sampled with a matrix of 512(*v*) x 224 (ø) lines was used. High resolution, 1 NEX, images were the available every 10 seconds for accurate positioning of the device. Albeit somewhat slow, sub-millimeter resolution is important to ensure the precision of MR-guided endovascular procedures. Imaging twice as fast was obtained using the same field of view but with a matrix

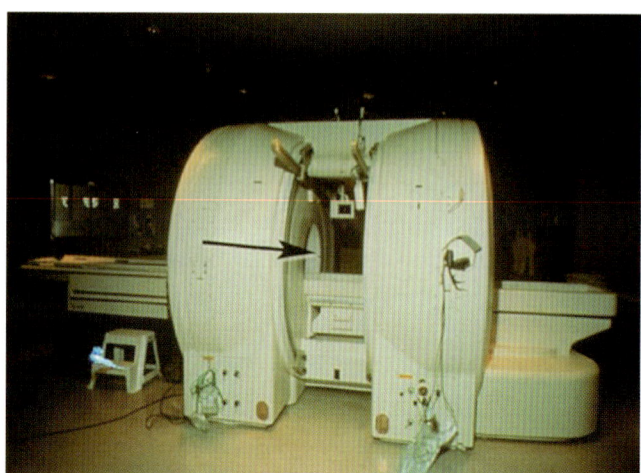

Figure 1. Interventional Magnetic Resonance Imaging Unit. Working area is shown by long arrow.

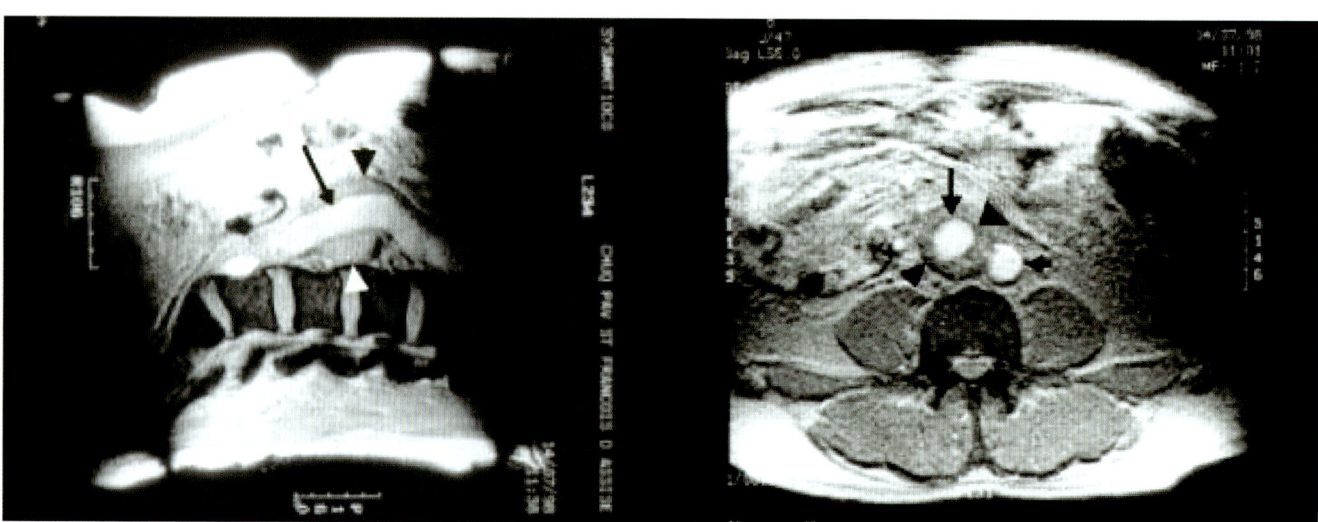

Figure 2. High-resolution near-real-time MR images of human infrarenal abdominal aortic aneurysm (AAA). a) Axial plane; b) Sagittal plane, which demonstrate lumen (long arrow) of the aorta surrounded by thrombus (arrowheads).

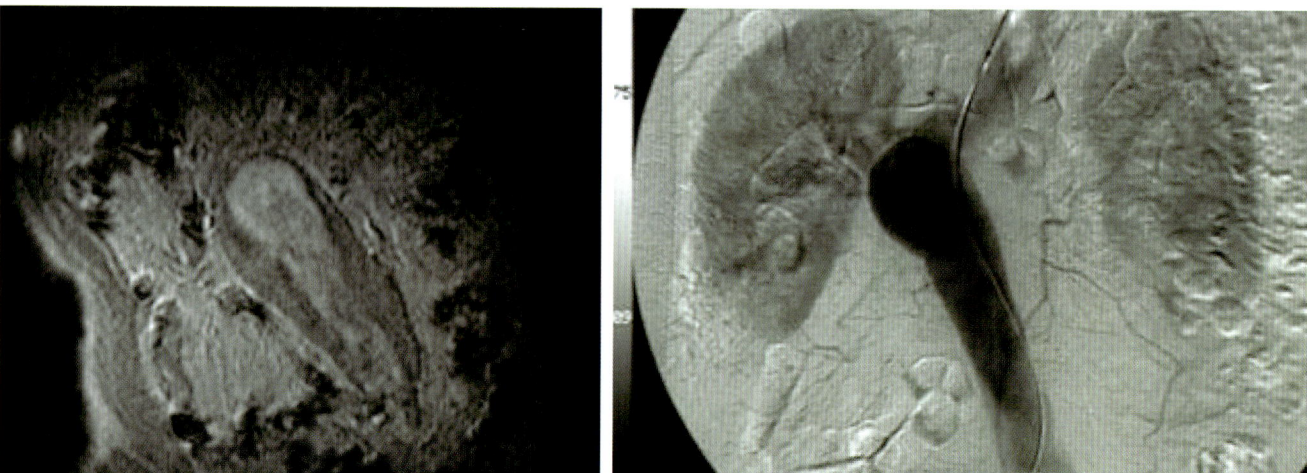

Figure 3. Images of human AAA. a) Coronal MR image showing aneurysm wall, thrombus, and its lumen; b) Corresponding X-ray contrast angiography.

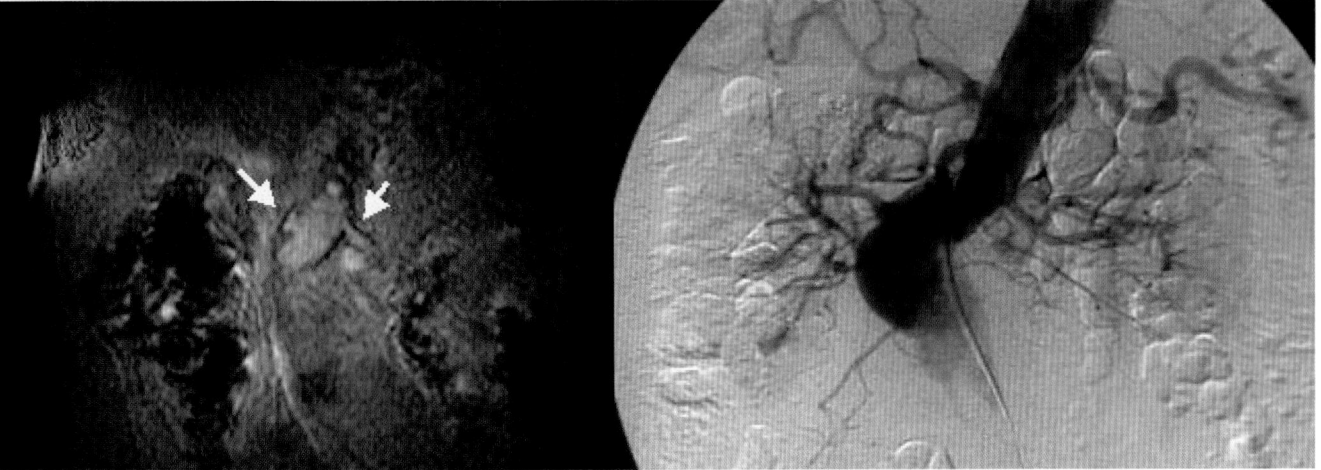

Figure 4. Images of human AAA. a) MR image of tortuous proximal aneurysm neck along with renal arteries (arrows); b) Corresponding X-ray contrast angiography.

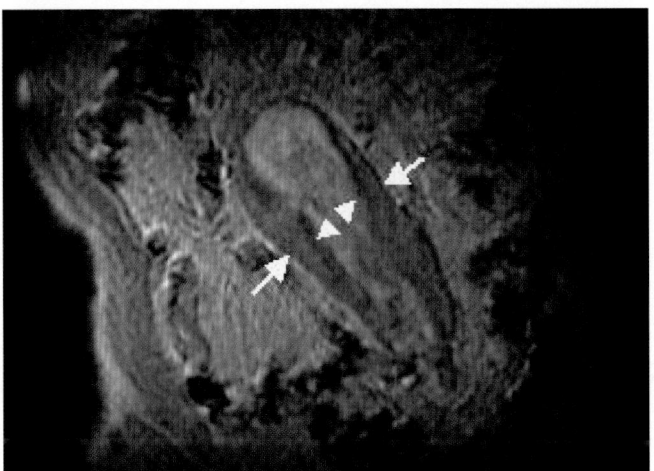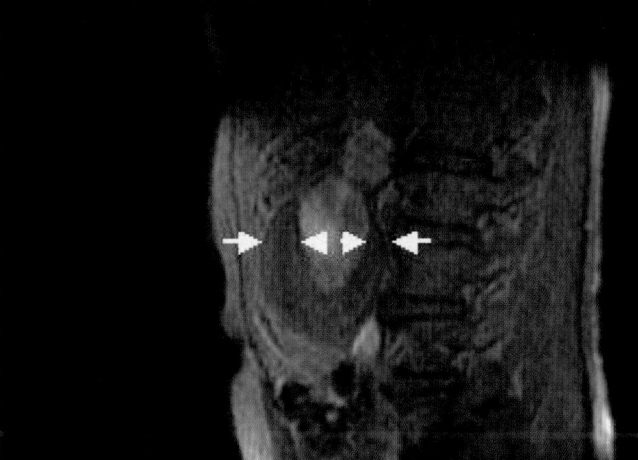

Figure 5. High-resolution near-real-time MR images of human AAA. a) Coronal plane; b) Sagittal plane; they demonstrate lumen (arrowheads) of the aorta, and wall of the aneurysm (arrows).

of 256 x 160 lines, providing 1 image every 5 seconds. Two different MR contrast agents were used. In the *in vitro* study, the phantom was perfused by water containing a 1% Gd-DTPA (Magnevist, Schering AG, Berlin, Germany) solution with a peristaltic pump, which provided a pulsatile flow. In the *in vivo* study, a MS325, long-lived blood pool MR contrast (AngioMARK™, EPIX Medical, Inc., Cambridge, MA) was used. This is a new blood pool MR contrast agent that binds reversibly to serum albumin following linkage of a diphenylcyclohexyl group to a Gadolinium chelate. MS-325 provides strong and persistent enhancement of blood vessels on MRI scans.[10]

Before performing these two sets of experiments, ten patients were imaged with abdominal aortic aneurysms (AAA) in order to verify the imaging quality with the iMRI system. On both axial and sagital planes, the AAAs' lumen and thrombus could be visualized accurately (Fig. 2). A good correlation was found between iMRI and X-ray CA in terms of blood flow (Fig. 3). Like X-ray CA, near-real-time imaging on our open-configuration MR system allows one to determine the origin of the renal arteries (Fig. 4). It also provides information regarding the location and size of the thrombus (Fig. 5).

IN VITRO MODEL

An anthropomorphic phantom was designed to reproduce an AAA and simulate MR-guided endovascular procedures (Fig. 6). This model consists of a 10-cm long aortic aneurysm lined with thrombus-like material (Fig. 7). The aneurysm's proximal and distal necks were 24 mm long; diameters of the aorta and renal arteries were 22 mm and 5 mm, respectively. The phantom was made of transparent tubing to allow accurate visual validation of the final catheter position. During the procedures, the phantom was hidden under an opaque lid. The introducer system of the Passager endovascular graft (Boston Scientific Corporation, Oakland, NJ, USA) was used. However, the metallic guidewire was replaced by a plastic optical fiber of the same diameter to ensure MR-compatibility of the entire introducer system. A nitinol hydrophilic-coated guidewire (Glide wire, Terumo, Somerset, NJ, USA), which is MR-compatible, also could have been used.

Our first goal was to demonstrate the accuracy with which the endovascular sheath could be placed at a target point located 5mm below the phantom's renal arteries. Although the renal arteries were clearly visible on MR images, it was decided to place a reference marker within them to allow determination of the final position of

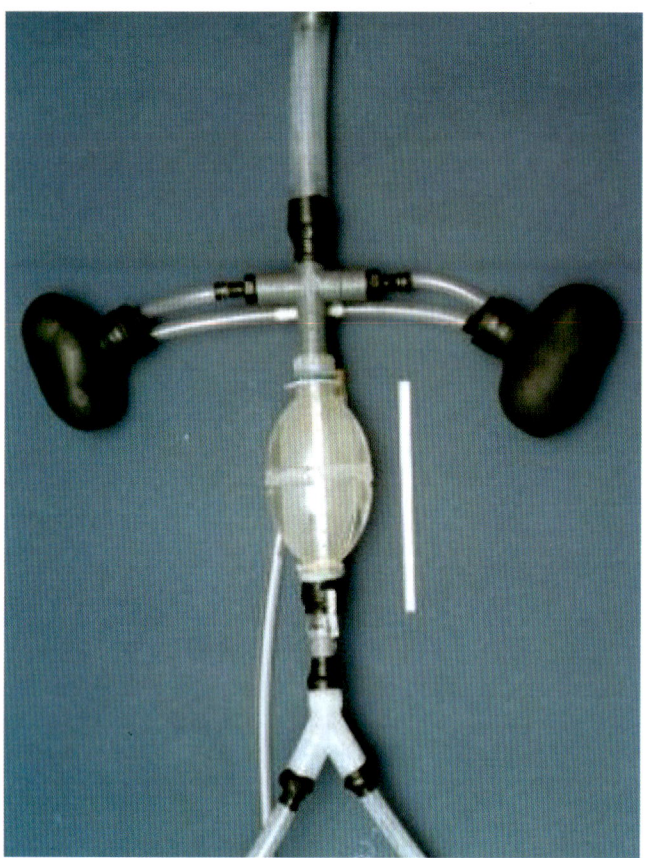

Figure 6. Anthropomorphic vascular phantom.

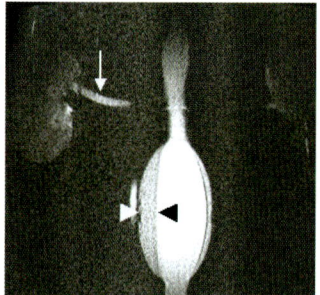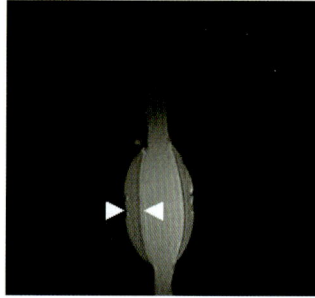

Figure 7. High-resolution near-real-time MR images of anthropomorphic vascular phantom (coronal planes), with visualization of right renal artery (long arrow), and thrombus-like material (arrowheads).

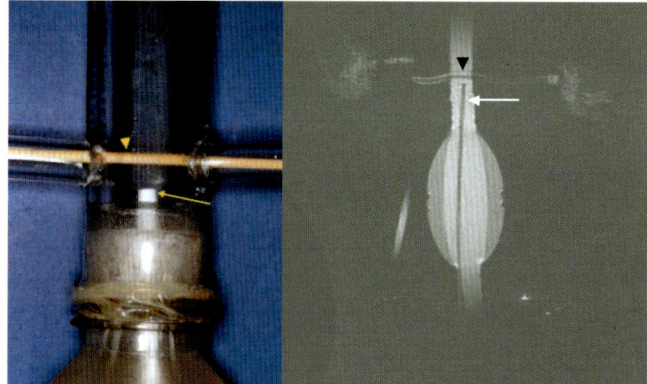

Figure 8. Catheter (long arrow) brought under MRI guidance 5 mm below origin of renal arteries, in which sharp wood stick (arrowhead) was placed. a) Direct view of phantom; b) High-resolution near-real-time MR image of phantom.

the introducer sheath by direct visual observation through the model (Fig. 8a). A similar image obtained in near-real-time allows the same observation (Fig. 8b). The target was determined to be on the MR image by a cursor seen on the magnet in-bore LCD display monitors (Fig. 9). The cursor was placed onto the target following measurements taken in the control room. To obtain independent and *de visu* measures of the position of the distal end of the introducer sheath, a millimeter-graduated catheter was inserted inside the sheath.

After the introducer sheath and catheter were brought onto the target, according to the images seen on the LCD display screen by the interventionist, the measures were demonstrated in two different ways. First, they were recorded from the high-definition operator console screen in the control room as well as from the LCD monitors used by the interventionist. The phantom's lid was then removed to allow for a direct visual reading of the location of the introducer sheath. The distance from the renal arteries was then judged by manually pushing the graduated catheter out of the introducer sheath until it touched the reference marker placed across the aorta in the renal arteries. Twenty procedures were performed; in 8 cases, a 1-mm difference was observed in measurements taken at the console in the control room compared to those obtained from the in-bore LCD monitors. This difference was attributed to the lower resolution of the in-bore LCD monitors (Fig. 10). When measurements taken from the screen were compared to those taken directly on the phantom with the graduated catheter, an average difference of 1mm was noted in 90% of the procedures (Fig. 11).

Our second goal was to evaluate the capacity of the iMRI to detect catheter displacement as the interventionist withdrew the introducer sheath. A 3-mm internal plastic catheter was used to replace the graduated catheter. The device was positioned under MR guidance as in the first technique; however, this time the introducer sheath was completely withdrawn while maintaining the catheter on the target. The final position of the catheter was measured on the Signa SPi operator console by the interventionist. Twenty-two procedures were performed, and the results were within -0.5 mm and +1.5 mm. The

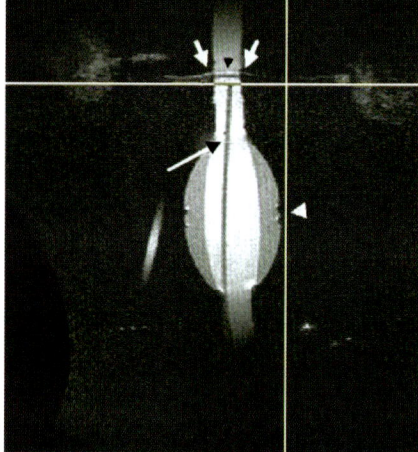

Figure 9. Target (small arrowhead), located 5 mm below renal arteries (short arrows), indicated on monitor by cross-wire cursor (large arrowhead) superimposed on MR image.

negative numbers indicate the catheter migrated upward toward the renal arteries, the positive numbers show that the catheter migrated distally.

IN VIVO MODEL

Five male piglets were used, three averaged 6 months of age and weighed between 70 and 77 kg, and two were 3

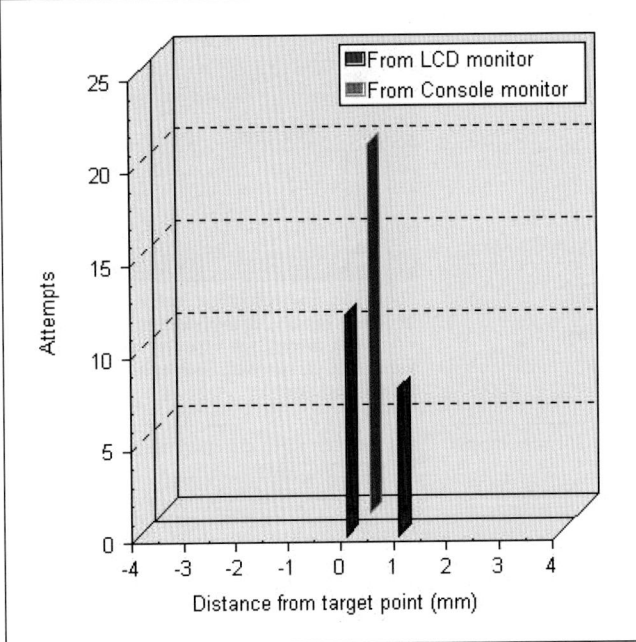
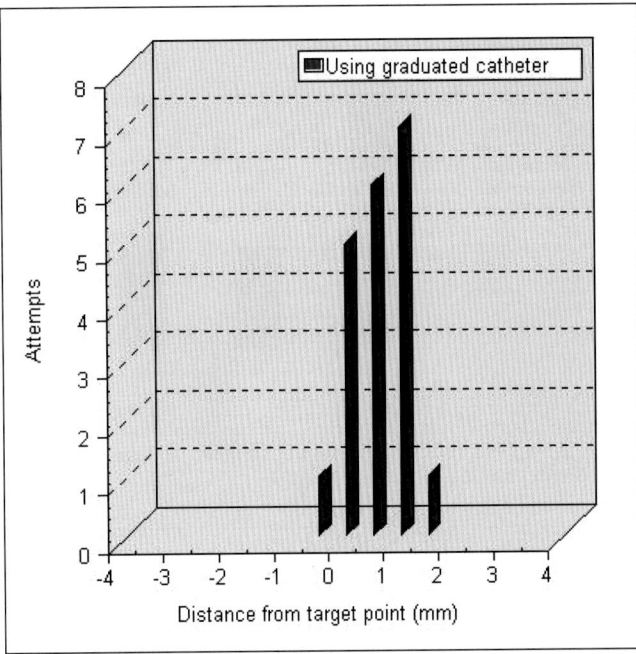

Figure 10. Distribution of distance between distal end of introducer sheath and its target as read by interventionist on iMRI LCD monitor screen (front row) and iMRI system console (back row). Readings from console considered as reference measures.

Figure 11. Distribution of distance between distal end of introducer sheath and its target as measured directly on phantom using graduated catheter.

months of age and weighed 40 to 44 kg.

Systemic heparinization (100 IU/kg) was provided, and a nitinol hydrophilic-coated guidewire was introduced through a right femoral arteriotomy. The piglet was then installed in the supine position in the iMRI system. A memotherm Sixty 8mm x 3cm or 8mm x 4cm iliac stent deployment system (Angiomed, Bard, Karlsruhe, Germany) was introduced into the femoral artery over the guidewire and positioned a few centimeters beyond the arteriotomy. A rectangular transmit/receive linear surface coil for MR imaging was used to cover the abdominal wall. To accurately visualize and localize the predefined targets, imaging of the abdominal vascular system was first achieved through Maximum Intensity Projections (MIPs). The targets were located at the level of the lowest renal artery in the aorta, and for the iliac artery at its origin. Using the high-resolution-dedicated near-real-time MR sequence, a permanent cursor was positioned at the target. The stent was brought to the target and deployed by the interventionist. The position of the stent was evaluated with coronal, sagittal, and axial views. The distance between the proximal extremity of the stent and target was measured on the MR screen. The animal was then sacrificed and position of the stent in relation to the target was measured with a millimetric ruler (Fig. 12).

Three stents were deployed at the level of the renal arteries in the aorta and two others in the right iliac artery below the aortic trifurcation. The mean duration of a procedure was 13 (12 to 15) minutes. The end position of the stent was 7.8 (0 to 22) mm away from the target. The large dispersion of the latter result is due to the migration of one stent because of a mismatch in diameter with the aorta. An axial view showed the mismatch between the stent diameter and the aorta diameter (Fig. 13). The migration was detected immediately with the near-real-time MR imaging system. Without this migration, the average distance between the end position of the stent and its target was 4.25 (0 to 9) mm. More importantly, the difference between the stent location as assessed by iMRIs and autopsy was found to be 0.6 (0 to 2) mm (Fig. 14), which confirms the reliability of the near-real-time MR imaging in accurately determining the end position of the stent.

DISCUSSION

Near-real-time MR images obtained from human volunteers demonstrated a satisfactory visualization of the AAA's lumen, thrombus, and wall.

To our knowledge, the *in vitro* study was the first to assess the accuracy of iMRI in the field of vascular surgery. The average 1-mm accuracy is comparable to the other existing interventional endovascular imaging techniques.[11]

With the *in vivo* model, data from this study demonstrated the feasibility of insertion of endovascular stents under open-field iMRI guidance and its precision. Despite the refresh rate of 5 to 10 seconds per image, the mean time to bring the stent to the target and deploy it was 13 minutes, which was quite rapid, although somewhat facilitated by the straight iliac arteries of the piglets. Ability of the interventionist increased noticeably during the course of the study. The first procedure was revealing. The stent migrated 22 mm away from the target, due to a preoperative, inadequate estimation of the aortic size. We could follow its migration and evaluate the stent position inside the artery as well as the flow, both inside and outside the stent. However, this incident allowed for demonstration that axial views provide accurate images of stent impaction on the vascular wall. Finally, the markers of the delivery system created artifacts at each end of the stent insertion kit, which we gradually learned to evaluate by taking the midpoint of the artifact as the reference point.

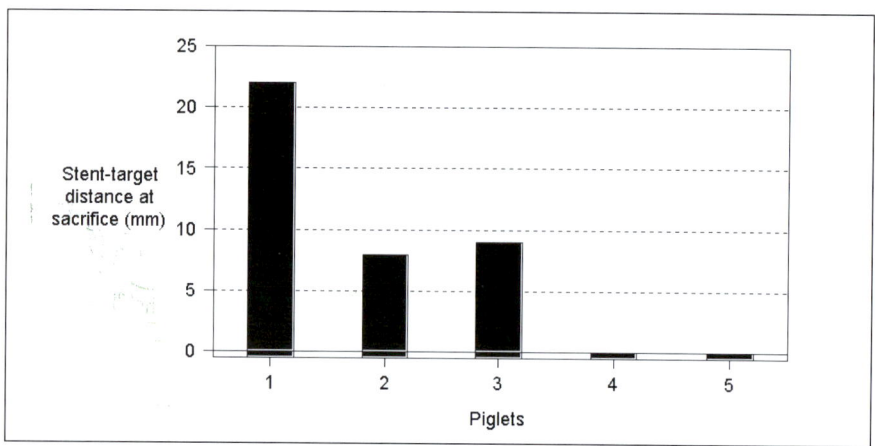

Figure 12. Distance from stent to target at sacrifice. Accuracy of stent positioning by operator ranges from 22 mm (stent that migrated) to 0 mm.

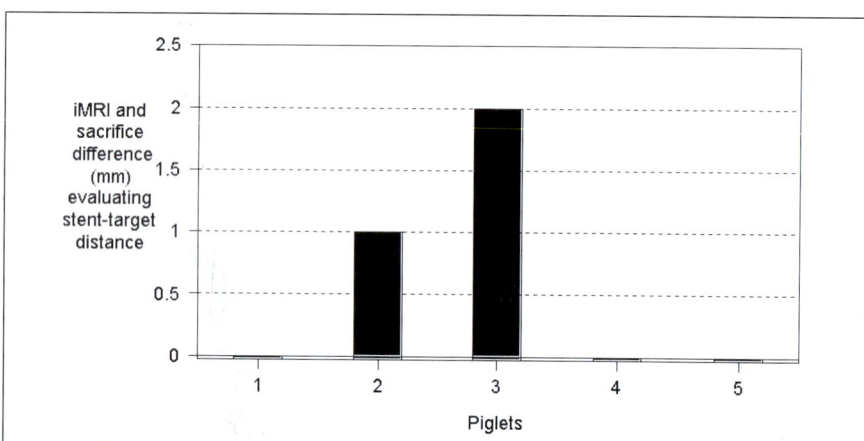

Figure 14. Difference between iMRI and sacrifice assessment of stent position in relation to target. Mean iMRI accuracy averaged 0.6 mm.

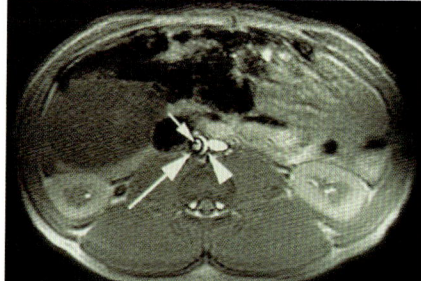

Figure 13. Low-resolution image, in axial plane, acquired rapidly, demonstrating stent as black ring (long arrow) not impacted on right side of aortic wall (arrowhead). Guidewire also visible in stent (short arrow).

Two approaches can be used to achieve MR tracking of endovascular devices: 1) active tracking and 2) passive tracking. Active tracking consists of using a miniature coil acting as a transmit/receive RF-antenna inserted at the distal end of the endovascular devices which facilitates navigation through tortuous vessels. However, current active-tracking catheters limit visualization to only the site where the endovascular device is located. Passive tracking, however, takes advantage of signal voids generated MR images by the magnetic susceptibility of catheters and guidewires. Currently, it is the easiest way to provide for visualization of a longitudinal segment of the vascular system while following progression of the endovascular device.

CT scan, CA, and IVUS are currently the technologies recommended to guide endografting procedures. However with recent advances, MRA is currently able to provide images of the lumen of an aneurysm as accurate as those from CA with eliminating parallax and projection error.[12] Like CTscan, MRA can allow measurement of the aneurysm and 3-D reconstruction. Axial views from MRA studies also have been shown to provide information similar to IVUS.[13] This technique further avoids the use of ionizing radiation and iodinated contrast agents. Renal complications are limited with MRI contrast agent.

Nevertheless, the refresh rate of 5 to 10 seconds is too long for clinical application, and improvement is warranted. One image every 2 seconds would be a favorable rate. Moreover, some feromagnetic elements currently exist on endovascular devices and are responsible for artifacts. Devices made of nitinol are MR compatible. Hikfiker and colleagues studied some plain and covered stent grafts and concluded that the ability to evaluate stents with contrast 3-D MRA is dependent on the type of stent.[14] Contraindications to examination or treatment under MR are related to the strength of the imager's magnet. Shellock published a pocket guide to MR procedures and metallic objects, which contains information about numerous materials from intravascular coils, filters, and stents to heart valves.[15]

FUTURE PERSPECTIVES

Data from this study demonstrated the accuracy of the iMRI system, which also combines diagnostic and therapeutic potentials. As the human iliac arteries are not as straight as piglet iliac arteries, dedicated navigation has to be designed to visualize them. To do so, we are currently developing a roadmap technique in an *in vitro* model. We anticipate, with the advance of technology in both hardware and software, endovascular procedures including endograft insertion will be feasible under iMRI in the near future with advantages for both patients and his physicians.

In summary, this *in vitro* study demonstrates the accuracy of this new imaging modality. Data from *in vivo* work confirm the feasibility of endovascular stenting under the guidance of an iMRI system.

REFERENCES

1. Slonim SM, Wexler L. Image production and visualization systems: angiography, US, CT and MRI. In: White RA, Fogarty TJ, eds. Peripheral endovascular interventions. 1st ed. St Louis; CV Mosby;1996. pp140-157.
2. Baum RA, Rutter CM, Sunshine JH, et al. Multicenter trial to evaluate vascular magnetic resonance angiography of the lower extremity. American College of Radiology Rapid Technology Assessment Group. Jama 1995;274(11):875-80.
3. Quinn SF, Sheley RC, Semonsen KG, et al. Aortic and lower-extremity arterial disease: evaluation with MR angiography versus con-

ventional angiography. Radiology 1998; 206(3):693-701.
4. Hertz SM, Baum RA, Owen RS, et al. Comparison of magnetic resonance angiography and contrast arteriography in peripheral arterial stenosis. Am J Surg 1993;166(2):112-6; discussion 116.
5. Wilson EP, White RA. Intravascular ultrasound. Surg Clin North Am 1998;78(4):561-74.
6. Martin AJ, Ryan LK, Gotlieb AI, et al. Arterial imaging: comparison of high-resolution US and MR imaging with histologic correlation. Radiographics 1997;17(1):189-202.
7. Schenck JF, Jolesz FA, Roemer PB, et al. Superconducting open-configuration MR imaging system for image-guided therapy. Radiology 1995;195(3):805-14.
8. Dion YM, Boudoux C, Ben EL, et al. In vitro evaluation of the accuracy of open-configuration MRI endovascular techniques. Surg Laparosc Endosc (accepted for publication).
9. Dion YM, Ben El Kadi H, Chafké N, et al. Endovascular procedures under near-real-time MRI guidance - an experimental feasibility study. J Vasc Surg (accepted for publication).
10. Caravan P, Bulte JWM, Dunham SU, Amedio J, Lauffer RB. T1 and T2 NMRD studies of Angiomark (MS 235). In: Proc. INMRM, 7thAnnual meeting. Philadelphia. 1999.
11. White RA, Donayre C, Kopchok G, Walot I, Wilson E, de Virgilio C. Intravascular Ultrasound: the ultimate tool for abdominal aortic assessment and endovascular graft delivery. J endovasc Surg 1997;4(1):45-55.
12. Beebe HG. Imaging modalities for aortic endografting. J Endovasc Surg 1997;4(2):111-23.
13. Levy MM, Baum RA, Carpenter JP. Endovascular surgery based solely on noninvasive preprocedural imaging. J Vasc Surg 1998;28(6):995-1003; discussion 1003-5.
14. Hilfiker PR, Quick HH, Debatin JF. Plain and covered stent-grafts: in vitro evaluation of characteristics at three-dimensional MR angiography. Radiology 1999;211(3): 693-7.
15. Shellock FG. Pocket guide to MR procedures and metallic objects: update 1997. Lippincott - Raven Publishers, Philadelphia - New York, p 123.

Use of Endovascular Stents in the Peripheral Circulation

Hanasoge T. Girishkumar, M.D., FACS
Attending in Surgery

Vellore S. Parithivel, M.D., FACS
Attending in Surgery

Satish C. Khaneja, M.D., FACS
Attending in Surgery

Paul H. Gerst, M.D., FACS
Attending in Surgery

Department of Surgery
Bronx-Lebanon Hospital Center
Bronx, NY

Renato Berroya, M.D., FACS
Attending in Surgery
St. Francis Hospital
Roslyn, NY

The concept of transluminal treatment of vascular obstruction by the percutaneous approach was introduced by Dotter and Judkins, in 1964.[1] Percutaneous transluminal angioplasty (PTA) developed rapidly into an extremely important therapeutic modality for relieving symptomatic obstructions in major arteries. However, it was not until 1969 that Dotter reported the successful placement of coiled stainless steel wire endarterial tube grafts, with the aid of a catheter, into the popliteal arteries of dogs.[2] This procedure stimulated the worldwide development and clinical application of endovascular stenting.

As PTA developed, it became apparent that occasional serious complications led to failure of the technique: acute vessel closure, extensive vessel wall (intimal and medial) dissection, as well as rapid restenosis of dilated lesions. In an effort to prevent these complications, stents, similar to those used for years by urologists and others to hold open ducts, were developed to be used in specific vascular cases. Originally used for failed PTA cases, or where the vessel closed off rapidly, it soon became apparent that in certain situations a stent should be used primarily (other than for failed PTA), when the surgeon or interventional radiologist believed the risk of complications was much greater than primary insertion of a stenting device.

ANGIOPLASTY: EARLY RESULTS

The first iliac angioplasty reported by Dotter in 1964 and 1965[1,2] was still patent 14 years later. In 1979, Tegtmyer and colleagues reported successful recanalization of an iliac occlusion, rather than the dilation of a stenosis.[3] However, in 1982, Ring and colleagues[4] reported poor results of angioplasty in iliac artery occlusion, with only a 50% success rate in traversing and dilating iliac occlusions, and a 40% incidence of distal embolization. This report dampened enthusiasm for PTA by itself. Other reports showed variable long-term angioplasty results: 85% patency at 7.5 years,[5] 90% at 7 years,[6] and 53% at 5 years.[7] Although angioplasty became popular for iliac artery occlusive disease, angioplasty of smaller-caliber vessels, such as superficial femoral artery (SFA), popliteal, and coronary vessels continued to pose a major challenge.[8] Early restenosis, calcified or eccentric plaque, as well as thrombotic complications appeared to limit the effectiveness of PTA alone for repair of small-vessel stenosis. Stenting, either following PTA or primarily implanted, has been shown to be an important addition to minimally invasive vascular surgery.

Currently, the main indications for endovascular stenting are obstructive and occlusive vascular disease, failed PTA, suboptimal balloon angioplasty (residual stenosis), and managing complications of angioplasty, such as acute occlusions (spasm, elastic recoil, thrombosis) and large intimal/medial dissections. In addition, primary stenting is often preferred for eccentric lesions, heavily calcified lesions, and ostial lesions, whereas balloon angioplasty by itself may not provide adequate vessel dilation and favorable long-term results.

Often, one cannot be sure in advance of the intra-procedural arteriogram of the necessity for a stent, or until an angioplasty has been attempted and a complication that requires a stent arises. "Bailout" stent insertion, where an angioplasty causes an acute occlusion and an emergent stent placement is required to restore circulation, is no longer the most common reason for stent insertion, but was originally the prime indication for placement of an endovascular stent.

TYPES OF STENTS

Currently, three types of endovascular stents are available: thermal-expansion, self-expanding, and balloon expandable. Some stents, such as the balloon-expandable tantalum stent[9] (Wiktor-Medtronic®, Medtronic, Inc., San Diego, CA), the WALLSTENT® (Boston Scientific/Meditech, Minneapolis, MN), or the Palmaz® (J&J International Systems, Warren, NJ) slotted-tube stent are metallic. Examples of non-metallic stents include the Slepian intravascular paving device[10] and the Mayo Clinic's biodegradable stents.

Thermal-Expansion Stents

The Nitinol® stent is an endoprosthesis made of thermal-shaped memory alloy Nitinol®, developed in the late 1970s and early 1980s. Nitinol® is an alloy of nickel and titanium, which can be annealed at high temperatures into a preferred shape, and then compressed into a much smaller shape for delivery (through a catheter) when maintained at a lower temperature; its original shape could be re-stored by heating it back up to body temperature, which requires ice water, heated saline infusion, or both, for placement. The initial reports of its use were discouraging because luminal narrowing developed within 4 to 8 weeks of placement,[11,12] despite antiplatelet therapy.[13] Nevertheless, newer stents with this thermal memory effect are being developed out of Nitinol®, such as the Cragg Endopro System® (Minteck, France), Symphony® (Boston Scientific, Natick, MA), and Memotherm® (Bard, Tempe, AZ).[14] However, they cannot be dilated up by balloon beyond their designed final diameter.

Self-Expanding Stents

Self-expanding stents made of spring steel spirals were reported first by Maass and colleagues in 1984,[15] and Wright and colleagues in 1985.[16] The spirals were stable and did not produce stenosis, thrombosis, or perforation, when an appropriate technique was used. However, these original stents required a cumbersome delivery system, and had a small expansion ratio; thus, they never reached clinical status. In 1987, Sigwart and colleagues introduced the spring-loaded meshwork stent.[17] This device was deployed by withdrawing a rolling membrane, which allowed the stent to increase its diameter.

Currently, the self-expanding stent used most commonly is the WALLSTENT® (Figs. 1 & 2), which consists of a preformed "knitted" meshwork of stainless steel filaments (or now other alloys) encased in a membrane. As the membrane is "peeled back" from the outer surface of the woven mesh, the WALLSTENT® expands into position, scaffolding the artery open; it continues to exert radial expansion forces until it reaches its pre-formed final diameter, so it may provide delayed dilation for stenosis/spasm after deployment. The WALLSTENT® is one of the few stents approved by the U.S. Food and Drug Administration for implantation in peripheral arteries. One major disadvantage of the WALLSTENT® is that its length shortens considerably (~20% to 30%) upon expansion, making for inaccurate placement across long lesions.[14] It also must be deployed in an already-dilated lesion, because a balloon is not used to expand this stent. However, many recommend a post-deployment balloon inflation inside the stent to further expand it and seat it into the arterial wall[18]; slight increases in diameter beyond that designed into the stent are possible with secondary intrastent balloon expansion. In addition, the WALLSTENT® is extremely flexible, and can conform to curved or bending segments

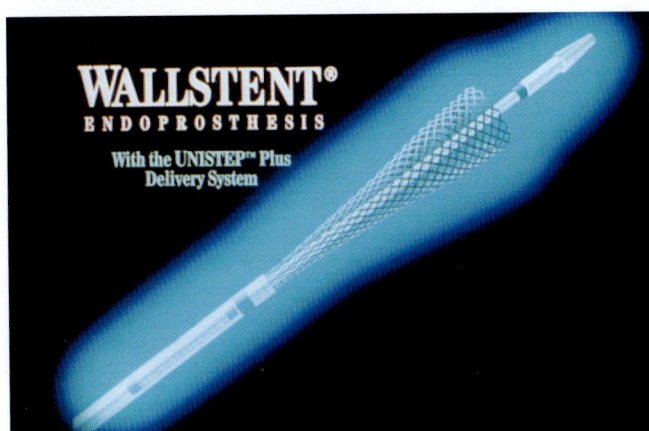

Figure 1. WALLSTENT®— an example of a self-expanding stent shown partially deployed by uncovering the stent.

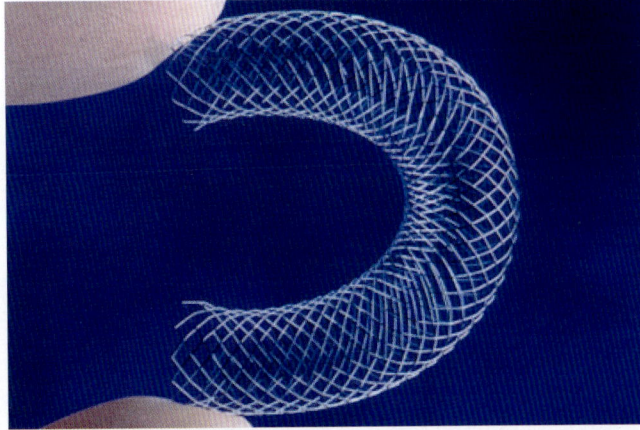

Figure 2. WALLSTENT® when fully uncovered and deployed. Photograph shows flexibility without kink.

of the artery; thus it can be inserted from a contralateral artery, and follow a tortuous guiding catheter path to its site of deployment, and stent open a curving portion of an artery.

Another stent being used is the self-expanding Gianturco-Z® (Cook, Bloomington, IN) stent, which has particular uses in large vessels, such as the vena cava or aorta, but requires a large (8F to 12F) introducer catheter.[14]

Balloon-Expandable Stents

In 1987, Roubin and colleagues reported a balloon-inflated stent developed by Gianturco®. Although the stent had a 95% success rate at delivery, it was associated with complications, which included a 12% rate of acute thrombosis and 10% rate of emergent repeat procedure.[19] However, a modified form was approved in 1993 for coronary artery stenting, and also has been used off-label for peripheral vascular lesions in the 2- to 3-mm artery size.[14]

Palmaz and colleagues, in 1985, revolutionized endovascular stenting by introducing expandable intraluminal stents (Figs. 3-6). These were designed to be placed in the stenotic lesion and used with balloon angioplasty.[20] The use of these endovascular stents included treatment of aorto-iliac, SFA, and popliteal artery lesions. About the same time, Strecker and colleagues reported a balloon-expandable vascular prosthesis that consisted of a flexible, knitted tantalum wire mesh tube.[21] Currently, the Palmaz® stent, which consists of a slotted tube that expands into an open mesh when dilated by the angioplasty balloon, is the stent used most commonly for peripheral vascular stenting; they also are being used extensively in coronary stenting. Unlike the WALL-STENT®, the Palmaz® is exceptionally rigid, and does not conform to tortuous arteries; it can, however, be dilated up to diameters greater than its design by further high-pressure balloon inflation.

"Experimental" Stents

Other concepts in intravascular stent placement were introduced: Gaspardt's temporary stent[22] (Lille, France); the tantalum stent by Wiktor-Medtronic®,[23] a relocatable stent from Tokorazawa[24] (Japan); and a removable stent developed at the University of Pennsylvania.[14]

Some investigators have suggested radioactive implants in the stent, to provide local radiotherapy to prevent cellular proliferation and neo-intimal hyperplasia, believed to be one of the major components to late stent restenosis.[25] However, this procedure remains experimental.

More recently, coated stents have become available. Three types are available: passive coatings, active coatings, *in-vitro* biologic coatings. Passive coatings include materials of decreased thrombogenecity such as gold, silicon carbide,[26] urethane, and carbon, as well as the thin layer of chromium dioxide obtained from electropolishing of stainless steel.[14] In addition, it is believed by some that the different metals may have different thrombogenic properties, due to variations in surface electrical charge; tantalum is believed to be less reactive than stainless steel.[14] Active coatings involve materials attached chemically to anticoagulants such as heparin, or have a meshwork structure

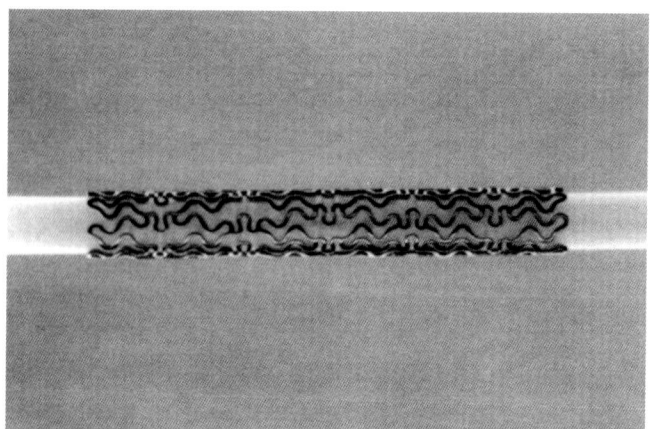

Figure 3. Palmaz®—Corinthian stent in its undilated state mounted over a balloon.

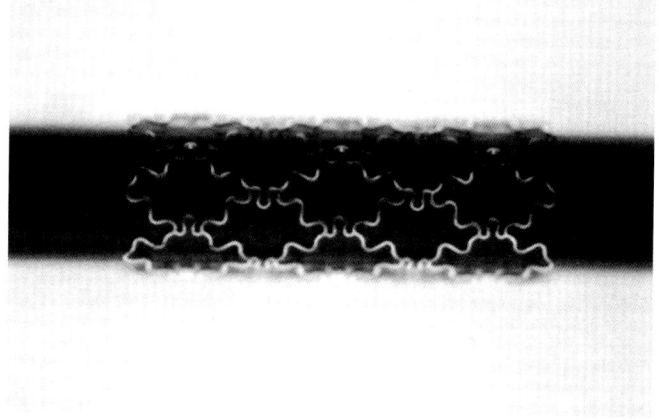

Figure 4. Palmaz®—Corinthian stent when dilated to a desired diameter.

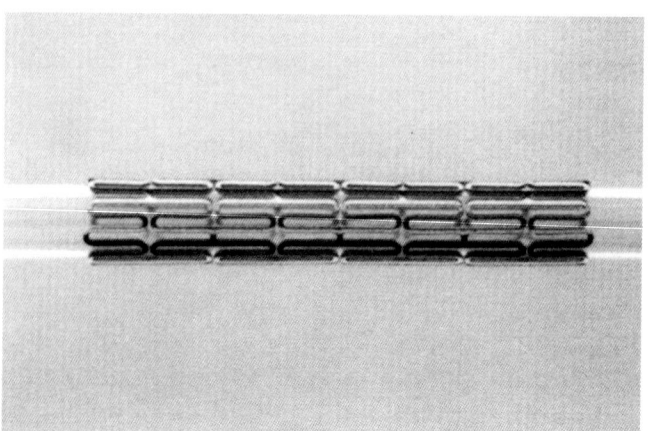

Figure 5. Shows another variety of balloon-expandable stent.

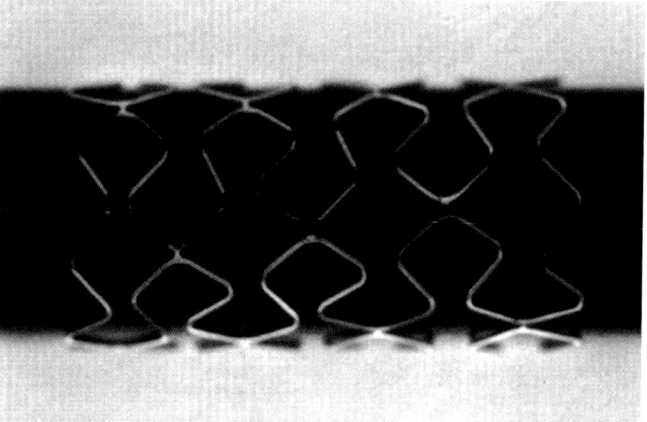

Figure 6. Balloon-expandable stent when expanded to its desired diameter.

that may incorporate active substances including anticoagulants and chemotherapeutic agents. *In-vitro* biologic coatings involve attaching endothelial cells to metal stents,[27] or stents genetically engineered to produce tissue plasminogen activator (TPA). Although these coated stents seem promising, there remain problems: the coating may slough off or peel off, and fluid may seep under the coating causing metal corrosion. Although the purpose of the coated stent is to reduce thrombus formation, coating may lead to delayed or incomplete endothelialization, defeating the purpose of its use. Long-term experimental studies are necessary before clinical application of these stents can begin.

The envelope stent, designed for occlusion of arteriovenous (AV) fistulas or saccular aneurysm, consists of a continuous envelope of silastic applied to balloon-expandable stents to render them impervious to flow through the stent mesh. So far, this stent has been used only in experimental models.

Covered endovascular stents were introduced in early 1990 to exclude localized true and false aneurysms. The devices consisted of polytetrafluorethylene (PTFE) stitched onto a Palmaz® stent. Mintec has also devised a Cragg Endopro System® in which a Nitinol® stent is covered with woven Dacron™.[28]

Stent-graft combinations were introduced to treat aneurysmal disease,[29] and are being tried for occlusive disease. However, discussion of these stent-grafts is beyond the scope of this manuscript. One recent review of this topic is by Marin and colleagues, in Surgical Clinics of North America 1998.[30]

ANTICOAGULATION/ANTIPLATELET AGENTS

As stents partially solve the problem caused by elastic recoil of the arterial vessel wall after balloon angioplasty, and hold up dissection flaps, they have been used to increase the primary success rate of failed or unsatisfactory angioplasties. However, addition of a foreign substance (the stent wall) into the bloodstream creates a new potential problem—that of thrombosis. Thus, some sort of anticoagulation regimen is usually required with the deployment of stents. As the intimal cracks created during balloon angioplasty also may lead to thrombosis, and the stent support may help to seal off these cracks, it has been difficult to dissect out how much potential for thrombosis is due to the stent, and how much from the vessel dilation; however, anticoagulation or antiplatelet drugs are used along with stents in many peripheral vascular sites.

As with usual balloon angioplasty, intravenous bolus heparin is usually administered before the procedure. Depending on the site of the lesion, full anticoagulation with heparin and then oral warfarin is advocated, particularly for smaller vessels, with lower blood flows, to prevent early stent thrombosis.[18] In larger vessels (such as the iliac), it appears warfarin is not necessary; many would still recommend antiplatelet agents such as aspirin, whereas for smaller vessels, a short course of warfarin may be used to prevent delayed stent thrombosis. Eventually, the stent should be covered with a thin layer of endothelium, and then there should be no further risk for thrombosis; however, the new intimal layer (neointima) may thicken, causing neointimal hyperplasia, which may lead to restenosis at the site of the stent. In addition, the atherosclerotic process also may cause restenosis if measures (such as lowering of serum lipids, stopping smoking, etc.) are not undertaken.

CONTRAINDICATIONS TO STENTING

Few formal contraindications exist to stenting. However, in the presence of an uncorrectable coagulation disorder, bacteremia, sepsis, or infection at the site of arterial access, the procedure should be deferred. The main contraindication is a judgment decision that the patient would benefit more from an open surgical procedure, or would do as well with conservative, non-operative therapies. Patients with long occlusions or stenoses (>10 cm), poor distal runoff, and diabetes tend to do worse, but often the angioplasty/stent procedure may be a good initial trial of therapy rather than a more extensive, open vascular procedure.

Early complications of stenting include, among others, failure to satisfactorily deploy the stent, inexact placement of the stent with respect to the stenosis, acute thromboses, cholesterol embolization, and embolization of atheromatous material. Delayed complications include stent misplacement, subacute thrombosis, and neointimal hyperplasia or atherosclerotic restenosis.

CURRENT CLINICAL APPLICATION OF ENDOVASCULAR STENTS

Iliac Artery Occlusive Disease

The first successful implantation of an endovascular stent in humans was performed in the iliac arteries.[17,31] Large-diameter, high flow rate, and easy access route through the femoral artery make the iliac artery a favorable site for endovascular stenting. Although most reports suggest iliac artery stenting has a high success rate, low complication rate, and high patency rate (at both 1 and 3 years), there has been only one randomized trial that compared PTA with stenting.[32] In this study, 247 patients were randomized, 123 to the stent group and 124 to the PTA group. The initial success rate was 98% for stenting and 90% for PTA. The patency rate at 4 years was 92% for stenting and 74% for PTA. In 1993, Johnston[33] analyzed 82 patients treated by PTA alone and noted a clinical success rate of 76% at 1 month and 48% at 3 years. Retrospective analysis by Dyet[34] suggests stenting in suitable patients provides results as good as surgery at approximately one-third the cost.

Iliac stenting is a safe and effective procedure, with the generally accepted indications being chronic occlusion, severe diffuse atheroma, and failure of previous angioplasty; short, isolated lesions have yielded the best result.[35]

Since the development of hydrophilic guidewires and stents, an increasing percentage of iliac artery occlusions can be transversed successfully, and, therefore, are amenable to primary stenting. Balloon angioplasty alone has been shown to have a higher failure rate than primary stenting in this setting, and randomized clinical trials have shown better long-term patency with the use of stents. For simple stenosis, there may not be any advantage to stenting over angioplasty alone, as long as PTA complications (such as elastic recoil or a large dissection) require insertion of an unplanned stent.

Other Peripheral Vascular Beds

In addition to iliac disease, stenting has become used commonly for SFA lesions, and even more distal lesions of the lower-extremity arteries. Using coronary artery stents, lesions of vessels as small as the peroneal artery have been stented successfully.[18] However, few trials exist to evaluate the actual role of stenting, versus more conventional, open procedures such as in-situ venous bypass, and so much of the developments have been empiric case reports and small series.

Renal Artery Disease

Renal artery stenosis is an established cause of hypertension, and bilateral renal artery stenoses, or stenosis of a renal artery to a single kidney, can promote renal failure.[36] Significant renal artery stenosis (60% or more) is followed frequently by renal parenchymal loss,[37] which justifies aggressive therapy for the renal artery stenoses. Mailloux and colleagues suggested that, in patients with renal artery stenosis, preservation of renal function may be a more important indication for intervention than the therapy for hypertension.[38]

In 1990, Baert and colleagues reported poor results of renal ostial angioplasty alone,[39] and Rodriguez-Perez and colleagues[40] confirmed this view in 1994. However, these poor results may be due to technical difficulties: an anterior or posterolaterally located ostium appears more proximal in the renal artery due to overlap with the aorta; thus, a stent intended to deal with ostial stenosis may be positioned too far distally. This problem may lead to subsequent recurrence of the lesion, or the lesion may be missed entirely if only a single anterior-posterior (AP) projection is used during the procedure. Such a situation may be avoided by performing an oblique aortogram before stent delivery.

Dyet suggested that renal artery angioplasty should be the first line of treatment for renal artery stenosis,[34] and the results were better in fibromuscular hyperplasia than with atherosclerotic disease. Recently, The Cleveland Clinic has reported favorable results with endovascular stents for renal ostial disease (unpublished data). Van de Ven and colleagues[41] reported on a randomized trial of PTA versus primary stenting in renal ostial atherosclerosis. They showed similar outcomes, but with a greater requirement for reintervention or secondary stenting after primary angioplasty alone, thus favoring primary renal ostial stenting. Results in renal ostial stenosis showed improvement or control of hypertension as well as improvement or stabilization of renal function.[41] Current consensus is to treat all renal ostial lesions and failed renal angioplasty with endovascular stents.

Stenting of renal artery ostial stenosis is performed currently with balloon-expandable stents just long enough to cover the lesion, to minimize the area of metal exposed to the vessel, thus reducing the likelihood of re-stenosis. Although an accepted mode of treatment, renal artery ostial stenting is not free of complications. Immediate complications include malposition, renal artery rupture, and acute thrombosis, whereas late complications include re-stenosis. Six-month patency rates after renal vessel stenting varies between 75% and 92%.[42]

Carotid Artery Disease

The efficacy of surgical endarterectomy for carotid artery disease has been proved in both symptomatic and asymptomatic patients. Since publication of the clinical alert from the North American Symptomatic Carotid Endarterectomy Trial (NASCET),[43] the standard of care has been to offer open surgical endarterectomy to patients with carotid atherosclerosis. Stenting and angioplasty are presumed to be unproven compared to the clearly beneficial open surgical procedure, so angioplasty and stenting in the carotid distribution have been relegated to patients not surgical candidates for formal endarterectomy. For patients judged to be at high risk, PTA plus stent implantation may be an alternative to conservative medical therapy (anticoagulation, antiplatelet therapy, or both). However, for special situations, stenting in the carotid or vertebrobasilar trees may have an important role for select patients.

When trauma to the artery produces a pseudoaneurysm or dissection of the carotid, many authors have advocated use of stenting to repair the aneurysm without the need for open surgery. In 1996, Huang and colleagues reported the first case of a false aneurysm of the internal carotid artery repaired by endovascular stenting.[44] Shames and colleagues[45] reported a similar case as well as a review of the literature for pseudoaneurysmal stent repairs, whereas Coldwell and colleagues recently reported a series of 14 patients with traumatic carotid pseudoaneurysms treated successfully with stenting; no strokes were observed in their series of 16 procedures.[46]

Patients with true aneurysms also have been treated successfully with endovascular stenting, often with adjunctive use of Guglielmi detachable coils.[47] Lanzino and colleagues have used stents to scaffold the parent vessel, and deployed the coils into the aneurysm by passing the catheter through the expanded mesh of the stent; the stent keeps the microcoils from dislodging and embolizing, while promoting thrombosis inside the aneurysm.[48] In their series of 12 patients, no permanent complications were noted, and significant aneurysmal occlusion was obtained in all the patients treated with stents and coils, whereas in four patients treated with stenting alone, no evidence of aneurysmal thrombosis was present. Fessler and colleagues reported on the use of stenting to trap a partially extruded microcoil before it embolized distally.[49]

For lesions not amenable to open surgery, such as stenoses in the intracranial artery segments, PTA plus stenting has been used successfully to treat symptomatic stenosis in the distal carotid, using flexible coronary stents, to avoid the complication of arterial dissection.[50] Morris and colleagues reported three successful cases using coronary artery stents.[51] Even the petrous portion of the carotid has been stented successfully,[52] as has the vertebrobasilar artery.[53]

For patients at high risk for open endarterectomy, who nevertheless have symptomatic carotid artery disease, PTA has been used, usually with a stent inserted after the lesion has been dilated. Dissections of the carotid have been treated by percutaneous stenting rather than open endarterectomy.[54,55]

Lanzino and colleagues reported 25 procedures in 21 patients of carotid stenting for patients who had developed restenosis after an successful, initial open carotid endarterectomy, rather than performing a repeat open procedure. Initially, PTA alone was performed, but suboptimal results and rapid recurrence of restenosis led to the use of stents; restenosis during follow up (from 6 to 57 months) was seen in only 1 of 18 arteries stented. In their series, no major cerebrovascular events or mortalities occurred, but one patient required a repair of a pseudoaneurysm at the femoral access site, and one developed a transit ischemic attack

(TIA), which suggested PTA and stent placement is a viable alternative to repeat endarterectomy.[56]

Some surgeons have used both procedures together, particularly for tandem lesions,[57] whereas others have reserved stenting for areas not reachable with conventional surgery, such as the carotid siphon[58] or intracranial carotid,[51] in which Morris and colleagues implanted coronary stents successfully into three symptomatic patients.

The role of carotid artery stenting, however, remains controversial. The presumed advantages of endovascular stenting include avoidance of general anesthesia, lack of cervical incision and cranial nerve damage, and shortened hospital stay. Disadvantages include cerebral embolization and stroke, stent deformation, and recurrent stenosis. Early results from the carotid angioplasty versus surgery in symptomatic carotid stenosis (CAVATAS)[59] trial, in which stenting is allowed for failed angioplasty, suggest that no more intracerebral complications occur in the angioplasty O group than in the surgical O group. However, long-term patency results of this trial are not available. Another European trial reported recently, the CAST I study, with 99 patients, similarly concluded that carotid stenting produces excellent results, with 97% initial technical success, 98% one-year patency, and 4% TIA rate with 1% minor stroke and no mortality or major stroke.[60]

In 1997, Wholey and colleagues reported that endovascular stenting for treatment of carotid artery disease appears effective in the short term, and without excessive risk of periprocedural stroke.[61] In this large series, 108/114 (95%) lesions were treated successfully with carotid stents. Two (2%) major and 2 (2%) minor strokes occurred, with one death in the stroke group. Five (4%) TIAs and two (2%) brief seizure episodes occurred during the procedure. The total stroke or death rate was 5%. A 1% re-stenosis rate was noted at six-month mean follow up. In a follow-up review in June, Whorley and colleagues reviewed 3129 carotid stent procedures, with a 2% TIA rate, 2% minor stroke rate, and 1% major stroke and 0.96% mortality rate.[62]

However, some immediate complications have been reported with carotid stenting. McCabe and colleagues reported one fatality after reperfusion hemorrhage in a 68-year-old man following carotid stenting.[63] Similarly, Ho and Cheung[64] and Chamorro and colleagues[65] also recently reported fatalities after carotid stenting. Noteworthy is that currently, surgical carotid endarterectomy remains the "gold standard" for treatment of carotid artery disease. PTA and endovascular stenting for carotid artery disease remain currently in the investigational or experimental category. New and colleagues[66] recently published a comprehensive review of the use of carotid stenting, particularly for patient in whom the risk of standard endarterectomy was high.

Brachiocephalic artery PTA and endovascular stenting have been used in treatment of occlusion of the brachiocephalic vessel, the innominate, common carotid, and subclavian arteries. Although preliminary results show these vessels are readily amenable to such therapy, long-term data are not available. The results of angioplasty in subclavian artery occlusions have not been encouraging;[67] stenting of these lesions has led to better outcome in terms of initial patency rates.[68]

Arterial Trauma

Endovascular stents have been used to manage blunt injuries of the carotid artery.

Duke and colleagues reported a small series of six such patients in 1977.[69] Michaels and colleagues also reported a series of patients with blunt trauma to the abdominal aortic in which two of the patients were treated successfully with endovascular stent placement.[70] Miyachi and colleagues reported a case of successful endovascular stenting of a traumatic dissecting aneurysm of the extra cranial internal carotid artery.[71] Nevertheless, as long-term results of endovascular stenting in trauma cases are not yet available, endovascular stenting for arterial trauma should be undertaken only by experienced persons in the appropriate clinical setting.

Venous Disease

Endovascular stent placement provides an option for reestablishment of flow in the venous system in patients with benign, as well as malignant, venous obstruction.[72]

Venous stenoses often are difficult to dilate and have a high frequency of recurrence.[73]

Zollikofer and colleagues successfully stented four of four venous lesions; all were patent after 4 to 12 months.[73] The largest experience with stenting in the large veins was reported with the Gianturco Z® stents.[74] The device was used mainly in patients with advanced neoplastic disease that caused superior or inferior vena cava (IVC) obstruction. Experience with Palmaz® and WALLSTENT® in large veins also is encouraging. Although stents in these venous locations may not prolong life, they can provide satisfactory palliation at an acceptable complication rate.[75]

Currently, stents in the venous system also are used for decompression of portal vein obstruction. The procedure, transjugular intrahepatic portosystemic stent shunt (TIPSS), is used to create a conduit interposed through the liver parenchyma between the portal vein and one of its major branches, and a hepatic vein. Early experience with three patients at the University of Freiburg showed a 100% success rate.[76] Richter and colleagues[77] reported 89% technical success, with 100% patency at the end of one month. Three (6%) deaths and four (8%) gastrointestinal bleeds occurred within 30 days of the procedure. No patient developed encephalopathy.

Latimer and colleagues recently reported an 88%, four-year patency rate of TIPSS.[78] However, 41% of the patients showed signs of stenosis, the majority of which (72%) were attributed to neointimal hyperplasia in the hepatic venous aspect of the shunt.

Animal studies have shown it is possible to insert PTFE-encapsulated endovascular stent-graft for TIPSS.[79] It is anticipated that with time and training, technicians will use these devices more commonly, and accumulating data will enhance our knowledge and use of endovascular stenting.

This procedure is recommended currently for patients with advanced liver disease and severe coagulopathy. It also is claimed to be adequate and appropriate for patients with failed surgical portosystemic shunt, and is a temporizing measure for patients awaiting liver transplantation.

Endovascular stents also have been used in the SVC to treat obstruction due to extravascular malignant lesion. Crowe and colleagues, in 1995, reported a primary success rate of 85% with symptom relief.[80] Post-procedure survival ranged from 5 to 243 days. Forty-six percent of patients had some recurrence of symptoms, which were further treated with thrombolysis, stenting, or both.

Endovascular stents also have been used to treat benign and malignant pelvic venous obstruction.[81] In a series of 56 lesions reported by Nazarian and colleagues,[82] endovascular stents were shown to be useful in reestablishing venous flow and relieving symptoms (IVC-10, common iliac vein-31, external iliac-vein-46, common femoral vein-27, superficial femoral vein-4). One-year patency rates after primary and secondary procedures were 50% and 81%, respectively. These values were 50% and 75% at the end of four years. Major complications occurred in only 7% of the patients.

Coronary Artery Disease

Discussion of stenting for coronary artery disease is beyond the scope of this article.

FUTURE OF ENDOVASCULAR STENTING

The use of intravascular stents as an adjunct to balloon angioplasty has facilitated the treatment of many complex stenotic and occlusive vascular lesions. Work is ongoing in developing new materials and techniques. Currently, stents removable or relocatable, as well as biodegradable, heparin-coated stents, and stents with drug-delivery capacity are being tested or are on trial.[83] Although the latter three are used mainly in coronary vessels, they may, in the future, be used to treat peripheral vascular disease as well.

Endovascular stenting is being tested currently to manage AV fistulae. It also may have a place in trauma surgery to assist in managing blunt carotid artery and aortic injuries and other major vascular trauma. Dissecting aneurysms of the aorta also may be treated successfully with endovascular stents.

The future of carotid stenting is encouraging. It is apparent that the delivery systems for stents are becoming more user-friendly, and intravascular ultrasound (in combination with endovascular stents) may further improve treatment by this modality. Intraoperative use of this technique also may provide benefits. However, complications of endovascular stents also are becoming apparent. An unusual complication, a midaortic pseudoaneurysm following extensive endovascular stenting,[84] was reported in 1997. Nevertheless, the advantages of obtaining restored blood flow distal to obstructing arterial lesions without the need for major, open vascular surgery has created an important role for intravascular stenting and angioplasty for patients with peripheral vascular diseases.

REFERENCES

1. Dotter CT, Judkins MP. Transluminal treatment of arteriosclerotic obstruction. Circulation 1964;30:654-70.
2. Dotter CT. Transluminally placed coilspring endarterial tube grafts. Invest Radiol 1969;4:329-32.
3. Tegtmeyer CH, Moore TS, Chandler JG, et al. Percutaneous transluminal dilation of a complete block in the right iliac artery. Am J Radiol 1979;133:532-5.
4. Ring EJ, Freiman DB, McLean GK, et al. Percutaneous recanalization of common iliac artery occlusions: an unacceptable complication rate. Am J Radiol 1982;139:587-9.
5. Tegtmeyer CJ, Hartwell GD, Selby JB, et al. Iliac artery angioplasty-long-term results. Circulation 1991;83:I53-60.
6. van Andel GJ, van Erp WFM, Krepel VM, et al. Percutaneous transluminal dilatation of the iliac artery: long-term results. Radiology 1985;321-3.
7. Johnston KW, Rae M, Hogg-Johnston SA, et al. 5-year results of a prospective study of percutaneous transluminal angioplasty. Ann Surg 1987;206:403-13.
8. Yang XM, Manninen H, Matsi P, et al. Percutaneous endovascular stenting development, investigation and application. Eur J Radiol 1991;13:161-73.
9. Buchwald A, Unterberg C, Werner G, et al. Initial clinical results with the Wiktor stent. Clin Cardiol 1991;14:374-9.
10. Slepian MJ, Schindler A. Polymeric endoluminal paving/sealing: a biodegradable alternative to intracoronary stenting. Circulation 1988;78:II-409 (Abstract).
11. Simon M, Kaplow R, Salzman E, et al. A vena cava filter using thermal shape memory alloy. Radiology 1977;125:89-94.
12. Dotter CT, Buschmann RW, McKinney MK, et al. Transluminal expandable nitinol coil stent grafting: preliminary report. Radiology 1983;147:259-60.
13. Cragg AH, Lund G, Rysavy JA, et al. Percutaneous arterial grafting. Radiology 1984;150:45-9.
14. Mattos MA, Hodgson KJ, Hurlbert SN, et al. Vascular stents. Curr Prob Surg 1999; 36:920-1033.
15. Maass D, Zollikofer CL, Largiader F, et al. Radiological follow-up of transluminally inserted vascular endoprostheses: an experimental study using expanding spirals. Radiology 1984;152:659-63.
16. Wright KC, Wallace S, Charnsangave J, et al. Percutaneous endovascular stents: an experimental evaluation. Radiology 1985; 156:69-72.
17. Sigwart U, Puel J, Mirkovitch V, et al. Intravascular stents to prevent occlusion and restenosis after transluminal angioplasty. N Engl J Med 1987;316:701-6.
18. Wholey MH, Nussbaum AJ, Wholey M. Angioplasty and interventional vascular procedures in the peripheral renal, visceral and extracranial circulation. In: Topol EJ, ed. Textbook of interventional cardiology, 3rd ed. Philadelphia: WB Saunders; 1999. p 920-1033.
19. Roubin GS, Robinson KA, King SB, et al. Early and late results of intracoronary arterial stenting after coronary angioplasty in dogs. Circulation 1987;76:891-7.
20. Palmaz JC, Sibbitt RR, Reuter SR, et al. Expandable intraluminal graft: a preliminary study. Radiology 1985;156:73-7.
21. Strecker EP, Liermann D, Barth KH, et al. Expandable stents for the treatment of arterial occlusive diseases; experimental and clinical results-work in progress. Radiology 1990;175:97-102.
22. Manke C, Geissler A, Seitz J, et al. Temporary Strecker stent for management of acute dissections in popliteal and crural arteries. Cardiovasc Interv Radiol 1999;2:141-3.
23. Serruys P, De Jaegere P, Betrand M, et al. Morphologic change in coronary artery stenosis with Medtronic Wiktor stent. Cathet Cardiovasc Diagn 1991;24:237-45.
24. Irie T, Furui S, Yamauchi T, et al. Relocatable Gianturco expandable metallic stents. Radiology 1991;178:575-8.
25. Liermann D, Bottcher HD, Kollath HJ, et al. Prophylactic endovascular radiotherapy to prevent intimal hyperplasia after implantation femoropopliteal arteries. Cardiovasc Intervent Radiol 1994;17:21-7.
26. Kutryk MJB, Serruy S. Stents: the menu. In: Topol EJ, ed. Textbook of interventional cardiology, 3rd ed. Philadelphia: WB Saunders; 1999. p 342-60.
27. Dichek DA, Neville RF, Zweibel JA, et al. Seeding of intravascular stents with genetically engineered endothelial cells. Circulation 1989;80:1347-53.
28. Goodwin AT, Swift RJ, Lewis JD, et al. Percutaneous endovascular covered stenting of a distal superficial femoral artery occlusion. J R Soc Med 1995;88:477-8.
29. Moore WS, Vescera CL. Repair of abdominal aortic aneurysm by transfemoral endovascular graft placement. Ann Surg 1994;220:331-41.
30. Marin ML, Hollier LH, Avrahami R, et al. Varying strategies for endovascular repair of abdominal and iliac artery aneurysms. Surg Clin North Am 1998;73(4):631-45.
31. Palmaz JC, Richter GM, Noeldge G, et al. Intraluminal stents in atherosclerotic artery stenosis: preliminary report of a multicenter study. Radiology 1988;168:727-31.
32. Tetteroo E, van der Graaf Y, Bosch JL, et al. Randomized comparison of primary stent placement versus primary angioplasty followed by selective tent placement in patients with iliac-artery occlusive disease. Dutch Iliac Stent Trial Study Group. The Lancet 1991;351:1153-9.
33. Johnston KW. Iliac arteries: reanalysis of

results of balloon angiplaty. Radiology 1993;186:207-12.
34. Dyet JF. Review: endovascular stents in the arterial system-current status. Clin Radiol 1997;52:83-108.
35. Haji-Aghaii M, Fogarty TJ. Balloon angioplasty, stenting and role of atherectomy. Surg Clin North Am 1998;78:59-61.
36. Rimmer JM, Gennari FJ. Atherosclerotic renovascular disease and progressive renal failure. Ann Int Med 1993;118:712-9.
37. Guzman RP, Zierler RE, Isaacson JA, et al. Renal atrophy and arterial stenosis. Hypertension 1994;23:346-50.
38. Mailloux LU, Napolitano B, Bellucci AG, et al. Renal vascular disease causing end-stage renal disease, incidence, clinical correlates, and outcomes: a 20-year experience. Am J Kidney Dis 1994;24:622-9.
39. Baert AL, Wilms G, Amery A, et al. Percutaneous transluminal renal angioplasty: initial results and long-term follow-up in 202 patients. Cardiovasc Intervent Radiol 1990;13:22-8.
40. Rodriguez-Perez JC, Plaza C, Reyes R, et al. Treatment of renovascular hypertension with percutaneous transluminal angioplasty: experience in Spain. J Vasc Interv Radiol 1994;5:101-9.
41. van de Ven PJG, Kaatee R, Beutler JJ, et al. Arterial stenting and balloon angioplasty in ostial atherosclerotic renovascular disease: a randomized trial. The Lancet 1999; 353: 282-6.
42. Dorros G, Jaff J, Jain A, et al. Follow-up of primary palmaz-schatz stent placement for atherosclerotic renal artery stenosis. Am J Cardiol 1995;75:1051-5.
43. Nascet Investigations. Clinical alert: benefit of carotid endarterectomy for patients with high-grade stenosis of the internal carotid artery. Stroke 1991;22:816-7.
44. Huang A, Baker DM, Al-Kutoubi A, et al. Endovascular stenting of internal carotid artery false aneurysm. Eur J Vasc Endovasc Surg 1996;12;375-7.
45. Shames ML, Davis JW, Evans AJ. Endoluminal stent placement for the treatment of traumatic carotid artery pseudoaneurysm: case report and review of the literature. J Trauma 1999;46:724-6.
46. Coldwell DM, Novak Z, Ryu RK, et al. Treatment of posttraumatic internal carotid arterial pseudoaneurysms with endovascular stents. J Trauma 2000;48:470-2.
47. Mericle RA, Lanzino G, Wakhloo AK. Stenting and secondary coiling of intracranial carotid artery aneurysm: technical case report. Neurosurgery 1999;43:1229-34.
48. Lanzino G, Wakhloo AK, Fessler RD, et al. Efficacy and current limitations of intravascular stents for intracranial internal carotid, vertebral and basilar artery aneurysms. J Neurosurg 1999;91:538-46.
49. Fessler RD, Ringer AJ, Qureshi AI, et al. Intracranial stent placement to trap an extruded coil during endovascular aneurysm treatment: technical note. Neurosurgery 2000;4:248-53.
50. Al-Mubarak N, Gomez CR, Vitek JJ, et al. Stenting of symptomatic stenosis of the intracranial internal carotid artery. Am J Neuroradiol 1998;19:1949-51.
51. Morris PP, Martin EM, Regan J, et al. Intracranial deployment of coronary stents for symptomatic atherosclerotic disease. Am J Neuroradiol 1999;20:1688-94.
52. Fessler RD, Lanzino G, Guterman LR, et al. Improved cerebral perfusion after stenting of a petrous carotid stenosis: technical case report. Neurosurgery 1999;45:638-42.
53. Malek AM, Higashida RT, Phatouros CC, et al. Treatment of posterior circulation ischemia with extracranial percutaneous balloon angioplasty and stent placement. Stroke 1999;30:2073-85.
54. Liu AY, Paulsen RD, Marcellus ML, et al. Long-term outcomes afer carotid stent placement treatment of carotid artery dissection. Neurosurgery 1999;45:1368-74.
55. Bejjani GK, Monsein LH, Laird JR, et al. Treatment of symptomatic cervical carotid dissections with endovascular stents. Neurosurgery 1999;44:755-61.
56. Lanzino G, Mericle RA, Lopes DK, et al. Percutaneous transluminal angioplasty and stent placement of recurrent carotid artery stenosis. J Neurosurg 1999;90:688-94.
57. Pappada G, Marina R, Fiori L, et al. Surgery and stenting as combined treatment of a symptomatic tandem stenosis of the carotid artery. Acta Neurochir (Wein) 1999;141:1171-81.
58. Gomez CR, Misra VK, Campbell MS, et al. Elective stenting of symptomatic middle cerebral artery stenosis. Am J. Neuroradiol 2000;21:971-3.
59. Sivaguru A, Venables GS, Beard JD, et al. European carotid angioplasty trial. J Endovasc Surg 1996;3:16-20.
60. Bergeron P, Becquemin JP, Jausseran JM, et al. Percutaneous stenting of the internal carotid artery: the European CAST I Study. J Endovasc Surg 1999;6:155-9.
61. Wholey MH, Holwy MH, Jarmolowski CR, et al. Endovascular stents for carotid artery occlusive disease. J Endovasc Surg 1997;4:326-38.
62. Wholey MH, Wholey MH, Eles G. Cervical carotid artery stent placement. Semin Interv Cardiol 1998;3:105-15.
63. McCabe DJ, Brown MM, Clifton A. Fatal cerebral reperfusion hemorrhage after carotid stenting. Stroke 1999;30:2483-6.
64. Ho DS, Cheung RT. Fatal cerebral hemorrhage after carotid stenting. Stroke 2000;31:793-4.
65. Chamorro A, Vila N, Obach V, et al. A case of cerebral hemorrhage early after carotid stenting. Stroke 2000;31:792-3.
66. New G, Roubin GS, Iyer SS, et al. Carotid artery tenting: rationale, indications and results. Compr Ther 1999;25:438-45.
67. Mathias KD, Luth I, Haarmann P. Percutaneous transluminal angioplasty of proximal subclavian artery occlusions. Cardiovasc Intervent Radiol 1993;16:214-8.
68. Hadjipetrou P, Cox S, Piemonte T, et al. Percutaneous revascularization of atherosclerotic obstruction of aortic arch vessels. J Am Coll Cardiol 1999;33:1238-45.
69. Duke BJ, Ryu RK, Coldwell DM, et al. Treatment of blunt injury to the carotid artery by using endovascular stents: an early experience. J Neurosurg 1997;87:825-9.
70. Michaels AJ, Gerndt SJ, Taheri PA, et al. Blunt force injury of the abdominal aorta. J Trauma 1996;41:105-9.
71. Miyachi S, Ishiguchi T, Taniguchi K, et al. Endovascular stenting of a traumatic dissecting aneurysm of the extracranial internal carotid artery-case report. Neurol Med Chir (Tokyo) 1997;37:270-4.
72. Nazarian GK, Austin WR, Wegryn SA, et al. Venous recanalization by metallic stents after failure of balloon angioplasty or surgery: four-year experience. Cardiovasc Intervent Radiol 1996;19:227-33.
73. Zollikofer CL, Largioder I, Bruhlmann WF, et al. Endovascular stenting of veins and grafts: preliminary clinical experience. Radiology 1988;167:707-12.
74. Palmaz JC, Rivera FJ, Encarnacion C. Intravascular stents. In: {Editor Needed}. Advances in vascular surgery, Vol 1. St. Louis, MO: Mosby-Year Book, Inc.; 1993. p 282-31.
75. Laing AD, Thomson KR, Vrazas JI. Stenting in malignant and benign venous caval obstruction. Australs Radiol 1998;42:313-7.
76. Richter GM, Noeldge G, Palmaz JC, et al. Transjugular intrahepatic portacaval stent shunt: preliminary clinical results. Radiology 1990;174;1027-30.
77. Richter GM, Noeldge G, Roessle M, et al. Three-year results of use of transjugular intrahepatic portosystemic stent shunt (Abstract). Later published in German: Richter GM, Roeren T, Brado M, et al. Long-term results after TIPSS with the Palmaz stent. Radiologe 1994;34:178-82.
78. Latimer J, Bawa SM, Rees CJ, et al. Patency and reintervention rates during routine TIPSS surveillance. Cardiovasc Intervent Radiol 1998;21:234-9.
79. Haskal ZJ, Davis A, McAllister A, et al. PTFE-encapsulated endovascular stent-graft for transjugular intrahepatic portosystemic shunts: experimental evaluation. Radiology 1997;205:682-8.
80. Crowe MTI, Davies CD, Gaines PA. Percutaneous management of superior vena cava occlusions. Cardiovasc Intervent Radiol 1995;18:367-72.
81. Carlson JW, Nazarian GK, Hartenbach E, et al. Management of pelvic venous stenosis with intravascular stainless steel stents. Gynecol Oncol 1995;56:362-9.
82. Nazarian GK, Austin WR, Wegryn SA, et al. Venous recanalization by metallic stents after failure of balloon angioplasty of surgery: four-year experience. Cardiovasc Intervent Radiol 1996;19:227-33.
83. Tanguay JF, Zidar JP, Phillips HR III, et al. Current status of biodegradable stents. Cardiol Clin 1994;12:699-713.
84. Cutry AF, Whitley D, Patterson RB. Midaortic pseudoaneurysm complicating extensive endovascular stenting of aortic disease. J Vasc Surg 1997;26:958-62.

Visit our Website at www.ump.com

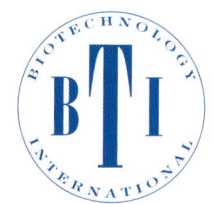

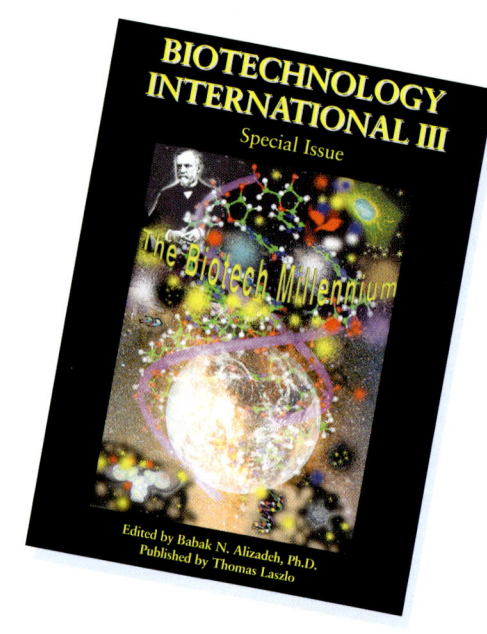

Tomorrow's Technologies At Your Fingertips!

"Biotechnology is well positioned for the 21st century, and publication of a volume devoted to its past accomplishments and challenges for the next millenium is well timed."

Stanley N. Cohen, MD, Stanford University School of Medicine, Palo Alto, CA.

- **Biannual coverage of the most recent advances in Biotechnology**
- **Written by internationally renowned scientists and researchers**
- **Offers the most concise, up-to-date information**
- **Over 300 pages in full color**
- **Saves time and money - no need to sort through magazines and articles**
- **Order a 3-year subscription now and get 50% off the bookstore price!**

Foreword by Stanley N. Cohen, M.D., Stanford University School of Medicine, Palo Alto, CA

Topics include:

A Preview of the Post-Genomic Era
Karl A. Thiel, DoubleTwist, Inc., Berkeley, CA

Viral Vectors for Gene Delivery
Alejandro R. Sica, M.D.; and Warren S. Pear, M.D., Ph.D., University of Pennsylvania School of Medicine

New Developments in Cancer Therapeutics
Hope S. Rugo, M.D.; and Debu Tripathy, M.D., UCSF, San Francisco, CA

Challenges for Bioinformatics
Philippe Rigault, Aventis Pharmaceuticals

Tissue Engineering and Cell Transplanation in the 21st Century
Boris A. Nasseri, M.D.; and Joseph Vacanti, M.D., Harvard Medical School, Boston, MA

and more...

Yes, please enter my subscription to Biotechnology International for:

Institutional: ☐ 3 years: $285.00, ☐ 2 year : $215.00   ☐ 1 year: $145.00

Individual: ☐ 3 years: $225.00   ☐ 2 year : $150.00   ☐ 1 year: $75.00

Please add 10% for shipping & handling per year on U.S. order
International orders, please add $46 for shipping & handling per year.   ISBN #: 1-890131-02-4

☐ Check enclosed*   ☐ Bill me   ☐ AMEX   ☐ MasterCard   ☐ VISA

Card Number: ☐☐☐☐ ☐☐☐☐ ☐☐☐☐ ☐☐☐☐

Signature: _____   Expiration Date: _____

Name: _____   Institution: _____

Address: _____

City: _____   State: _____   Zip: _____

Country: _____   Phone/Fax: _____

Please send to: Universal Medical Press, Inc., 2443 Fillmore Street, #229, San Francisco, CA 94115, USA, or FAX YOUR ORDER TO: (415) 436-9791. Telephone: (415) 436-9790 E-mail: info@ump.com Website: www.ump.com

* Make checks payable to **Universal Medical. Press, Inc.** California residents, please add applicable state sales tax.

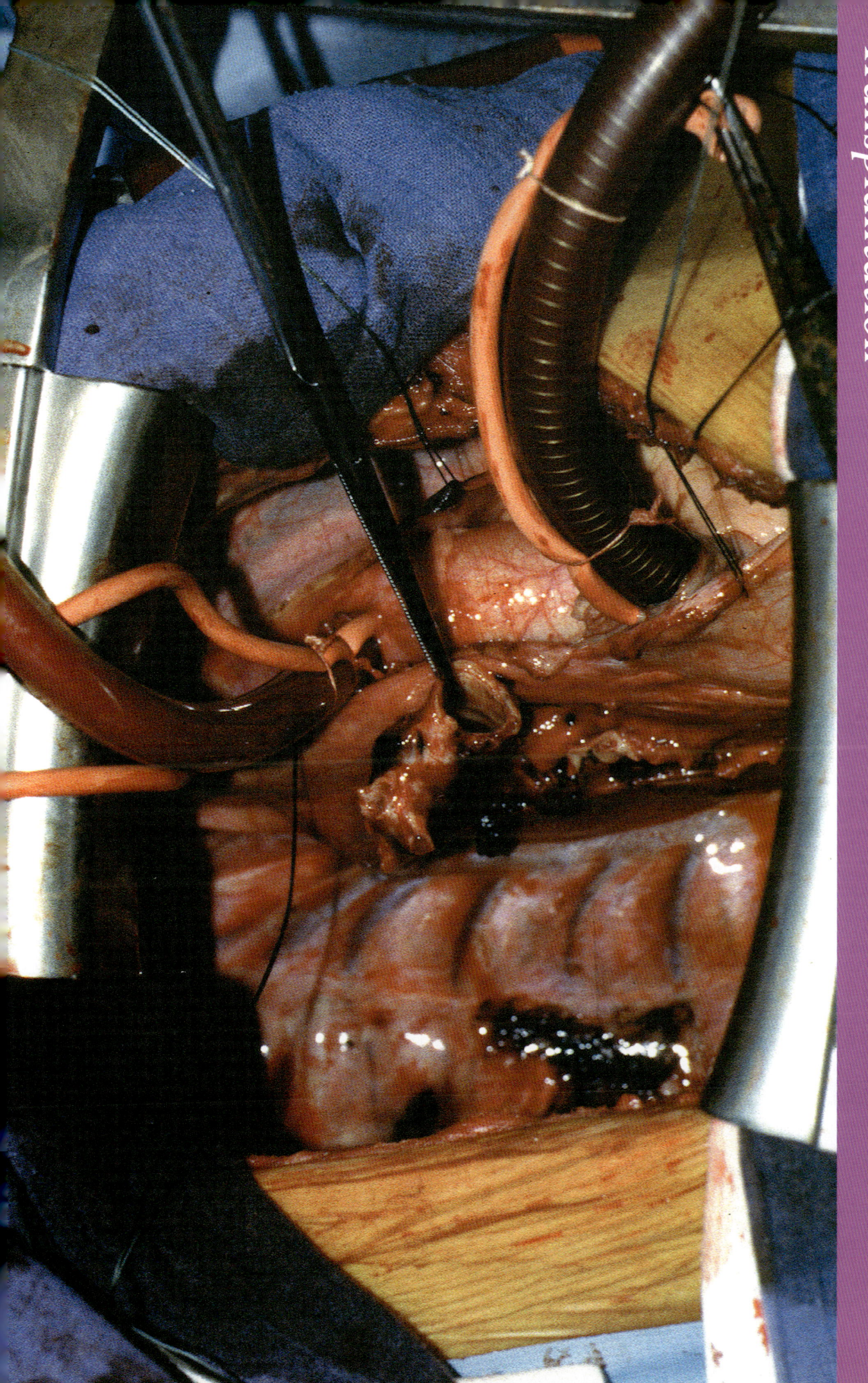

Transplantation

Human Heart, Lung, and Heart-lung Transplantation

CARSTEN SCHRÖDER, M.D.
PAOLO MACCHIARINI, M.D., PH.D.

DEPARTMENT OF THORACIC AND VASCULAR SURGERY
HEIDEHAUS HOSPITAL
HANNOVER MEDICAL SCHOOL
HANNOVER, GERMANY

Compared to other organ transplantations, lung and heart-lung transplantations have the following peculiarities: (1) bacterial colonization of the bronchi or lung parenchyma is almost constant because of the contact of donor's and recipient's lungs to the air through the intubation tube; (2) the lung is a particularly fragile organ and sensitive to the hemodynamic modifications in the donor following brain death; (3) the lung is the only organ transplanted without systemic revascularization, which increases the risks of bronchial ischemia, bronchomalacia, and mucociliary dysfunction; and (4) the lung has a large amount of lymphoid tissue, rendering it particularly immunogenic.

Over time, the understanding of these problems and those involving transplant technique, recipient and graft protection, physiology, pathology, and immunosuppression have disclosed the widespread and successful application of the heart, lung, and heart-lung allotransplantation.

HEART TRANSPLANTATION

Orthotopic cardiac transplantation is the only realistic opportunity of survival for many patients with terminal heart insufficiency. Since the first clinical transplantation in 1967, the number of operations had risen to 70 cases by 1980, with variable success. However, since the introduction of cyclosporine-based immunosupression in 1981, the number of successful cardiac transplantation procedures increased rapidly and is now a widely accepted therapeutic option for end-stage cardiac failure, with more than 2,700 procedures performed annually (Table 1).[1]

Evaluation of patients with end-stage heart disease and selection of potential candidates for cardiac transplantation are undertaken by a multidisciplinary committee to ensure an equitable, objective, and medically justified allocation of the limited donor organs to patients with the greatest chance of postoperative survival and rehabilitation. Eligibility criteria have been expanded significantly contributing to the escalating donor shortage, complicating the selection process, and perhaps jeopardizing the results of future procedures. Inclusion and exclusion criteria are evolving guidelines, and variations exist between transplantation centers. The basic objective of the selection process is to identify those relatively healthy patients with irreversible cardiac disease not amenable to other therapy, who are likely to resume a normal active life and be compliant with the rigorous medical regimen postoperatively. Accumulating transplant experience facilitates optimal donor organ allocation through improved risk stratification of potential recipients and prediction of successful outcomes for cardiac transplantation.

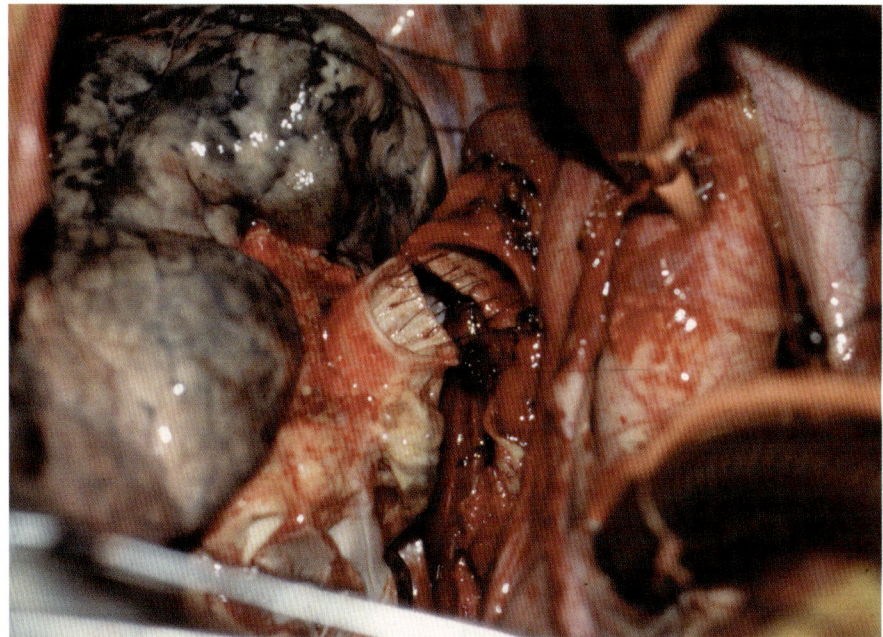

Figure 1. Telescoping technique used for bronchial anastomosis during SLT under cardiopulmonary bypass. Running suture on the membranous posterior portion is shown.

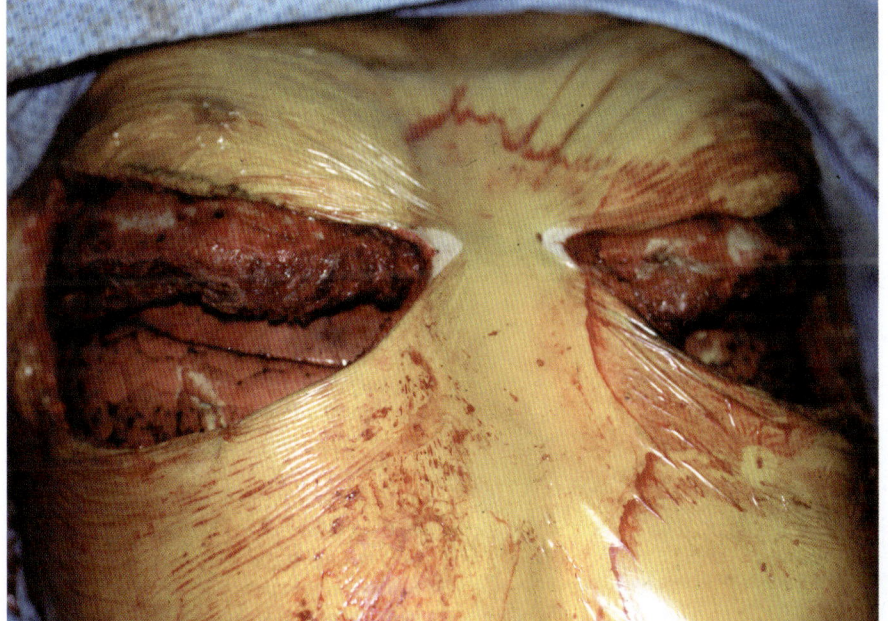

Figure 2. Intraoperative view following BSLT using a bilateral anterolateral thoracotomy to avoid the clamshell incision-associated complications.

Selection of recipients and donors

Absolute indications for transplantation include peak VO_2 less than 10 mL/kg/min with achievement of anaerobic metabolism, severe ischemia limiting routine activity not amenable to angioplasty or bypass surgery, and recurrent symptomatic ventricular arrhythmias refractory to all accepted therapeutic interventions. Relative indications include peak pO_2 less than 14 mL/kg/min and major limitation of daily activities, recurrent unstable ischemia not amenable to standard interventional measures. The following criteria are not indications for transplantation: ejection fraction less than 20%, history of functional class III symptoms of heart failure, previous ventricular arrhythmias, and maximum VO_2 more than 15 mL/kg/min without other indications.

Potential donors should be less than 45 years of age and free of anamnestic heart diseases and malignant neoplasm except low-grade osteocytoma. Special attention should be given toward ABO blood group compatibility of the recipient and donor, as well as a negative lymphocyte cross match.

Standard Standford Technique

The surgical technique of the orthotopic heart transplantation, described by Lower and Shumway in 1961, had essentially not been modified until the early 1990s due to its efficiency and simplicity. This technique is known as "biatrial technique for cardiac transplantation".[2]

The recipient is prepared for cardiopulmonary bypass using a median sternotomy incision. Venous drainage cannulae are placed in both venae cavae; arterial cannulation is by way of the ascending aorta. The heart is excised, retaining the posterior portions of both atria. The great vessels are divided just above their respective valves. Simultaneously, the donor heart is prepared by suture ligation of the superior vena cava; incision of the lateral right atrial wall from the inferior vena cava to right atrial appendage, avoiding the major internodal pathways; and preparation of the left atrium by incision between the pulmonary venous openings to a common and wide cuff. The final implantation is accomplished by suturing the left atrial wall, atrial septum, and right atrial wall continuously (3-0 polypropylene), and anastomosing the pulmonary artery and aorta (4-0 polypropylene). The procedure is completed by rewarming and de-airing the heart.[3] However, atrial arrhythmia, tricuspid and mitral valve regurgitation, and thromboembolism occurred frequently, due to the enlarged atrium.[2]

Alternative techniques for Ortotopic Heart Transplantation

Two alternative techniques for orthotopic heart transplantation have gained popularity over the past several years.[4-8] Total heart transplantation involves complete excision of the recipient heart with bicaval end-to-end anastomoses and bilateral pulmonary venous anastomoses. The Wythenshawe bicaval technique is performed in a similar fashion, except the recipient's left atrium is prepared as a single cuff with all four pulmonary vein orifices.

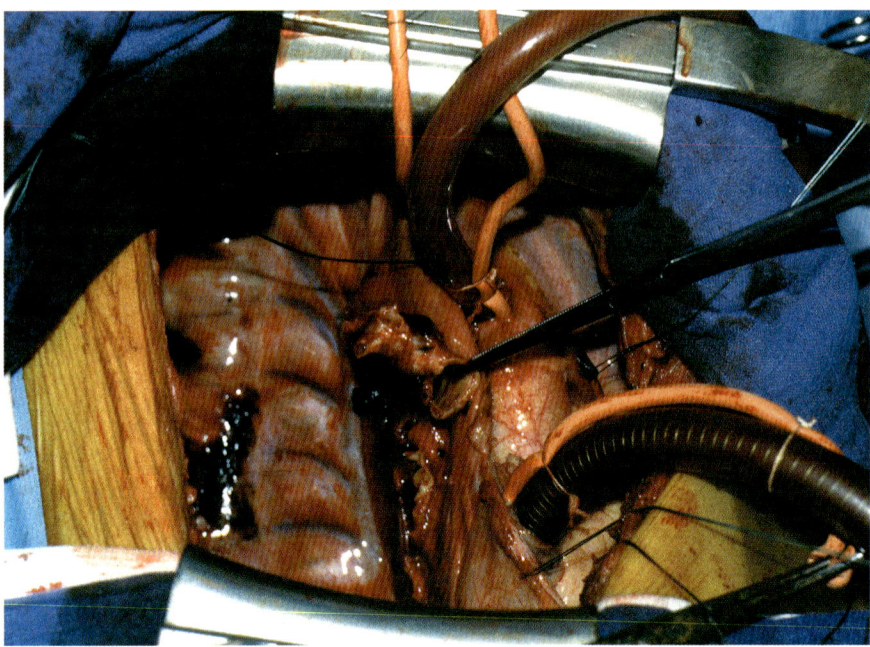

Figure 3. Intraoperative view using cardiopulmonary bypass during SLT. Thorax opened through a right anterolateral thoracotomy; recipient's right lung resected; right lower lobe bronchus is hold with forceps.

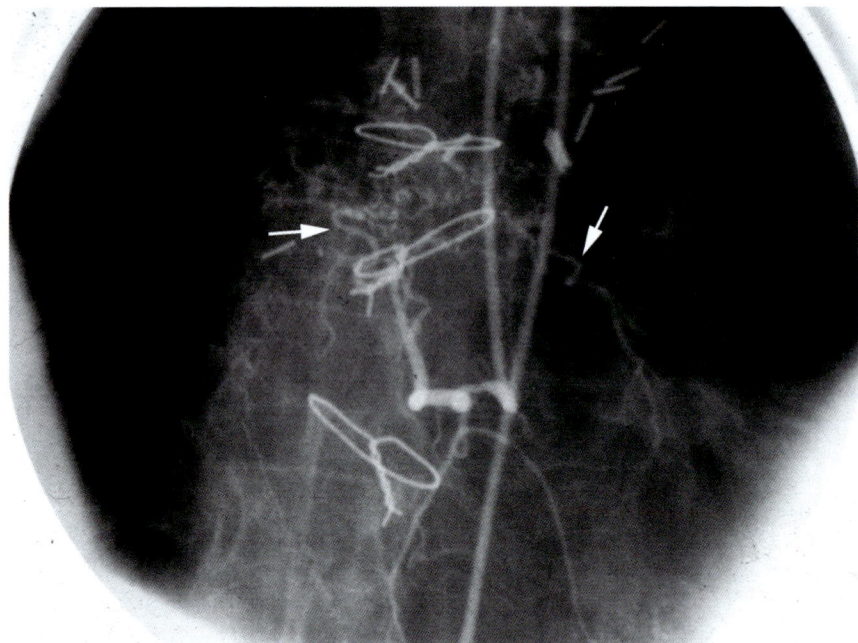

Figure 4. Postoperative angiography showing the coronary-carinal collaterals following heart-lung transplantation to assure nutrition of distal part of tracheal anastomosis.

Although these procedures are more technically difficult than standard orthotopic transplantation, preliminary series using these techniques have reported shorter hospital stays, reduced postoperative dependence on diuretics, in addition to lower incidences of atrial dysrhythmias, conduction disturbances, mitral and tricuspid valve incompetence, and right ventricular failure. The efficacy of these alternative techniques remains to be determined.

LUNG TRANSPLANTATION

Progress in lung transplantation was not as rapid as transplantation of other solid organs. Attempts in the 1990's years to perform single lung transplantation (SLTx) were disappointing because of the early graft failure and death or complications related to bronchial anastomotic healing.[9] Introduction of cyclosporin and the technique of bronchial omentopexy contributed to the initial success of isolated lung transplantation performed by Cooper and colleagues from the University of Toronto.[10-11] As experience has increased, surgical techniques have evolved, indications have broadened, and outcome has improved.

Selection of recipients

The selection criteria, in general, are end-stage pulmonary parenchymal or vascular disease with a life expectancy of less than two years. In addition, the patient should be at a New York Heart Association functional level of at least class 3 or 4, and have rehabilitation potential. Some of the specific diseases considered for lung transplantation include: idiopathic pulmonary fibrosis, cystic fibrosis, pulmonary hypertension (with symptoms), and emphysema (with a post-bronchodilator forced expiratory volume in 1 second [FEV_1] of <25% predicted).

Major indications for bilateral transplantation are cystic fibrosis, bronchiectasis, and 1-antitrypsin deficiency, as well as obliterative bronchiolitis and primary pulmonary hypertension. In the presence of infectious end-stage disease, all contaminated tissue must be replaced at the time of transplantation. Contraindications are the presence of a significant infectious component or severe bullous emphysema. Patients with primary pulmonary hypertension should receive a bilateral transplantation (BLTx) when the left heart function is preserved. Otherwise, a combined heart-lung transplantation is indicated. SLTx for primary pulmonary hypertension yields the worst late results.[12-14]

The majority of multiple organ donors do not have lungs suitable for transplantation because of pneumonia, bronchitis, or pulmonary edema. Occasionally, some donors have unilateral lung dysfunction, so that an aggressive approach to evaluation can be helpful to increase the number of available organs. Also, slit lungs technique and living donors are a reasonable way to optimize the number of potential lung donors.[15-17]

Single lung transplantation (SLTx)

Choice of transplant side depends on

Table 1. Indications of Adult Heart Transplantation.

Disease Category	Number	Percent (%)
Cardiomyopathy	18,602	46
Coronary artery disease	18,599	46
Valvular disease	1,298	3.4
Retransplantation	891	2.2
Congenital disease	646	1.6
Miscellaneous	646	1.6
TOTAL	48,541	100

Data obtained from the ISHLT (April, 1999)

the nature of recipient's disease and relative contribution of each lung to the overall pulmonary function. For patients with parenchymal lung disease, the side with poorer lung function is transplanted more commonly, so the "better" lung remains intact. Patients with primary pulmonary hypertension usually receive a right lung side transplant because of its larger vascular surface area and the easier institution of cardiopulmonary bypass. For patients with patent ductus arteriosus or Eisenmenger's syndrome, a left lung transplant is preferred because further interventions such as division of the ductus can be done more easily. Cardiopulmonary bypass should be available for all patients undergoing SLTx because recipients' pneumonectomies can be associated with ventilatory insufficiency or hypoxemic failure, as well as right ventricular failure related to elevated pulmonary vascular resistance. These recipients often require cardiopulmonary bypass to unload the right ventricle.

The posterolateral thoracotomy is the preferred incision for most SLTx. The recipient's pneumonectomy awaits the arrival of the donor lung; meanwhile, the vessels are dissected and encircled. To preserve bronchial vascularity, dissection is minimized. After the donor organ has arrived, pneumonectomy is done using a vascular stapler for the pulmonary artery distal to the upper lobe artery takeoff, as well as for both veins. The donor lung is positioned in the chest, and anastomoses (bronchus, pulmonary artery, and left artrium) can then be performed. The 'gold standard' for bronchial anastomosis is the telescoping technique (Fig. 1). This technique usually contains a running suture on the membranous portion and interrupted sutures on the anterior portion using 4-0 polypropylene, so the donor bronchus is telescoped into the recipient bronchus;[12,18] non-telescoping techniques can be done but is associated with a higher incidence of bronchial stenotic complications.[19,20]

Bilateral sequential lung transplantation (BSLTx)

As double-lung transplantation with a tracheal anastomosis led to irreversible airway complications because of the tracheal anastomotic ischemia and necrosis, the BSLTx with separate bronchial anastomoses has been developed. Currently, the usual incision for BSLTx is bilateral anterolateral thoracotomy without division of the sternum (Fig. 2). Although the working field is smaller and approach for cardiovascular bypass more difficult (Fig. 3), the sternum division complications and restrictive respiratory syndrome are avoided, as observed with the former clamshell incision.[21]

Both native lungs are mobilized and dissected before arrival of the donor lungs. The lung with the least amount of blood flow is removed first, based on a preoperative quantitative pulmonary perfusion scan. The right lung is replaced first, if perfusion is balanced. The need of cardiopulmonary bypass is tested by one lung ventilation or pulmonary artery clamping. Vessels are divided using vascular staplers. To avoid contamination of the pleural space by bronchial secretion, the bronchus is divided last after endobronchial suction. Bronchial anastomosis is done by telescoping technique, followed by pulmonary artery and left atrial anastomoses. When hemostasis and ventilation with positive end-expiratory pressure is achieved in the first transplanted lung, the second lung is implanted. Wrapping the bronchial anastomoses with omentum, pericardium or intercostal muscle is no longer done. Instead, the techniques of minimally dissecting the bronchi have been improved in protecting the native vascularization.[22-24]

HEART-LUNG TRANSPLANTATION

A total of 2510 heart-lung transplants had been reported by the Registry of the International Society for Heart and Lung Transplantation (ISHLT) by 1998. Heart-lung transplantation was developed initially for patients suffering from severe pulmonary vascular disease, specifically, primary pulmonary hypertension (PPH) and Eisenmenger's syndrome secondary to congenital heart disease. Over time, indications for this procedure have broadened to include patients with intercurrent end-stage lung disease and cardiac dysfunction, as well as patients with septic lung disease.

Primary pulmonary hypertension with severe right-sided heart failure is the most common indication for heart-lung transplantation and was the diagnosis in 31.5% of the heart-lung transplants reported to the ISHLT Registry. During the past several years, there has been a shift away from heart-lung transplantation to SLTx and BLTx for pulmonary hypertension without right-sided heart decompensation. This shift resulted from the relative shortage of heart-lung blocs and recognition that right-sided heart function could recover if pulmonary vascular resistance was decreased. However, the long-term outcome of patients with pulmonary hypertension treated with SLTx and BLTx is unknown. Graft-related mortality is significantly greater and overall functional recovery significantly lower at one year in SLTx versus BLTx lung and heart-lung recipients transplanted

Table 2. Indications and Contraindications of Adult Heart Transplantation.

Indications	• End-stage heart disease not amenable to medical or other surgical therapy
	• New York Heart Association Class III or IV symptoms on optimal medical therapy
	• Prognosis for 1-year survival without transplantation of <75% Eligibility Criteria
	• Age <55-65 (center-specific)
	• Healthy apart from heart disease
	• Compliant with medical advice
	• Psychosocially stable, supportive family or companions
Absolute Contraindications	• Severe irreversible pulmonary hypertension
	• Active systemic infection
	• Irreversible renal or heparhic dysfunction
Potential Contraindications	• Chronic obstructive pulmonary disease
	• Peripheral vascular or cerebrovascular disease
	• Peptic ulcer disease
	• Insulin-dependent diabetes mellitus with end-organ damage
	• Malignancy
	• Recent and unresolved pulmonary infarction
	• Current or recent diverticulitis
	• Other systemic illness likely to limit survival or rehabilitation
	• Cachexia
	• Alcohol or drug abuse
	• History of noncompliance or psychiatric illness likely to interfere with long-term compliance
	• Absence of psychosocial support

Edmunds LH. Cardiac surgery in the adult 1999

for pulmonary hypertension. Uncorrectable congenital heart disease with severe Eisenmenger's syndrome is the second most frequent diagnosis encountered in heart-lung transplantation. Congenital cardiac lesions that may lead to severe Eisenmenger's syndrome include atrial and ventricular septal defects, patent ductus arteriosus, and truncus arteriosus. Other complex congenital defects treated successfully with heart-lung transplantation include univentricular heart with pulmonary atresia and aortic atresia-hypoplastic left heart syndrome.

The balance of heart-lung transplants are performed for a variety of cardiac and pulmonary disease processes. Septic lung disease, particularly cystic fibrosis and bronchiectasis, and severe emphysema have been treated successfully with heart-lung transplantation. Others include simultaneous end-stage coronary disease with severe emphysema, primary parenchymal lung disease with right-sided heart decompensation (e.g., idiopathic pulmonary fibrosis, lymphangioleiomyomatosis, sarcoidosis, and desquamative interstitial pneumonitis), and cardiomyopathy with pulmonary hypertension. In patients in whom right ventricular function is relatively preserved, SLTx or BLTx should be considered.[14]

Technique

A median sternotomy is usually used for heart-lung transplantation. The patient is placed on bicaval cardiopulmonary bypass. Sequentially, the heart and each lung are removed. The great vessels are divided just above their respective valves, the right atrium is incised from the coronary sinus to the aortic root removing the appendage, and bilateral phrenic nerve pedicles are created. First, the pulmonary vessels are divided on each side at the hiliar level. Both bronchi are isolated and then occluded using a bronchial stapler; lungs are removed and; the trachea is cut just above the carina taking care of its blood supply.

The trachea of the donor heart-lung block is cut one cartilaginous ring above the carina. The heart-lung block is passed under the phrenic pedicles and right atrial cuff. First, the tracheal anastomosis is done using a running suture posterior wall and interrupted sutures on the anterior portion with 3-0 polypropylene. Alternatively, a single running suture can be done. The tracheal healing is compared to the bronchial anastomoses protected by natural coronary-tracheal collaterals

Table 3. Disease specific Guidelines for Lung Transplantation.

Emphysema
- FEV1 <25%
- PaCO2 >55 mm Hg
- Cor pulmonale
- Preference: elevated $PaCO_2$, progressive deterioration, use of long-term oxygen

Idiopathic Pulmonary Fibrosis
- Symptomatic, progressive disease with failure to keep or improve lung function while on corticosteroid or immunosuppressive drug therapy
- Symptomatic patients with VC 60-70% and/or DC 50-60%

Cystic Fibrosis and other Bronchiectatic Diseases
- FEV1 <30% or rapid deterioration with FEV1 >30%
- Resting $PaCO_2$ >50 mm Hg
- Young female with rapid deterioration

Pulmonary Hypertension with no Congenital Heart Disease
- symptomatic, progressive disease despite optimal therapy
- Pre-transplant: Cardiac Index <2L/min/m²
- Right atrial pressure >35 mm Hg and Mean arterial pressure >55 mm Hg

Eisenmenger´s Syndrome
- Severe, progressive symptoms with NYHA III or IV level despite optimum medical management

J Resp Crit Care 158: 335-9, 1998

Table 4. Indications of Adult Single Lung Transplantation.

Disease category	Number	Percent (%)
Emphysema	2,164	45
Idiopathic pulmonary fibrosis	1,049	22
Miscellaneous	614	13
Alpha-1-antitrypsin deficiency	514	11
Primary pulmonary hypertension	224	5
Cystic fibrosis	133	3
Retransplantation	96	2
TOTAL	5,347	100

Data obtained from the ISHLT (April, 1999)

(Fig. 4). The atrial or bicaval anastomoses are done next using 3-0 or 4-0 polypropylene sutures. The aorta is then anastomosed in an end-to-end fashion. Usually, a single layer is adequate. After rewarming, de-airing and discontinuing the cardiopulmonary bypass, the posterior anastomosis on each side is checked.[12]

Difficulties during the procedure depend on preexisting diseases: in patients with patent ductus arteriosus the ductus is occluded by a balloon catheter by way of the opened pulmonary artery after establishing cardiopulmonary bypass. The abundant bronchial collaterals due to secondary pulmonary hypertension may result in extensive bleeding in the posterior mediastinum after removing the native

Table 5. Indications of Adult Bilateral Double Lung Transplantation.

Disease Category	Number	Percent (%)
Cystic fibrosis	1,017	33
Emphysema	601	19
Miscellaneous	555	18
Alpha-1-antitrypsin deficiency	331	11
Primary pulmonary hypertension	306	10
Idiopathic pulmonary fibrosis	225	7
Retransplantation	63	2
TOTAL	3,751	100

Data obtained from the ISHLT (April, 1999)

Table 6. Indications of Adult Heart-Lung Transplantation.

Disease category	Number	Percent (%)
Congenital disease	511	27
Primary pulmonary hypertension	492	26
Miscellaneous	347	18
Cystic fibrosis	296	16
Emphysema	78	4
Retransplantation	50	3
Idiopathic pulmonary fibrosis	51	3
Alpha-1-antitrypsin deficiency	46	2
TOTAL	2,510	100

Data obtained from the ISHLT (April, 1999)

organs; therefore, the mean arterial bypass pressure is kept to 70 mm Hg to detect any bleeding points. Patients with primary pulmonary hypertension have large pulmonary arteries and right heart dimensions. Large cannulae and, occasionally, pledgeted sutures are useful to avoid bleeding at the thin-walled right atrium. More time is needed for dissection, because of infection-associated reactions in patients with cystic fibrosis such as dense adhesions, large lymph nodes, and purulent cystic pockets exist.[12,14]

Domino Procedure

To address the severe shortage of thoracic organs for transplantation, the so-called "domino operation" has been developed. This approach involves the use of explanted hearts from patients undergoing heart-lung transplantation for primary lung disease for a second recipient in need of a heart transplant. More than 50 % of heart-lung transplant recipients have hearts with normal or near-normal left ventricular function and some degree of right ventricular hypertrophy resulting from elevated pulmonary artery pressures. The use of hearts explanted from patients with pulmonary hypertension has theoretic appeal in that the right ventricle is already adapted to elevated pulmonary vascular resistances; therefore, the likelihood of acute donor right-sided heart failure is decreased in recipients with preexisting pulmonary hypertension.

In preparing the heart-lung recipient for cardiopulmonary bypass, the venous cannulas are placed into the inferior vena cava extrapericardially close to the diaphragm and high superior vena cava at least 4 to 5 cm above the sinoatrial node. This modification enables excision of the domino heart high on the superior vena cava to preserve the sinoatrial node for the domino recipient.

CONCLUSION

The evolution of intrathoracic organ transplantation from rudimentary laboratory experimentation to its current prominence as an accepted therapy for end-stage cardiopulmonary diseases is a product of ingenuity, resolution, skill, and audacity. Many debilitated patients, both adult and pediatric, currently have an opportunity to resume full and active lifestyles after heart, heart-lung, and lung transplantation. Nevertheless, significant barriers have yet to be overcome, particularly graft rejection, infection, and the limited donor supply. Important advances in the future include transplantation between different species (xenotransplantation), improved immunosuppression, induction of immunologic "tolerance" to foreign tissue, and improved organ-preservation techniques.

REFERENCES

1. The registry of the international society for heart and lung transplantation: sixteenth annual data report-1998. April 1999.
2. Trento A, Czer LS, Blanche C. Surgical technique for cardiac transplantation. Semin Thorac Cardiovasc Surg 1996;8(2):126-32.
3. Schwartz SI, Shires GT, Spencer FC, et al. Principles of surgery 4th edition. Singapore: McGraw-Hill Book Company; 1984.
4. Blanche C, Nessim S, Trento A, et al. Heart transplantation with bicaval and pulmonary venous anastomoses. A hemodynamic

analysis of the first 117 patients. J Cardiovasc surg (Torino) 1997;38(6):561-6.

5. Sievers HH, Weyand M, Bernhard, et al. An alternative technique for orthotopic cardiac transplantation, with preservation of the normal anatomy of the right atrium. Thorac Cardiovasc Surg 1991; 39(2):70-2.

6. Aziz T, Burgess, Yonan N, et al. Bicaval and standard techniques in orthotopic heart transplantation. J Thorac Cardiovasc Surg 1999;118(1):115-22.

7. Blanche C, Tsai TP, Trento A, et al. Superior vena cava stenosis after orthotopic heart transplantation: complication of an alternative surgical technique. Cardiovasc Surg 1995;3(5):549-52.

8. Freimark D, Czer LS, Siegel RJ, et al. Improved left atrial transport and function with orthotopic heart transplantation by bicaval and pulmonary venous anastomoses. Am Heart J 1995;130(1):121-6.

9. Egan TM, Kaiser LR, Cooper JD. Lung transplantation. Curr Probl Surg 1989;26:675-751.

10. The Toronto Lung Transplantation Group. Unilateral lung transplantation for pulmonary fibrosis. N Engl J Med 1986;314:1140-5.

11. The Toronto lung transplantation group. Experience with single-lung transplantation for pulmonary fibrosis. JAMA 1988;259: 2258-62.

12. Shumway SJ, Shamway NE. Thoracic transplantation. Blackwell Science;1995.

13. Speich R, Boehler A, Weber W. Lung transplantation in advanced pulmonary emphysema. Ther Umsch 1999;56(3):161-5.

14. Chapelier A, Vouhe P, Lafont D, et al. Comparative outcome of heart-lung and lung transplantation for pulmonary hypertension. J Thorac Cardiovasc Surg 1993;106(2):299-307.

15. Puskas JD, Hirai T, Christie N, Mayer E, Slutsky AS, Patterson GA. Reliable thirty-hour lung preservation by donor lung hyperinflation. J Thorac Cardiovasc Surg 1992;104:1075-83.

16. Artemiou O, Birsan T, Klepetko W, et al. Bilateral lobar transplantation with split lung technique. J Thorac Cardiovasc Surg 1999;118(2):369-70.

17. Baron O, Haloun A, Despins P, et al. Mucoviscidosis: lung transplantation is always in order. Press Med 1999;28(30):1676-9.

18. Shumway SJ, Hertz MI, Petty MG, et al. Liberalization of donor criteria in lung and heart-lung transplantation. Ann Thorac Surg 1994;57:92-95.

19. Griffith BP, Magee MJ, Gonzalez IF, et al. Anastomotic pitfalls in lung transplantation. J Thorac Cardiovasc Surg 1994;107:743-54.

20. Taghavi S, Birsan T, Klepetko W, et al. Initial experience with sequential anterolateral thoracotomies for bilateral lung transplantation. Ann Thorac Surg 1999;67(5):1440-3.

21. Macchiarini P, Ladurie FL, Dartevelle P, et al. Clamshell or sternotomy for double lung or heart-lung transplantation? Eur J Cardiothorac Surg 1999;15(3):333-9.

22. Pattersson G, Norgaard MA, Svendsen UG, et al. Direct bronchial artery revascularization and en bloc double lung transplantation-surgical techniques and early outcome. J Heart Lung Transplant 1997;16(3):320-33.

23. Jenkinson SG, Levine SM. Lung transplantation. Dis Mon 1994;40(1):1-38.

24. Norgaand MA, Olsen PS, Pettersson G, et al. Revascularization of the bronchial arteries in lung transplantation: an overview. Ann Thorac Surg 1996;62(4):1215-21.

Preoperative Imaging of Donor Patients for Adult Right-Lobe Liver Transplantation

Ihab R. Kamel, M.D., Ph.D.
Jonathan B. Kruskal, M.D., Ph.D.
Gisele Warmbrand, M.D.
Kevin F. Reynolds, R.T.R.
Vassilios Raptopoulos, M.D.
Abdominal Imaging Section
Beth Israel Deaconess Medical Center and Harvard Medical School
Boston, MA

A major discrepency exists between the number of available cadaveric livers and patients requiring liver transplants, which has resulted in the innovative procurement of liver segments taken from healthy donors being implanted into cirrhotic patients. Most recently, liver surgeons have started resecting the entire right lobe (segments V-VIII) from healthy adult donor livers, and implanting these segments into recipients where the graft is able to sustain and maintain metabolic function and fully regenerate.

As part of the complex, yet rigorous, evaluation of healthy donors, cross-sectional imaging has an essential role because important anatomic variants must be identified that preclude the patient from undergoing surgery. From our recent experience with use of a multidetector helical computed tomography (CT) scanner, we describe the important imaging steps that should be performed when evaluating the donor liver, and illustrate the additional necessary information provided to the surgeon to facilitate surgical planning and the hepatectomy incision.

IMAGING EQUIPMENT

A variety of strategies and technologies exist for imaging the donor liver. Essential information that must be obtained includes identification of the origin of the artery supplying segment IV, accurate depiction of anatomic portal vein variants, and total and lobar volumetric measurements of the liver. Traditionally, parenchymal and volumetric determinations have been made using CT scanning, with arterial evaluation obtained using conventional angiography. When comparing the relative advantages of different imaging techniques, magnetic resonance imaging (MRI) offers the potential to evaluate the extrahepatic bile ducts non-invasively, but newer contrast agents being evaluated may permit CT to depict important intrahepatic ducts. In addition, major recent improvements in CT technology now permit high-resolution vascular anatomic detail to be provided, and obviate the need for an invasive angiogram for imaging important segmental hepatic arteries. These advances have been brought about with development of the multidetector helical CT scanner, in which at least four separate detector arrays rotate continuously around the patient during image acquisition. This process permits thin (1.25-mm) slices to be obtained as a continuous volume of data, allowing accurate reconstructions to be made of crucial vascular anatomy.

SCANNING TECHNIQUE

Using a multidetector CT scanner

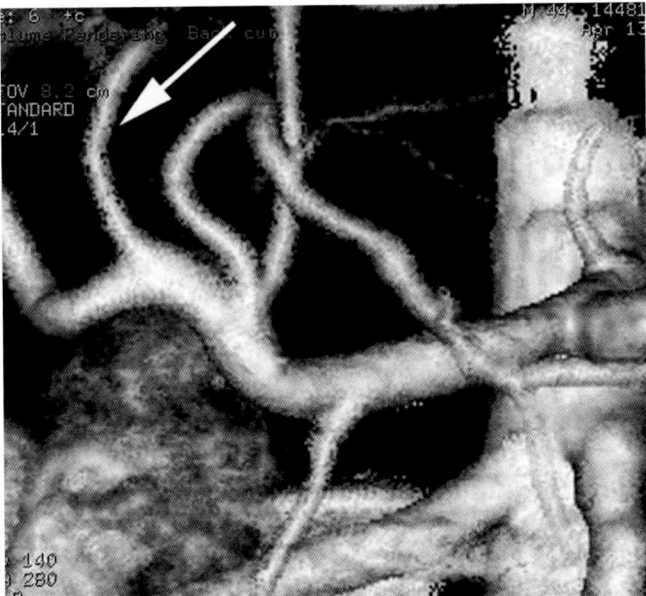

Figure 1. Volume-rendered image with shaded surface display of hepatic arteries. Arrow demonstrates the artery supplying segment IV of the liver, an important anatomic structure that must be documented before surgery to prevent ischemic injury to the left lobe of the liver remaining in the healthy donor patient.

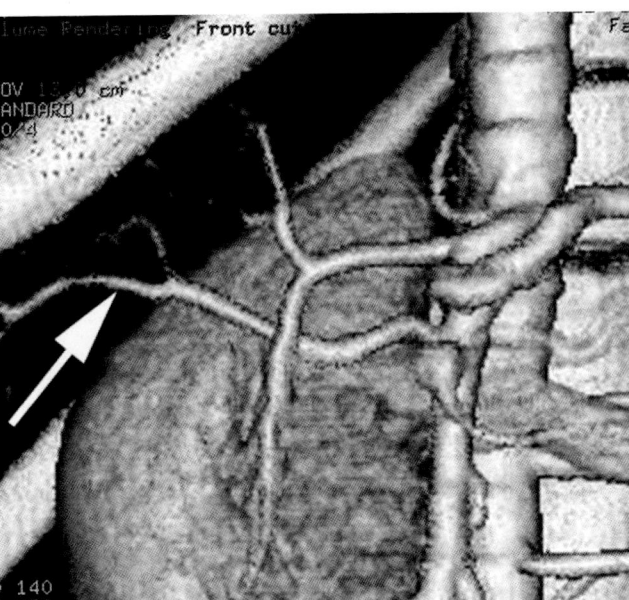

Figure 2. Replaced right hepatic artery. This volume-rendered image demonstrates a replaced right hepatic artery (arrow) originating from the anterior surface of the superior mesenteric artery. When replaced right hepatic arteries are present, the surgeon should be made aware to facilitate surgical planning and ensure the artery is removed in its entirety when removing the right lobe of the liver.

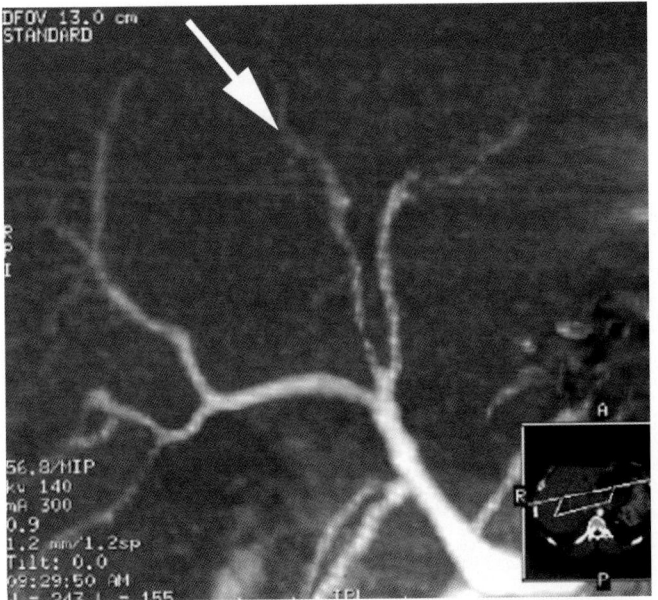

Figure 3. MIP image of hepatic arteries. This MIP image demonstrates the artery to segment IV (arrow) arising from the proximal left hepatic artery and coursing into the liver parenchyma.

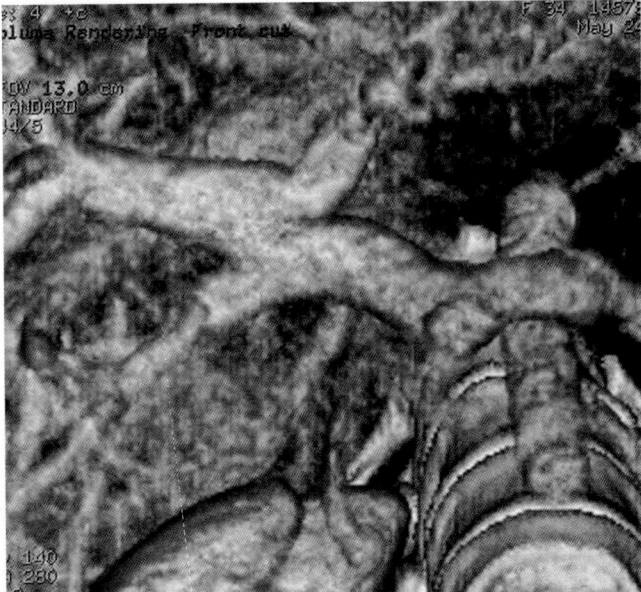

Figure 4. Trifurcation of the portal vein. This volume-rendered image of the portal venous system demonstrates trifurcation of the main portal vein, with a separate branch supplying the posterior segment of the right lobe of the liver. Depending on experience of the surgeons, resection of separate portal branches supplying the anterior and posterior portions of the right lobe of the liver may be technically challenging and the surgeons should be fully aware of this anatomy before undertaking a right lobectomy.

(GE Medical Systems, Milwaukee, WI), patients are administered a rapid bolus (5 mL/sec) of intravenous contrast material, and images are acquired during single breath-holds of both the bolus (hepatic arterial) and non-equilibrium (portal venous) phases. The data are transferred to a commercially available workstation (Advantage Windows, GE Medical Systems, Milwaukee, WI) where post-processing occurs. This process permits three-dimensional (3-D) models to be constructed of the hepatic arteries, portal veins, hepatic veins, and liver segments, and accurate volumetric determinations to be obtained. In addition, to facilitate the surgical incision, a curved avascular plane is identified between the left and right lobes to perform a preoperative "virtual hepatectomy" incision.

PARENCHYMAL EVALUATION

The multiphasic CT scan permits full evaluation of the liver parenchyma to identify and charaterize unexpected

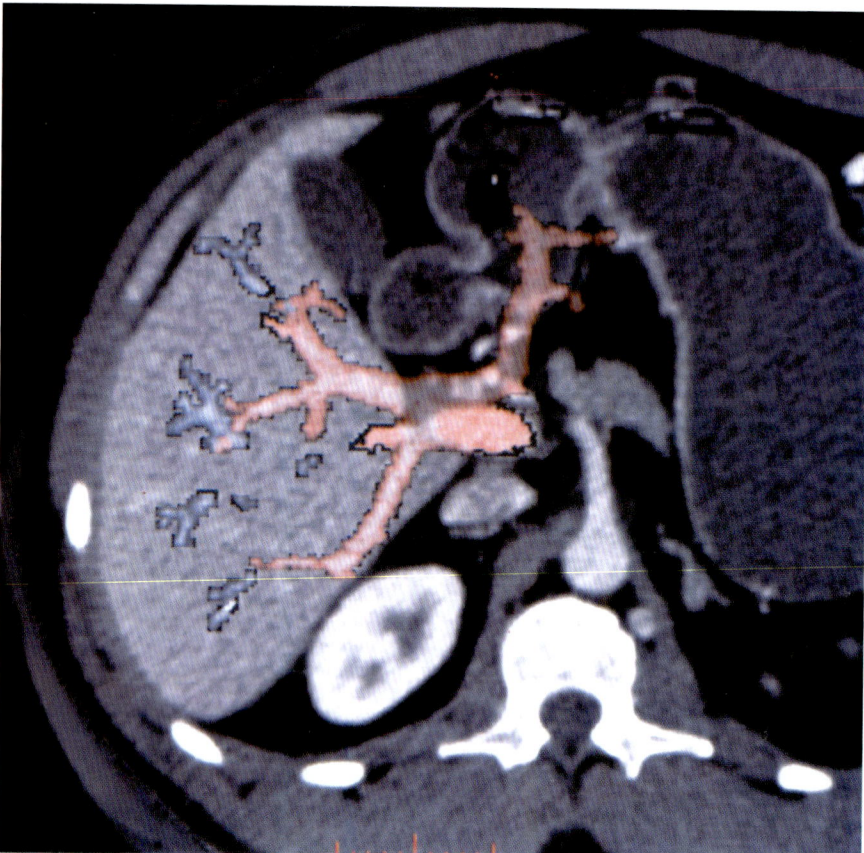

Figure 5. 3-D image of the hepatic venous anatomy superimposed on the liver parenchyma. This 3-D image with a superior cut demonstrates separate color assignment to the portal veins in red and hepatic veins in blue, used by the surgeons to plan their hepatectomy incision.

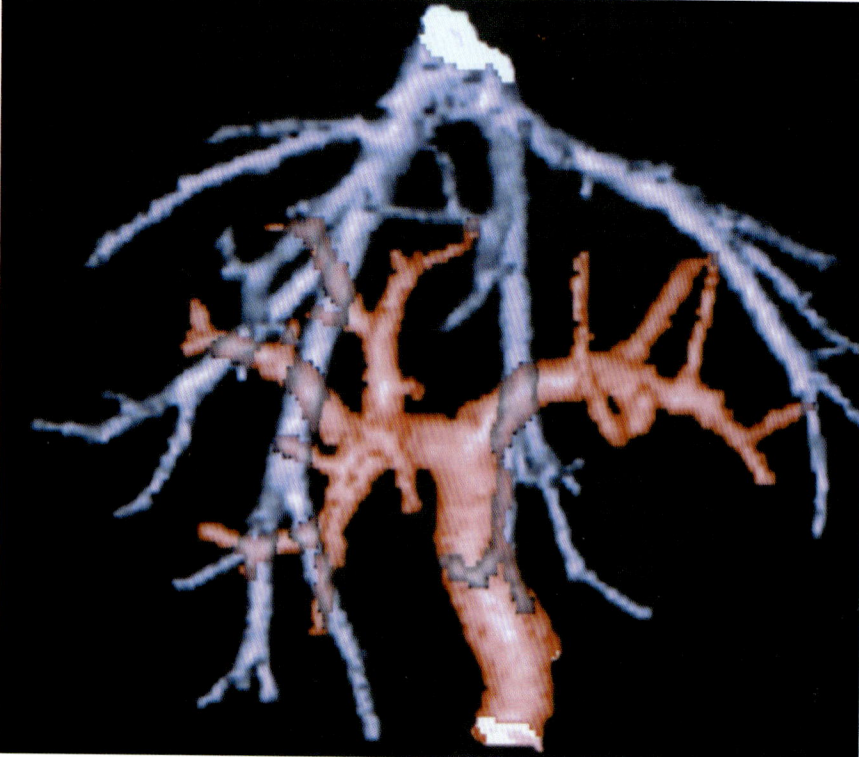

Figure 6. Portal and hepatic venous anatomy. This 3-D image of the portal venous system in red and hepatic veins in blue demonstrates a cast of the major vascular structures, used both to facilitate the surgical incision and depict the important relationship between segments of the liver and major branching points of the vessels.

traindication to graft procurement. The authors use a dual energy technique in which changes in liver attenuation (with variations in KVp) approximate the fat content. Many surgeons choose to biopsy the donor liver before surgery to exclude fatty change.

HEPATIC ARTERIES

A 3-D, volume-rendered model is created of the hepatic arteries (Fig. 1). Whereas not contraindications to surgery, many surgeons prefer to be aware of the presence of replaced or accessory right or left hepatic arteries, both of which are well depicted with volume rendering (Fig. 2). Most important, however, is to document the precise origin of the artery supplying segment IV (Fig. 3). As the right lobe is being removed leaving segment IV behind, arterial supply to segment IV from the right hepatic artery would remove the vascular supply to a large portion of the remaining liver, compromising liver function and even survival in the healthy donor. Clearly, identification of the origin of this small artery is important, and can be performed using the multidetector CT scanner. To evaluate this artery, we use the images acquired during the bolus phase and create multiplanar reformatted images in a plane parallel to the main portal vein. This procedure allows us to identify the origin and follow the course of the artery supplying segment IV.

PORTAL VEINS

Depending on the experience of the surgeons, several anatomic portal vein variants may be relative or absolute contraindications to surgery. These include separate origin of the vein supplying the posterior right lobe, and a portal vein trifurcation (Fig. 4). Using images acquired during the non-equilibrium phase, 3-D models are created of the portal veins, which are then superimposed on the 3-D liver model (Figs. 5 & 6). These models are created from the axially acquired data and allow the surgeon to visualize the veins in multiple planes to plan the surgical incision. The 3-D model also is used to perform the virtual hepatectomy incision.

HEPATIC VEINS

Using the axial images acquired dur-

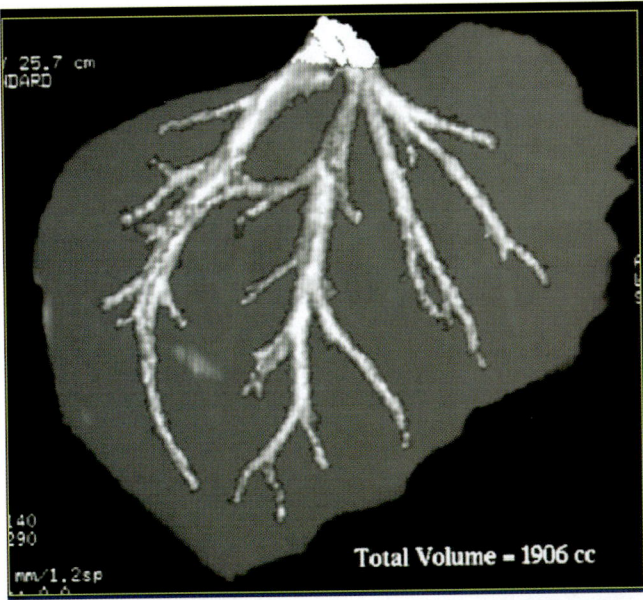

Figure 7. 3-D image of the hepatic veins. This 3-D cast of the hepatic veins has been superimposed on the liver volume to demonstrate the relative anatomy of the hepatic venous structures to the liver segments. It also is used as a guide to the surgeons to identify the major branching points along the right side of the middle hepatic vein, where the surgical incision is undertaken.

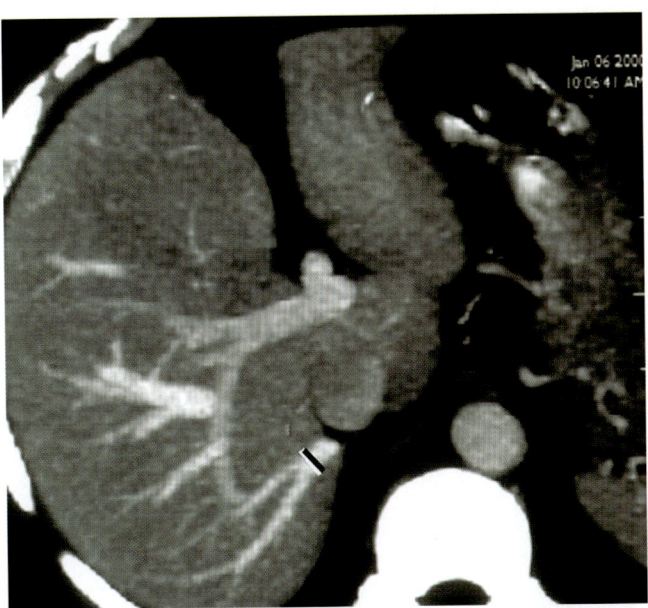

Figure 8. Accessory inferior right hepatic vein. This thick slab axial reformat of the portal and hepatic veins superimposed on liver parenchyma demonstrates a small, early branching accessory inferior right hepatic vein with its separate confluence into the adjacent retrohepatic vena cava. The surgeons prefer to have the diameter of the vessel measured before surgery to facilitate planning. In addition, the angle of the inferior accessory hepatic vein relative to the right hepatic vein facilitates surgical planning.

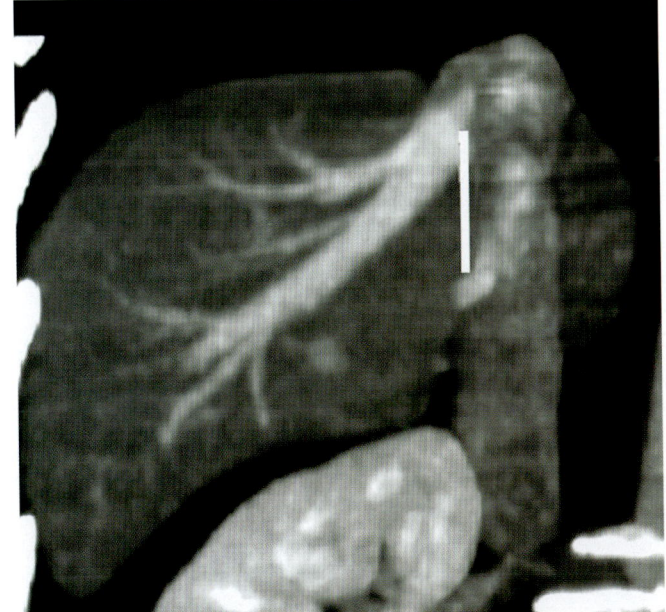

Figure 9. Accessory inferior right hepatic vein. Coronal image through the liver in this healthy donor with an inferior accessory right hepatic vein demonstrates how image processing is used to depict and measure the distance of the inferior accessory right hepatic vein to the site of confluence of the right hepatic vein into the vena cava.

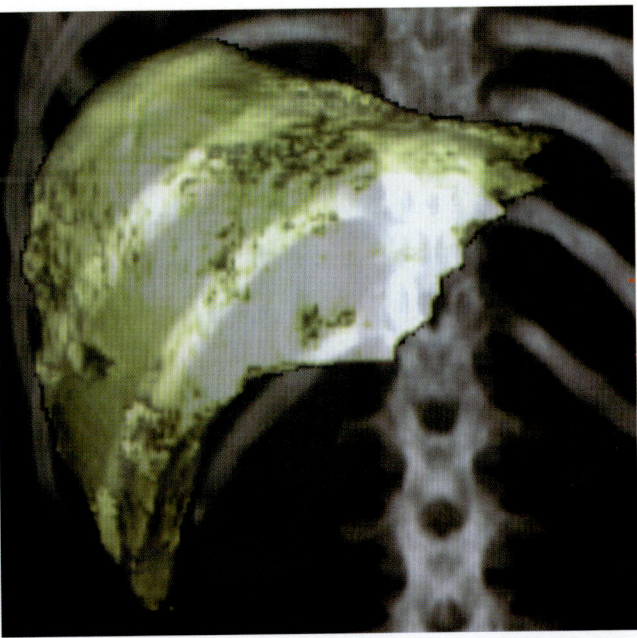

Figure 10. 3-D volume of the liver. After hand-tracing the liver outline from the axial images, a 3-D model of the liver is generated automatically and can be superimposed on important anatomic structures, such as the ribs and stomach. This 3-D model is then used for superimposition of vascular structures to facilitate performance of a virtual hepatectomy, and can be rotated into different planes to demonstrate the relative size and shape of different segments of the liver.

ing the non-equilibrium phase of scanning, a 3-D model is created of the hepatic veins to demonstrate the exact relationship between the middle and right hepatic veins (Fig. 7). To facilitate surgery, the site of bifurcation of the middle hepatic vein is identified, which allows the surgeon to anticipate when larger venous structures need to be transected. Common anatomic variants that alter the surgical approach much be depicted, such as an accessory inferior right hepatic vein (Figs. 8 & 9). When this is present and larger than 1 cm in diameter, the sagittal distance from, and relative angle to, the main right hepatic vein are illustrated in the coronal plane.

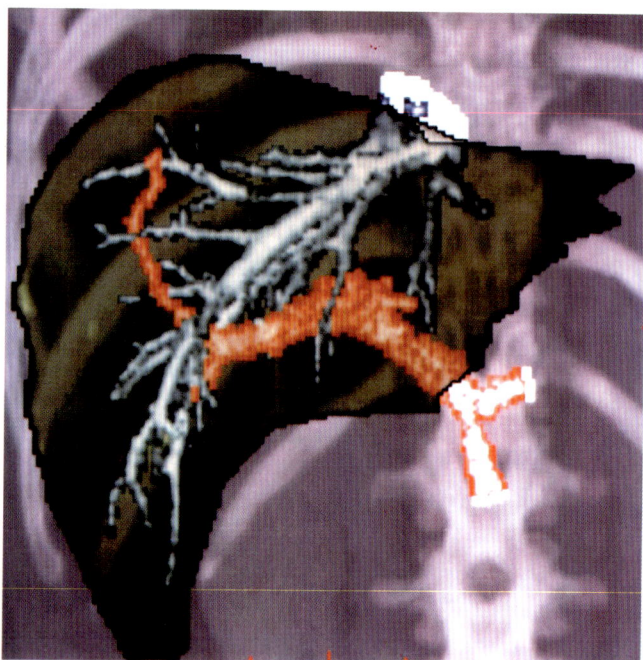

Figure 11. Portal and hepatic veins superimposed on 3-D of the liver. The color-assigned portal veins (red) and hepatic veins (blue) have been superimposed on the 3-D model of the liver. These images can be rotated separately at a work station and used to identify the relatively avascular plane lying immediately to the right of the middle hepatic vein.

Figure 12. 3-D model of the liver and vessels. A superior cut has been performed to remove liver parenchyma from the superior aspect of this image to demonstrate the important anatomic relation between portal and hepatic venous branches.

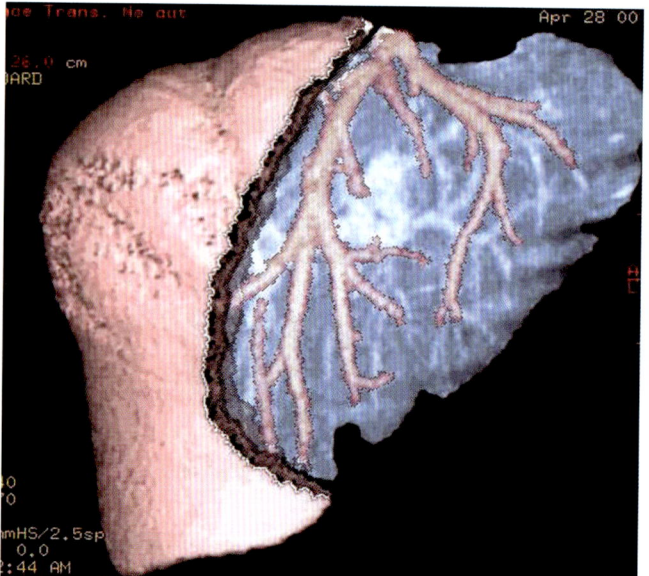

Figure 13. Virtual hepatectomy plane. By rotating the 3-D model of the liver with superimposed vascular structures, a curved virtual hepatectomy plane is obtained approximately 1 cm to the right of the middle hepatic vein. The plane not only depicts major vascular branches traversing this plane, of which the surgeons must be aware, but also is used to separately generate segmental liver volumes for important preoperative planning information.

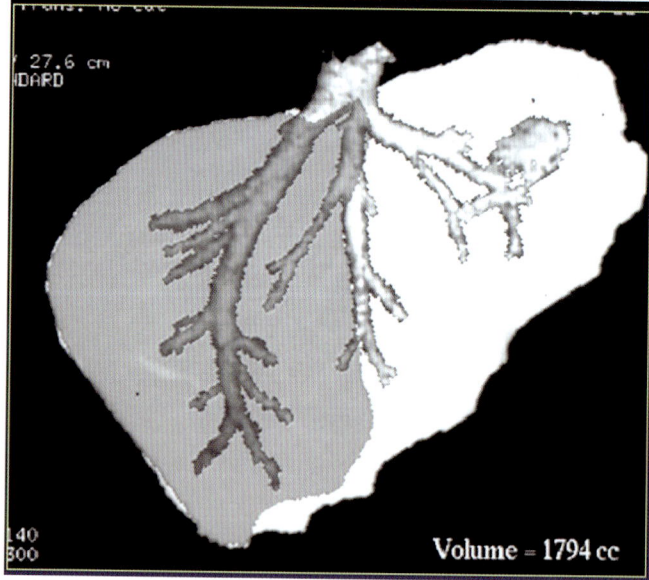

Figure 14. 3-D cast of hepatic veins with gray scale assignments to left and right lobes of liver. The hepatic venous structures depicted in three dimensions are superimposed on the liver, and the curved virtual hepatectomy plane has been created immediately to the right of the middle hepatic vein. By automatically calculating separate volumes for the left and right lobes of the liver, the hepatectomy plane can be adjusted interactively to identify an optimal avascular site whereby suitable liver volume can be left *in situ* in the healthy donor and implanted into the recipient.

VIRTUAL HEPATECTOMY

To serve as a guide to the liver surgeon, we are able to identify a curved plane that traverses the relatively avascular plane lying approximately 1 cm to the right of the middle hepatic vein, made possible by superimposing a 3-D model of the vessels on the 3-D model of the liver (Figs. 10-12). This plane should approximate the intended surgical plane and be decided upon in conjunction with the surgeons. This plane usually traverses the gallbladder fossa, caudate lobe, and extends through the bifurcation of the main portal vein. By "incising" through this plane, the left and right lobes of the liver can be sepa-

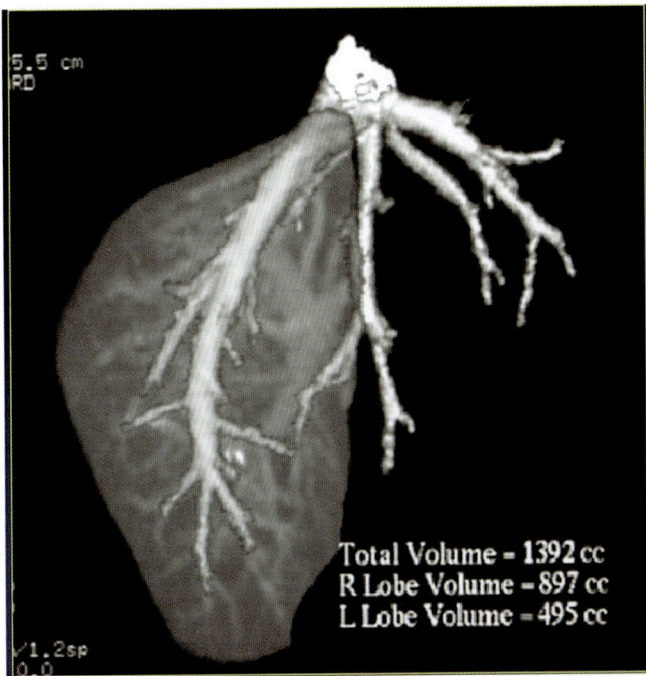

Figure 15. Hepatic veins superimposed on the right lobe graft. This 3-D model of the hepatic veins has been superimposed on the right lobe of the liver to facilitate surgical planning. This model of the liver provides the surgeon important information as to the size and shape of the planned graft to be implanted into the recipient. This model also depicts important venous structures that traverse the planned hepatectomy plane.

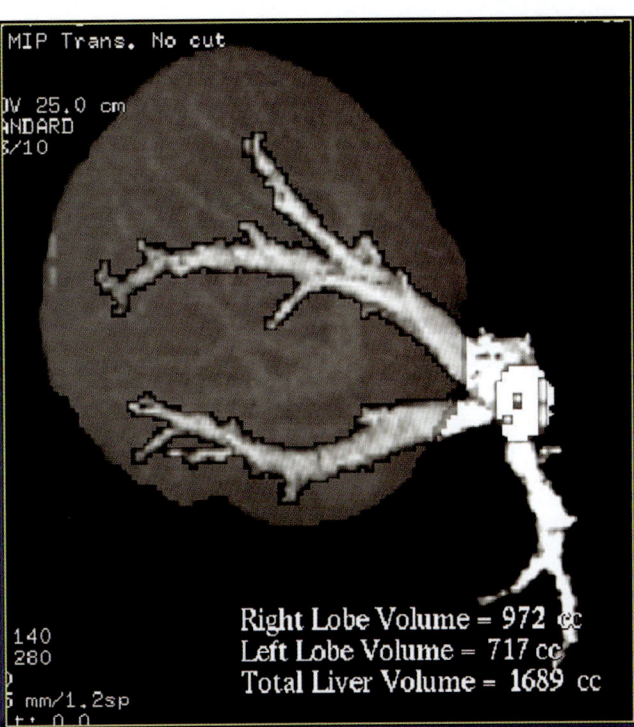

Figure 16. Superior view of right lobe of liver. This superior view of the liver, rotated to depict the hepatic vein confluence into the vena cava, demonstrates the curved nature of the planned hepatectomy plane. The model can be rotated into any angle and used by the surgeons during preoperative planning.

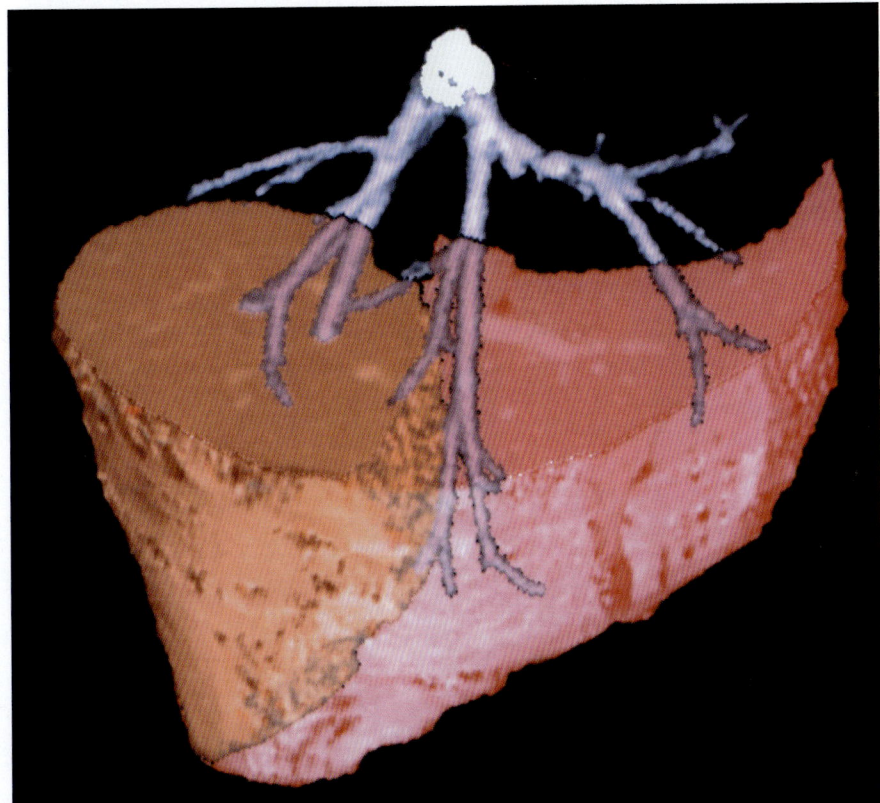

Figure 17. Superior cut of liver to separately demonstrate the color-assigned right and left lobes of the liver relative to the hepatic veins. This 3-D cast of the hepatic veins superimposed on the color-assigned left and right lobes of the liver demonstrates the anticipated hepatectomy plane immediately to the right of the middle hepatic vein. This model is used by the surgeons in an interactive manner during the preoperative planning stages.

rated and used both to guide surgery and obtain accurate volumetric measurements of the separate lobes of the liver (Figs. 13-17).

VOLUMETRIC MEASUREMENTS

To sustain metabolic function, accurate volumetric measurements must be made to implant sufficient volume into the recipient and leave sufficient liver in the donor. This procedure requires measurements of both total and right lobe liver volumes. Using a paintbrush technique and axially acquired images, we trace a hand-drawn line around the liver carefully excluding the gallbladder, fissures, vena cava, and intrahepatic main portal vein. These data are applied to software, which automatically calculates liver volume. The right lobe volume is determined from the "virtual incision."

In conclusion, recent advances in CT scanner technology permit thin section scans to be obtained as a volume during a single breathhold. This procedure allows high-resolution 3-D models to be created of vascular anatomy. These data are essential for preoperative evaluation of healthy adults undergoing evaluation for potential right lobe liver transplantation.

Reach for 13 years of clinical experience with Solution System®.

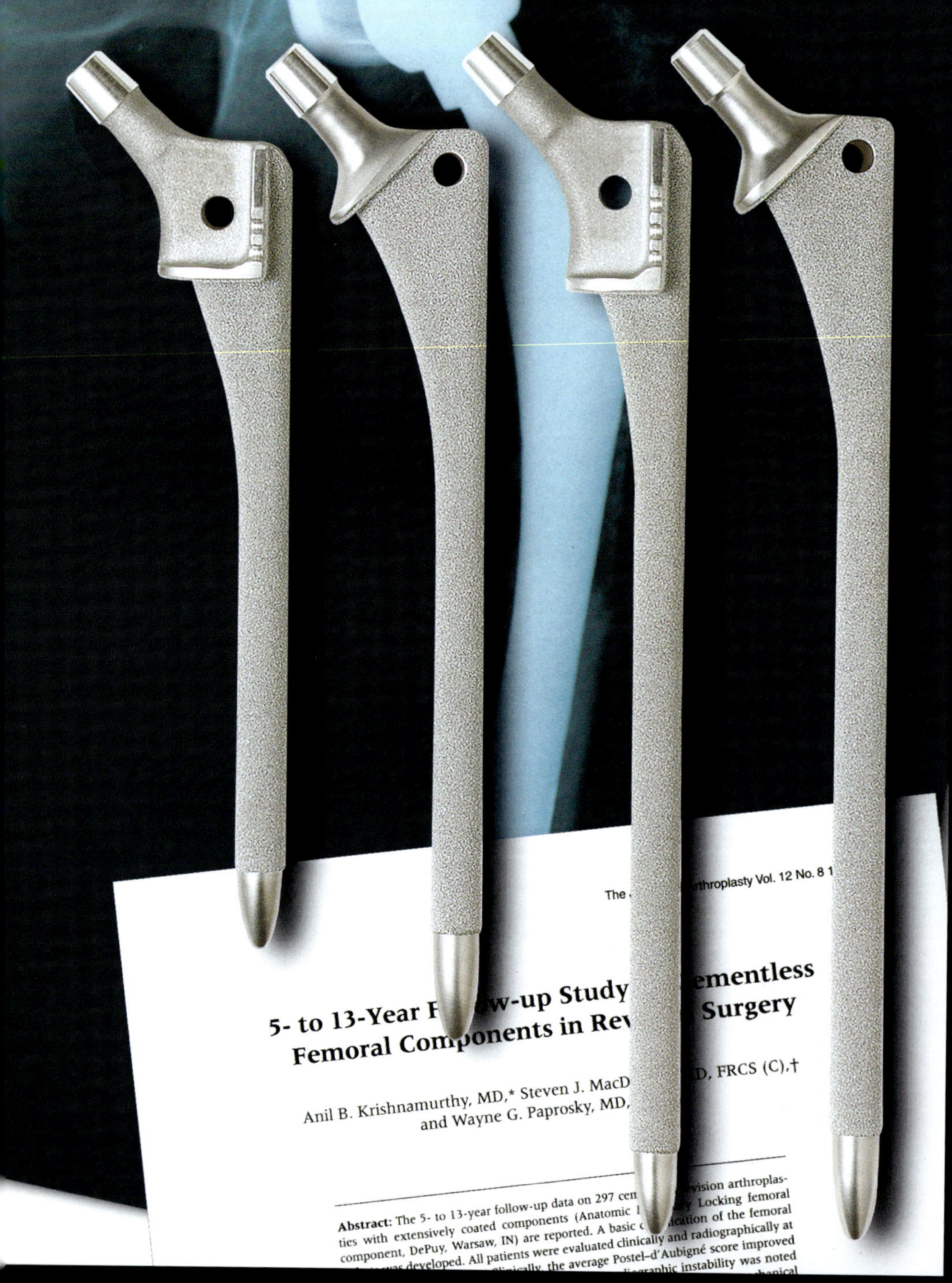

SOLUTION SYSTEM®

THE REVISION HIP

SYSTEM WITH A

97.6% SURVIVORSHIP

AT 5 TO 13 YEARS.[1]

For more information, contact your DePuy representative, call (800) 366-8143 or visit our web site at www.depuy.com.

THE SOLUTION SYSTEM® REVISION SURGERY

1. Krishnamurthy, A.B., MacDonald, S.J. and Paprosky, W.G.: 5- to 13-Year Follow-up Study on Cementless Femoral Components in Revision Surgery. ***Journal of Arthroplasty,*** Vol. 12, No. 8, 1997.

Solution System® is a trademark of DePuy Orthopaedics, Inc.
©1999 DePuy Orthopaedics, Inc.

DePuy
a Johnson & Johnson company

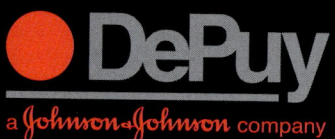

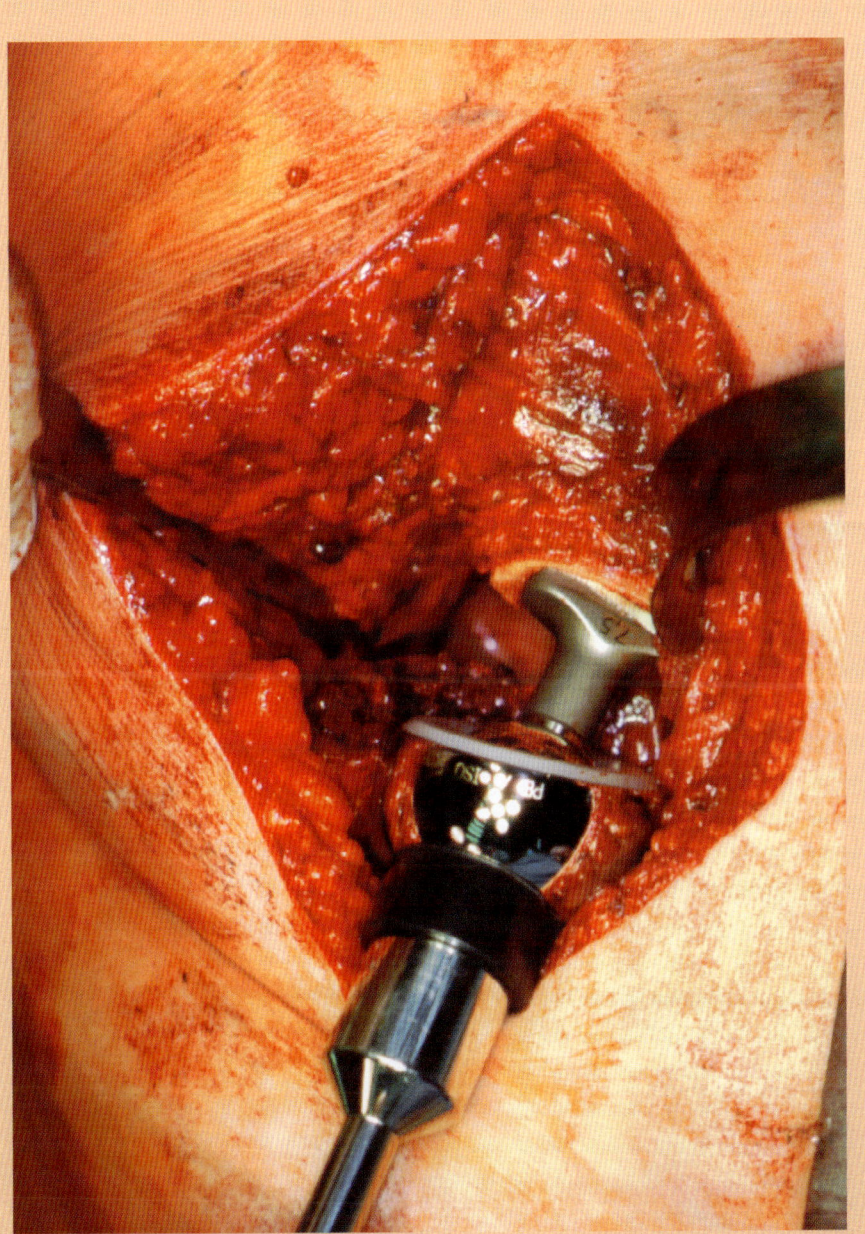

Orthopaedic Surgery

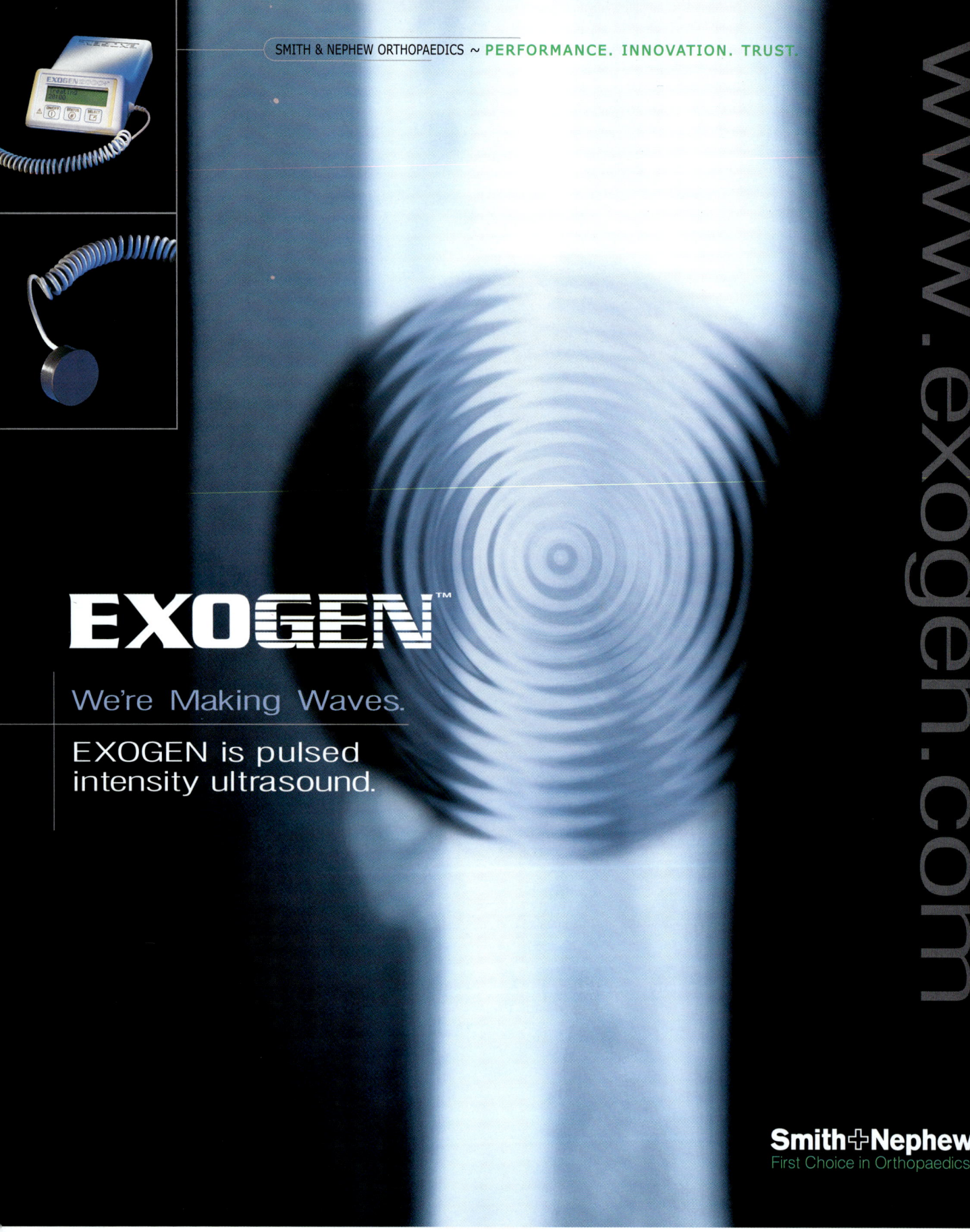

Management of Non-Union with Pulsed, Low-Intensity Ultrasound Therapy – International Results

VICTOR H. FRANKEL, M.D., PH.D., K.N.O.
PRESIDENT EMERITUS, HOSPITAL FOR JOINT DISEASES ORTHOPAEDIC INSTITUTE
PROFESSOR, ORTHOPAEDIC SURGERY, NEW YORK UNIVERSITY
NEW YORK, NEW YORK

KOSAKU MIZUNO, M.D., PH.D.
PROFESSOR & CHAIRMAN, DEPARTMENT OF ORTHOPAEDIC SURGERY
KOBE UNIVERSITY SCHOOL OF MEDICINE
HYOGO, JAPAN

In prospective, randomized, double-blind, placebo-controlled, multi-center clinical studies, pulsed, low-intensity ultrasound has been proven to be effective in decreasing the time to heal in both fresh diaphyseal (tibia) and metaphyseal (distal radius) fractures. It also decreases the likelihood of a delayed union (>150 days to heal) in tibia fractures and loss of reduction in distal radius fractures. World-wide clinical studies, using pulsed, low-intensity ultrasound for treatment of non-union in a self-paired control study design, have demonstrated a heal rate of 88% with an average treatment time of 4.5 months in non-unions and an average fracture age of 23 months. The therapy is safe and non-invasive, and is used by the patient at home for a 20-minute treatment session per day.

Stratification of the study data included gender, age, number of previous operations, failed previous electromagnetic stimulation, pre-existing smoking status, systemic disease conditions, and medication comparisons and did not show a statistically significant difference among variable strata regarding the heal rate. The age of the non union showed a strong trend ($p=0.06$) toward influencing the heal rate. Use of pulsed, low-intensity ultrasound in treating non-unions showed a heal rate that ranged from 83% to 91% in The Netherlands, Germany, France, Japan, and the United States (83%). In comparison with surgery, pulsed, low-intensity ultrasound in non-unions has the same success rate as surgery but without the local or systemic complications. In addition, a comparison of the heal rate in treating non-unions was significantly higher with pulsed, low-intensity ultrasound as compared to electrical stimulation.

INTRODUCTION

The use of pulsed, low-intensity ultrasound in fresh, closed, and Grade I open tibial diaphysis fractures resulted in a 38% decrease in healing time by clinical and radiologic criteria. At 150 days (delayed union), Heckman et al. showed that 36% of the controls were not healed compared to only 6% of the treated fractures.[1] In fresh, distal, radial metaphysis factures, Kristiansen et al. demonstrated that heal time was reduced by 38% in the ultrasound-treated compared to placebo control.[2] Also, a 115% less loss of reduction of the fracture was noted in the ultrasound-treated group.

Through these double-blind, randomized, prospective studies and the more recent study of fresh scaphoid fracture, the efficacy of pulsed ultrasound in management of fresh fractures was established.[3] In 1998, a description of the method and results in fresh fractures, early delayed unions, late delayed unions, and non-unions was presented in this journal by one of the authors.[4] The pulsed, low-intensity ultrasound therapy device provided a signal with a frequency of 1.5 MHz in a signal burst width of 200 μsec followed by an off time of 800 μsec (modulating repetition rate of 1 kHz) at an intensity of 30 mw/cm^2 (spatial average/temporal average). This intensity is equivalent to that used for fetal sonograms and provides a force to the tissue of less than 3 mg/cm^2. The patient administered the treatment at home with one daily 20-minute treatment (Fig. 1). A thorough review of the in-vivo animal, in-vitro and clinical results was presented by Rubin et al.[5]

The purpose of this paper is to present the results of the international use of pulsed, low-intensity ultrasound for management of non-unions in a United States study; in studies conducted in The Netherlands, Germany, and France; and in post-market registry databases maintained in Japan and the United States. In February 2000, use of pulsed, low-intensity ultrasound for non-unions was approved by the United States Food and Drug Administration. With the exception of the skull and spine, all bones that demonstrated non-union by radiologic and clinical assessment were considered candidates for this therapy. Non-union can be defined as the point when healing has stopped and does not proceed without some type of intervention. Currently, non-unions are treated by various surgical techniques including bone grafting and internal and external fixation. Invasive and non-invasive electric or electromagnetic stimulation and ultrasound stimulation have been used in management of non-union. The regulatory signals emanating from these mechanical and electrical stimuli can affect bone tissue positively.

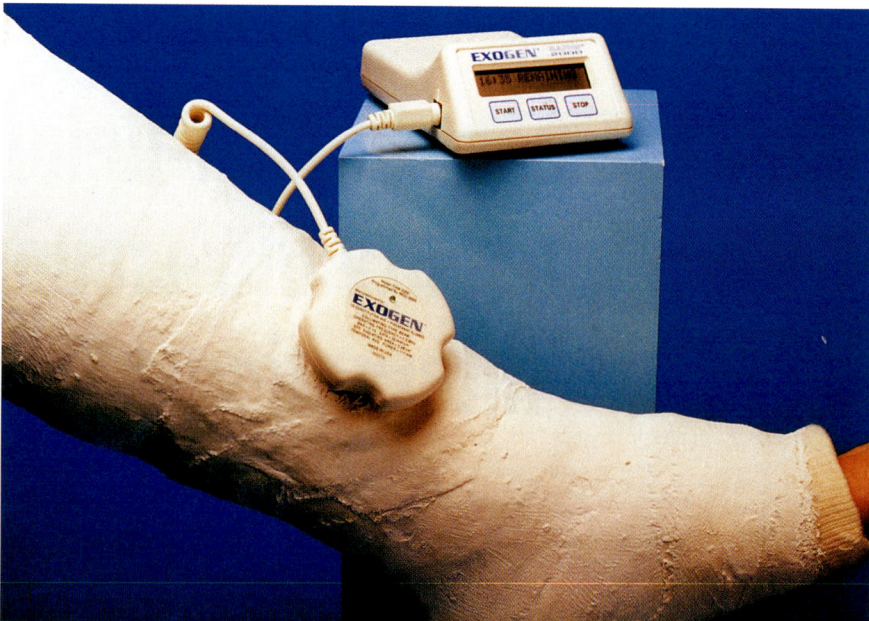

Figure 1. SAFHS 2000 Pulsed, Low-Intensity Ultrasound Stimulator shown in a tibia application (Smith+Nephew/Exogen, Memphis, TN, USA)

MATERIALS AND METHODS

The study design for cases of non-union has certain restraints. A prospective, randomized, double-blind, placebo-controlled study, the so-called "gold standard" of medical research, is not appropriate in these patients. In established non-unions, the control group side of a study has no chance of healing. It is also unethical to take a patient with a 2- to 3-year-old non-union and expose that patient to a double-blind study. Another alternative study design is surgical treatment versus ultrasound treatment, which might not be in the patients' best interest as many of them have had two or more operations before establishment of the non-union. A third possible methodology comparing ultrasound to electrical stimulation also would not be a proper double-blind study. Pulsed, low-intensity ultrasonic stimulation requires 20 minutes a day, whereas certain electrical and electromagnetic stimulation therapies take from 3 to 24 hours a day. In addition, the devices are different physically and in the way they are attached at the non-union site.

An appropriate study design for treatment of non-unions used to date is to consider each patient as his own self-paired control. In this type of design, a period exists to allow for normal fracture healing; there must be a latent period in which no surgical procedure is performed and no healing progress is observed before ultrasound treatment, and the results are evaluated by radiologic and clinical examination. In the international studies reported here, the minimum fracture age for diagnosis of non-union was at least 6 months from the initial fracture date in France and The Netherlands, 8 months in Germany, and 9 months in the United States. In France, The Netherlands, and the United States, the minimum period with no surgical intervention before initiation of pulsed, low-intensity ultrasound treatment was 3 months, and in Germany, 4 months. This minimum latent period assured that surgical procedures would not bias the effect of the ultrasound in healing of the non-union. The efficacy results were established by the healing rate as determined by clinical healing and radiologic healing (at least 3 bridged cortices for long bones and complete endosteal bridging for other bones). The time from the initial fracture date to the start of ultrasound treatment (fracture age) of the fracture and duration of treatment also was noted in these studies.

RESULTS

The above entry criteria were used in a study by Heppenstall et al. of United States for established non-unions, which resulted in a heal rate of 80% (249/313) (in italics in Table 1).[6] The data from that study were stratified by several covariates, as shown in Table 2. The stratification results by bone indicate heal rates varied from 89% in foot bones—such as the metatarsal—to 78% in the femur (non-significant comparison, $p=0.12$). Patient age groups were compared for heal rate and patients aged 18 through 29 had an 85% heal rate versus 74% for those 65 years of age or older (non-significant comparison, $p=0.71$). The time from fracture to the start of pulsed, low-intensity ultrasound (fracture age) was stratified and indicated a heal rate of 84% in patients 9 to 12 months from fracture, compared with the lowest heal rate of 64% for non-unions with a fracture age of 5 years or greater ($p=0.06$). The heal rate by the number of prior failed surgical procedures was compared to determine whether repetitive failed procedures affected the heal rate achieved with pulsed, low-intensity ultrasound therapy, and showed a non-significant comparison of $p=0.23$, with a heal rate for no failed procedures of 83% compared to 71% for the 76 patients with three or more prior failed surgeries. As none of the patients in the non-union study group had a surgical procedure either within 3 months or at the start of ultrasound therapy, the fixation or immobilization present during the pulsed, low-intensity ultrasound treatment period was compared for its heal rate to the group that did not have this fixation. The fixation comparisons (ORIF, external fixation, or cast) were not significant except for intramedullary rod fixation. This comparison was significant at $p=0.0005$ with 66% of patients with rod fixation healed versus 84% for those without rod fixation. Several of the patients in the study group had prior failed electrical stimulation. Treatment with pulsed, low-intensity ultrasound resulted in a 72% heal rate for patients with prior failed electrical stimulation versus 81% for those without electrical stimulation (a non-significant comparison, $p=0.21$).

Table 1. International Low-Intensity Ultrasound Treatment of Non-Unions–June 2000

Country	Totals	#Healed	%Healed
Netherlands Study*	29	25	86%
Germany Study*	67	57	85%
France Study*	44	39	89%
*U.S. Study**	*249*	*313*	*80%*
Japan**	3,313	3,000	91%
U.S.A.**	1,546	1,283	83%
Totals	4,999	4,404	88%

* Prospective, self-paired study; ** Post-market registry study--Italics numbers are in U.S.A numbers [9]

Table 2. Stratification of United States Non-Union Study—Patient and Non-union Characteristics

Covariate Strata		#Healed	#Failed	%Healed	Exact p-value
Bone:					
Tibia		96	22	81%	
Femur		35	10	78%	
Radius		19	3	86%	0.12
Humerus		27	13	68%	
Foot Bones		39	5	89%	
Scaphoid		17	4	81%	
Other		16	7	70%	
Patient Age:					
<17		14	3	82%	
18-29		39	7	85%	
30-49		113	27	81%	0.71
50-64		51	16	76%	
> 65		32	11	74%	
Fracture Age (months):					
9-12		107	20	84%	
>12 to 24		100	24	81%	0.06
>24 to 60		33	15	69%	
>= 60		9	5	64%	
No. Prior Failed Surgical Procedures:					
0		90	18	83%	
1		63	15	81%	0.23
2		42	9	82%	
>=3		54	22	71%	
Fixation in Place Before, at Start, and During Ultrasound Treatment:					
IM Rod	No	167	32	84%	
	Yes	37	19	66%	0.0005
ORIF	No	179	49	79%	
	Yes	70	15	82%	0.53
External Fixation	No	185	45	84%	
	Yes	19	6	76%	0.61
Cast	No	182	47	80%	
	Yes	67	17	80%	1
Prior Failed Electrical Treatment:					
	No	221	3	81%	
					0.21
	Yes	28	11	72%	

A post-market registry of all prescription use of the pulsed, low-intensity ultrasound therapy has been maintained with prescribing physician input from the date of the first use in Japan and the United States.[7,8] The previously described United States non-union study data are included in the United States post-market registry numbers.[9] The United States post-market summary data are presented in Table 3 for the 3,865 non-union patients treated with the low-intensity ultrasound therapy as of June 2000. The resulting heal rate in the completed cases was 83% (1,283/1,546), with an average treatment time of 136 days and an average fracture age of 23 months. The data are stratified by bone in Table 2 and shows a variation of heal rate from a high of 89% in the metatarsal bone to a low of 70% in the humerus.

Additional stratification of the United States data demonstrates the effect of other confounding factors (Table 4). Comparison by gender indicates little difference in heal rates for males (84%) and females (81%). A comparison of heal rates for patient age groups shows a slight difference in heal rates ranging from 88% in patients 30 years of age or younger to 79% in those 50 years of age or older. Fracture age groups are stratified and indicate a slight decrease in heal rates as the fracture age increases, with the heal rate remaining at 80% in the 91 non-unions with a fracture age of 5 years or more. Although the smoking status of the non-union patient has been shown to affect the healing of non-unions seriously,[8] no significant difference exists in this series among smoking-status strata. This result indicates pulsed, low-intensity ultrasound for treatment of non-unions, as in fresh fractures, affects the outcome and reverses deleterious effects of smoking in the non-union patient positively. The results in patients with diseases associated commonly with healing failures also are stratified. Many of these patients are poor surgical candidates because of the concomitant disease processes, and results indicate pulsed, low-intensity ultrasound is a good alternative non-union therapy. Various medications have been shown to slow bone healing, and this stratification demonstrates ultrasound can maintain an acceptable healing rate in non-unions even in the presence of medications that have a strong negative effect

Table 3. Non-Union Post-Market Registry United States Completed Cases—June 2000

Non-Union Total	3,865
Deceased	8
Lost to Follow Up	300
Non-Compliant/Withdrawn	332
In Treatment	1,679
Completed Cases	1,546
Healed	1,283
Failed	263
Heal Rate	83%
Avg. Heal Time	136 days
Avg. Fracture Age	692 days

Table 4: Stratification of United States Post-Market Registry—Patient and Non-Union Characteristics

Covariate Strata	#Healed	#Failed	%Healed	Heal Time (days)	Fracture Age (days)
Bone:					
Tibia	568	108	84%	124	661
Femur	278	56	83%	157	730
Radius/Ulna	75	11	87%	98	486
Humerus	126	53	70%	138	593
Metatarsal	109	14	89%	113	506
Scaphoid	126	23	85%	107	568
Patient Gender:					
Male	702	132	84%	133	650
Female	575	131	81%	140	743
Patient Age:					
<30	291	40	88%	129	523
31-49	525	106	83%	147	724
50-64	306	80	79%	173	654
>= 65	169	44	79%	185	642
Fracture Age (months):					
9-12	491	73	87%	124	302
>12 to 24	492	114	81%	139	499
>24 to 60	227	58	80%	148	1080
>= 60	73	18	80%	134	3375
Smoking Status:					
Currently	230	62	79%	133	776
Stopped	209	47	82%	142	705
Never	629	119	84%	137	618
Disease Type:					
Alcoholism	23	4	85%	140	925
Diabetes	71	16	82%	142	640
Osteoporosis	32	9	78%	163	900
Renal	15	3	83%	120	1167
Vascular Problem	31	9	78%	158	908
Medication Type:					
NSAID	131	38	78%	137	712
Anti-coagulants	34	7	83%	182	693
Steroids	36	8	82%	127	665
Calcium Channel Blockers	24	11	69%	119	759

NSAID = nonsteroidal anti-inflammatory drug

Table 5. Non-unions in Japan–Post-Market Registry–6/15/2000

Bone	Totals	#Healed	#Failed	%Heal Rate
Clavicle	212	168	44	89%
Femur	822	726	96	88%
Humerus	472	403	69	85%
Foot	120	106	14	88%
Metacarpal	9	9	0	100%
Metatarsal	37	36	1	97%
Other	295	272	23	92%
Radius/ulna	151	146	5	97%
Scaphoid	33	25	8	76%
Tibia	1,019	960	59	85%
Totals	3,313	3,000	313	91%

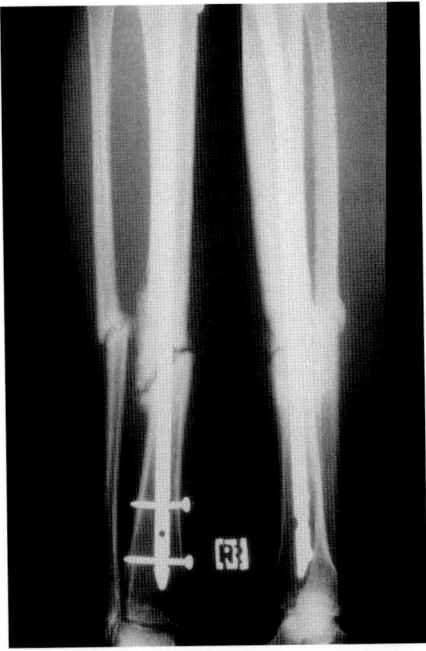

Figure 2a. 41-year-old man, hypertrophic non-union at 268 days after poly-trauma. Start of ultrasound treatment (Courtesy of E. Mayr, M.D.).

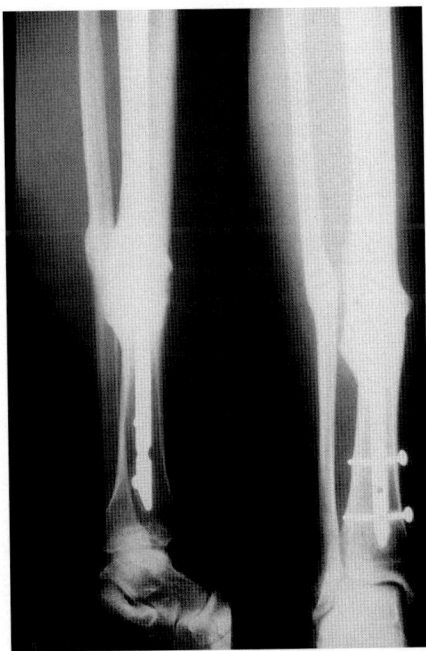

Figure 2b. Healed fracture after 108 days of pulsed, low-intensity ultrasound treatment.

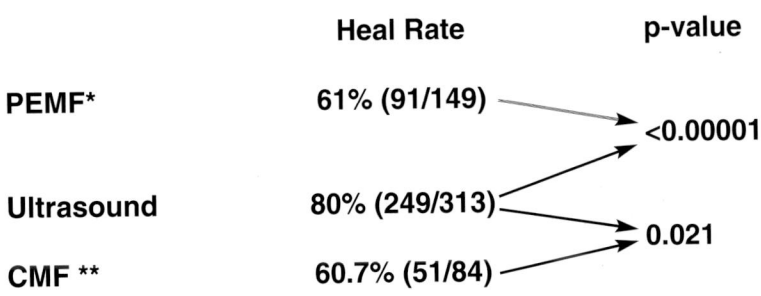

Table 6. PEMF vs. Low-Intensity Ultrasound vs. CMF

	Heal Rate	p-value
PEMF*	61% (91/149)	<0.00001
Ultrasound	80% (249/313)	
CMF **	60.7% (51/84)	0.021

- Heckman, et al. JBJS, 1981[13]: ** Longo. Surgical Technology International VII, 1997[14]
- PERF = pulsed electromagnetic fields; CMF = combined electromagnetic fields

on bone metabolism.

The start and end of treatment radiographs of an established non-union patient treated by pulsed, low-intensity ultrasound are shown in Figures 2a and 2b. The case report describes a 41-year-old man who suffered from polytrauma on 8/25/95 consisting of a fractured right tibia, fractured left humerus, liver rupture, thoracic trauma, and kidney contusion. Intramedullary fixation of the tibia on the day of injury was performed. Six weeks later, on 10/10/95, a bone-graft procedure was performed. On 1/16/96, the patient suffered a coronary occlusion. On 4/19/96, a diagnosis of hypertrophic non-union was established and treatment was started with pulsed, low-intensity ultrasound (Fig. 2a). On 9/4/96, fracture healing was complete (Fig. 2b). Due to the patient's coronary occlusion, he was a poor risk for further surgery.

Self-paired studies of established non-unions were conducted in The Netherlands,[10] France,[11] and Germany[12] following the strict entry criteria described previously. In the United States post-market registry data, the minimum fracture age of a non-union was 9 months (Table 3).[8] For the Japanese post-market registry of intractable fractures, a fracture was considered a non-union when the surgeon determined the diagnosis of non-union and stated that further treatment was necessary to heal the established non-union.[7] Table 5 presents the Japanese non-union data by bone.

DISCUSSION

These international studies have established the efficacy of pulsed, low-intensity ultrasound in management of non-unions with heal rates of 86% in The Netherlands, 85% in Germany, 89% in France, 91% in Japan, and 83% in the United States (Table 1). A comparison may be made of the efficacy of pulsed, low-intensity ultrasound to electromagnetic fields (PEMFs) and combined magnetic fields (CMF) (Table 6).[13,14]

Heppenstall et al. presented the data for the pulsed, ultrasound treatment of non-union in the United States at the AAOS in 1999.[6] The data for the use of PEMFs by 5 orthopaedic surgeons was reported by Heckman et al. in 1981.[13] Results of a multi-center study of CMF therapy for non-union was reported by Longo et al. in 1997.[14] In addition to the significant difference in the efficacy of pulsed, low-intensity ultrasound compared to the other modalities, the short duration of ultrasonic stimulation (20 minutes/day) compared to the lengthier periods (3 to 24 hours/day) for electrical stimulation makes pulsed, low-intensity ultrasound acceptable to and for the patient.

SUMMARY

Pulsed, low-intensity ultrasound has been demonstrated to be effective in treatment of non-union in several international clinical studies. The percentage of healed patients averaged 88%, but varied with bone location. The mean fracture age was 696 days, and average treatment time was 120 days. This report demonstrates that pulsed, low-intensity ultrasound can provide similar outcomes in treating non-union as operative intervention without the associated risks and complications of surgery.

REFERENCES

1. Heckman JD, Ryaby JP, McCabe J, et al. Acceleration of tibial fracture healing by non-invasive low-intensity pulsed ultrasound. J Bone Joint Surg (Am) 1994; 76A(1):26-34.
2. Kristiansen TK, Ryaby JP, McCabe J, et al. Accelerated healing of distal radial fractures with the use of specific, low-intensity ultrasound. J Bone Joint Surg (Am) 1997; 79A:961-73.
3. Mayr E, Rudzki M-M, Rudki M, et al. Acceleration by pulsed, low-intensity ultrasound of scaphoid fracture healing. Handchir Mikrochir Plast Chir 2000; 32:115-22.
4. Frankel VH. Results of prescription use of pulse ultrasound therapy in fracture management. In: Szabó Z, Lewis JE, Fantini GA, et al. Surgical Technology International VII. San Francisco: University Medical Press; 1998. p 389-93.
5. Rubin C, Bolander M, Ryaby JP, et al. The use of low-intensity ultrasound to accelerate the healing of fractures. J Bone Joint Surg (Am) 2000 (Accepted for Publication).
6. Heppenstall RB, Frey JJ, Ryaby JP, et al. Non-invasive nonunion treatment by pulsed low-intensity ultrasound. Presented at the American Academy of Orthopaedic Surgery (AAOS), 66th Annual Meeting, Anaheim, CA, February 1999.
7. Mizuno K. Current topics on fracture treatment with ultrasound. Orthop Surg Traumatol 2000, 43 (3):213-23.
8. Hashmi MA, Ali A, Rigby A, et al. Fracture healing in non-unions population—effects of smoking. Int Soc Fracture Repair Proc 2000 Sept. 20-23; Hong Kong, 4E.
9. Exogen Post-Market Registry. June 2000.
10. Albers RGH, Patka P, Janssen IMC, et al. An effective therapy for non unions—low-intensity ultrasound. J Bone Joint Surg.(Br) 1999; 81-B(Supp II):247.
11. Moyen B, Mainard D, Azoulai JJ, et al. Delayed and nonunions—a safe and effective treatment. J Bone Joint Surg (Br) 1999; 81B(Supp II):247.
12. Gebauer D, Mayer E, Orthner E, et al. Non-unions treated by pulsed low-intensity ultrasound. J Orthop Trauma 2000; 14:154.
13. Heckman JD, Ingram AJ, Loyd RD, et al. Nonunion treatment with pulsed electromagnetic fields. Clin Orthop Rel Res 1981; 161:58-66.
14. Longo JA. Successful treatment of recalcitrant nonunions with combined magnetic field stimulation. In: Szabó Z., et al, eds. Surgical Technology International VI. San Francisco: University Medical Press; 1997. p 397-403.

Prosthetic Design and Early Clinical Results of the TRAC® (Two Radii Area Contact) Knee Prosthesis

LAWRENCE A. POTTENGER, M.D., PH.D.
ASSOCIATE PROFESSOR

LOUIS DRAGANICH, PH.D.
ASSOCIATE PROFESSOR

UNIVERSITY OF CHICAGO
SECTION OF ORTHOPAEDIC SURGERY
CHICAGO, IL

Patients with 75 TRAC® (Biomet, Inc., Warsaw, IN) knees have been observed for one year with the following results: average flexion 117 degrees, HSS score 88.4, Knee Society scores 92.2 (knee), and 76.8 (function). Early results of the TRAC® knee appear promising.

CONSIDERATIONS OF KNEE PROSTHETIC DESIGNS

The TRAC® (Biomet, Inc., Warsaw, IN) knee was designed with the premise that the design of the normal human knee is flawed. The normal knee has menisci prone to degenerate with age. Loss of meniscal function decreases contact areas greatly between the femoral condyles and tibial plateau, leading to premature osteoarthritis. Anterior cruciate ligaments frequently rupture during athletic events with resultant anterior instability. The posterior cruciate ligament does not function normally when the anterior cruciate ligament is absent.[1] Instead of pulling the femoral condyles posteriorly during flexion to increase quadriceps efficiency, lone posterior cruciate ligaments allow the condyles to move forward on the tibia.

The need for cruciate ligaments and menisci stems from the fact that knees flex and rotate at the same surface, where the femoral condyles contact the tibial plateau. Rotation requires relatively flat surfaces on the plateau, whereas maintaining a large contact area to reduce pressure across the joint in flexion requires the contact surfaces of the condyles and tibial plateau be relatively congruent. The menisci act as wedges to fill in for the lack of congruency, whereas the cruciate ligaments, located at the sagittal center of the knee, allow axial rotation.

A routine total knee prosthesis typically consists of metal caps on the end of the distal femur and proximal tibia with an intervening polyethylene bearing attached to the tibial cap (baseplate). The articular surface of the patella also may be replaced with a polyethylene bearing. Attempting to create knee prostheses that emulate the anatomy of a normal knee leads to carry over of the design flaws in the normal knee. However, none of the prostheses have menisci anatomically similar to natural menisci, and the vast majority of prostheses require removal of the anterior cruciate because their tibial baseplates cover the surface of the plateau where the anterior cruciate attaches.

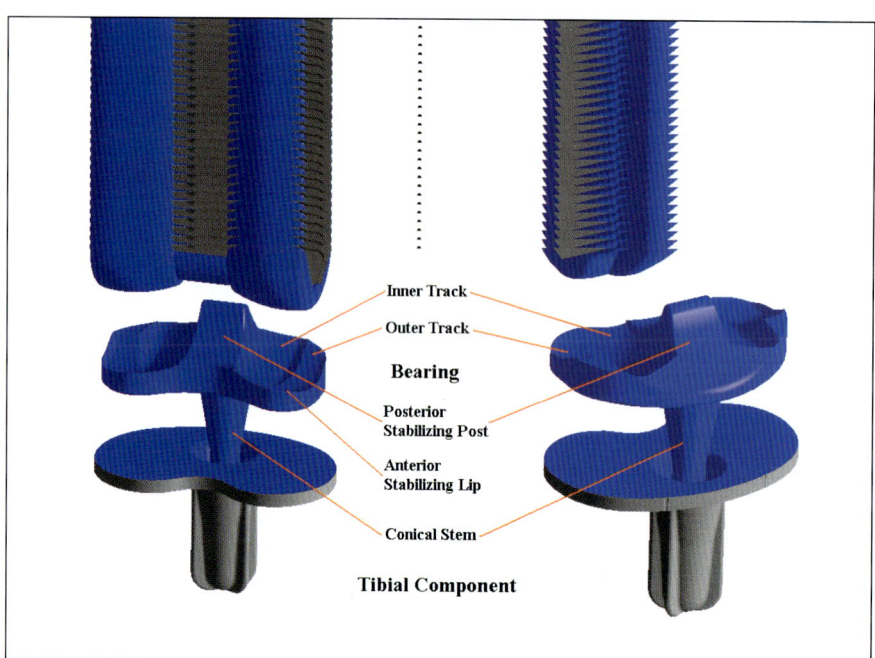

Figure 1. Anterior and posterior oblique views of the tibial, polyethylene-bearing and femoral components. The tibial and femoral components are made of cobalt chrome.

As a result of the above considerations, prostheses with anatomic designs tend to have a low surface area for contact between the condyles and tibial polyethylene bearing. They do not have consistent "roll-back" of the condyles on the polyethylene with flexion, to provide quadriceps efficiency, and they often roll forward,[2] making it difficult to climb stairs and rise from chairs. If the prosthesis is implanted with the posterior cruciate too loose, or the posterior cruciate becomes stretched after implantation, the prosthesis will be unstable,[3] whereas prostheses implanted with the posterior cruciate too tight have increased polyethylene wear from high pressures across the knee.[4] Small contact areas and the high contact pressures lead to excessive polyethylene wear that reduces the life of the prosthesis. Unless the collateral ligaments are tight, lack of an anterior cruciate ligament leads to feelings of instability, especially when descending stairs. Improvements on the "anatomic" design have concerned attempts to substitute for posterior cruciate ligament function and create broader surfaces for weight bearing on the polyethylene.

Substitution for the posterior cruciate ligament is effected by raising areas anteriorly on the polyethylene bearing which impinge upon the femoral component to prevent anterior movement of the femoral component at a certain point on the bearing.[5] The elevated polyethylene areas can impinge upon the condyles directly, or they can impinge upon bars between the condyles of the femoral components. When bars between the femoral condyles are used, impingement between the bars and polyethylene can create femoral rollback with progressive flexion. The position of the bar determines the point at which the posterior stabilizer engages. Engagement early in flexion creates early femoral rollback with increased quadriceps efficiency for activities such as walking. The normal knee starts rollback with the initiation of flexion, and most of the rollback is accomplished within the first 20 degrees of flexion.

The area of contact between the femoral condyles and polyethylene bearing surface is limited if both flexion and rotation occur on the same surface of the bearing. "Mobile" bearings have been created that rotate on the tibial baseplate, thus allowing pure flexion/extension at the upper surface of the tibial bearing with the potential for greater congruity between the femoral component and bearing.[6]

Only recently have mobile knees been designed and contain posterior stabilizers and enforce rollback. If the stabilizer post is on the polyethylene bearing, the bearing, itself, must be stabilized through a connection with the tibial baseplate that prevents the mobile bearing from moving anteriorly, so the bearing can push the femur posteriorly. An alternative possibility is to have the posterior stabilizer on the tibia, with a hole in the bearing that allows the bearing to move in the sagittal plane. In this case, the bearing would be captured by the femoral condyles and move passively as the stabilizer on the tibial baseplate pushes the condyles posteriorly with flexion.

Even the presence of a mobile bearing and posterior stabilizer does not necessarily create large areas of contact for weight bearing. If the posterior stabilizer is on the mobile bearing, a large area of contact between the femur and bearing throughout the range of motion requires the condyles to go from one area of contact to another as the condyles roll back. If the posterior stabilizer is on the tibial plate and the bearing is only passively drawn posteriorly by the femoral component with flexion, the arcs of curvature of the femoral condyles in the sagittal plane must be segments of circles. The authors choose to have the posterior stabilizer on the bearing because that mechanism appeared more adjustable with regard to the arcs of curvature of the femur and areas of contact. In addition, a bearing that passively moves between the femoral and tibial components could not, by itself, produce anterior stability.

PROSTHETIC DESIGN OF THE TRAC® KNEE

The TRAC® knee was designed to have the following attributes:
- Unrestricted flexion and rotation
- A large area of weight bearing on the polyethylene bearing throughout its entire range of motion
- Anterior and posterior stability in the absence of anterior and posterior cruciate ligaments
- Enforced rollback of the femoral omponent on the polyethylene bear-

Table 1. Summary of the one-year follow up of 75 TRAC® knee implantations.

Original demographcs

Prostheses in females	47
Prostheses in males	28
Dx Rheumatoid arthritis	7
Dx Osteoarthritis	68

	Average	Range	
Age (yr.)	65	44-78	
Height (in.)	66	59-76	
Weight (lb.)	194	106-280	

Clinical Results at 1 year	Average	Range	Average Change from Preop.
HSS* score	88.4	61-98	30.2
Knee Society (knee)	92.2	52-100	34.8
Knee Society (function)	76.8	28-100	34.6
Flexion contracture (deg.)	1.1	0-15	-2.4
Flexion (deg.)	117.0	79-135	11.1
Not using a cane (%)	89.1		30.8
Negative anterior drawer	91.5		15.9

* HSS = Hospital for Special Surgery

ing early in flexion to improve quadriceps muscle efficiency when walking up hills, climbing stairs, and rising from chairs.

The lower surface of the TRAC® polyethylene bearing has a conical stem that fits into the stem of the tibial prosthesis (Fig.1). The surfaces of the tibial component that touch the bearing are polished to allow free, unrestricted rotation of the bearing with minimal wear. The raised surfaces on the top of the bearing prevent axial rotation between the femur and bearing, thus allowing only flexion and extension on the upper surface of the bearing.

To have large areas of contact in both flexion and extension with rollback, it was necessary to spread the areas of contact sagittally across the bearing in the form of tracks. The center of the bearing contains a posterior stabilizer. On each side of the stabilizer, two tracks, inner tracks and outer tracks are present. The femoral component has contact with the inner tracks from 5 degrees of hyperextension to 8 degrees of flexion. At 8 degrees, the femoral component simultaneously contacts both sets of tracks and the posterior aspect of the posterior stabilizer, through a common tangent point. With further flexion, the femoral component lifts off the inner tracks and rollback occurs because the center of rotation of the outer tracks and posterior stabilizer are posterior to the center of rotation of the inner track. The rollback occurs early in flexion to assist the quadriceps during walking in addition to stair climbing. The femoral component remains on the outer tracks and posterior aspect of the posterior stabilizer throughout further flexion. As the femoral component remains on the lateral tracks that have a single arc of curvature in the sagittal plane, only rotation and no sliding of the femoral prosthesis is present and, thus, anterior stability can be obtained merely by raising the posterior lips of the outer tracks.

The bearings are mated in size to the femoral components rather than to tibial baseplates, as is the case in non-mobile bearing knees. Contact areas between the femoral components and bearings increase proportionately with the size of the femoral components. The 65-mm femoral component has a theoretical area for weight bearing of 1077 mm^2 in extension and 674 mm^2 in flexion.

CLINICAL OUTCOMES

The TRAC® knee is currently under Federal Drug Administration investigation and is not available for routine implantation in the United States. In its present form, it has been implanted on an experimental basis for four years. Table 1 shows the results of a prospective study of 75 TRAC® knees in 64 patients. The patients were relatively non-selected. They tended to be obese with multiple arthritic joints that lowered the "functional" parts of their scores (distance walking and stair climbing). X-rays of the knees showed no progression of radiolucent lines indicative of loosening.

DISCUSSION

Understanding the effect of area contact on prosthesis longevity requires more years of study. With the TRAC® prosthesis, the area of contact between the femoral component and bearing during flexion and extension is always along straight lines, whereas that of axial rotation between the bearing and tibial plate follows the same circular lines. The authors believe the simple motions and broad surfaces for weight bearing will substantially reduce polyethylene wear and, therefore, be particularly suitable for young patients who need total knee arthroplasties.

Using longevity to evaluate prostheses is impractical because most prostheses become obsolete before their longevity is determined. In addition, clinical scores too subjective and study populations too diverse to differentiate any but the worst prostheses. Instead, we believe more scientific evaluations are needed. Better knee simulators, more fluoroscopic studies, stair-climbing studies, and mechanical studies are needed to predict the potential success of prostheses.

In a previous study to determine knee motion and stability[7], 17 patients with TRAC® prostheses for at least one year and 18 age-matched controls with normal knees were evaluated with a Genucom knee ligament-testing machine. Results showed no significant differences between TRAC® prostheses and normal knees with respect to collateral ligament laxity, medial/lateral horizontal (axial) rotation, and anterior/posterior translation at 90 degrees of flexion. At 30 degrees of flexion, anterior/posterior translation of the TRAC® prostheses was reduced significantly compared to controls, suggesting the TRAC® affords more stability because of firmer endpoint of the polyethylene stabilizer compared to the cruciate ligaments.

Although no knee prosthesis can compare to a well-functioning, normal knee, early results of total knee arthroplasty with the TRAC® knee prosthesis suggest near normal postoperative stability and no loosening are present. In addition, the "mechanical" aspects of the TRAC® appear to duplicate knee function better than prostheses that emulate normal knee anatomy. We are currently studying the TRAC® patients in our gait laboratory, to evaluate walking and stair climbing.

REFERENCES

1. Draganich LF, Andriacchi TP, Andersson GBJ. Interaction between intrinsic knee mechanics and the knee extersor mechanism. J Orthop Res 1987;5:539-47.
2. Stiehl JB, Komistek RD, Dennis DA, et al. Fluoroscopic analysis of kinematics after posterior-cruciate- retaining knee arthroplasty. J Bone Joint Surg [Br] 1995;77-B:884-9.
3. Pagnano MW, Hassen AD, Lewallen DG, et al. Flexion instability after primary posterior cruciate retaining total knee arthroplasty. Clin Orthop 1998;365:39-46.
4. Swany MR, Scott RD. Posterior polyethylene wear in posterior cruciate ligament-retaining total knee arthroplasty. J Arthroplasty 1993;8:439-46.
5. Colizza WA, Insall JN, Scuderi GR. The posterior stabilized total knee porsthesis. Assessment of polyethylene damage and osteolysis after a ten-year minimum follow-up. J Bone Joint Surg [Am] 1995;77:1713-20.
6. Buechel FF, Pappas MJ. Long-term survivorship analysis of cruciate-sparing versus cruciatesacrificing knee prostheses using meniscal bearings. Clin Orthop Rel Res 1990;260: 162-9.
7. Draganich LF, Pottenger LA. The TRAC PS mobile-bearing prosthesis: design rationale and in vivo 3-dimensional laxity. J Arthroplasty 2000;15:102-12.

The ABG II Hip System Implantation Technique

CHRISTIAN NOURISSAT, M.D.
CLINIQUE DU RENAISON
ROANNE, FRANCE

JOSE ADREY, M.D.
POLYCLINIQUE ST ROCH
MONTPELLIER, FRANCE

DANIEL BERTEAUX, M.D.
CLINIQUE DE LA PRESENTATION
ORLEANS, FRANCE

CHRISTIAN GOALARD, M.D.
POLYCLINIQUE ST ROCH
MONTPELLIER, FRANCE

WILLIAM WALTER, M.D.
MATER MISERICORDIAE HOSPITAL
SYDNEY, AUSTRALIA

Articles in the literature about hydroxyapatite-coated hip prostheses show both the clinical and radiological results are extremely satisfactory in the short and medium term.[1-5] They bear out the reliability, constancy, and durability of bio-active fixation.[6] As in the case of cemented prostheses, results are tempered by the emergence of complications linked with the particles produced by polyethylene wear, a particular cause of osteolysis in the femur or acetabulum. The ABG II HA hip prosthesis was designed with the aim of reducing this type of complication while maintaining the principle of bio-active fixation. Implantation of the system is subject to certain requirements; in particular, a preoperative radiologic assessment is required and the surgical technique must be strictly followed to optimize the biomechanical functioning of the implanted hip.

ABG II HIP SYSTEM

Designed for cement-free implantation, the ABG II prosthesis is made of titanium alloy with a precise, thin coating of hydroxyapatite (HA) (Fig. 1). The design rationale stresses the need for excellent initial stability, due to the "anatomic" shape of the implant, as the prerequisite for good secondary fixation to be provided by the hydroxyapatite.

The femoral component is "anatomic" with an extensive range of right and left implants that provide metaphyseal fixation in sizes 1 to 8. The stem fea-

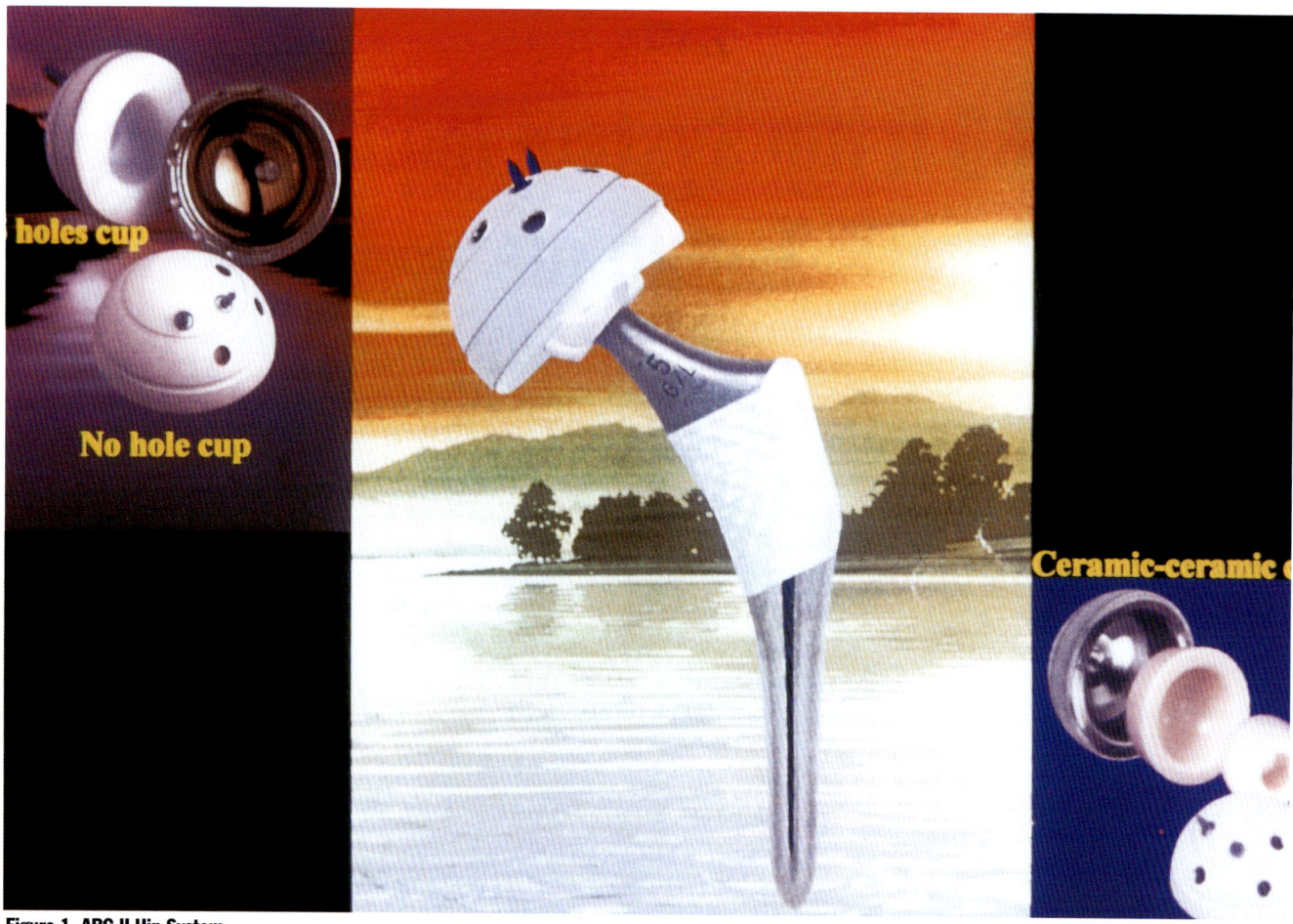
Figure 1. ABG II Hip System

tures an anteroposterior curve, which straightens out distally, with a cervico-diaphyseal angle of 128°, an anteversion of 7°, and an antetorsion of 5°.

The stem is anchored only in the metaphysis; this accounts for the proximal flare as opposed to shortness and small diameter of the distal section designed to avoid any contact between the implant and diaphyseal cortex that might be a source of postoperative pain.

The flare is both transverse and antero-posterior, thus ensuring auto-stereo-stability in the frontal and sagittal planes, as well as in rotation. This stability is strengthened by the metaphyseal surface effect created by the presence of anterior, posterior, and medial surface scales. The scales vary in diameter with size of the prosthesis, and their thickness decreases from top to bottom to prevent the stem subsiding during weight-bearing; they convert shear stresses into compressive forces and have a role in long-term osteo-integration of the prosthesis as the hydroxyapatite is resorbed. The hydroxyapatite is coated around this metaphyseal area.

The taper of the V40 femoral component can be fitted with cobalt chrome or zirconia heads in sizes 22.2 mm to 28 mm. The heads have a variable neck length: short, medium, or long.

The acetabular component is hemispheric in shape. The initial fixation of the implant is achieved by impacting the cup into the subchondral bone of the acetabulum, which has been prepared by using progressively larger sizes of reamer to obtain an "exact fit." The shape ensures an even distribution of compressive forces across the acetabulum, thus providing for perfect stability from the outset. Screwing one or two TA6V spikes, additionally, into the cup increases initial fixation because they act against the shear stresses as the hip joint moves.

The two types of acetabular component are:

- *A no-hole cup*, to reduce the risk of polyethylene particle migration, the 8-mm spikes being fixed to the outside of the cup.
- *A 5-hole cup*, generally used in revision surgery, with 7- or 9-mm spikes fixed to the inside of the cup. When insufficient initial stability of the cup is present for anatomic reasons, especially in revision surgery, the spikes may be replaced by 6.5 mm diameter cancellous screws; they have an anti-recoil thread enabling them to be joined to the cup, thus ensuring autocompression.
- The convex side of the implant has a number of circular grooves to improve bone ongrowth; this side has the hydroxyapatite and provides secondary fixation.

A standard or hooded insert (with a 7°3 gradient) made of high-density polyethylene and matched size for size to the cup, provides the head-cup interface. An ABG II cup with an alumina ceramic insert is also currently being evaluated.

For the secondary fixation of the prosthesis, we opted for a biologic sur-

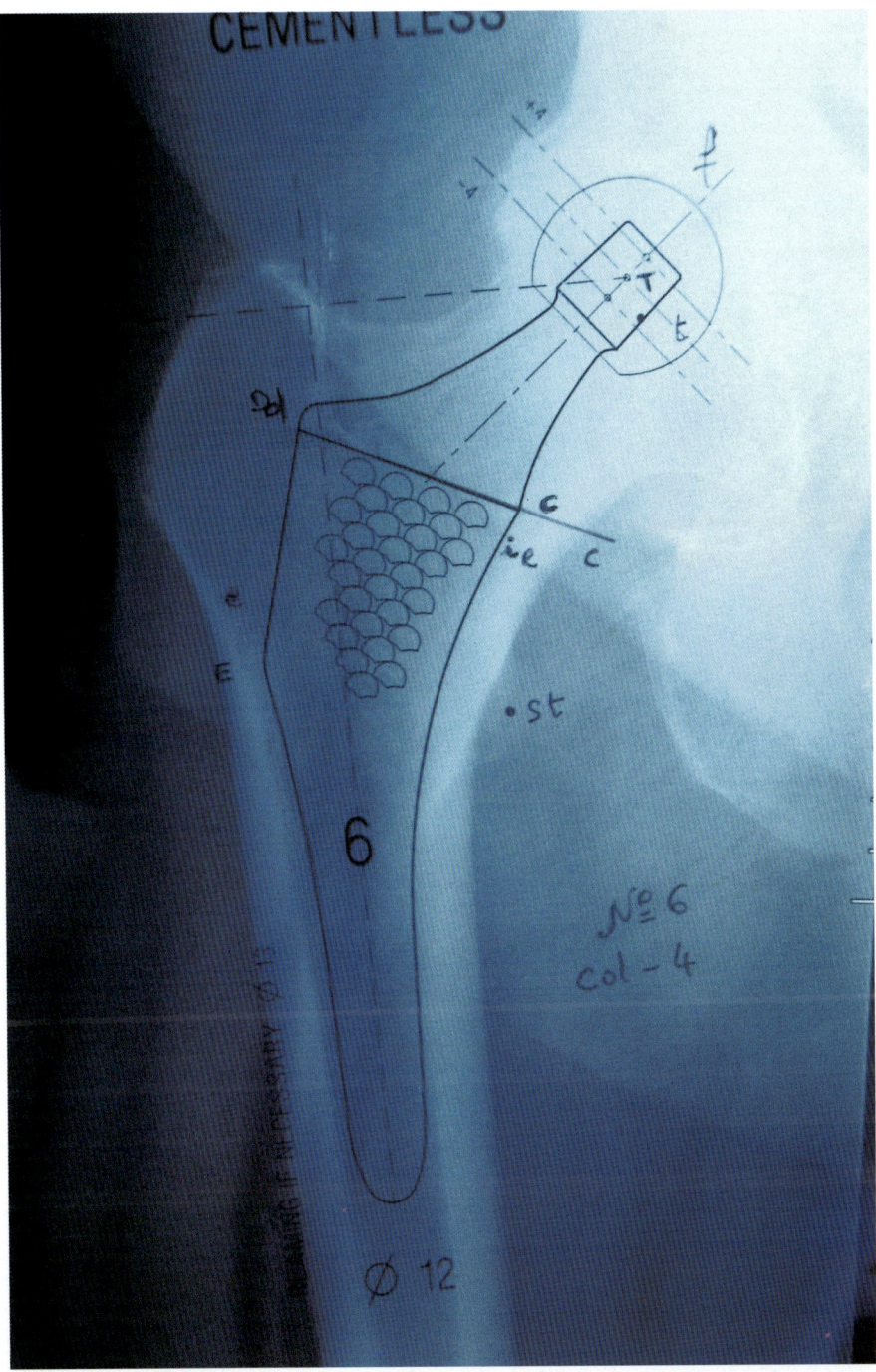

Figure 2. Preoperative planning

face effect using hydroxyapatite; because of its properties of osteoconduction, it ensures early solid bone fixation without the interposition of a fibrous layer, culminating in osteo-integration of the prosthesis. We use a sintered HA powder with 75% crystallinity and less than 10% porosity; low porosity ensures the coating is as compact as possible, which would suppose a lower risk of resorption. The average thickness of the HA coating is 60 microns. The HA is applied to the prosthesis by vacuum plasma spray.

PREOPERATIVE PLANNING

Preoperative planning is essential and done with templates placed on an AP radiograph of the femur (Fig. 2).

The implant is selected with the aid of three landmarks:

1) Diaphyseal: the axis of the prosthesis on the template must match the axis of the femoral diaphysis.

2) Vertical positioning is defined by the digital point (D): shoulder of the prosthesis (d) must be flush with the digital fossa (D)

3) The inferolateral point of the greater trochanter (E): inferolateral portion of the prosthesis (e) must rest on the inferolateral portion of the greater trochanter, with a minimum 3-mm thickness of cancellous bone.

The implant must be chosen to ensure maximum metaphyseal fill whilst preserving as much of the calcar as possible. A number of basic checks must be made:

- There must be optimum metaphyseal fill: if a choice exists between two implant sizes, it is better to opt for the smaller size as long as the intraoperative trial broach is absolutely stable.
- The centre of the head (t) must be on a level with the horizontal line that runs through the tip of the greater trochanter. Leg length can be adjusted precisely by choosing one of the various types of head.
- There should be no diaphyseal contact between the stem and cortical femur. If contact exists, the trial implant indicates the minimum reaming to be carried out.

The neck osteotomy line can then be drawn on the radiograph from the digital point at an angle of approximately 30° to the horizontal. The vertical osteotomy line runs parallel to the axis of the femoral diaphysis, from the digital fossa toward the tip of the greater trochanter.

SURGICAL TECHNIQUE

Approach

Any approach may be used for insertion of the ABG prosthesis, but approaches requiring a trochanterotomy should be avoided. The following is a description of a posterolateral approach.

The patient is placed on an ordinary operating table in lateral decubitus; the pelvis is immobilised in a strict lateral position using pubic and gluteal supports, but ensuring flexion, adduction, and medial rotation remain possible in the limb to be operated, while protecting the contralateral brachial plexus.

The skin incision is centred on the tip of the greater trochanter, extending lengthwise for 10 cm over the diaphy-

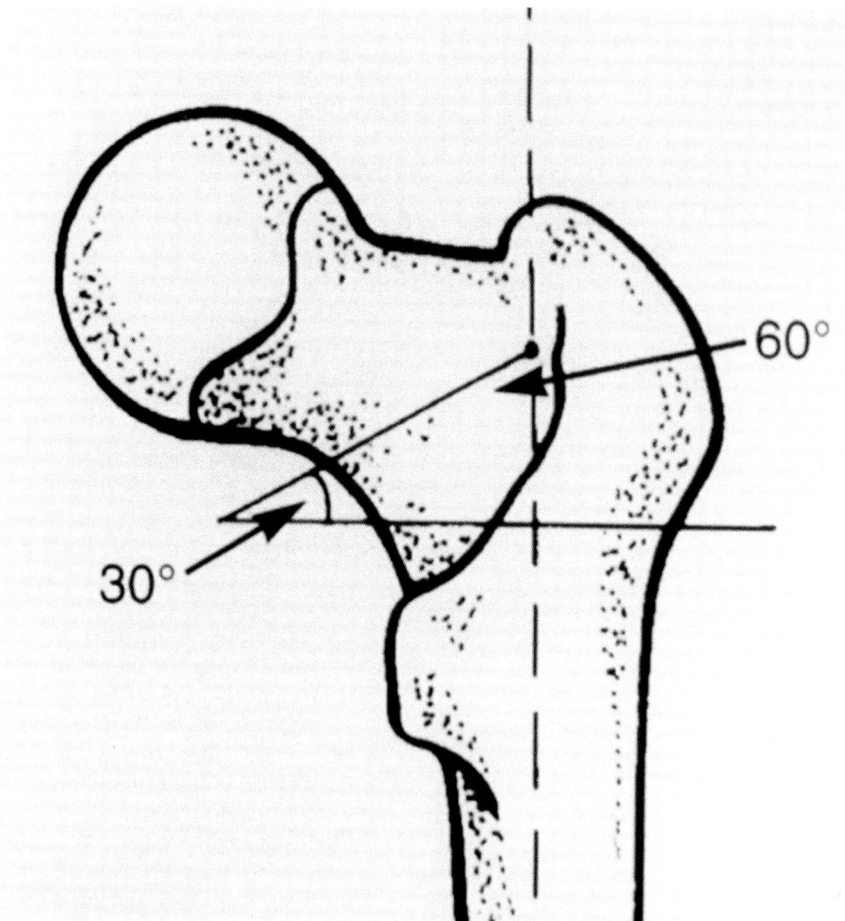

Figure 3. Neck osteotomy

seal area of the femur, and at a slight angle upwards and backwards toward the posterosuperior iliac spine over a further 10 cm. After incision of the fascia lata, the gluteus maximus is dissected in the direction of its fibres and a self-retaining retractor inserted. The pelvi-trochanteric muscles are sectioned flush with the posterior aspect of the femoral neck, as is the aponeurotic extension of the gluteus maximus. However, it is extremely important to conserve the posterior head of the gluteus medius, holding it on a retractor. The joint capsule is then incised.

Dislocation of the Hip

The femoral head and neck are then exposed using flexion, adduction and medial rotation, and a beaked retractor slipped under the femoral neck. The digital fossa is exposed and an oblique line can be drawn on the neck at an angle of 60° to the axis of the femoral diaphysis.

Neck Osteotomy (Fig. 3)

The osteotomy is performed in two planes with an oscillating saw:
- The first cutting plane follows the oblique line on the posterior aspect of the neck; no anteversion of the cut is required.
- The second cutting plane is perpendicular to the medial aspect of the greater trochanter, running proximally from the digital fossa.

The complete head and neck is then removed, releasing the capsule inferiorly and anteriorly over the neck and preserved in a cup containing saline (grafts may be used during the surgical procedure).

INSERTION OF THE CUP

Exposure of the Acetabulum

Insertion of the cup requires excellent exposure of the acetabulum. After a conservative capsulectomy, the anterior and posterior horns are removed. The transverse ligament of the acetabulum is excised and any osteophytes at the bottom removed. The hollow chisel is then used to expose the bottom and upper rim of the obturator hole. Frequently, areas of sclerotic bone require freshening. In these instances, the smallest reamer (40-mm diameter) is used vertically to complete this stage of the preparation.

Reaming

The acetabular cavity is reamed out to allow implant of the cup in subchondral bone, by far the preferred solution to achieve good biologic fixation. The acetabulum is prepared using reamers of increasing size (by 2-mm increments) at an angle of about 40 to 45 degrees, and with approximately 15° of anteversion. Reaming continues into bleeding subchondral bone until the trial cup is stable and covered adequately by acetabular bone. When using the last reamer, excessive rotation should be avoided, to not oversize the acetabular cavity.

Insertion of the Trial Cup

The trial cup, identical in diameter to that of the last reamer ("exact fit" effect), is impacted into the acetabulum at the same angle and with the same anteversion as the reamer. The trial cup must be absolutely stable in the cavity; the holes in the cup enable proper contact with the acetabular bone to be verified. The diameter should be the same as the definitive implant.

If the trial cup is unstable, one must ensure no soft tissue or capsular tissue overhangs the acetabulum, which might make it difficult to impact the cup. However, instability is sometimes due to insufficient reaming; stability can be improved by further limited reaming of the acetabulum, beginning with a 2- to 4-mm smaller reamer and continuing up to the size of the templated trial cup. The stability should be checked again; then the trial cup is removed. Any subchondral cysts should be excavated, curetted, and filled with cancellous bone from the femoral head.

Insertion of the No-Hole ABG II cup (Fig. 4)

This cup is preferable for use in primary surgery. After opening the inner blister, the cup is grasped by means of the cup holder; two 8-mm spikes are generally used to provide additional primary stability. Using the spikedriver, the spikes must be screwed into the row of holes closest to the apex, in two adjacent holes.

edge of the metal cup must be flush with the upper rim of the obturator hole). The stability of the cup is then checked.

One or more obturator plugs can be screwed into the unused holes. They have been designed to seal the cup and, thus, reduce the risk of particle migration. If inadequate stability is present, one should check to determine no capsular or soft tissue is interposed between the cup and the reamed bone.

In some primary surgery cases of instability, or in revision surgery, the spikes can be replaced by 6-mm cancellous screws. A drill guide is available and its tip is screwed into the selected insertion hole using the screwdriver. A drill bit of the required length is placed in the drill guide to drill into the cancellous bone. The drill guide is then removed and gauge used to measure the length of the screw to be inserted with the universal screwdriver. One must ensure the screw, firmly attached to the cup due to its double screw threads, has been impacted adequately and it does not project from its seating to avoid any conflict with the definitive insert. One or more screws may be used. The cup impactor is removed and a trial insert introduced.

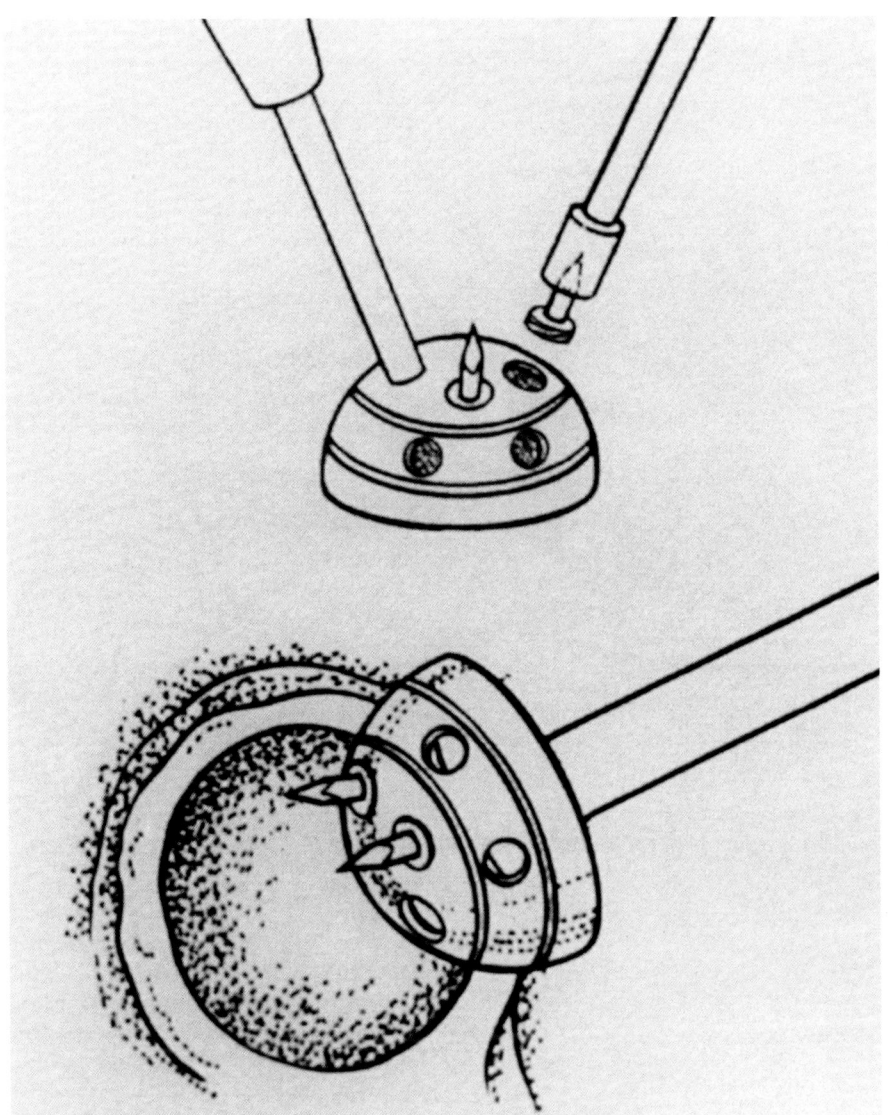

Figure 4. Spikes fixation and insertion of no-hole cup

The spikes must be screwed down as tightly as possible. The cup is then fixed onto the cup impactor and the cup holder removed.

The cup is impacted into the acetabulum at an angle of 45° and an anteversion of about 15°, achieved by inserting the cup so the spikes penetrate the acetabulum superiorly at 11 o'clock and 1 o'clock position. The cup is then impacted with the hammer until it has engaged with the acetabulum correctly (the bottom edge of the metal cup must be flush with the upper rim of the obturator hole). The stability of the cup is then checked. The cup impactor is removed and a trial insert introduced.

Insertion of the 5-Hole ABG II Cup

This cup can be used in primary surgery, but is especially of use in revision surgery. After opening the inner blister, the cup is fixed onto the cup holder. Two 7-mm or 9-mm spikes are generally used; they must be screwed inside the cup, by means of the hexagonal screwdriver, into the holes closest to the apex, in two adjacent holes. The spikes must be screwed down as tightly as possible. The cup is then fixed onto the cup impactor and the cup holder removed.

The cup is impacted into the acetabulum at an angle of about 45° and an anteversion of about 15°; this process is achieved by inserting the cup so the spikes penetrate the acetabulum superiorly at 11 o'clock and 1 o'clock positions. The cup is then impacted with the hammer until it has engaged with the acetabulum correctly (the bottom

PREPARATION OF THE FEMUR

The leg is dislocated by flexion, adduction and medial rotation. With the aid of a hollow chisel, the remainder of the anterior and superior portion of the femoral neck is removed and the metaphyseal compartment prepared to receive the implant. Using the box chisel of appropriate size for the prosthesis, a core of cancellous bone is removed from the metaphysis, preserving as much of the calcar as possible.

If preoperative planning shows the possibility of a contact between the prosthetic stem and diaphyseal cortex, reaming is required; the reaming guide and then flexible reamers are inserted up to the size indicated on the preoperative template. The broaches are then introduced, beginning with the smallest and conserving as much of the calcar cancellous bone as possible, until the diameter indicated at the time of the preoperative planning is reached.

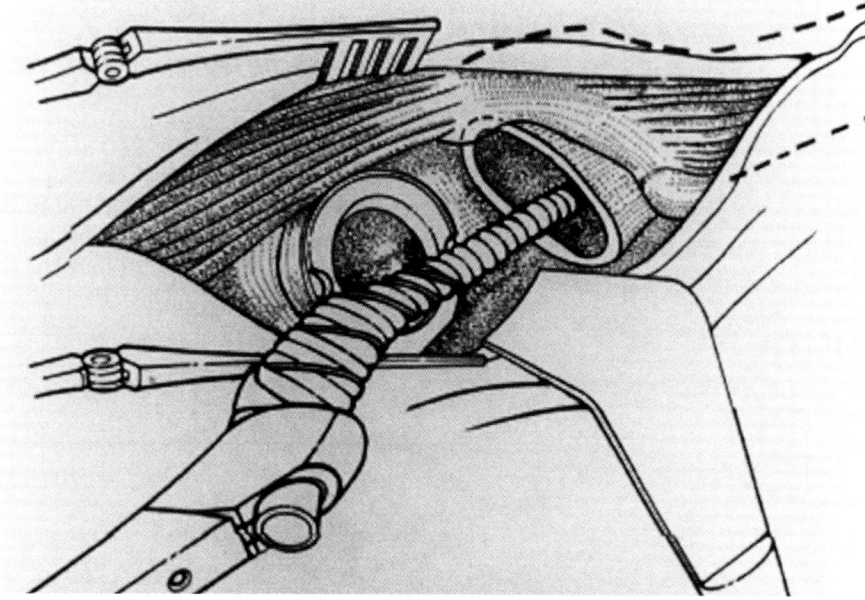

Figure 5. Insertion of trial broach

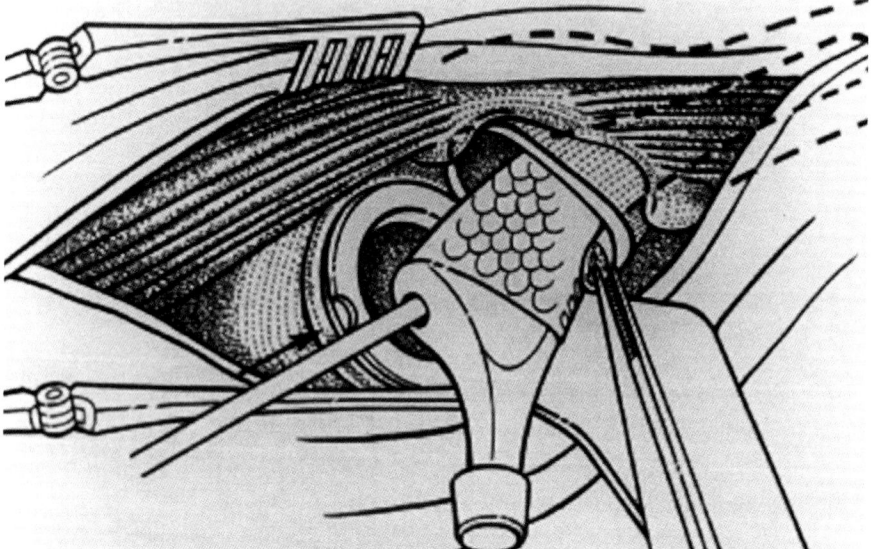

Figure 6. Implantation of femoral stem

Insertion of the broaches (Fig. 5)

The trial broach determines the final size of the implant if two conditions are met:

1. The broach must be driven down to the right level; i.e., the shoulder of the broach must be on a level with the digital fossa.

2. The broach must be absolutely stable in the transverse direction (varus-valgus) and also in rotation.

If, despite correct reaming, a trial broach smaller than the size chosen at the planning stage is absolutely stable in rotation (especially if anteroposterior narrowness of the neck exists), one should not try to use a larger size because of the risk of a metaphyseal crack or fracture.

Conversely, if the trial broach is unstable, three possible solutions are:

1. Take the next larger broach, as long as the reamer is used first on the basis of the templated data:

2. Stabilise the implant with a cortico-cancellous graft using material from the resected part (but a graft should rarely be depended on to ensure implant stability)

3. Cement an ABG II vitallium stem.

With the broach still in position, a trial head is fitted onto the spigot.

Checking the Stability of the Hip

The hip is reduced by deflexion, traction, lateral rotation, and abduction. The following should be checked:

1. Leg-length adjustment using the trial heads with a short, medium, or long neck, and a diameter to match the insert.

2. Stability of the hip.

IMPLANTATION OF THE DEFINITIVE INSERT

The hip is again dislocated, and the trial head, broach, and trial insert are removed. The cup is cleaned and a standard or hooded insert impacted using the insert impactor. The stability of the insert in the cup is checked.

IMPLANTATION OF THE FEMORAL STEM

Insertion of the ABG II HA stem should be performed, avoiding contact between the hydroxyapatite and gloves. The distal end of the stem is put into the medullary canal and before impaction, placing part of the core of cancellous bone (removed by the box chisel) between the calcar and medial border of the prosthesis is often useful to counter varus positioning (Fig 6). The prosthesis is inserted into the femur with the aid of the stem impactor until the shoulder of the prosthesis is flush with the digital fossa. Leg length adjustment can be checked again using the trial heads and after reduction.

IMPLANTATION OF THE HEAD

Washing and drying the spigot is essential before implanting the definitive head. Whether made of cobalt chrome or zirconia, the head should not be struck, simply pushed onto the spigot.

REDUCTION

After abundant lavage of the joint cavity with saline solution, the hip is reduced for the last time. The posterior capsular ligaments are closed with great care to reduce the risk of postoperative dislocation.

POSTOPERATIVE MANAGEMENT

Postoperative management of the

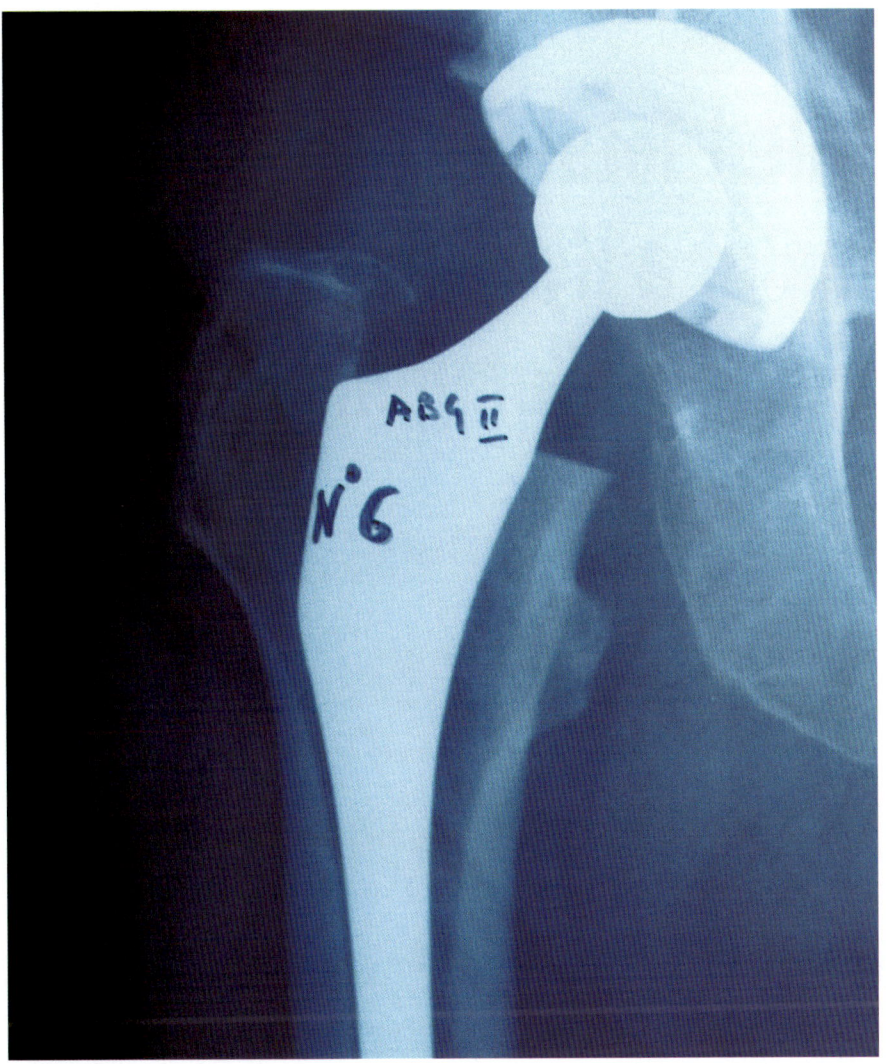

Figure 7. Two years postoperative X-rays

ABG II HA prosthesis is the same as for cemented prostheses, with immediate weight-bearing using two crutches recommended for the first month following the operation. One-legged weight-bearing is generally achieved approximately the 13th day (Fig. 7).

REFERENCES

1. Epinette JA, Geesink RGT, eds. Hydroxyapatite coated hip and knee arthroplasty. Cahiers d'Enseignement de la SOFCOT No. 51. Paris: Expansion Scientifique Française; 1995. p 376.
2. Nourissat C, Adrey J, Berteaux D, et al. The ABG Standard hip prosthesis: five-year results. In: Epinette JA, Geesink RGT, eds. Hydroxyapatite coated hip and knee arthroplasty. Cahiers d'Enseignement de la SOFCOT No. 51. Paris: Expansion Scientifique Française; 1995. p 227-38.
3. Rossi P, Sibelli P, Fumero S, et al. Short-term results of hydroxyapatite-coated primary total hip arthroplasty. Clin Orthop 1995; 310: 98-102.
4. Tonino AJ, Romanini L, Rossi P, et al. Hydroxyapatite-coated hip prostheses. Clin Orthop 1995; 312: 211-25.
5. Nourissat C. et al. ABG Scientific Group. The use of Hydroxyapatite-Coated implants in revision surgery for acetabular component loosening: Surgical Technology International VII 1998.
6. Tonino, AJ, Thèrin M, Doyle C. Hydroxyapatite-coated femoral stems. J. Bone Joint Surg. (Br), 1999; 81-B(1); 148-54.

Revision of Failed Total Hip Prosthesis with Insertion of a Hydroxyapatite-Coated Femoral Component

Jordi Casas-Sabater, M.D.
Chief, Department of Orthopaedic Surgery

Marc Cots-Pons, M.D.
Chief, Section of Hip and Knee Surgery

Félix Castillo-García, M.D.
Consultant, Department of Orthopaedic Surgery

Hospital General de Catalunya
Barcelona, Spain

Ernane Dodero Reis, M.D.
Assistant Professor, Department of Surgery
The Mount Sinai Medical Center
New York, NY, USA

Joaquim Rodriguez-Miralles, M.D., Ph.D.
Professor, Department of Human Anatomy
Consultant, Department of Orthopaedic Surgery
Barcelona University
Barcelona, Spain

As the population ages, primary total hip arthroplasty (THA) is becoming one of the most common orthopedic procedures. Therefore, revisions for mechanical loosening after THA should also increase in future years. Loosening is a progressive phenomenon that, along with intracortical granuloma, causes bone destruction. The main concern in total hip revision surgery is the reduced bone stock, which makes it difficult to obtain optimal stability of the femoral stem (Case 1: Figs. 1 a, b).

Femoral revision arthroplasty aims at relieving pain and restoring bone integrity (to ensure stable fixation of the component) and biomechanical function. Adequate function requires correction of the limb-length discrepancy and femoral offset. To obtain stability of the revision implant, one alternative is to fill bone defects with metal or cement, often in large amounts. This strategy invariably leads to further bone destruction and, as a result, rates of reoperation within 10 years after revision THA with cement have ranged from 9% to 29%.[1-4] Another alternative is to seal the bone defect with the prosthesis itself, inserting a cementless implant for metaphyseal stabilisation (Case 2: Figs. 2 a, b, c). Rates of repeat revision after revision arthroplasty without cement using an uncovered

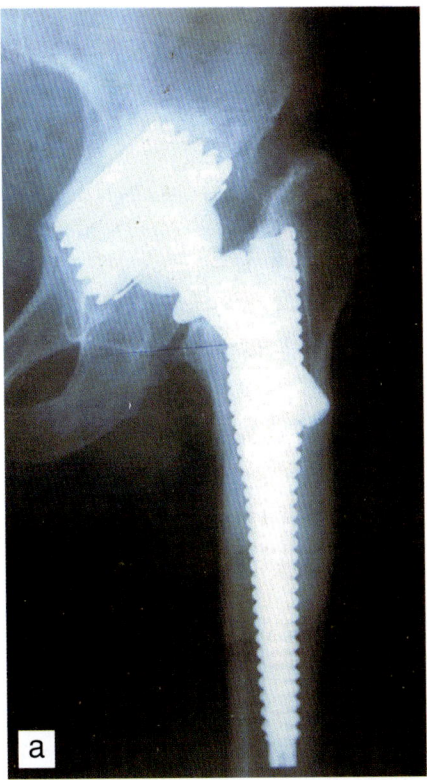
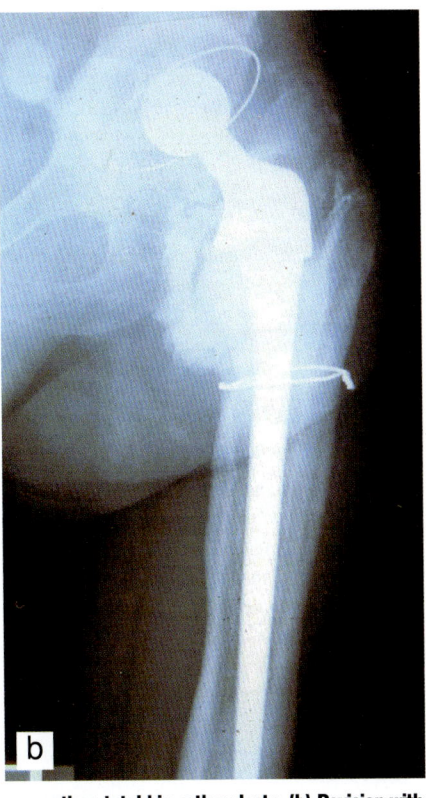

Figure 1. (a) X-ray of femoral loosening at the site of a cementless total hip arthroplasty. (b) Revision with a cemented femoral component three years after the primary procedure.

stem are lower, ranging from 2% to 7% after three to six years.[5-7]

Covering of the femoral stem with active biomaterials has been developed recently. The earliest clinical series using hydroxyapatite (HA) coating were reported by Furlong and Osborn in 1991,[8] Geesink in 1990,[9] and the Artro group in 1993.[10] In Spain, the GESPHA group, of which we are a part since the foundation in 1987, was the first to use HA-coated prostheses in primary THA, obtaining encouraging results.[11] However, the behavior of HA-coated implants has not been evaluated thoroughly in the setting of revision surgery, where a deficit of bone stock exists.

Calcium phosphates, such as HA and tricalcic phosphate (TCP), promote the bony response and facilitate close contact between bone and implant. Such properties are important in preventing development of a fibrous matrix around the prosthesis,[12-15] with associated loosening and eventual bone loss. HA ($Ca10$ $[PO4]6$ $[OH]2$) is synthesized from inorganic phosphate in solution, and calcium nitrate in alkaline buffer. The crystalline structure is identical to that of the min-

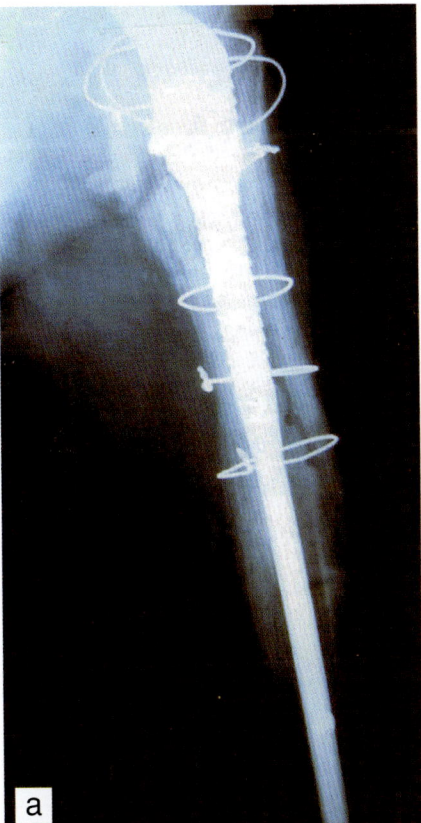
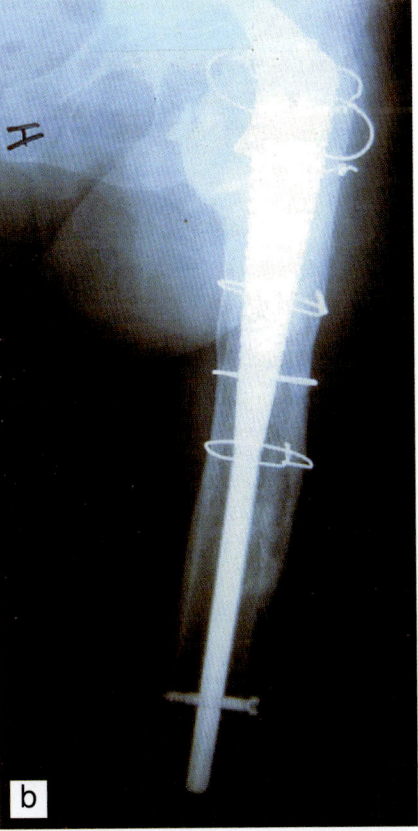
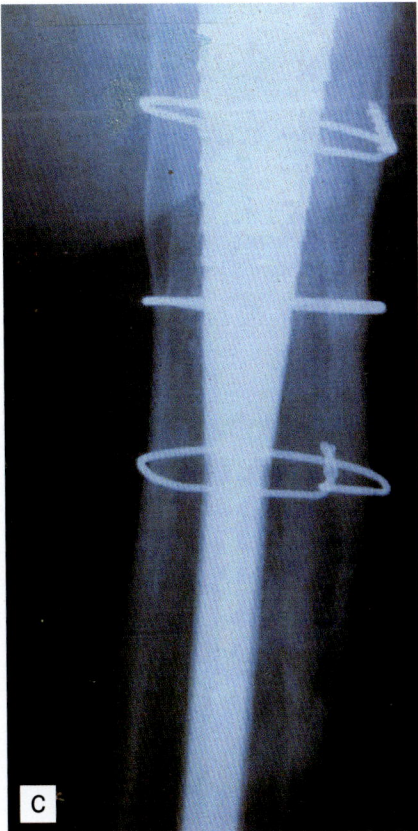

Figure 2. Second revision with a HA-coated femoral component (REEF), two years after the primary procedure. An extended trochanteric osteotomy was performed to facilitate removal of the cement. (a) Anteroposterior X-ray made three months postoperatively. (b and c) Anteroposterior and magnified X-rays made one year postoperatively show the presence of endosteal bone in contact with HA-coated stem, with absence of the radiolucent lines and cortical alterations or reactive lines.

eral component of bone. HA has slower absorption and is less soluble than TCP in physiologic pH, thereby being more widely used as a biomaterial.[16]

In primary cementless hip arthroplasty using HA-coating, the survival rate of femoral stems is between 95% to 98%, with up to nine years of follow up.[11,17,18] Densitometric analysis has demonstrated excellent preservation of bone stock.[19] Our group has performed operations using HA-coated devices in revision surgery since 1987, which allows for 11 years of follow up.[20,21] In our experience, the failure rate after revision THA with HA-coated implants ranges from 2% to 8%, after 3 and 6 years, respectively.[20,21] Bone-ingrowth fixation of the prosthesis has been approximately 94% at two years.[20,21]

Properties of Hydroxyapatite

HA has excellent biocompatibility; composed only of Ca and P ions, it causes no local or systemic toxicity.[22] HA also has good osteoconduction, allowing bone to grow onto the surface of the implant. Bone growth of 2 mm can be achieved with HA coating, in contrast with approximately 300 microns obtained by stuffed porous implant.[23-25]

Bone fixation to HA-coated implants involves biologic fixation, the process by which the components of the prosthesis become bound to the bone by growth or apposition, without the use of any cement.[26] Given the main advantage of using HA coating is to obtain a rapid biologic fixation to the bone, important to consider is the mechanism underlying this fixation.[13,14,26,27] The process, termed "osteointegration,"[28] can be divided into several steps: partial dissolution of HA, increase of Ca and P concentrations in the microenvironment of the bone-implant interface, formation of apatite carbonate (AC) microcrystals, binding of AC to the bone matrix, and induction of bone growth. Although osteointegration of HA implants has long been known, inadequate mechanical properties of the coated metallic surfaces limited their use in human surgery. As it is established that HA behaves like a "biologic cement," the concept of 'bioactive,' instead of 'uncemented,' prosthesis has evolved.

Application of Hydroxyapatite Coating to the Metallic Substrate

Several procedures are available currently to apply HA to the metallic substrate–plasma spray considered the most satisfactory.[29] Coating can be obtained by the following methods:[30]

(1) Atmospheric Plasma Spray (APS)– Heat projection by atmospheric plasm consists of depositing a substrate of mineral particles in a highly exothermic gaseous vector. These particles are vaporized at temperatures up to 29727°C, having high kinetic energy, and are thereby projected at high speed over the metallic substrate.

(2) Vacuum Plasma Spray (VPS)–The plasma chamber is maintained at a low pressure before introducing a mixture of hydrogen and argon. This gas mixture goes through two electrodes, and induces an ionization effect that generates flux of particles at high velocity and temperature (5000°C). HA particles, subjected to this temperature for a short time, are finally projected against the prosthesis. This method is superior to ASP because the flame is more laminar and easily controllable, working temperature is lower, and speed is higher.[31]

(3) High-Velocity Oxyfuel (HVO)–Compared to the plasma spray method, in high-speed O_2, HA particles are heated at lower temperatures but applied over the substrate at higher speed. With this method, the coating obtained is more stable chemically, although the strength of its binding to the metal is less optimal.[32]

Analysis of the coating density produced by the different methods has shown the most compact padding was obtained by APS, followed by VPS and HVO; however, no clear clinical differences have been noted among patients treated with the first two methods.[33]

A number of chemical, mechanical, and biologic properties of the coating depend on the methods used for delivery.[30] To limit HA decomposition into TCP, Ca oxide, and tetracalcic phosphate, the bioactive powder used should be 100% pure.[31] The chemical composition of the powder, or the way it is applied to the metallic substrate, do not effect the biocompatibility of the final coating. However, subtle changes in the HA coating could effect its biodegradation kinetics.[31]

An ideal deposition has the following characteristics:[34] crystal index of 50% to 70%; Ca/P quotient, 1.6 to 1.8; porosity index below 5%; and a coating depth of 50 to 250 (mean: 150) microns. Degradation kinetics of the bioactive coating is among the most important factors that influence the eventual outcome of the surgical procedure. Fast degradation of the coating greatly increases the risk of osteolysis,[35] whereas a slow and progressive decay can help the formation of a barrier and hinder the foreign-body reactions usually observed in the presence of non-reabsorbable particles such as polyethylene and metacrylate.[26,36-38]

Reabsorption of the Hydroxyapatite Coating

HA coating shrinks and eventually disappears by reabsorption.[39,40] This process is mediated primarily by osteoclasts, which induce osteo-aposition, or contact of bone with the microstructures of the metallic implant.[41,42] The prosthesis is fixed long-term by progressive replacement of the bioactive coating by bone (reabsorption-reconstruction).[43] Therefore, the HA component should be stable sufficiently to be reabsorbed slowly, but also be capable of rapid linking to the bone.[14,44,45] This favorable context can only be achieved by a well-designed and appropriately inserted prosthesis.[26,46,47] Suitable implantation provides a bone-prosthesis interface free of fibrosis, inflammatory reaction, and osteoclasts, facilitating formation of new bone in contact with the HA. This configuration results in an increased resistance to extirpation with absence of fibrous intrusions, and reduces the time needed to achieve strongest fixation. A poorly designed prosthesis, however, cannot be corrected by the bioactive coating.

PATIENTS AND METHODS

Between 1988 and 1998, 36 patients (37 hips) were operated in our unit for the indication of mechanical failure of a cemented or cementless femoral component. Only femoral components are included in this study. Excluded from the database were three patients (4 hips), who either died or were lost to follow up; therefore, the remaining 33 hips are analyzed.

Mean duration of follow up was 59 (range: 12 to 127) months. Mean age of the patients at the time of operation was 63 (range: 35 to 84) years. Eighteen (54%) of the 33 stems were

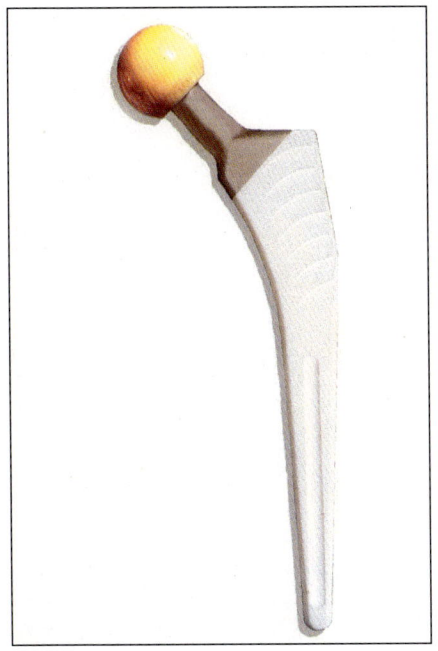

Figure 3. The Karey HA-coated femoral stem.

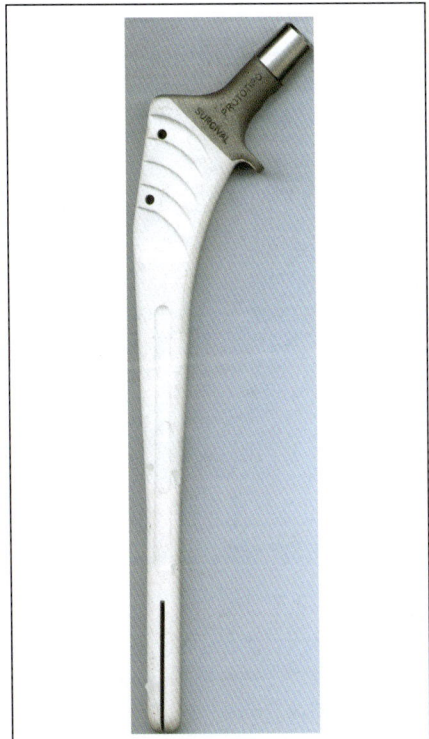

Figure 4. The Karey-R HA-coated femoral stem. Note the two holes in the proximal region for reattachment of the trochanteric fragments.

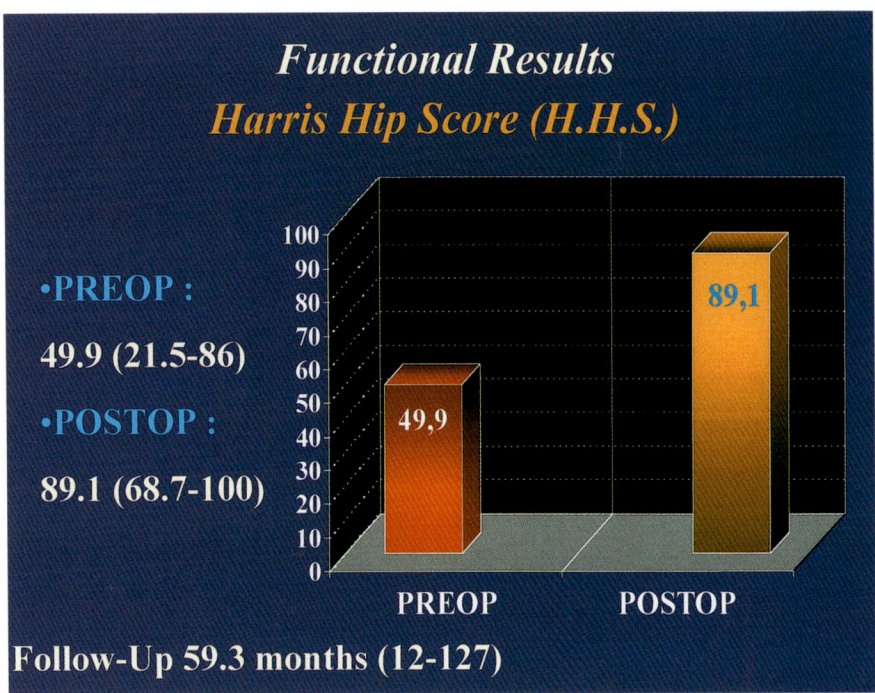

Figure 5. Functional results. Distribution of Harris Hip Score preoperative and postoperative period.

implanted in men and 15 (46%) in women; 26 (78%) consisted of a first implant revision, six (18%) of a second revision, and one (3%) of a third revision. Of the revised femoral components, 22 (67%) were performed because of failure of a cemented femoral component, and 11 (33%) because of loosening of an uncemented component.

A posterolateral surgical approach was used in all patients. Extended trochanteric osteotomy[48] was used in 8 patients—when the total extraction of cement or fibrous interface was not achieved—without having to vary significantly the postoperative protocol. The Dall-Miles cable-claw system (Stryker Howmedica Osteonics, Allendale, NJ) or cerclage wires were used for reattachment of the trochanteric osteotomy fragments.

According to the Paprosky et al. classification of bone stock damage,[49] eight patients had neck femoral damage only (Type I), 22 had intertrochanteric damage (Types IIA, IIB and IIC), and three had proximal and femoral shaft damage (Type III).

Choice of the stem to be implanted was made as a function of the bone stock damage, using as reference the Paprosky et al. classification: Type I-IIA: Corail7 (De Puy [Johnson and Johnson], Warsaw, Indiana) or Karey7 (Karey-Surgival, Valencia, Spain) (Fig. 3) in eight patients; Type II A,B,C: KAR7 (De Puy [Jonhson and Jonhson]) or Karey-R7 (Karey-Surgival, Valencia, Spain) (Fig. 4) in 21 patients; Type III: REEF7 (De Puy [Johnson and Johnson]) in three patients. The ARTRO group designed the Corail7, KAR7, and REEF7 stems, and the GESPHA group designed the Karey7 and Karey-R7 stems. Only the Karey and Karey-R stems are used currently.

All implants were made of forged titanium alloy (Ti-Al6-V4). The HA coating specifications were the same for all implants, all using APS. The HA coating thickness is 130 to 150 μm, with a purity of 97%, porosity below 5%, and 70% crystallinity. The coating is applied to the entire stem, to prevent the release of metal ions, provide maximal osseointegration at the interface, and prevent interposition of a fibrous membrane around the distal portion of the stem. All implants are macrotextural, a feature that enhances primary mechanical stability.

In the patients in whom proximal femoral stability could not be obtained (Type III of Paprosky) distal fixation of the implant with two screws (REEF7 stem) was performed. Bone graft augmentation was used in 10% of the hips, with either heterologous or autologous bone.

Management included a 24-hour course of prophylactic intravenous antibiotics and peri- and postoperative prophylactic anticoagulation for six weeks. In uncomplicated cases, early full weight-bearing with crutches was allowed. If mechanical stability was poor, weight-bearing was restricted for at least six weeks.

Before operation, all patients were evaluated clinically according to the Harris Hip Score (HHS) system,[50] and the Postel-Merle d'Aubigné, Pain-

Motion-Activity (PMA) rating,[51] using the original definitions of pain, motion, and activity rating and comparison scores.

RESULTS

Complications

Intraoperative complications occurred in three patients; all were trochanteric fractures, and were reattached using the Dall-Miles cable-claw system.

Early postoperative complications (within 3 months) occurred in two patients. One patient had a fracture of the proximal third of the femur (diagnosed on postoperative radiology), and later had three episodes of dislocation that required surgical intervention. The other patient had a fracture of the femoral shaft below the stem line, also diagnosed on postoperative X-rays, and was postponed weight-bearing for three weeks. No sequelae occurred as a result of these fractures.

One (3%) *late complication* occurred, a deep joint infection (Staphylococcus epidermidis), which required removal of the component 25 months postoperatively. (As in this case, extraction of the implant may be difficult in revision surgery.) No femoral component required revision because of aseptic loosening.

Two *reoperations* were required, for septic failure, and reorientation of the stem because of recurrent dislocation. Both of these revisions had satisfactory clinical results. No reoperations were related to the HA coating.

Clinical Outcomes

The mean preoperative HHS was 50 (range: 21 to 86). After operation, mean HHS was 89 (range: 69 to 100), with a follow up of 59 (range: 12 to 127) months (Fig. 5).

In 18 hips with follow up of more than five years (mean: 81 [range: 60 to 127] months), the HHS went from 53 (range: 21 to 86) preoperatively, to 87 (range: 72 to 100) postoperatively (Fig. 6).

Loss of points occurred in the walking and activity portions (walking up stairs). Decrease in HHS for pain was from 41 to 40; for walking, 42 to 40; for deformities, 3.5 to 3.0; and for mobility, 4.3 to 3.7 (Fig. 7). The decrease of 2.4 points in the HHS could be explained by an increase in patient's age, with poorer general condition and higher incidence of degenerative osteoarthritis.

The mean PMA score was 9.5 preoperatively, and rose to 15.7 at the last postoperative follow up. Early disappearance of pain occurred in all patients. Patients with a first-time revision had a significantly better range of motion and better ability to walk. After one year, no differences were noted in terms of HHS and PMA ratings between the different groups.[49]

Radiographic Results

An anteroposterior view of the lower pelvis and a lateral view of involved hip were taken at each postoperative visit. X-rays were evaluated by Gruen's zones of the stem[52] for signs of endosteal bone formation (spotwelds), reactive lines formation in bone around

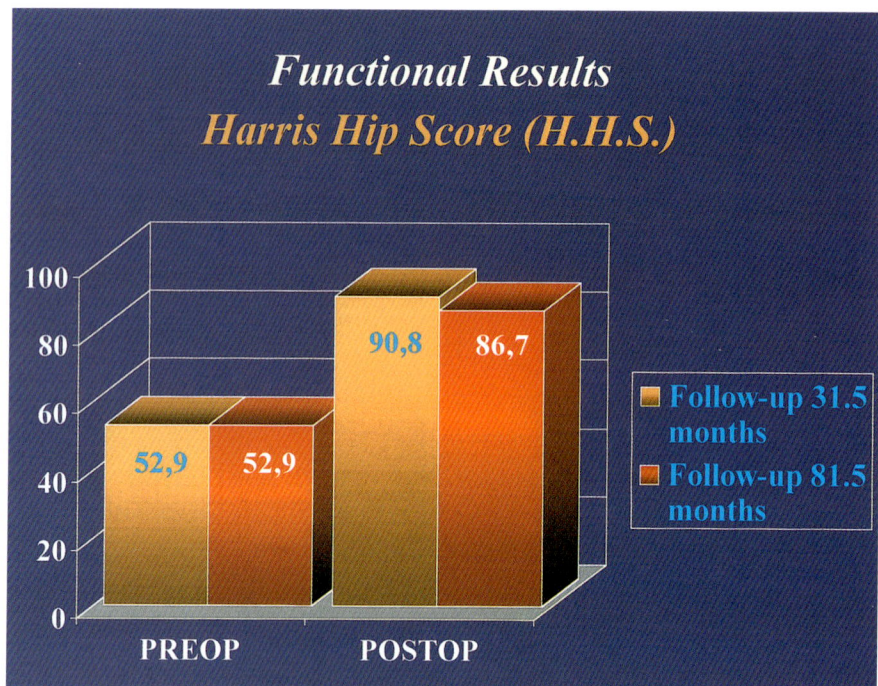

Figure 6. Functional results. Comparison of time-related evolution of Harris Hip Score.

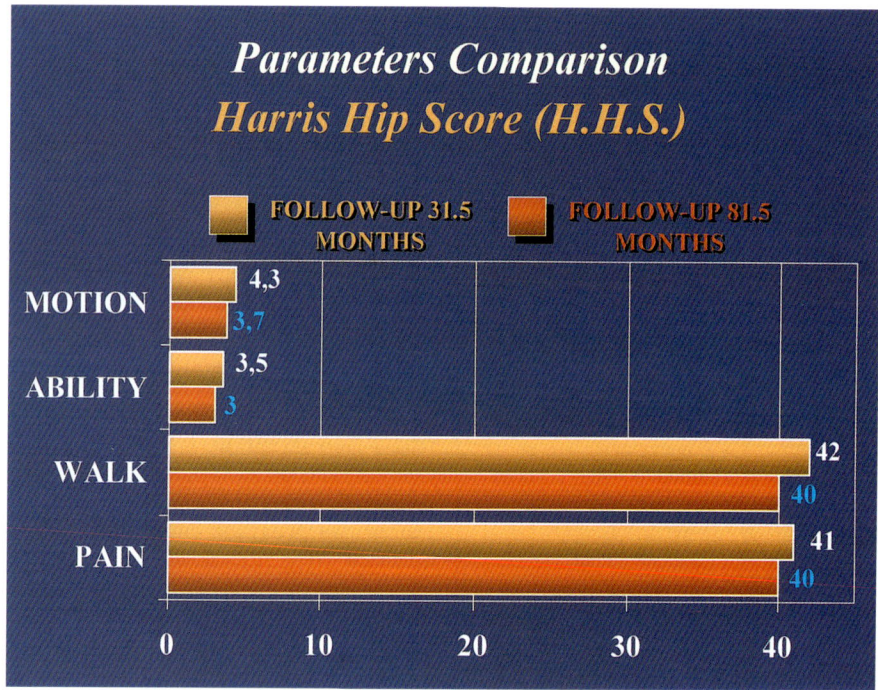

Figure 7. Distribution of time-related evolution of Harris Hip Score parameters.

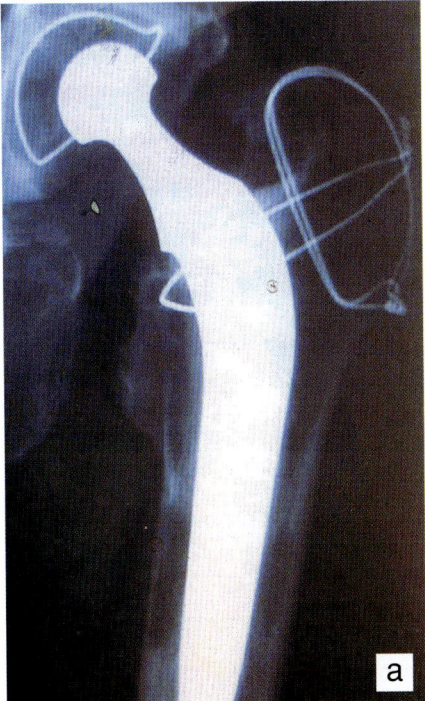 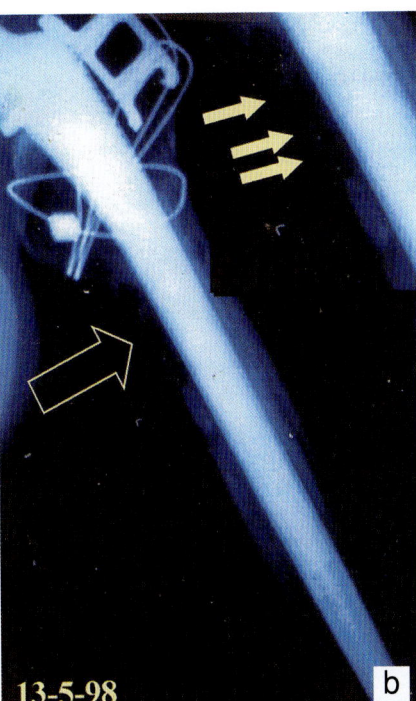 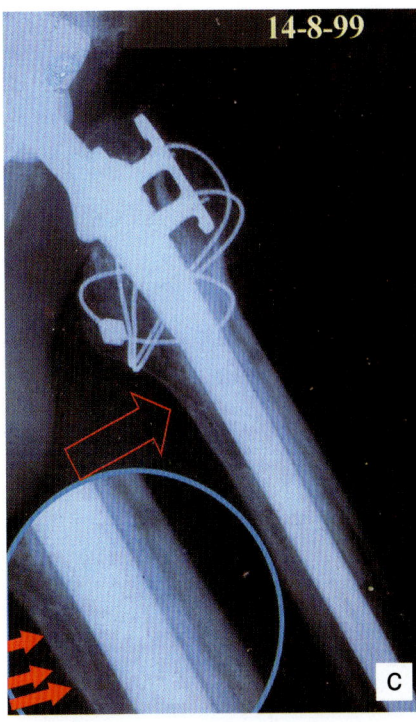

Figure 8. (a) X-ray of a patient who had a femoral osteolysis and loosening at the site of a cemented total hip arthroplasty. (b) Revision with a HA-coated femoral component (KAR stem), 12 years after the primary procedure. Lateral X-ray made three months postoperatively showing the presence of osteolysis area in femoral shaft, zone 13 (arrows, magnified inside box). (c) Lateral X-ray made 15 months postoperatively with signs of newly formed cancellous bone all along the stem, and presence filling in the osteolysis areas in zone 13 (arrows, magnified inside box). Absence of radiolucent lines and cortical alterations.

coated implant, periosteal bone reactions, cortical remodelling, osteolysis, and pedestal formation.

The radiologic aspects of osteointegration of femoral stem appeared within six months after surgery, and increased later until two to three years (Case 2: Figs. 8 a, b, c). Condensation of endosteal bone around the HA-coated stem increased between 6 and 12 months after surgery, extending proximally and distally. Bone ingrowth with apposition was observed in Gruen zones 1, 3, 4, and 5 over the medial and lateral parts of the stem.

Cancellous densification produces bridging between implant and the host bone. The pattern of this newly formed bone and radiographic signs observed depend on the general conditions at the site (cancellous bone, medullar cavity, cortical bone), as well as distance between the stem tip and femoral shaft. Bone bridging is most clearly seen in zone IV, a phenomenon that should not be confused with pedestal formation.

Signs of bone growth were noted in 88% and calcar resorption in 55% of patients at five years. Periprosthetic lucency (a radiolucent line surrounding the implant) and reactive lines is rarely seen. We have not noted any formation of femoral cortical reactive lines or any areas of osteolysis at five years follow up.

Stem migration was uncommon (3.8%), and was greater than 2 mm in only 3.2% of the hips. Migration occurs during the first six months following surgery and stabilizes later. Stem sinking has no clinical translation regarding the functional results. One patient was noted to have radiographic failure of the femoral component and may require revision for septic loosening.

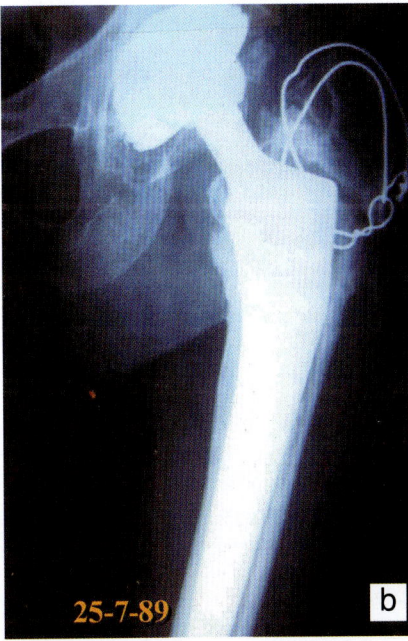

Figure 9. (a) X-ray of a man who had a femoral loosening at the site of a cementless total hip arthroplasty. (b) Revision with a HA-coated femoral component (Corail stem), nine years after the primary procedure. Anteroposterior X-ray made three months postoperatively.

DISCUSSION

Adequate primary stability of the revision femoral stem may be difficult to obtain due to the loss of bony stock

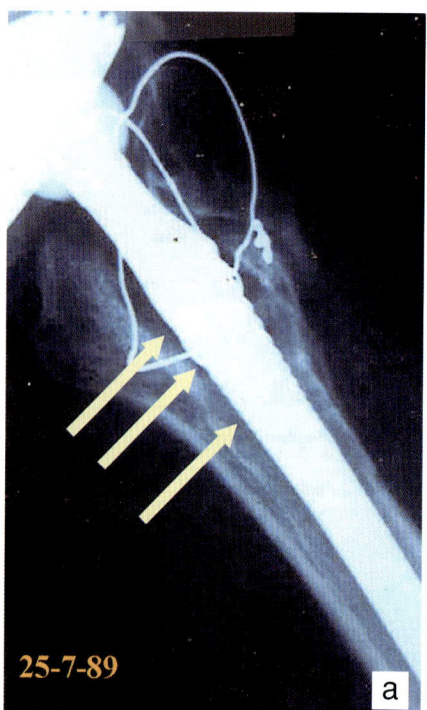
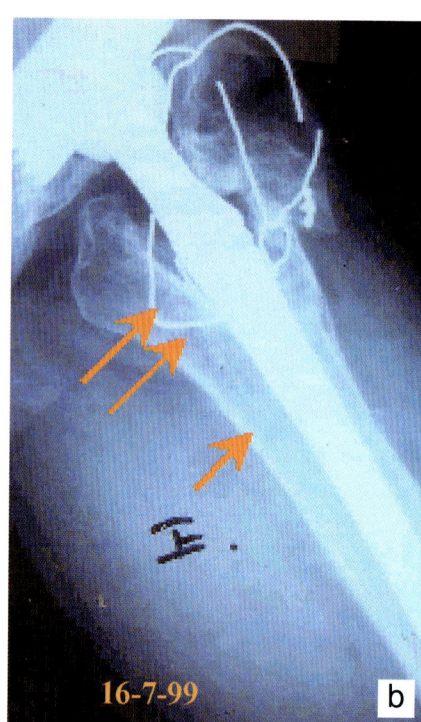

Figure 10. (a) Lateral X-ray taken three months postoperatively showing the presence of radiolucent and reactive lines (yellow arrows). (b) Lateral X-ray taken ten years postoperatively with signs of presence of newly formed cancellous bone along the stem. Absence of radiolucent lines and cortical alterations (orange arrows).

(Case 3: Fig. 9 a, b). The unique characteristics of the HA-coated hip prosthesis have led to using this type implant in revision THA. The results of HA-coated implants in revision surgery obtained in this series of patients are similar or superior to those published for other hip prosthesis coated with HA.[20,21] In addition, these results are comparable to the best results of cementless[5-7, 53-55] or cemented[1-4, 56-59] application with the same length of follow up.

Studies on the behavior of HA coating in settings of osteoporosis or bony atrophy[60-62] have shown capabilities of filling bony defects of up to 2 mm,[25,63] and facilitating the incorporation of bony implants, which can help filling the defects. Consequently, these features help improve the primary stability of revision implants[64] (Case 3: Figs. 10 a, b).

The histology of well-fixed components is of special interest. Postmortem studies of HA-coated prosthetic components obtained from ten days to five years have shown bone ingrowth into the HA coating varying from 10% of the surface after 3 weeks to 78% after 5 to 25 months; the same rates noted in primary as in revision THA.[15,40]

The radiologic documentation in the current series demonstrates the cure of lesions caused by the intracortical granuloma and eventual recovery of the bone stock. Another study has shown HA coating can inhibit the migration of polyethylene particles along the bone-implant interface, and may reduce the incidence of osteolytic lesions and the later failure of the implant.[65] In the long term, these effects could be important in reducing the incidence of osteolytic lesions and the later failure of the implant.

HA has properties of biocompatibility and osteoconduction that confer the implants possibilities of osteointegration and consequent long-term function of the arthroplasty. The behavior of these covered prostheses—first in primary surgery of the hip, and later in revision surgery—has been favorable consistently. Excellent clinical outcomes, even after more than 12 years of close follow up, suggest HA coating associated to a coherently designed prosthesis currently represents the best means for implanting without cement, both in primary and revision surgery of the hip.

REFERENCES

1. Callaghan JJ, Salvati EA, Pellici PM, et al. Results of revision for mechanical failure after cemented total hip replacement, 1979 to 1982. A two to five-year follow-up. J Bone Joint Surg 1985; 67A:1074-85.
2. Estok DM II, Harris WH. Long-term results of cemented femoral revision surgery using second-generation techniques. An average 11.7 year follow-up evaluation. Clin Orthop 1994;299:190-202.
3. Kersaw CJ, Atkins RM, Dodd CAF, et al. Revision total hip arthroplasty for aseptic failure. A review of 276 cases. J Bone Joint Surg 1991;73B:564-8.
4. Pellici PM, Wilson PD Jr, Sledge CB, et al. Long-term result of revision total hip replacement. A follow-up report. J Bone Joint Surg 1985;67A:513-6.
5. Engh CA, Massin P. Cementless total hip arthroplasty using the anatomic medullary locking stem. Clin Orthop 1989;249:141-58.
6. Gustilo RB, Pasternak HS. Revision total hip arthroplasty with titanium ingrowth prosthesis and bone grafting for failed cemented femoral component loosening. Clin Orthop 1988;235:111-9.
7. Hungerford DS, Jones LC. The rationale of cementless revision of cemented arthroplasty failures. Clin Orthop 1988;235:12-24.
8. Furlong RJ, Osborn JF. Fixation of hip prostheses by hydroxyapatite coatings. J Bone Joint Surg 1991;73B:741-5.
9. Geesink RGT. Hydroxyapatite-coated total hip prostheses. Two-year clinical and roentgenographic results of 100 cases. Clin Orthop 1990;261:39-58.
10. Vidalain JP. La prothèse Corail: 5 années d'éxpérience du group ARTRO. Acta Orthop Belg 1993;59(Suppl 1):165-9.
11. Casas-Sabater J, Cots Pons M, Rodriguez-Miralles J. Hydroxyapatite coated (HAC) femoral components. In: Szabó Z, Lewis Je, Fantini GA, Salvagi RS (eds), Surgical Technology International VII. Universal Medical Press, Inc., San Francisco, USA; 1998. p 369-76.
12. Cook SD, Thomas KA. Hydroxyapatite-coated porous titanium for use as an orthopaedic biologic attachment system. Clin Orthop 1988;230:303-12.
13. Cook SD, Thomas KA, Kay JF, et al. Hydroxyapatite coated titanium for orthopedic implant applications. Clin Orthop 1988;232:225-43.
14. Geesink RGT, De Groot K, Klein CPA. Chemical implant fixation using HA coatings: the development of a human total hip prosthesis for chemical fixation to bone using coatings on titanium substrates. Clin Orthop 1987;225:147-70.
15. Hardy DCR, Frayssinet P, Guilhem A, et al. Bonding of hydroxyapatite-coated femoral prostheses. Histopathology of specimens from four cases. J Bone Joint Surg 1991;73B:732-40.
16. De Groot K, Wolke JGC, Geesink RGT, et al. Plasmasprayed coatings of hydroxyapatite. Aus Abstracts Jahrestagung der Europäischen Gesellschaft für biomaterialen, Bologna (Italia), 1986.
17. Vidalain JP and ARTRO Group. HA coating. Ten year experience with the Corail System in primary THA. Acta Orthop Belg 1997;63 (Suppl 1):93-5.

18. Geesink RGT, Hoefnagels NHM. Eight years results of HA-coated primary total hip replacement. Acta Orthop Belg 1997;63 (Suppl 1):72-5.
19. Scott DF, Shubin-Stein K, Geesink RGT, et al. Seven years radiographic and densitometric results of hidroxyapatite-coated femoral component. Transactions of the AAOS.1995;1:1.
20. Machenaud A, et le groupe ARTRO. Le système Corail dans les révisions fémorales. Justifications. Stratégie. Résultats. In: Epinette JA, Geesink RGT (eds), Hydroxyapatite et Prothèses articulaires, Cahiers d'enseignement de la SOFCOT. Paris, Expansion scientifique française; 50, 1994. p 265-72.
21. Geesink RGT, Hoefnagels NHM. Revision total hip arthroplasty using hydroxyapatite-coated implants. Acta Orthop Belg 1997;63 (Suppl 1):77-80.
22. Geesink RGT, Manley MT (eds). Hydroxyapatite Coatings in Orthopaedic Surgery. New York, Raven Press, 1993.
23. Martens M. Interax Conference. London, February 1992.
24. Munuera L. Principios básicos del diseño de las prótesis totales de rodilla. Rev Orthop Trauma 1992;36(Suppl I):77-81.
25. Soballe K, Hansen ES, Rasmussen H, et al. Hydroxyapatite coating enhances fixation of porous coated implants. A comparison between press fit and non-interference fit. Acta Orthop Scand 1990;61(4):299-306.
26. Jaffe WL, Scott DF. Total hip arthroplasty with hidroxyapatite-coated prostheses. J Bone Joint Surg 1996;73A:1918-34.
27. Geesink RGT, De Groot K, Klein CPA. Bonding of bone to apatite-coated implants. J Bone Joint Surg 1988;70B(1):17-21.
28. Legeros RZ, Orly I. Substrate surface dissolution and interfacial biological mineralization. In: Davids JE (ed), The Bone-Biomaterial Interface. Toronto, University of Toronto Press; 1991. p 76-88.
29. D'Angelo C, El Joundi H. Reliable coatings via plasma arc spraying. Adv Mat Proc 1988;134:641-4.
30. Wolke JGC, De Groot K, Kraak TG. The characterisation of HA coatings sprayed with VPS, APS and DJ systems. In: Thermal Spray Coatings: Properties, Processes and Applications. Materials Park, Ohio, ASM International; 1991. p 481-90.
31. Doyle C. Hydroxyapatyte. Traitement et propriétés. Les facteurs "P". In: Epinette JA, Geesink RGT (eds), Hydroxyapatite et Prothèses articulaires, Cahiers d'enseignement de la SOFCOT. Paris, Expansion scientifique française 1994; 50, p 26-8.
32. Haman JD, Lucas LC, Crawmer D. Characterization of high velocity oxy-fuel combustion sprayed hydroxyapatite. Biomaterials 1995;16:229-37.
33. De Groot K, Jansen J, Wolke JGC, et al. Developments in bioactive coatings. In: Geesink RGT, Manley MT (eds), Hydroxyapatite Coatings in Orthopaedic Surgery. New York, Raven Press; 1993. p 49-61.
34. De Bruijn JD, Flach JS, De Groot K, et al. Analysis of the bony interface in vitro. In: De Bruijn JD (ed), Calcium Phosphate Biomaterials: Bone-Bonding and Biodegradation Properties. Thesis, Leidin 1993.
35. De Groot K, Klein CPAT, Driessen AA. Calcium phosphate bioceramics. Head Neck Pathol 1985;4:90-3.
36. D'Antonio JA, Capello WN, Jaffe WL. Hydroxyapatite-coating hip implants. Multicenter three-year clinical and roentgenographic results. Clin Orthop 1992;285:102-15.
37. D'Antonio JA, Capello WN, Manley MT. Remodeling of bone around hydroxyapatite coated femoral stems. J Bone Joint Surg 1996;78A:1226-33.
38. Capello WN, D'Antonio JA, Feinberg JR, et al. Hydroxyapatite-coated total hip femoral components in patients less than fifty years old. J Bone Joint Surg 1997;79A:1023-29.
39. Geesink CPAT, De Groot K, Klein CPAT. Revêtements d'hydroxyapatite: caractéristiques d'ancrage, expérimentation animale. In: Hydroxyapatite et Prothèses articulaires. Cahiers d'enseignement de la SOFCOT. Epinette JA, Geesink RGT (eds). Paris, Expansion Scientifique Française, 50; 1994. p 54-60.
40. Bauer TW, Geesink CPAT, Zimmermann R, et al. Hydroxyapatite-coated femoral stems. Histological analysis of components retrieved at autopsy. J Bone Joint Surg 1991;73A:1439-52.
41. Munting E. Improved biological fixation with macroporous hydroxiapatite coated implants. In: Harmand MF (ed), Les Publications de Biomat, Biomat, 87; 1987. p 137-46.
42. Munting E, Verhelpen M, Li F, et al. Contribution of hydroxyapatite coatings to implant fixation. In: Yamamuro T, Hench L, Wilson J (eds), Handbook of Bioactive Ceramics, CRC Press, Boca Raton, Florida, 2; 1990. p 143-8.
43. Epinette JA, Geesink RGT. Hydroxyapatite: bilan et perspectives d'avenir. In: Epinette JA, Geesink RGT (eds), Hydroxyapatite et Prothèses articulaires. Cahiers d'enseignement de la SOFCOT. Paris, Expansion Scientifique Française, 50; 1994. p 299-313.
44. De Groot K. HA coatings for implants in surgery. In: Vicencini P (ed), High Tech Ceramics. Amsterdam, Elsevier Science; 1987. p 381-6.
45. De Groot K, Geesink RGT, Klein CPAT, et al. Plasma sprayed coatings of hydroxyapatite. J Biomed Mater Res 1987;21:1375-81.
46. Hughes SS, Furia JP, Smith P, et al. Atrophy of the proximal part of the femur after total hip arthroplasty without cement. A quantitative comparison of cobalt-chromium and titanium femoral stems with use of dual x-ray absorptiometry. J Bone Joint Surg 1995;77A:231-9.
47. Pritchett JW. Femoral bone loss following hip replacement. A comparative study. Clin Orthop 1995;314:156-61.
48. Younger TI, Bradford MS, Magnus RE, et al. Extended proximal femoral osteotomy: a new technique for femoral revision arthroplasty. J Arthroplasty 1995;10:329-38.
49. Paprosky WG, Bradford MS, Younger TI. Classification of bone defects in failed prostheses. Chir Organi Mov 1994;79:285-91.
50. Harris WH. Traumatic arthritis of the hip after dislocation and acetabular fractures: treatment by mold arthroplasty. J Bone Joint Surg 1969;51A:737-55.
51. Aubigné RM, d'Postel M. Functional results of hip arthroplasty with acrylic prosthesis. J Bone Joint Surg 1954;36A:451-75.
52. Gruen TA, McNeige GM, Amstutz HC. Modes of failure of cemented stem type femoral components. A radiographic analysis of loosening. Clin Orthop 1979;141:17-27.
53. Cameron HU. The two to six year results with a proximally modular noncemented total hip replacement used in hip revisions. Clin Orthop 1994;298:47-53.
54. Engh CA, Glassman AH, Suthers KE. The case for porous-coated hip implants. Clin Orthop 1990;261:63-81.
55. Lawrence JM, Eng CA, Macalino GE, et al. Outcome of revision hip arthroplasty done without cement. J Bone Joint Surg 1994;76A:965-73.
56. Izquierdo RJ, Northmore-Ball MD. Long-term results of revision hip arthroplasty. J Bone Joint Surg 1994;76B:34-9.
57. Pierson JL, Harris WH. Cemented revision for femoral osteolysis in cemented arthroplasties. Results in 29 hips after a mean 8.5 year follow-up. J Bone Joint Surg 1994;76B:40-4.
58. Raut VV, Siney PD, Wroblewsky BM. Cemented Charnley revision arthroplasty for severe femoral osteolysis. J Bone Joint Surg 1995;77B:362-5.
59. Raut VV, Siney PD, Wroblewsky BM. Revision for aseptic stem loosening using the cemented Charnley prosthesis. A review of 351 hips. J Bone Joint Surg 1995;77B:23-7.
60. Soballe K, Hansen ES, Rasmussen HB, et al. Gap healing enhanced by hydroxyapatite coated in dogs. Clin Orthop 1991;272:300-7.
61. Soballe K, Hansen ES, B-Rasmussen H, et al. Fixation of titanium - and hydroxyapatite-coated implants in arthritic osteopenic bone. J Arthrop 1991;6(4):307-16.
62. Soballe K, Pedersen CM, Odgaard A, et al. Physical bone changes in Carragheenin-induced arthritis evaluated by quantitative computed tomography. Skel Radiol 1991;20:345-52.
63. Stephenson PK, Freman MAR, Revell PA, et al. The effect of a hydroxyapatite coating on ingrowth of bone into cavities in an implant. J Arthrop 1991:651-8.
64. Soballe K, Hansen ES, B-Rasmussen H, et al. Bone graft incorporation around titanium alloy and hydroxyapatite coated implants in dogs. Clin Orthop 1992;274:282-93.
65. Rahbeck O, Obergaard S, Soballe S, et al. Hydroxyapatite coating might peri-implant particle migration: a pilot study in dogs. Acta Orthop Scand 1996;67(Suppl 267):58-9.

FOR UNIQUE ADVANCES IN HUMAN ENGINEERING

Dynamic biarticular head with safety clip Self-Centric®

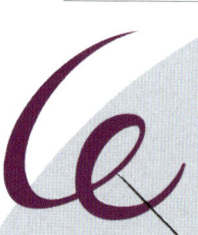
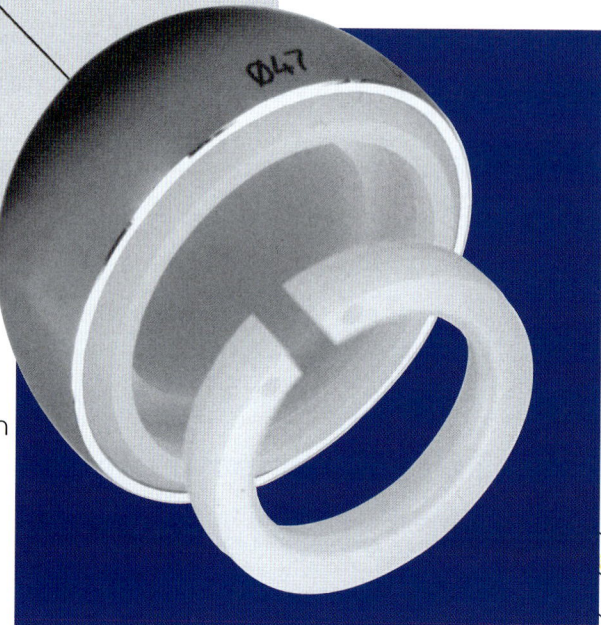

2 mm positive excentricity leading to dynamic stand up of the cup and having a self-adjustment effect. This prevents tilting.

Permanent maximum contact with bone and extensive range of motion.

Little reaction of the acetabulum to the implant because the main articulation has been transferred to the head and polyethylen inlay.

Traction and pressure are aligned in one axis.

Luxation prevention through clip with a diameter 3 mm smaller than the head.

Multiple bodyweight is needed for violent separation.

Polyethylen inlay safely fixed in the metallic shell preventing micro movements and wear.

Simple handling and assembling.

Simple disassembling with special clamp and possibility of converting to total artroplasty without having to replace the femoral stem.

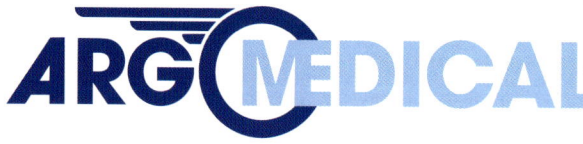

Argomedical AG, Gewerbestrasse 5, CH-6330 Cham/Schweiz, Tel. ++ 41 (0)41-741 40 18, Fax ++ 41 (0)41-741 40 19
Argomedical GmbH, Brucknerweg 2, D-38518 Gifhorn, Tel. ++49 (0) 5371-93 52 44, Fax ++49 (0) 5371-93 52 45
Argomedical Italia s.r.l., Via Giambellino 1, I-30174 Zelarino (Ve) Italia, Tel. ++39 041-952 815, Fax ++39 041-950 252
e-mail info@argomedical.ch, www.argomedical.ch

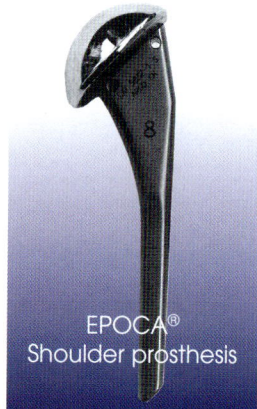

EPOCA®
Shoulder prosthesis

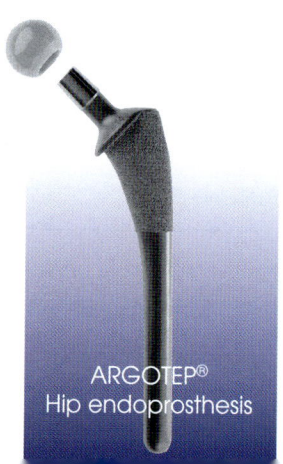

ARGOTEP®
Hip endoprosthesis

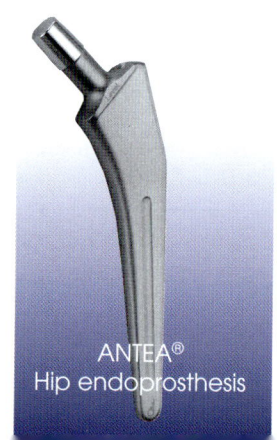

ANTEA®
Hip endoprosthesis

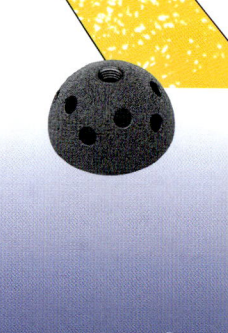

ARGOCUP®
Pressfit Cup

Bipolar Hemiarthroplasty for Treatment of Femoral Neck Fractures in Geriatric Patients—Surgical Technique and Outcome

HANS JOSEF ERLI, M.D.
SENIOR SURGEON

PETER KLEVER, M.D.
SENIOR SURGEON

OTHMAR PAAR, M.D.
PROFESSOR
DEPARTMENT. OF TRAUMA SURGERY
UNIVERSITY HOSPITAL OF THE RWTH
AACHEN, GERMANY

Fractures of the femoral neck are frequent in the elderly population. The reduced general health status and presence of concomitant diseases, in many cases, make the treatment of these patients demanding. Early mobilization is mandatory to avoid secondary infections, which were often lethal in the past. Surgical intervention has become the standard treatment for these patients. Only a few patients with stable fracture-types allow early mobilization without operation.

Internal fixation using lag screws or special plate systems, well established in the treatment of younger patients, are not recommended for the elderly population. Geriatric patients need a longer period of reduced load-bearing after an operation for internal fixation, with immediate full load-bearing during the rehabilitation period. Other problems such as the risk of nonunion and late segmental collapse of the femoral head caused by ischemia, which lead to persistent pain and sometimes the need to reoperate, are not to be tolerated for the geriatric patient.[1-3]

For these reasons, consensus is to treat fractures of the types, Pauwels II–III or Garden III–IV in geriatric patients using alloarthroplastic procedures.[4] What remains under discussion is whether total replacement of the joint or hemiarthroplasty should be favored in cases that show no concomitant coxarthrosis and allow replacement of only the fractured femoral portion without expanding surgery to the non-injured acetabulum. As hemiarthroplasty with unipolar Moore-type systems have shown acetabular erosion and protrusion of the femoral head into the

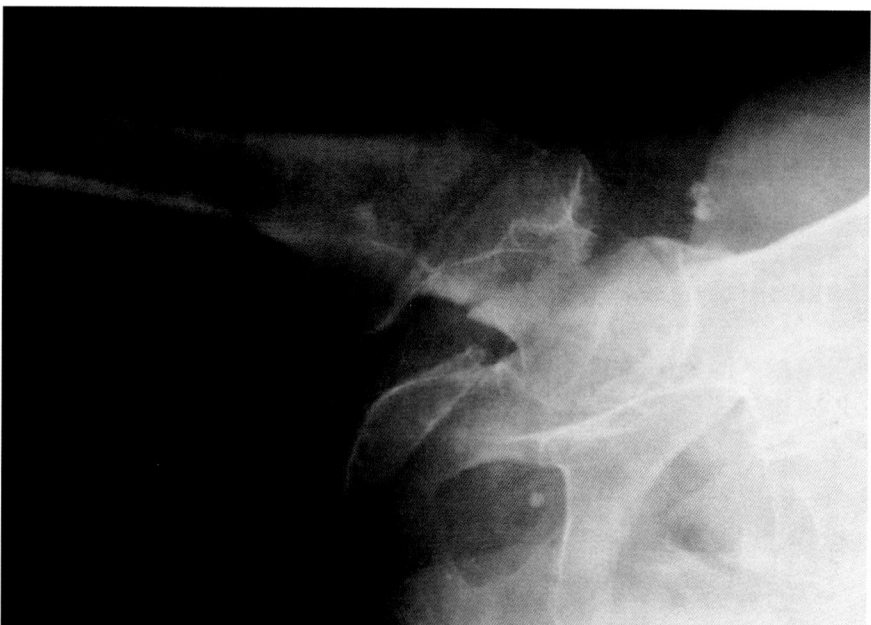

Figure 1a. Radiograph showing proximal femur of an 87-year-old female patient after femoral neck fracture type Pauwels II, Garden III.

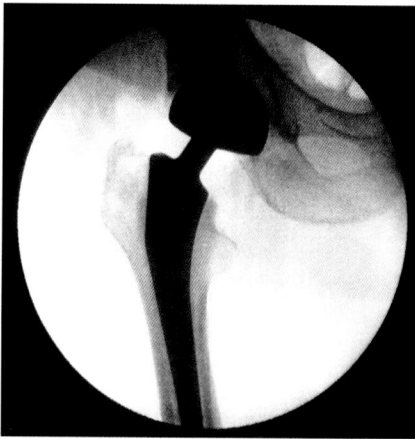

Figure 1b. Intraoperative radiograph of the same patient in 1a after implantation of a bipolar prosthesis. The positive eccentric cup is self-aligning to avoid varus position, which can lead to wear and dislocation in concentric cup-constructions

acetabulum, the bipolar construction of the femoral head as described by Bateman[5] and Giliberty[6] a method was devised to avoid this complication, thereby providing this type of arthroplasty for a wider range of clinical applications.[7-8]

Advantages of hemiarthroplasty meet the needs of the geriatric patient by shortening operating time significantly while reducing blood-loss and operative trauma. Therapy-register statistics show operating time for hemiarthroplasties is 20 minutes shorter than for total hip replacement. Ekkernkamp and colleagues reported that of 3,857 patients with femoral neck fractures from the therapy register of Westphalia-Lippe 43.3% of the hemiarthroplasties were performed in less than one hour, whereas only 15.5% of the total replacements were completed in that time. Blood loss was significantly higher for total replacement; 53.5% of the patients needed blood supply compared to 39.2% of those treated by hemiarthroplasty. Early postoperative complication rates showed no significant difference between the two groups.[9]

Polyethylene-wear with consecutive aseptic inflammatory reaction and loosening of the implant were complications of bipolar heads with the polyethylene-layer facing the acetabular cartilage. These problems could be overcome by using a metal outer cup covering the polyethylene layer. The first bipolar systems used a concentric structure of the cup, which could not avoid mal-positioning of the cup in varus, led to an impingement of the femoral neck on the polyethylene cup with particle wear, cup breakage and dislocation of the prosthesis in up to 18%. To reduce these complications, a positive eccentric cup construction was introduced and yielded better results.[10-13] Currently, the dislocation rates after hemiarthroplasties are below that of total replacements and are reported to be below 1%.[9]

SURGICAL TECHNIQUE

At the University Hospital in Aachen we have been performing bipolar hemiarthroplasty in the treatment of geriatric patients with fractures of the femoral neck since 1994, using positive eccentric bipolar cups and a modular prosthesis-system, both provided by Argomedical AG, Cham, Switzerland. Taking biologic age into consideration in patients older than 70 years, fractures of the Garden I type receive a functional treatment without operation. Garden II or Pauwels I fractures are treated by internal fixation using lag screws. Fractures of the Pauwels II-III or Garden III-IV types are treated by arthroplasty, using bipolar hemiarthroplasty in cases with no major degenerative changes of the joint, whereas total arthroplasty is performed in patients with concomitant coxarthrosis.

Surgery is performed within the first 24 hours after admittance to the hospital, following diagnosis of a femoral neck fracture in an elderly patient—as long as no short-term improvement of the general state indicates a delay for surgery and no severe general contraindications are present. Surgery is performed with the patient in the supine position, using an anterolateral approach, which minimizes muscular trauma, important for early mobilization. After opening the joint by a T-shaped cut, a portion of the anterior capsule is resected to facilitate implantation. Osteotomy of the femoral neck is then performed, followed by the extraction of the femoral head. After calibrating the size of the cup, using the patient's fractured femoral head, the acetabulum is checked for degenerative changes, which are a contraindication to performing hemiarthroplasty.

In adduction and outside-rotation of the thigh, the femur is then prepared for implantation using osteoprofilers. To facilitate this procedure, a small indentation of the gluteal muscles may be necessary. As cemented arthroplasty is always used in geriatric patients to allow immediate full load bearing postoperatively, the stem size is chosen one size below the last osteoprofiler. After cement-fixation of the stem, the bipolar head is assembled using the implant sizes resulting from the measurement. The femoral head of the prosthesis is inserted into the cup and secured by a polyethylene-locking ring placed in a notch of the polyethylene inlay. To bal-

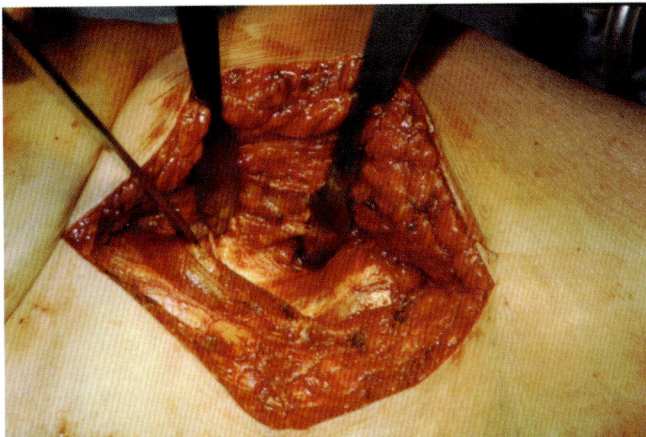

Figure 2. Anterolateral approach to the hip joint, exposing the articular capsule, before opening by a T-shape incision, which allows access to the fractured femoral neck.

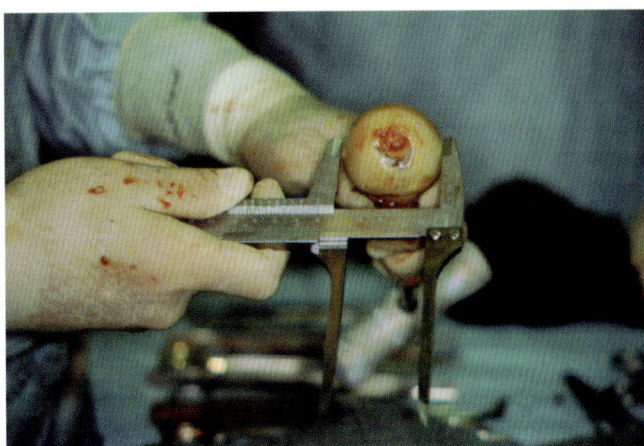

Fig. 3. The extracted femoral head is used for calibrating the cup size. Measurement in different diameters is necessary because of the slightly elliptic shape of the femoral head.

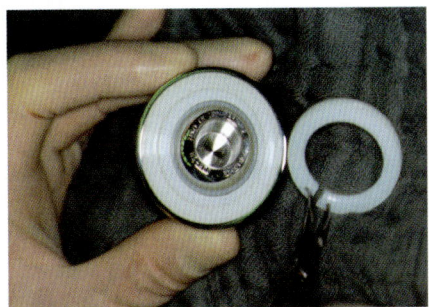

Figure 4a. Inserting the head into the cup with the locking-ring removed assembles cup and head of the prosthesis. After insertion of the head, the ring is placed in the notch of the polyethylene-inlay of the cup.

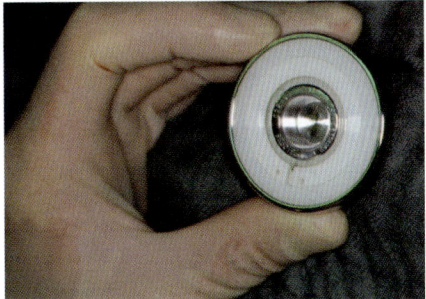

Figure 4b. The bipolar head, ready for the in-situ assembly to the cone of the prosthesis' stem, which is implanted into the proximal femur.

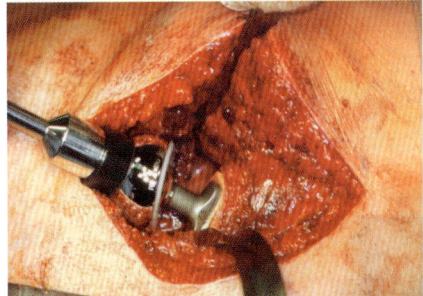

Figure 5. Repositioning the hemiprosthesis into the acetabulum, directing the prosthesis' head, while an assistant performs the reposition maneuver.

ance resection level and length of the femoral neck, different heads can be used. Connecting the bipolar head to the stem and repositioning of the joint are the final steps to completion of the implantation. After controls for dislocation, muscular tension, and length of the limb, the wound is closed, leaving several vacuum drains which are removed after 48 hours.

POSTOPERATIVE CARE

Most patients can return to the ward immediately after operation; in cases of severe concomitant diseases, the patient spends the first day in the intensive care unit. Mobilization begins under the supervision of physiotherapists from the first postoperative day. The patient begins assuming seated and prone positions for short periods on the first day, followed by taking the first steps after wound drains are removed the second or third day. On approximately the 10th day, patients who had lived alone or with their families before hospitalization are transferred to a rehabilitation unit, where further training takes place. During this time, social assistance or nursing care are then organized in preparation for discharge from the hospital.

MATERIAL AND METHODS

To evaluate the results in elderly patients, the authors performed a retrospective outcome study on all types of fractures of the femoral neck and pertrochanteric region, in which patients who had been treated by hemiarthroplasties and by total hip-replacement were evaluated as therapy-groups. Female patients of more than 60 years of age at the date of the injury, who had suffered from fractures of the proximal femur were included in this study. Those who had suffered more than one fracture were excluded.

Focusing on long-term outcome and quality-of-life after-treatment, patients in the study had to have been living alone before the injury without need for nursing help; they all had to pass a four-week stay in a rehabilitation unit (or longer), and had to be able to answer the questionnaires. To exclude demented patients, a minimal mental state screening test was applied.

In the study were patients who had been dismissed from the rehabilitation unit between January 1997 and December 1998, with an interval between operation and investigation of at least six months. Of the patients selected for the investigation, only 4% were able to attend; 96% had to be visited in their homes where the investigation was performed.

The study consisted of a clinical investigation and the review of radiographies. For evaluation purposes, the hip-scores of Harris[14], Iselin[15] and Charnley[16] were applied. Quality-of-life as an outcome measure was evaluated by generic Quality-of-Life questionnaires as the Spitzer Index and a visual

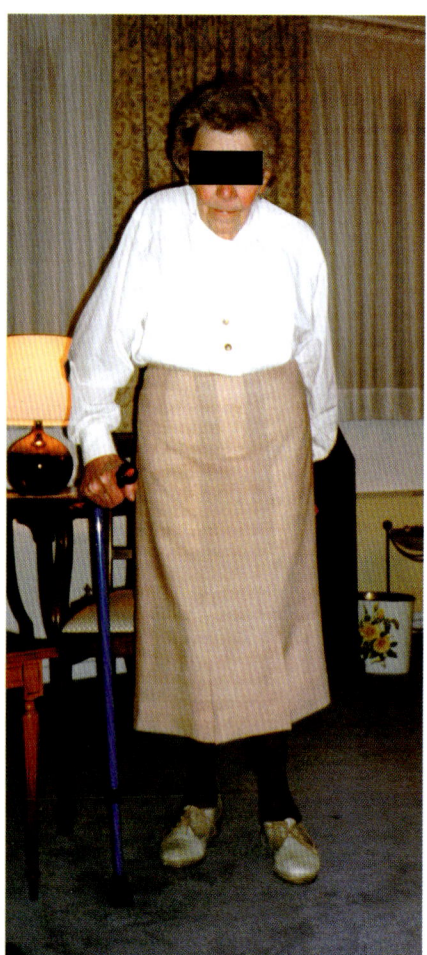

Figure 6. 83-year-old patient, visited in her home for the investigation of the outcome study 18 months after implantation of a bipolar hemiprosthesis for femoral neck fracture. The patient lives alone and receives social help for housekeeping; no nursing help is needed.

analog scale (VAS).

RESULTS

Of the 78 patients included in the study, 67 (86%) were alive at the time of investigation. Three patients had to be excluded because of dementia, another ten refused to participate in the study, and three patients had unknown residences. The remaining 51 patients (65%) could be investigated; 51% of the fractures were on the right, 49% on the left side. The average age at the time of the injury was 78.2 years for all patients; in the group treated with hemiarthroplasties, 80.2 years; in the group with total hip replacement, 78.2 years.

Arthroplasties had been performed primarily in 41% of the patients, half as total replacement and half as hemiarthroplasties. In two patients after primary internal fixation, reoperation was necessary with arthroplasty performed in the second operation.

Primary hospital stays were shorter for the hemiarthroplasty-group, an average of 20.9 days, compared with 35.9 days for the patients with total replacement.

Concerning complications, no wound infection or dislocation of the prosthesis as noted in the two joint replacement groups; no thrombembolic complications occurred. One patient after total hip replacement could not be mobilized with full load bearing in the first weeks, because stem implantation had led to a fissure of the femoral shaft.

Time spent in the rehabilitation unit after discharge from the surgical department showed no differences in the two groups, whereas the total replacement patients received more therapy units than the other group (57.2 therapy-units compared to 46 units after hemiarthroplasty). The average time between dismissal from the rehabilitation unit and investigation was 19.9 months after total hip replacement and 18.6 months after hemiarthroplasty.

At the time of the investigation, all patients lived in their own apartments except one, who had moved into an institution. Before the injury, if walking without devices was possible for all patients, by the time of the investigation 60% needed a device regardless of the arthroplastic procedure.

The hip-score ratings for the hemiarthroplasty-group were good; i.e., over 80% in the scores of Iselin,[14] Harris,[15] and Charnley.[16] In all scores, the hemiarthroplasty ratings were higher than those of the total replacement group.

The quality-of-life measures yielded higher ratings after hemiarthroplasty compared to total hip replacement. The VAS as a global measure for quality of life was significantly higher after hemiarthroplasty, with a value of 68.4 compared to 53.8 after total replacement.

The Spitzer-Index rated higher for hemiarthroplasty in the scales, "Activity," "Health," "Social Contact," and "Future." In the scale, "Everyday Life" ratings were higher for total hip replacement.

DISCUSSION

The modern bipolar hip prostheses, providing a positive eccentric cup design, have been shown to minimize acetabular erosion and the tendency to dislocate, reported in up to 18 % after implantation of systems containing a concentric cup.[10] Although the different procedures remain controversial, most authors view advantages for the bipolar arthoplasty, as treatment of femoral neck fractures in the elderly.[2,17-19]

Bipolar systems have been implanted by some authors not only in geriatric patients, but also in those without limitation of age after destruction of the femoral head due to trauma or ischemia, as long as the acetabulum was not damaged.[20-21] For these patients Takeshi and colleagues report a high rate of aseptic inflammatory reactions, with loosening of the stem after cementless implantation of the bipolar hemiarthroplasties. The average age of patients in their study was 41 (21–66) years. They noted that the loosening takes place due to polyethylene wear particles, caused by impingement of the polyethylene cup against the stem of the prosthesis.[21] Kim and colleagues reported similar results, using hemiarthroplasty in young patients with an average age of 48.4 years.[20] The phenomenon is clinically relevant only in biologically younger patients with a wider range of motion in the hip-joint and higher degree of daily activity, compared to elderly patients in this study and of others who report good to excellent results after hemiarthroplasty.[22-24]

The impingement phenomenon must be taken into consideration in the technologic construction of bipolar heads, to meet the demands of a wide range of motion between cup and head of the prosthesis, and a specially designed contact area between cup and stem to minimize friction and wear.

In this study, hemiarthroplasty yielded superior results in all score systems compared to total hip replacement, which may have been partially caused by the concomitant coxarthrosis in the total replacement group that created a more complex situation. It also may have been of some influence–considering the small number of patients–that the two patients who had to be reoperated after primary internal-fixation, were treated by total replacement, as inferior results after secondary arthroplasty after internal fixation of femoral neck fractures have been reported.[25] The extremely low number of complications and good reintegration results in this study compared to others justified the strict limitations for patients to be included in the study.[10,13,19,22,23] However, the limitations were necessary to make a quality-of-life evaluation possible and reduce the variances of influence.

Broos states that in 32% of the elderly patients in this study, a femoral neck fracture indicated a serious additional impairment.[23] This situation must be taken into consideration when health costs are calculated. The high number of patients in this study who could return to their preoperative daily life circumstances, underlines the importance of special rehabilitative measures.[18,19,26] Only the combination of surgery, which takes into consideration the bodily condition of the elderly, and a good rehabilitation and reintegration are able to keep the patient's quality of life on a level close to the pre-injury state. To evaluate surgical procedures regarding this aim, including reducing the long-term health costs, one should measure the quality-of-life aspect, (i.e., the subjective result), in the same fashion as clinical outcome.[27]

CONCLUSION

Given that there was coxarthrosis was a complicating factor in the total replacement group, our results show that hemiarthroplasty yields favorable results after femoral neck fractures in elderly patients. Considering the advantages of hemiarthroplasty—shorter operation time, reduced blood-loss and lower dislocation rate—the authors view see this procedure as the treatment of first choice for elderly patients with no or only moderate degenerative changes of the acetabulum, if surgical treatment of a femoral neck fracture is indicated. Considering the high loosening rate reported for younger patients, the authors restrict this method to patients over 70 years of age.

REFERENCES

1. Lo W-H, Chen W-M, Huang C-K, et al. Bateman Bipolar Hemiarthroplasty for Displaced Intracapsular Femoral Neck Fractures. Clin.Orthop 1994;302: 75-82.
2. Hudson JI, Kenzora JE, Hebel JR et al. Eight-year outcome associated with clinical options in the management of femoral neck fractures. Clin Orthop 1998;(348): 59-66.
3. Lindequist S. An algorithm for preoperative prediction of reoperation risk after internal fixation of femoral neck fractures. Comput Methods Programs Biomed 1998; 57(3): 187-199.
4. Siebler G, Edler G, Kuner EH. Zur Totalendoprothese bei der Schenkelhalsfraktur des alten Menschen. Unfallchirug 1988; 91: 291.
5. Bateman JE. Single assembly total hip prosthesis: Preliminary report. Orthop Digest 1974; 2: 15-22.
6. Giliberty R.P. A new concept of a bipolar endoprosthesis. Orthop Rev 1974; 3: 40-45.
7. Phillips TW. Thompson Hemiarthoplasty and Acetabular Erosion. J.Bone Joint Surg.Am. 1989; 71A: 913-917.
8. Devas M, Hinves B. Prevention of Acetabular Erosion after Hemiarthroplasty for Fractured Neck of Femur. J.Bone Joint Surg. 1983 ; 65 B: 548-551.
9. Ekkernkamp A, Overbeck S, Haeske-Seeberg H. Total- oder Hemiprothese - Kann die externe Qualitätssicherung zur Entscheidung beitragen? Breyer H-G, editor. Bipolare Hüftgelenksendoprothetik. Reinbek, Einhorn-Presse Verlag GmbH; 1996. 62-66.
10. Möllers M, Stedtfeld HW, Paechtner S et al. Hemiarthroplastik des Hüftgelenks: Konzentrische oder positiv exzentrische (selbstzentrierende) Duokopfprothese. Unfallchirurg 1992; 95: 224-229.
11. Herzenberg JE, Harrelson JM, Campbell II D.C. et al. Fractures of the polyethylene bearing insert in Bateman bipolar hip prostheses. Clin.Orthop. 1988; 228: 88-93.
12. Ekkernkamp A, Ostermann PAW, Muhr G. Die selbstausrichtend-bipolare Prothese–prospektive Evaluation eines neuen Systems. Breyer H-G, editor. Bipolare Hüftgelenksendoprothetik. Reinbek, Einhorn-Presse Verlag GmbH; 1996. 105-112.
13. Möllers M, Schätzler A. Klinische Erfahrungen mit 1133 bipolaren Duokopfprothesen. Breyer H-G, editor. Bipolare Hüftgelenksendoprothetik Reinbek, Einhorn-Presse Verlag GmbH; 1996. 113-115.
14. Iselin M. Metallprothesen nach Schenkelhalsfrakturen. Nachuntersuchung von 75 Prothesen. Arch.Orthop.Trauma Surg. 1968; 63: 52-64.
15. Harris WH. Traumatic arthritis of the hip after dislocation and acetabular fractures:treatment by Mold arthroplasty. J.Bone Joint Surg.Am. 1969 ; 51-A: 737-755.
16. Charnley J. The long-term results of low-friction arthroplasty of the hip performed as aprimary intervention. J.Bone Joint Surg. 1972 ; 54-B: 61-76.
17. Burns RB, Moskowitz MA, Ash A et al. Do hip replacements improve outcomes for hip fracture patients? Med Care 1999; 37(3): 285-294.
18. Cornell CN, Levine D, O'Doherty J et al. Unipolar versus bipolar hemiarthroplasty for the treatment of femoral neck fractures in the elderly. Clin Orthop 1998;(348): 67-71.
19. Kenzora JE, Magaziner J, Hudson J et al. Outcome after hemiarthroplasty for femoral neck fractures in the elderly. Clin Orthop 1998;(348): 51-58.
20. Kim YH, Kim JS, Cho SH. Primary total hip arthroplasty with a cementless porous-coated anatomic total hip prosthesis: 10- to 12-year results of prospective and consecutive series. J Arthroplasty 1999; 14(5): 538-548.
21. Nishii T, Sugano N, Masuhara KT. Bipolar Cup Design may lead to Osteolysis around the Uncemented Femoral Comonent. Clin.Orthop. 1995; 316: 112-120.
22. Maricevic A, Erceg M, Gekic K. [Treatment of femoral neck fractures with bipolar hemiarthroplasty]. Lijec Vjesn 1998; 120(5): 121-124.
23. Broos PL. Prosthetic replacement in the management of unstable femoral neck fractures in the elderly. Analysis of the mechanical complications noted in 778 fractures. Acta Chir Belg 1999; 99(4):190-194.
24. Matsuno T. Geriatric femoral neck fractures--how to regain prefracture ambulatory status. Hokkaido Igaku Zasshi 1997; 72(4): 377-380.
25. Perka C, Ludwig R, Stern S. Total endoprosthetic management of the hip joint after failed osteosynthesis of para-articular hip fracture. Z Orthop Ihre Grenzgeb 2000; 138(1): 39-45.
26. Chamberlin B, Laude F, Rolland E et al. Evaluation of the direct cost of trochanteric fractures in the elderly. Rev Chir Orthop Reparatrice Appar Mot 1997; 83(7): 629-635.
27. Knahr K, Kryspin-Exner I, Jagsch R et al. Evaluating the quality of life before and after implantation of a total hip endoprothesis. Z Orthop Ihre Grenzgeb 1998; 136(4):321-329.

Management of Venous Thrombosis and Thromboembolism: Prevention and Treatment

RODGER L. BICK, M.D., PH.D., F.A.C.P.
CLINICAL PROFESSOR OF MEDICINE AND PATHOLOGY
UNIVERSITY OF TEXAS SOUTHWESTERN MEDICAL CENTER
DIRECTOR, DALLAS THROMBOSIS HEMOSTASIS & DIFFICULT HEMATOLOGY CLINICAL CENTER
DALLAS, TX

Thrombosis is a common cause of death in the United States. More than two million people die each year from an arterial or venous thrombosis, or the consequences thereof.[1] Approximately an equal number suffer non-fatal thrombosis; for example, deep venous thrombosis (DVT), non-fatal pulmonary embolus (PE), non-fatal cerebrovascular thrombosis (CVT), transient cerebral ischemic attacks (40% of these have a fatal or non-fatal CVT within one year),[2] non-fatal coronary artery thrombosis, retinal vascular thrombosis (RVT), and other non-fatal thrombotic deaths. These numbers emphasize the scope of the problem. By contrast, approximately 550,000 people will die this year in the United States from cancer; thus, fatal thrombosis is approximately four times as prevalent as fatality from malignancy.[1] Thrombosis, therefore, accounts for extraordinary morbidity, mortality, and cost of medical care.[1]

Many, if not most, episodes of thrombosis can be prevented by appropriate primary antithrombotic therapy, and most instances of recurrence can be prevented by appropriate choice of secondary therapy.[3] Approximately 80% to 90% of all unexplained episodes of venous thrombosis (non-traumatic and non-surgical), and approximately 65% of arterial thrombosis are associated with a blood coagulation protein or platelet defect that can now be defined with respect to cause.[3,4] Of these, approximately 50% of all patients harbor a congenital and 50% harbor an acquired blood coagulation protein or platelet defect that caused the thrombotic event.[1,3]

To better understand the scope of the problem, specific examples are: the incidence of DVT in the United States is approximately 159/100,000, or 450,000/year. The overall incidence of PE in the United States is approximately 139 cases/100,000, or 355,000 cases/year (clinical data); the incidence of fatal PE in the United States is 94/100,000, or approximately 240,000 deaths (autopsy data).[5-7] The incidence of fatal and non-fatal thrombotic events are summarized in Table 1.

The causes of hypercoagulability and overt thrombosis are becoming more clear and often definitive, with enhanced knowledge of hemostasis and development and extended use of testing systems for evaluating patients with thrombotic and thromboembolic disorders.[8] Using these test systems, in conjunction with careful clinical assessment of patients, approximately 80% to 90% of patients with thrombosis will have defined etiologic findings.[1,3,4] Many of these will have an obvious clinical condition that leads to thrombosis, and at least 50% to 80% will have an underlying hereditary or acquired blood protein/platelet defect that causes or contributes to thrombosis.

Many clinical conditions are associated with an increased risk of arterial or venous thrombosis and thromboembolism; the more common of these and blood coagulation protein/platelet defects associated with thrombosis are summarized in Table 2.[1] However, in many instances a clinical situation associated with thrombosis, particularly surgery or trauma, serves to unmask a congenital or acquired blood coagulation protein/platelet defect.

Cost-containing[9] and effective management of thrombosis, and reducing morbidity, mortality, and costs center around three interrelated areas: (1) clear definition of the cause of thrombosis, (2) appropriate secondary prevention (prevention of recurrence), and (3) appropriate primary (prophylactic) therapy for first events.

DEFINITION OF ETIOLOGY

Many instances of venous thrombosis are unexplained (unassociated with surgery, trauma, cardiac emboli, etc.).

The more common and rarer blood coagulation protein/platelet defects that lead to thrombosis are summarized in Table 2. Of major importance is to define persons who harbor these defects, to allow for: (1) appropriate secondary antithrombotic therapy to decrease risks of recurrence, (2) determining length of time the patient must remain on therapy for secondary prevention, and (3) testing of family members in those who harbor a hereditary blood-coagulation protein or platelet defect (~50% of all coagulation and platelet defects mentioned above), thus allowing for primary prevention in appropriate relatives. The prevalence of many of these defects is high.[3,4,10]

Thrombosis should no longer be viewed as a generic diagnosis; approaching thrombosis improperly probably accounts for many treatment failures. Failure to make a specific diagnosis accounts for enhanced morbidity and mortality and exorbitant, unnecessary medical costs for recurrent episodes.

Prophylaxis of Venous Thromboembolism

Numerous studies have provided evidence that patients who undergo surgery or trauma are at significant risk for developing venous thromboembolic complications, including PE, and general medical patients also are at risk. Thus, an important task for the medical profession is to prevent DVT and its complications and morbid sequelae (PE, chronic venous insufficiency, compartmental compression syndromes, other morbidity and mortality). Therefore, it is important to define risk groups, by quantifying risk(s) when possible, where prophylaxis must be considered.

Unfortunately, the attitudes and opinions, and occasionally "myths," regarding prophylaxis show immense regional variability.[11] Variations include the definition of risk groups, numbers of patients receiving prophylaxis, and prophylactic modalities used. For this reason, various "consensus conference" groups have been formed in attempts to alleviate these problems. Formerly, at least three consensus conference groups existed: American College of Chest Physicians (ACCP, begun in 1986),[12] European Consensus Conference Groups (begun in 1991),[13] and Scandinavian Consensus Conference Group (begun in 1995).[14] Since then, the International Consensus Conference group, derived from the European Group, has been formed and encompasses experts from the other groups.[11,15] The primary purpose of consensus guidelines is to provide optimal direction to the prac-

Table 1. Incidence of thrombosis in USA

DISEASE	USA INCIDENCE/100,000	TOTAL IN USA/YEARS (CASES)	DEFINABLE REASON
DEEP VEIN THROMBOSIS (DVT)	159/100,000	450,000	≅80%
PULMONARY EMBOLUS (PE)	139/100,000	355,000	≅80%
FATAL PULMONARY EMBOLUS	94/100,000	240,000	≅80%
MYOCARDIAL INFARCTION (AMI)	600/100,000	1,500,000	≅67%
FATAL MYOCARDIAL INFARCTION	300/100,000	750,000	≅67%
CEREBROVASCULAR THROMBOSIS (CVT)	600/100,000	1,500,000	≅30%
FATAL CEREBROVASCULAR THROMBOSIS	396/100,000	990,000	≅30%
TOTAL SERIOUS THROMBOSES IN USA	1498/100,000	5,785,000	≅50%
TOTAL DEATHS FROM ABOVE THROMBOSES	790/100,000	1,990,000	≅50%
ALL CANCER IN USA 1996	544/100,000	1,359,150	
CANCER DEATHS IN USA 1996	222/100,000	554,740	

Table 2. Causes of thrombosis

CLINICAL CONDITIONS ARTERIAL	CLINICAL CONDITIONS VENOUS	BLOOD PROTEIN & PLATELET DEFECTS
ATHEROSCLEROSIS	GENERAL SURGERY	ANTIPHOSPHOLIPID SYNDROME
CIGARETTE SMOKING	ORTHOPEDIC SURGERY	APC RESISTANCE
HYPERTENSION	ARTHROSCOPY	FACTOR V LEIDEN
DIABETES MELLITUS	TRAUMA	STICKY PLATELET SYNDROME
LDL CHOLESTEROL	MALIGNANCY	PROTHROMBIN G 20210A
HYPERTRIGLYCERIDEMIA	IMMOBILITY	PROTEIN S DEFECTS
POSITIVE FAMILY HISTORY	SEPSIS	PROTEIN C DEFECTS
LEFT VENTRICULAR FAILURE	CONGESTIVE HEART FAILURE	ANTITHROMBIN DEFECTS
ORAL CONTRACEPTIVES	NEPHROTIC SYNDROME	HEPARIN COFACTOR II DEFECTS
ESTROGENS	OBESITY	PLASMINOGEN DEFECTS
LIPOPROTEIN (a)	VARICOSE VEINS	TPA DEFECTS
POLYCYTHEMIA	POST-PHLEBITIC SYNDROME	PAI-1 DEFECTS
HYPERVISCOSITY SYNDROMES	ORAL CONTRACEPTIVES	FACTOR XII DEFECTS
LEUKOSTASIS SYNDROMES	ESTROGENS	DYSFIBRINOGENEMIA
		HOMOCYSTINEMIA
		MTHFR MUTATIONS
		FACTOR V CAMBRIDGE
		IMMUNE VASCULITIS

LDL = low-density lipoproteins
APC = activated protein C
TPA = tissue plasminogen activator
PAI-1 = plasminogen activator inhibitor
MTHFR = methyltetrahydrofolate reductase

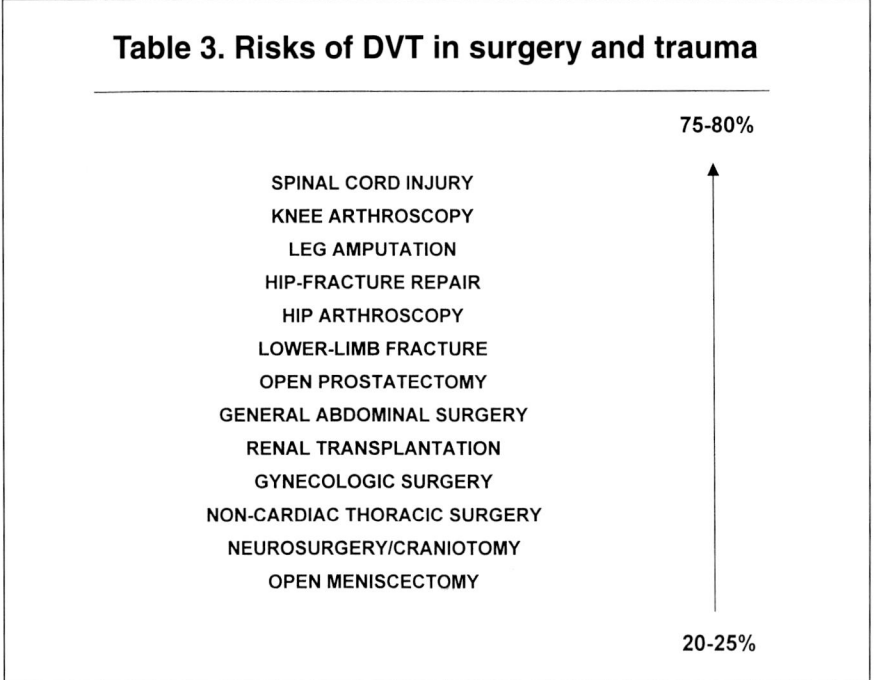

Table 3. Risks of DVT in surgery and trauma

75-80%

SPINAL CORD INJURY
KNEE ARTHROSCOPY
LEG AMPUTATION
HIP-FRACTURE REPAIR
HIP ARTHROSCOPY
LOWER-LIMB FRACTURE
OPEN PROSTATECTOMY
GENERAL ABDOMINAL SURGERY
RENAL TRANSPLANTATION
GYNECOLOGIC SURGERY
NON-CARDIAC THORACIC SURGERY
NEUROSURGERY/CRANIOTOMY
OPEN MENISCECTOMY

20-25%

Table 4. Levels of risk

TYPE OF THROMBOSIS	CALF (%)	PROXIMAL (%)	FATAL PE (%)
HIGH RISK (=3)	40-80	10-30	>1
MODERATE RISK (= 2)	10-40	1-10	0.1-1.0
LOW RISK (=1)	<10	<1	< 0.1

PE = PULMONARY EMBOLUS

ticing physician/surgeon. If practice guidelines generated are successful, clinicians are assisted in decision-making for individual patients and provided protection against unjustified malpractice actions.[16]

PE is responsible for approximately 150,000 to 240,000 deaths/year in the United States.[17-19] The incidence of DVT in the United States is approximately 160/100,000, or 450,000 cases/year; approximately 30% to 50% of undetected, untreated DVT will progress to PE and approximately 40% with DVT will develop chronic venous insufficiency, with the chances increasing approximately six-fold with each recurrent episode.[1,20,21] Despite significant advances in prevention and treatment of venous thromboembolism (venous thrombosis ± PE), PE remains the most common preventable cause of hospital death.[22] Venous thromboembolism often occurs in the setting of surgery, trauma, and other medical conditions, but also may affect ambulant, healthy people. Thus, prevention is major to reducing death and morbidity from venous thromboembolism. Effective and safe prophylactic measures to prevent DVT, PE, and attendant sequelae are currently available for most high-risk patients.[23-25] Table 3 lists the ascending probability of DVT with surgical procedures and trauma.[26] A recent study shows that despite innumerable consensus conference meetings and resultant publications, surgeons in the United States are apparently not yet offering appropriate prophylaxis to appropriate patients and appropriate numbers of patients.[27]

Surgical Prophylaxis

Without prophylaxis, the frequency of fatal PE ranges from 0.1% to 0.8% in patients who undergo elective general surgery,[17,28-32] 2% to 3% in those who undergo elective hip replacement,[33] and 4% to 7% in those who undergo surgery for a fractured hip.[34] Guidelines for risk assessment are defined in Table 4.[11] The risk of postoperative DVT can be identified as low, moderate, or high, depending on the surgical procedure and presence or absence of additional risk factors.[11,29] See Figures 1 and 2 for guidelines for assessing risk in general, orthopedic, and gynecologic surgery patients.

Surgery for major trauma or orthopedic surgery, followed by abdominal surgery, is associated with a risk rate of up to 30%.[17] However, the degree of risk is increased by predisposing risk factors, including age, morbidity, malignancy, obesity, prior history of thromboembolism, immobility, varicose veins, recent operative procedures, and hereditary or acquired thrombophilia.[11] These factors are further modified by general care, including duration and type of anesthesia, pre- and postoperative immobilization, level of hydration, and presence of sepsis.[11] Thus, the individual risk is determined by the type of surgery and an accumulation of predisposing factors; i.e., patients who undergo minor surgery, but bear several additional risk factors, also may be at high risk for thromboembolic complications.[11] As many medical patients may become surgical candidates, risk assessment for medical patients is shown in Figure 3.

APPROACHES TO THROMBOPROPHYLAXIS

The prophylactic measures used most commonly are low-molecular-weight heparin (LMWH), low-dose or adjusted-dose unfractionated heparin (UFH), oral anticoagulants [(a) International Normalized Ratio (INR) of 2 to 3, (b) fixed low dose, or (c) dose-adjusted to prothrombin time (PT) 1.3 to 1.5 seconds prolonged], intermittent pneumatic leg compression, and graduated compression stockings (GCS), in probable descending order of efficacy, depending on procedure and other clinical circumstances.[11] Other less common measures include the use of aspirin and intravenous (IV) dextran.[11]

It has become standard practice to commence prophylaxis (e.g., with low-dose heparin) before anesthesia in patients who undergo thoracic or abdominal surgery; in Europe, prophylaxis is started the night before surgery in patients who undergo total hip- or

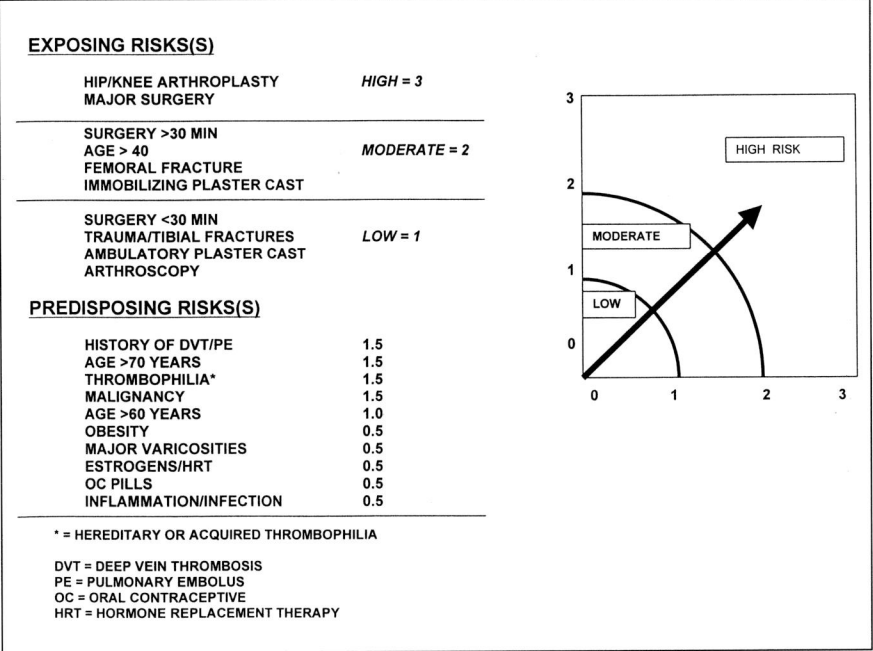

Figure 1. Guidelines for risk assessment – general and orthopedic surgery.

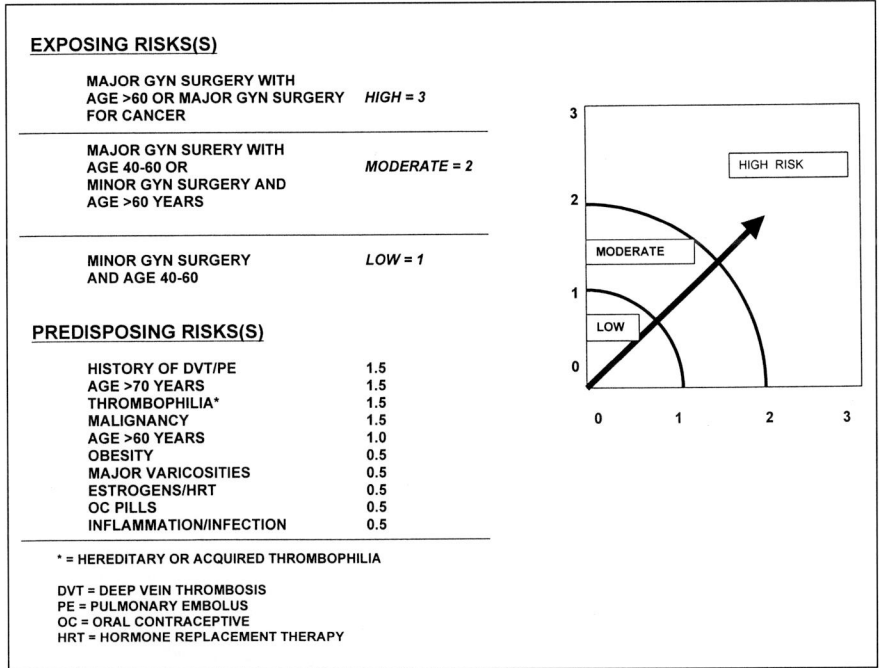

Figure 2. Guidelines for risk assessment – gynecologic surgery.

total knee-replacement surgery.[11] In North America, because of the concern related to perioperative bleeding, prophylaxis for patients who have total knee or total hip replacement has often been started postoperatively.[35,36] This difference in the patterns of practice may account for the differences in the rates of postoperative venous thrombosis in Europe and North America.[11] A recent randomized trial failed to note a significant difference in DVT or bleeding when LMWH was started preoperatively or postoperatively.[37]

Low-Dose Unfractionated Heparin (UFH)

The effectiveness of low-dose UFH for preventing DVT has been established by multiple randomized clinical trials.[23-25,30,38] Low-dose subcutaneous (s.c.) heparin is usually given in a dose of 5000 U 2 hours preoperatively, and then postoperatively every 8 or 12 hours. The incidence of major bleeding complications is not increased by low-dose heparin, but an increase in minor wound hematomas is present. The platelet count should be monitored every other day in all patients on low-dose heparin to detect heparin-induced thrombocytopenia.[39] Low-dose UFH is relatively inexpensive, easily administered, and does not require monitoring, except mandatory platelet counts.

Low-Molecular-Weight Heparin (LMWH)

A number of LMWH fractions have been evaluated by randomized clinical trials in general surgical patients.[39-48] In randomized clinical trials that compared LMWH with UFH, the LMWH given once or twice daily are as effective or more effective in preventing thrombosis.[39-48] The incidence of bleeding is significantly lower in patients receiving LMWH versus UFH by noting a reduction in wound hematomas, severe bleeding, and those who required repeat surgery for bleeding.[41]

Although the number of patients who undergo total knee replacement currently, equals those who undergo total hip replacements, fewer trials have been conducted in this patient population.[49-52] The incidence of DVT with LMWH is significantly lower than those with warfarin.[49-51,53] Recent studies have shown that LMWH is superior to UFH in patients who suffer multiple trauma.[53]

Oral Anticoagulants

Warfarins can be started preoperatively, at the time of surgery or in the early postoperative period; however, if started at the time of surgery or in the early postoperative period they may not prevent small venous thrombi from forming during surgery, or after surgery, as an antithrombotic effect is not achieved until the third or fourth postoperative day.[11,17] However, oral anticoagulants may be effective in inhibiting the extension of thrombi and potentially preventing otherwise clinically significant venous thromboembolism.[11,17]

Low-dose warfarin, however, does not provide protection against DVT following hip or knee replacement.[54]

Intermittent Pneumatic Leg Compression

Intermittent pneumatic leg compression is effective for preventing DVT in moderate-risk general surgical patients,[55] in patients who undergo neurosurgery,[56] and cardiac surgery.[57] In patients who undergo hip surgery, intermittent pneumatic compression (IPC) of the calf is ineffective for proximal vein thrombosis.[58]

Graduated Compression Stockings (GCS)

GCS are a simple, safe, and moderately effective form of thromboprophylaxis. GCS are recommended in low-risk patients, and only as an adjunct in those with medium and high risk.[11] The only major contraindication is peripheral vascular disease. However, no conclusive evidence exists that GCS are effective in reducing the incidence of fatal and nonfatal PE.[11]

SPECIFIC RECOMMENDATIONS FOR PROPHYLACTIC MODALITIES IN VARIOUS SURGICAL PATIENTS [11,15]

Low-Risk General Surgical Patients (e.g., minor surgery without risk factors)

The data are insufficient to make any recommendations. On the basis of risk:benefit ratio and extrapolation from studies in moderate-risk patients, the practice in some countries is to use GCS in addition to early ambulation and adequate hydration.[11,15]

Moderate-Risk General Surgical Patients (e.g., major surgery, age >40 years, or surgery >30 minutes without additional risk factors)

The use of LMWH or UFH is recommended for all moderate-risk patients. An alternative recommendation is IPC used continuously until the patient is ambulant, graduated elastic compression stockings, or a combination of both. These are grade A recommendations based on Level I or Level II data.[11,15]

Further studies are needed to assess the effect of using GCS, IPC, or both, in addition to pharmacologic methods and the combined effects of different pharmacologic methods such as heparin plus aspirin versus heparin alone.

High-Risk General Surgical Patients (e.g., major surgery, age >60 years or presence of additional risk factors)

All should receive prophylaxis, as for moderate-risk patients (Grade A recommendation).[11,15] In addition to single modalities such as LMWH or UFH, combined modalities of pharmacologic (LMWH or UFH) and mechanical methods should be considered, as they may be more effective (Grade B recommendation).[11,15]

In moderate- and high-risk patients, dextran and aspirin are not the methods of choice because of their limited efficacy for DVT prevention, the anaphylactoid reactions, and danger of cardiac overload associated with the former, the high dose of aspirin (1000 to 1500) mg/day required, and the fact that oral medications are not possible for several days in patients who have abdominal surgery.[11,15]

Guidelines for scoring risk assessment, in general, and orthopedic surgical patients are summarized in Figure 1.

Neurosurgery

Neurosurgery patients should be considered for mechanical methods of

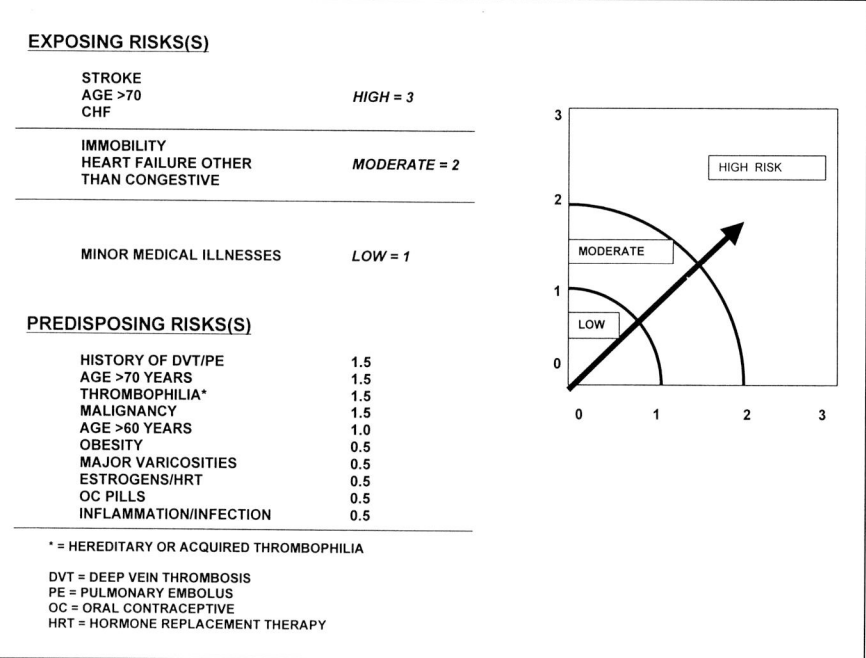

Figure 3. Guidelines for risk assessment – medical patients.

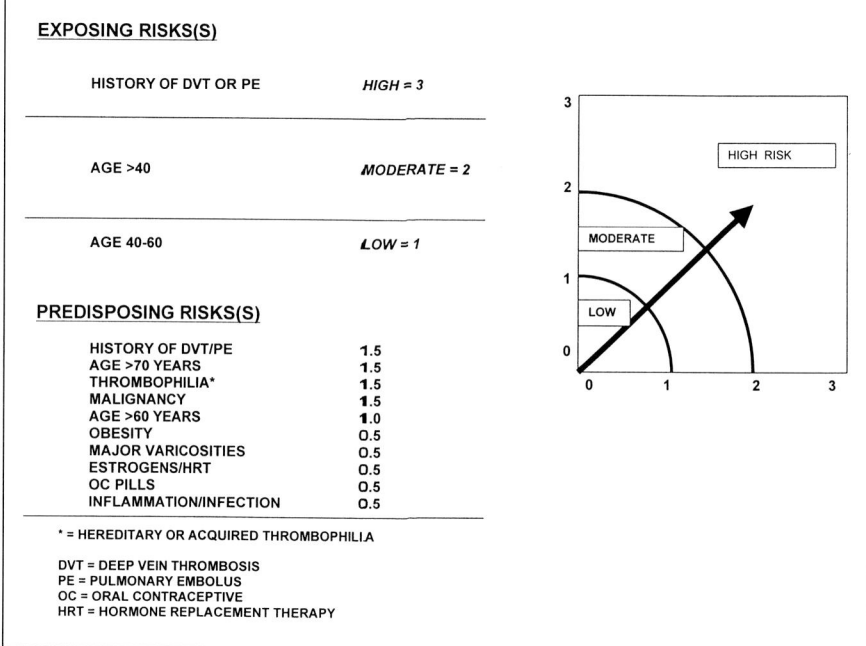

Figure 4. Guidelines for risk assessment – obstetrics.

prophylaxis. In three randomized controlled studies involving a total of 422 patients, the incidence of DVT was reduced from 21.3% in controls to 6.0% in the prophylactic groups using IPC (relative risk, 0.28; 95% CI: 0.16 to 0.51); (Grade A recommendation).[11,15]

Orthopedic Surgery and Trauma
Elective Hip Replacement

Fixed, low-dose UFH, 5000 IU every 8 or 12 hours, is effective for reducing DVT (Level I data) and PE (Level II data) in patients who have elective hip replacement. Increasing the dose leads to a greater risk of bleeding.[11,15]

LMWH appears superior to UFH in reducing both DVT and PE for hip-replacement surgery, but more studies are needed.[11,15] Fixed "mini-dose" oral anticoagulant therapy is not effective.[11,15,36]

Antiplatelet therapy (mainly aspirin) in elective hip surgery is only moderately effective for protection against DVT (relative risk, 0.70; 95% CI: 0.61 to 0.82); (Level II evidence), but the observed reduction in the risk of PE is substantial (relative risk, 0.49; 95% CI: 0.26 to 0.92); (Level II evidence).[11,15] The effect of aspirin on PE needs confirmation.

The incidence of efficacy of graduated elastic compression alone after hip-replacement surgery has not been well described in the literature, but its use in orthopedic surgery is supported by data extrapolated from general surgery (Grade C recommendation). IPC is effective (Level I evidence).[11,15]

Elective Knee Replacement

Fewer studies are available on prophylaxis after knee replacement. Data from hip replacement should not be extrapolated to knee replacement.[11]

IPC is effective (Level I evidence). Evidence exists that LMWH is more effective than warfarin, and more effective than UFH (Level I evidence).[11,15] Some data exist to support the combined use of regional anesthesia with graduated elastic compression. In most randomized controlled trials, after knee replacement, the absolute risk of DVT remains high despite prophylaxis.[11]

Duration of Prophylaxis in Elective Orthopedic Surgery

The optimal duration of prophylaxis in elective orthopedic surgery has not been established. As intraoperative risk factors are probably important, prophylaxis should ideally be started before surgery. A randomized comparison of preoperative and postoperative commencement of pharmacologic prophylaxis is necessary.

Most trials have studied prophylaxis for 7 to 10 days, or until the patients are ambulatory; however, three recent randomized controlled studies in patients who have hip arthroplasty indicate more prolonged thromboprophylaxis with LMWH decreases the frequency of venographically detected DVT.[11,15]

Emergency Orthopedic Surgery

The risks of DVT/PE, including fatal PE, are high in patients with hip fractures. Prophylaxis should be started as soon as possible after diagnosis, and should be the same as recommended for elective hip surgery. The best results so far have been obtained from studies using LMWH.[11,15] LD-UFH is effective in reduction of DVT, and although an overview of trials has not demonstrated a significant reduction in total PE, the observed effect was not different from that noted in general surgery and a significant reduction was noted in fatal PE.[11,15]

Guidelines for risk assessment in orthopedic patients also are summarized in Figure 1.

Multiple Trauma

Multiple-trauma patients are at high risk for thrombosis and LMWH represents the prophylaxis of choice.[15,45,59] IPC may be used when feasible, as this is unassociated with any bleeding risk. Other alternatives include low-dose UFH or warfarin based on extrapolation from other high-risk situations such as hip-fracture and hip-replacement surgery. Insertion of an inferior vena cava filter may be considered for high-risk situations in which anticoagulants may be contraindicated. However, recent randomized trials have questioned the efficacy of caval filters and suggest these devices may increase the incidence of DVT while not protecting against PE in some people.[60,61]

Acute Spinal Cord Injury Associated With Paralysis

LMWH is the most effective prophylaxis.[62] Adjusted-dose heparin also has been shown to be effective. Low-dose heparin and IPC are less effective. Combining IPC with LMWH or adjusted-dose heparin may provide additional benefit, but this is not supported by data.

GYNECOLOGIC SURGERY

Low-Risk Patients

Low-risk patients may receive prophylaxis. Turner et al. reported a Level I study that demonstrated a lower DVT rate with the use of graduated elastic compression (0% vs. 4%; $p<0.05$).[63] On the basis of this study, the risk:benefit ratio, and extrapolation from moderate-risk patients, GCS may be used in addition to early ambulation and adequate hydration.

Moderate-Risk Patients

LMWH and low-dose UFH (5000 U every 12 hours) are effective prophylaxis in medium-risk gynecologic surgery patients (Grade A recommendation based on Level I data).[11,15] By extrapolation from other types of surgery, IPC also should be considered because it is effective in higher risk patients (Grade A recommendation). Adjusted-dose warfarin is not recommended for routine prophylaxis, but may have a role when UFH/LMWH is contraindicated (a history of heparin-induced throm-bocytopenia) (Grade A recommendation).[11,15]

High-Risk Patients

Low-dose UFH (5000 U every 8 hours) or IPC used continuously for at least 5 days provides effective prophylaxis (Grade A recommendation). When these two modalities were compared in a randomized trial, their efficacy appeared to be equal, but more bleeding complications were associated with use of low-dose heparin. Data evaluating LMWH and GCS in high-risk gynecologic surgery patients are currently insufficient, but extrapolation from other high-risk surgical popu-lations suggest LMWH is effective prophylaxis.[11,15]

Guidelines for DVT/PE risk assessment for gynecologic surgical patients are summarized in Figure 2.

OTHER CONDITIONS

Pregnancy

Low-dose heparin prophylaxis is used commonly in pregnant patients at high risk for DVT and PE such as previous

DVT or PE and certain thrombophilias (see below), although data regarding efficacy from controlled trials are lacking (Grade C recommendation). Insufficient data are available on both the optimum timing and dosing schedule of low-dose heparin prophylaxis. Substantial evidence is present for safety with low-dose aspirin use in pregnancy. Although no direct evidence exists regarding aspirin in preventing DVT or PE in pregnancy, its efficacy in other settings suggests it may be worth considering (Grade C recommendation).[11,15]

Oral anticoagulants are contraindicated for prophylaxis of venous thromboembolism in the first trimester due to increased risk of embryopathies; warfarin is associated with increased fetal and maternal-fetal bleeding in the second and, particularly, the third trimester. In the presence of contraindications to LMWH/UFH, oral anticoagulants may be considered, when justified, for prophylaxis in the second trimester because bleeding is uncommon at this stage (Grade C recommendation).

The benefits of prophylaxis have not been demonstrated in patients who undergo Cesarean section and do not have additional risk factors. Perioperative and postpartum prophylaxis should be considered if risk factors are present, particularly: age over 35 years, obesity, previous DVT or PE, or thrombophilia (Grade C recommendation).

Dextran should be avoided in pregnancy, as an anaphylactoid reaction may precipitate acute fetal distress. Dextran should be withheld during Cesarean section until after delivery.

Insufficient data on the use of LMWH or mechanical methods in pregnancy are insufficient. The need exists for multicenter trials that compare standard heparin with LMWH in high-risk pregnant patients to assess efficacy, safety, and possible side effects, such as osteoporosis.

Women who develop thromboembolism during pregnancy should be treated with therapeutic levels of adjusted-dose s.c. heparin, which should be continued throughout pregnancy, labor, and delivery. Higher doses are required in late pregnancy, but the s.c. dose should be reduced in labor or before Cesarean section to decrease the risk of hemorrhage during delivery.

Anticoagulation is usually continued for at least 6 weeks postpartum, but the optimal duration of antithrombotic therapy has not been established in this setting.[11,15]

Patients who develop thromboembolism during pregnancy or the puerperium should be referred for hematologic consultation. Management of thrombophilic conditions through pregnancy usually requires LMWH or adjusted-dose UFH, with monitoring of the heparin effect and platelet counts.[11,15]

Combination Estrogen Containing Oral Contraceptives

A combination of estrogen containing oral contraceptives may be associated with increased risk of DVT in patients who undergo gynecologic surgery. Discontinuation of oral contraceptives 4 to 6 weeks before surgery should be considered, but balanced against the risk of unwanted pregnancy. In the absence of other risk factors, insufficient evidence exists to support a policy of stopping the combined pill routinely before major surgery. LMWH/UFH prophylaxis is advisable when oral contraceptives have not been discontinued and additional risk factors are present. For emergency surgery, thromboprophylaxis should be provided in women who take the combined pill, as the risk of DVT is greater (Grade C recommendation).[11,15]

Hormone Replacement Therapy (HRT)

In the absence of other risk factors, insufficient evidence exists currently to support a policy of routinely stopping HRT before surgery. Although no data are available, LMWH/UFH prophylaxis is advisable when HRT has not been discontinued before surgery. In practice, most patients who receive HRT have additional risk factors, particularly age, which alone would be indications for thromboprophylaxis (Grade C recommendation). Obstetric and pregnancy risk assessments are summarized in Figure 3.

TREATMENT OF DEEP VEIN THROMBOSIS (DVT)

Cost-Effective Treatment of DVT/PE

DVT is common, accounts for significant morbidity and moderate mortality through development of PE, and is associated with high costs of care as delineated previously. Cost-effective, excellent care is possible by considering several important principles of therapy. This section is divided into cost-effective inpatient care for DVT ± PE versus "early discharge"/outpatient care for DVT. Sufficient information is not available currently to provide guidelines for outpatient management of PE. In general, calf thrombosis should be treated the same as proximal vein thrombosis.[64] Although the majority of PE arise from proximal vein thrombosis, approximately 25% of PE arise from isolated calf vein thrombosis.[65] Additional problems with calf vein thrombosis include propagation to proximal deep veins (30% of calf thrombi), destruction or damage to venous valves, and late sequelae of chronic venous insufficiency.[66] The goals of therapy for DVT are arresting of thrombus growth; prevention of recurrence, limiting swelling, which may lead to compartmental compression syndrome with resultant interference with venous and arterial flow with gangrene/loss of limbs; and prevention of embolization, which may lead to significant morbidity (pulmonary hypertension, etc.) or mortality.[64] The mainstay of initial treatment of DVT/PE is heparin/LMWH in some form.[65] Thrombolytic therapy may be indicated for extensive or recurrent DVT/PE, as it is clearly associated with reduction in incidence of chronic venous insufficiency.[66] However, costs and hemorrhagic complications limit indications for thrombolysis, which have been reviewed.[67,68]

Inpatient Management of Acute DVT/PE

In general, the initial therapy for inpatient care of DVT/PE is porcine mucosal UFH or fixed-dose LMWH. UFH may be given by the IV route or a dose-adjusted s.c. route; the dose-adjusted s.c. route has been shown clearly to be equal to, or better than, the IV route.[69-72] IV UFH is given by IV bolus, followed by infusion to maintain an activated partial thromboplastin time (aPTT) prolongation, equivalent to a therapeutic range of 0.30 to ≈1.0 anti-Xa U.[64,69] Reliance of simple prolongation of the aPTT to 1.5 to 2.0 times baseline is no longer reliable with cur-

Table 5. Results using low-molecular-weight heparin versus unfractionated heparin

(RESULTS FROM 13 RANDOMIZED TRIALS)

38.5% REDUCTION IN RECURRENCE	(7.8% - 4.8%)
45.1% REDUCTION IN MAJOR BLEEDS	(2% - 1.1%)
24.7% REDUCTION IN MORTALITY	(7% - 5.2%)

rent hypersensitive reagents and inconsistencies between collection in 3.2% versus 3.8% citrate; thus, all laboratories must calibrate the particular aPTT reagents used to a therapeutic anti-Xa range as defined above.[11] Warfarin is started at the same time as IV UFH; UFH is continued for ≥ 5 days; and stopped when the INR is ≈ 2.0 for at least 48 hours.[11] Dose-adjusted s.c. UFH is given as a s.c. injection every 12 hours, aiming for the same aPTT as mentioned above and initiating warfarin therapy as defined above. It should be noted that if using IV or dose-adjusted UFH for initial therapy for DVT/PE, it is imperative to reach a therapeutic range, as defined above, within 24 hours; if not achieved, the late recurrence is increased markedly.[73] DVT/PE also may be treated by LMWH; in this instance, the dose is fixed and given every 12 hours or every 24 hours, the aPTT is not used to assess therapy, and the dose is not varied.[64] Thus, an aPTT is not needed. In general, heparin assays by anti-Xa assay also are unnecessary unless clinical changes suggest too much (hemorrhage) or too little (recurrence) LMWH or if the patient is unusually obese or small. With both modes of therapy (UFH or LMWH), frequent platelet counts are required to assure quick detection of heparin-induced thrombocytopenia, a rare complication of UFH or LMWH therapy, and much less common with LMWH than UFH.[74]

Thirteen well-controlled, double-blind randomized trials have been conducted that compared UFH (IV or dose-adjusted s.c.) with LMWH for treatment of active DVT/PE.[75-87] In all such trials, objective methods were used for initial diagnosis and confirmation of recurrence. These trials have used a variety of LMWH preparations given once or twice a day, depending on brand. Results of these trials are summarized in Table 5. An analysis of these trials demonstrates clear superiority of LMWH over UFH for treatment of active DVT.[88] The recurrence rates are reduced significantly with LMWH, major hemorrhage [defined as intracranial bleeding episode, retroperitoneal, required transfusion(s), caused disruption of therapy, necessitated surgery, or fatality] is significantly less, and mortality is reduced significantly. As some of the studies included patients with PE and others excluded PE, risk reduction of PE cannot be assessed adequately in analysis of these trials.

In summary, major cost containment and a major impact on quality of life through reduction of recurrence, reduction of bleeding episodes, and reduction in development of chronic venous insufficiency can be achieved by use of LMWH for inpatients with DVT ± PE. Further cost containment is achieved by choosing appropriate, long-term therapy for those patients who harbor hereditary or acquired blood coagulation protein/platelet defects causing DVT ± PE. It is unjustified and cost wasteful to place DVT/PE patients on long-term warfarin after initial UFH or LMWH if they harbor a causative defect refractory to warfarin (e.g., antiphospholipid syndrome, sticky platelet syndrome).

Outpatient/"Early Discharge" Management of Acute DVT/PE

Recent studies have suggested another major question: What is the role of outpatient management for deep vein thrombosis? Particularly in North America, where cost-containment-often driven by managed care-is of primary concern and clinicians are under increasing pressure to decrease costs through decreased hospital admissions, recent publications that state results of LMHW in randomized trials that demonstrated the clear safety and efficacy of home treatment or "early-discharge" management of DVT have become of major interest.[89-93] These studies are too recent to have been considered in consensus conferences, and firm guidelines have not yet been established. Three well-designed, randomized trials were conducted to assess inpatient treatment of DVT/PE with UFH versus outpatient management of DVT/PE with LMWH.[91-93] These trials have included 1104 patients; 550 treated in the outpatient LMWH group and 554 in the inpatient group. Thirty-two (5.8%) recurrences in the outpatient group and 37 (6.6%) in the inpatient group were noted, which represented a non-significant risk reduction rate of 12.2%. All bleeding was minor: 10 (1.8%) minor bleeds in the outpatient group, and 9 (1.6%) in the inpatient group.

When assessing the trials and DVT patients in general, realistically, only approximately 70% of DVT patients can be treated on an outpatient basis; the remaining 30% must be admitted because of comorbid conditions that require hospitalization, or must be admitted for 12 to 24 hours to initiate the items needed for successful outpatient management (e.g., those who arrive late in the day at the physician's office or hospital often need short-term admission to institute appropriate measures for successful outpatient therapy). Recent studies have suggested that selected patients with PE also may be treated safely at home with LMWH.[94,95] Obviously, if 70% of patients with DVT can be managed as outpatients, this represents a cost savings of approximately $4,900,000/1000 patients with DVT. The following general principles of outpatient or "early-discharge" management of DVT can be instituted, pending more results of randomized trials or consensus-driven recommendations provide additional information.

SUGGESTED GUIDELINES FOR OUTPATIENT OR "EARLY-DISCHARGE" MANAGEMENT OF DVT [11,96]

1. Admit for 24 hours if no comorbid condition, or treat as outpatient if no comorbid condition and all below can be accomplished.
2. Complete blood cell (CBC)/platelet count on admission.
3. PT and aPTT on admission.
4. Teach patient applicable anti-embolic exercises on admission (see below).

5. Start s.c. LMWH as:
   a. FRAGMIN (Dalteparin) @ 200 U/kg Q 24 hours (available as 2500 U/0.2 mL or 5000 U/0.2 mL or multidose vials of 95,000 U/9.5 mL): Lindmarker Regimen.[93]
   OR
   b. LOVENOX (Enoxaparin) @ 1 mg/kg Q 12 hours (=100 U kg Q 12 hours). (30 mg or 40 mg AMPS): Levine Regimen.[92]
6. Instruct patient in self-injection of s.c. LMWH in anterior/lateral-thighs or anterior abdominal wall (thighs preferred-use rotating injection sites).
7. Measure for medium compression panty hose, lower extremity (LE) or upper- extremity (UE) hose for use during waking hours only.
8. Start warfarin @ 5 mg/day if <70 kg total body weight or 10 mg/day if >70 kg total body weight (*see exceptions below).
9. Discharge at 24 hours if no co-morbid conditions or discharge as soon as co-morbid condition (not DVT) allows.
10. Arrange home health care if patient/family cannot self-inject LMWH.
11. Arrange outpatient PT/INR and CBC/platelet count at home on days 3 and 5.
12. Evaluate patient clinically (in office/clinic) on days 5 or 7; obtain PT and CBC/ platelet count days 5 and 7; stop LMWH when INR 2.0, then adjust warfarin dose accordingly.
13. See patient weekly until stable on long-term antithrombotic therapy.
14. If young aged patient (60) with unexplained DVT, consider evaluation for blood coagulation protein(s)/platelet defects leading to thrombosis.
15. While hospitalized, when patient is in bed, raise foot of bed-straight, with feet elevated 70 to 100 above hips; never put pillow(s) under popliteal fossae.
16. *Depending on clinical variables (thrombophilia, platelet defects, etc.), alternatives to oral anticoagulants may be indicated.

Ancillary Measures For Management of DVT

Several ancillary measures should, generally, be instituted for all patients with DVT of the extremities: use of medium-compression panty hose during waking hours for patients with LE DVT, medium-compression arm hose for those with UE DVT, and the teaching of antiembolic exercises and correct body positioning as summarized below. These modalities, particularly appropriate exercises and body positioning, of no-or minimal-cost and aid in preventing recurrence.[11,95]

Anti-Embolic Leg Exercises

The patient should be instructed in anti-embolic leg exercises consisting of dorsi-plantar flexion of each foot at a time with the legs supported at the feet, legs straight, and elevated above the hips 70 to 100. Continue these for 3 to 5 minutes, or until the calf muscle group is fatigued, with initiation of muscle pain; then the opposite leg exercised in a likewise manner. The patient should be told to do these exercises 4 to 6 times a day. The patient also should be instructed to not remain in a sitting position or indulge in other activities, such as car or airplane trips, with the thighs and knees bent tightly, for more than 20 minutes at a time without straightening the legs through brief ambulation or leg stretching for a few minutes.

Anti-Embolic Arm Exercises

The patient should be instructed in anti-embolic arm exercises consisting of palmar "squeezing" of each hand at a time, with the arms elevated and straightened above the head. Holding a tennis ball by the hand, while squeezing, is excellent for this exercise. These should continue for 3 to 5 minutes, or until the arm muscles are fatigued, with initiation of muscle pain; the opposite arm should then be exercised in a likewise manner. The patient should be told to do these exercises 4 to 6 times a day. The patient also should be instructed to not remain in a position or indulge in other activities with the arms bent tightly at the elbow or shoulder for more than 20 minutes at a time, without stretching the arms straight for a few minutes.

Recent studies have demonstrated that home therapy can be accomplished easily by 80% of patients with both safety and efficacy, and a high level of patient satisfaction is associated with home care of DVT.[97,98]

CONCLUSIONS

The principle factors to cost containment in management of DVT/PE is to: (a) define the cause (blood coagulation protein/platelet defect) and institute appropriate long-term therapy as indicated, and assess appropriate family members as indicated, if a hereditary defect is found; (b) use LMWH as inpatient management, saving a minimum of $210,000/1000 patients from cost-savings of recurrence, saving 17 lives/1000 patients, and saving exorbitant costs of care for patients recurring and developing chronic venous insufficiency. The use of outpatient LMWH saves $4,900,000/1000 patients if applied to the 70% of patients with DVT who fit criteria of no comorbid condition that requires hospitalization, and arrive with a diagnosis early enough to be sent home or hospitalized for 24 hours. The simple defining of defects that lead to unexplained thrombosis adds another $3,000,000 in savings/1000 patients with DVT.

REFERENCES

1. Bick RL, Fareed J. Current status of thrombosis: a multidisciplinary medical issue and major American health problem-beyond the year 2000. Clin Appl Thromb Hemost 1997;3(Suppl 1):1.
2. Heart and Stroke-1997. American Heart Association National Headquarters, Dallas, Texas, 1996.
3. Bick RL, Kaplan H. Syndromes of thrombosis and hypercoagulability: congenital and acquired causes of thrombosis. Med Clin North Am 1998;82:409.
4. Bick RL, Jakway J, Baker WF. Deep vein thrombosis: prevalence of etiologic factors and results of management in 100 consecutive patients. Semin Thromb Hemost 1992;8:267.
5. Bergqvist D, Lundblad B. Incidence of venous thromboembolism in medical and surgical patients. In: Bergqvist D, Comerota A, Nicolaides A, et al., eds. Prevention of venous thromboembolism. London: Med-Orion Press; 1994. p 3.
6. Silverstein MD, Heit JA, Mohr DN, et al. Trends in the incidence of deep vein thrombosis and pulmonary embolism: a 25-year population-based study. Arch Intern Med 1998;158:585.
7. Ramaswami G, Nicolaides AN. The natural history of deep vein thrombosis. In: Bergqvist D, Comerota A, Nicolaides A, et al., eds. Prevention of venous thromboembolism. London: Med-Orion Press; 1994. p 3.
8. Bick RL, Ancypa D. Blood protein defects associated with thrombosis: laboratory assessment. Clin Lab Med 1995;5:125.
9. MedPar: The MedStat Group Outcomes Analysis. MedPar, 1998. Nashville: Inforum, Medistat; 1998.

10. De Stefano V, Finazzi G, Mannucci PM. Inherited thrombophilia: pathogenesis, clinical syndromes and management. Blood 1996;87:3531.
11. Bick RL, Haas SK. International consensus recommendations: summary statement and additional suggested guidelines. Med Clin North Am 1998;83:613-34.
12. American College of Chest Physicians: Conference on Antithrombotic Therapy. Chest (Feb) 1986;89:1.
13. European consensus statement on the prevention of venous thromboembolism. Int Angiol 1992;11:151.
14. Treatment of venous thrombosis and pulmonary embolism. In: Waersted A, Westbye O, Beermann B, et al., eds. Oslo Norway: Norwegian Medicines Control Authority, 1995; Uppsala, Sweden: Medical Products Agency, 1995.
15. Prevention of venous thromboembolism. International consensus statement (Guideline according to scientific evidence). Int Angiol 1997;16:3.
16. McIntyre K. Medicolegal implications of consensus statements. Chest 1995;108:502.
17. Hull RD, Pineo GF. Prophylaxis of deep venous thrombosis and pulmonary embolus: current recommendations. Med Clin North Am 1998;82:477.
18. Dismuke SE, Wagner EH. Pulmonary embolism as a cause of death. The changing mortality in hospitalized patients. JAMA 1986;255:2039.
19. Dalen JE, Alpert JS. Natural history of pulmonary embolism. Prog Cardiovasc Dis 1975;17:257.
20. Prandoni P, Lensing AWA, Cogo A, et al. The long-term clinical course of acute deep venous thrombosis. Ann Intern Med 1996;125:1.
21. Baker WF. Diagnosis of deep venous thrombosis and pulmonary embolism. Med Clin North Am 1998;82:459.
22. Anderson FA, Wheeler HB, Goldberg RJ, et al. A population-based perspective of the hospital incidence and case-fatality rates of deep vein thrombosis and pulmonary embolism. Arch Intern Med 1991;151:933.
23. Clagett GP, Reisch JS. Prevention of venous thromboembolism in general surgical patients. Results of meta-analysis. Ann Surg 1988;208:227.
24. Collins R, Scrimgeour A, Yusef S, et al. Reduction in fatal pulmonary embolism and venous thrombosis by perioperative administration of subcutaneous heparin. N Engl J Med 1988;318:1162.
25. Nicolaides AN, Bergqvist D, Hull RD, et al. Prevention of venous thromboembolism. International consensus statement. Int Angiol 1997;16:3.
26. Nicolaides AN. Prevention of thromboembolism: European consensus statement. In: Bergqvist D, Comerota AJ, Nicolaides AN, et al., eds. Prevention of venous thromboembolism. Los Angeles: Med-Orion Publishing Co; 1994. p 445.
27. Bratzler DW, Raskob GE, Murray CK, et al. Underuse of venous thromboembolism prophylaxis for general surgery patients. Arch Intern Med 1998;158:1909.
28. Kakkar VV, Adams PC. Preventive and therapeutic approach to venous thromboembolism. Can death from pulmonary embolism be prevented? J Am Coll Cardiol 1986;8:146B.
29. Skinner DB, Salzman EW. Anticoagulant prophylaxis in surgical patients. Surg Gynecol Obstet 1967;125:741.
30. Shephard RM, White HA, Shirkey AL. Anticoagulant prophylaxis of thromboembolism in post-surgical patients. Am J Surg 1966;112:698.
31. International multicentre trial: prevention of fatal postoperative pulmonary embolism by low doses of heparin. Lancet 1975;2:45.
32. Bergqvist D. Prevention in individual patient groups: general surgery. In: Bergqvist D, Comerota AJ, Nicolaides AN, et al., eds. Prevention of venous thromboembolism. Los Angeles: Med-Orion Publishing Co; 1994. p 243.
33. Coventry MB, Nolan DR, Beckenbaugh RD. "Delayed" prophylactic anticoagulation: a study of results and complications in 2,012 total hip arthroplasties. J Bone Joint Surg 1973;55:1487.
34. Eskeland G, Solheim K, Skhorten F. Anticoagulant prophylaxis, thromboembolism and mortality in elderly patients with hip fracture: a controlled clinical trial. Acta Chir Scand 1986;131:16.
35. Kearon C, Hirsh J. Starting prophylaxis for venous thromboembolism postoperatively. Arch Intern Med 1995;155:366.
36. Hull RD, Pineo GF, Francis C, et al. Low-molecular-weight heparin prophylaxis using dalteparin in close proximity to surgery vs. warfarin in hip arthroplasty patients. Arch Intern Med 2000;160:2199.
37. Palareti G, Borghi B, Coccheri S, for the CITO Study Group. Postoperative versus preoperative initiation of deep-vein thrombosis prophylaxis with a low molecular weight heparin (Nadroparin) in elective hip replacement. Clin Appl Thromb Hemost 1996;2:18.
38. Hull RD, Hirsh J, Carter CJ, et al. Diagnostic efficacy of impedance plethysmography for clinically suspected deep-vein thrombosis: a randomized trial. Ann Intern Med 1985;102:21.
39. Walenga J, Bick RL. Heparin associated thrombocytopenia and other adverse effects of heparin therapy. Cardiol Clin (Ann Drug Ther) 1998;2:123-40.
40. Kakkar VV, Cohen AT, Edmonson RA, et al. Low-molecular-weight versus standard heparin for prevention of venous thromboembolism after major abdominal surgery. Lancet 1993;341:259.
41. Kakkar VV, Boeckl O, Boneau B, et al. Efficacy and safety of a low-molecular-weight heparin and standard unfractionated heparin for prophylaxis of postoperative venous thromboembolism: European multicenter trial. World J Surg 1997;21:2.
42. Bergqvist D, Matzsch T, Brumark U, et al. Low-molecular-weight heparin given the evening before surgery compared with conventional low-dose heparin in prevention of thrombosis. Br J Surg 1988;75:888.
43. Samama M, Bernard P, Bonnardot JP, et al. Low-molecular-weight heparin compared with unfractionated heparin in prevention of postoperative thrombosis. Br J Surg 1988;75:128.
44. The European Fraxiparin Study Group. Comparison of a low-molecular-weight heparin and unfractionated heparin for the prevention of deep vein thrombosis in patients undergoing abdominal surgery. Br J Surg 1988;75:1058.
45. Caen JP. A randomized double-blind study between a low-molecular-weight heparin Kabi 2165 and standard heparin in the prevention of deep-vein thrombosis in general surgery. A French multicentre trial. Thromb Haemost 1988;59:216.
46. Leizorovicz A, Picolet H, Peyrieux JC, et al. Prevention of perioperative deep vein thrombosis in general surgery: a multicentre double-blind study comparing two doses of logiparin and standard heparin. Br J Surg 1991;78:412.
47. Nurmohamed MT, Verhaeghe R, Haas S, et al. A comparative trial of a low molecular weight heparin (Enoxaparin) versus standard heparin for the prophylaxis of postoperative deep vein thrombosis in general surgery. Am J Surg 1995;169:567.
48. Bergqvist D, Burmark US, Flordal PA, et al. Low molecular weight heparin started before surgery as prophylaxis against deep vein thrombosis: 2500 versus 500 XaI units in 2070 patients. Br J Surg 1995;82:496.
49. Leclerc JR, Geerts WH, Desjardins L, et al. Prevention of deep vein thrombosis after major knee surgery-a randomized, double-blind trial comparing a low-molecular-weight heparin fragment (Enoxaparin) to placebo. Thromb Haemost 1992;67:417.
50. Leclerc JR, Geerts WH, Desjardins L, et al. Prevention of venous thromboembolism after knee arthroplasty-a randomized, double-blind trial comparing a low molecular weight heparin fragment (Enoxparin) to Warfarin. Thromb Haemost 1995;73(6):1103. [Abstract]
51. Heit J, Berkowitz S, Bona R, et al. Efficacy and safety of Normiflow (a LMWH) compared to warfarin for prevention of venous thromboembolism following total knee replacement: a double-blind, dose-ranging study. Thromb Haemost 1995;73(6):A739. [Abstract]
52. Nurmohamed MT, Rosendaal FR, Büller HR, et al. Low molecular weight heparin in the prophylaxis of venous thrombosis: a meta-analysis. Lancet 1992;340:152.
53. Geerts WH, Jay RM, Code KI, et al. A comparison of low-dose heparin with low-molecular-weight heparin as prophylaxis against venous thromboembolism after major trauma. N Engl J Med 1996;335:701.
54. Dale C, Gallus A, Wycherley A, et al. Prevention of venous thrombosis with minidose warfarin after joint replacement. Br Med J 1991;303:224.
55. Roberts VC, Sabri S, Beely AH, et al. The effect of intermittently applied external pressure on the hemodynamics of the lower limb in man. Br J Surg 1972;59:233.
56. Skillman JJ, Collins RR, Coe NP, et al. Prevention of deep vein thrombosis in neuro-

56. (reference continues) surgical patients: a controlled, randomized trial of external pneumatic compression boots. Surgery 1978;83:354.
57. Ramos R, Salem BI, Pawlikowski MP, et al. The efficacy of pneumatic compression stockings in the prevention of pulmonary embolism after cardiac surgery. Chest 1996;109:82.
58. Hull RD, Raskob G, Gent M, et al. Effectiveness of intermittent pneumatic leg compression for preventing deep vein thrombosis after total hip replacement. JAMA 1990;263:2313.
59. Geerts WH, Jay RM, Code KI. A comparison of low-dose heparin with low-molecular-weight heparin as prophylaxis against venous thromboembolism after major trauma. N Engl J Med 1996;335:701.
60. White RH, Zhou H, Kim J, et al. A population-based study of the effectiveness of inferior vena cava filter use among patients with venous thromboembolism. Arch Intern Med 2000;160:2033.
61. Decousus H, Leizorovich A, Parent F, et al. A clinical trial of vena cava filters in the prevention of pulmonary embolism in patients with proximal deep-vein thrombosis. New Engl J Med 1998;338:409.
62. Clagett GP, Anderson FA, Heit J. Prevention of venous thromboembolism. Chest 1995;108:312s,
63. Turner GM, Cole SF, Brooks JH. The efficacy of graduated compression stockings in the prevention of deep vein thrombosis after major gynecological surgery. Br J Obstet Gynecol 1984;91:588-91.
64. Haas SK. Treatment of deep venous thrombosis: current recommendations. Med Clin North Am 1998;82:495.
65. Philbrick JT, Becker DM. Calf deep vein thrombosis: a wolf in sheep's clothing? Arch Intern Med 1988;148:2131.
66. Baker WF, Bick RL. Deep vein thrombosis: diagnosis and management. Med Clin North Am 1994;78:685.
67. Murano G, Bell WR. Thrombolytic therapy. In: Bick RL, Bennett JM, Brynes RK, eds. Hematology: clinical and laboratory practice. St. Louis: Mosby; 1993. p 1633.
68. Bell WR. Thrombolytic therapy: agents, indications and laboratory monitoring. Med Clin North Am 1994;78:745.
69. Hoomes DW, Bura A, Mazzolai L, et al. Subcutaneous heparin compared with continuous intravenous heparin administration in the initial treatment of deep vein thrombosis: a meta-analysis. Ann Intern Med 1992;116:279.
70. Doyle DJ, Turpie AGG, Hirsh J, et al. Adjusted subcutaneous heparin or continuous intravenous heparin in patients with acute deep vein thrombosis. Ann Intern Med 1987;107:441.
71. Anderson G, Fagrell B, Holmgren K, et al. Subcutaneous administration of heparin: a randomized comparison with intravenous administration of heparin to patients with deep-vein thrombosis. Thromb Res 1982;27:631.
72. Hull RD, Raskob G, Hirsh J, et al. Continuous intravenous heparin compared with intermittent subcutaneous heparin in the initial treatment of proximal vein thrombosis. New Engl J Med 1986;315:1109.
73. Hull RD, Raskob GE, Brant RF, et al. The importance of initial treatment on long-term outcomes of antithrombotic therapy. Arch Intern Med 1997;157:2317.
74. Walenga JM, Bick RL. Heparin-induced thrombocytopenia, paradoxical thromboembolism, and other side effects of heparin therapy. Med Clin North Am 1998;82:635.
75. The Columbus Investigators. Low-molecular-weight heparin in the treatment of patients with venous thromboembolism. N Engl J Med 1997;337:657-62.
76. Duroux P. A collaborative European multicentre study: a randomized trial of subcutaneous low molecular weight heparin (CY216) compared with intravenous unfractionated heparin in the treatment of deep vein thrombosis. Thromb Haemost 1991;65:251.
77. Faivre R, Neuhart Y, Kieffer Y, et al. Un nouveau traitement des thromboses veineuses profondes: les fractions d'heparine de bas poids moleculaire. Etude randomisee. Presse Med 1988;17:197.
78. Fiessinger JN, Lopez-Fernandez M, Gatterer E, et al. Once-daily subcutaneous Dalteparin, a low molecular weight heparin, for the initial treatment of acute deep vein thrombosis. Thromb Haemost 1996;76:195.
79. Hull RD, Raskob GE, Pineo GF, et al. Subcutaneous low-molecular-weight heparin compared with continuous intravenous heparin in the treatment of proximal-vein thrombosis. N Engl J Med 1992;326:975.
80. Koopman MMW, Prandoni, P, Piovella, F, et. al. Treatment of venous thrombosis with intravenous unfractionated heparin administered in the hospital as compared with subcutaneous low-molecular-weight heparin administered at home. N Engl J Med 1996;334:682.
81. Levine M, Gent M, Hirsh J, et al. A comparison of low-molecular-weight heparin administered primarily at home with unfractionated heparin administered in the hospital for proximal deep-vein thrombosis. N Engl J Med 1996;334:677.
82. Lindmarker P, Holmstrom M, Granqvist S, et al. Comparison of once-daily subcutaneous Fragmin with continuous intravenous unfractionated heparin in the treatment of deep venous thrombosis. Thromb Haemost 1994;72:186.
83. Lopaciuk S, Meissner AJ, Filipecki S, et al. Subcutaneous low molecular weight heparin versus subcutaneous unfractionated heparin in the treatment of deep vein thrombosis: a Polish multicenter trial. Thromb Haemost 1992;68:14.
84. Luomanmaki K and the Finnish Multicentre Group. Low molecular weight heparin (Fragmin) once daily vs. continuous infusion of standard heparin in the treatment of DVT. Haemostasis 1994;24(Suppl. 1):248. [Abstract]
85. Prandoni P, Lensing AWA, Buller HR, et al. Comparison of subcutaneous low-molecular-weight heparin with intravenous standard heparin in proximal deep-vein thrombosis. Lancet 1992;339:441.
86. Simonneau G, Charbonnier B, Decousus H, et al. Subcutaneous low molecular weight heparin compared with continuous intravenous unfractionated heparin in the initial treatment proximal vein thrombosis. Arch Intern Med 1993;153:1541.
87. Simonneau G, Sors H, Charbonnier B, et al. for the THESEE Study Group. A comparison of low-molecular-weight heparin with unfractionated heparin for acute pulmonary embolism. N Engl J Med 1997;337:663.
88. van den Belt AGM, Prins MH, Lensing AWA, et al. Fixed dose subcutaneous low molecular weight heparins versus adjusted dose unfractionated heparin for venous thromboembolism. (Cochrane Review) In: The Cochrane Library, Issue 2. Oxford: Update Software; 1998.
89. Hull RD, Raskob GE, Pineo GF, et al. The treatment of proximal vein thrombosis with subcutaneous low molecular weight heparin compared with continuous intravenous heparin. The Canadian-American Thrombosis Study Group. Clin Appl Thromb Haemost 1995;1:151.
90. Shafer AI. Low-molecular-weight heparin-an opportunity for home treatment of venous thrombosis (Editorial). N Engl J Med 1996;334:724.
91. Koopman MMW, Prandoni P, Piovella F, et al. Treatment of venous thrombosis with intravenous unfractionated heparin administered in the hospital as compared with subcutaneous low-molecular-weight heparin administered at home. N Engl J Med 1996;334:682.
92. Levine M, Gent M, Hirsh J, et al. A comparison of low-molecular-weight heparin administered primarily at home with unfractionated heparin administered in the hospital for proximal deep-vein thrombosis. N Engl J Med 1996;334:677.
93. Lindmarker P, Holmstrom KM, Granquist S, et al. Comparison of once-daily subcutaneous Fragmin with continuous intravenous unfractionated heparin in the treatment of deep vein thrombosis. Thromb Haemost 1994;72:186.
94. Hull RD, Raskob GE, Brant RF, et al. Low-molecular-weight heparin vs heparin in the treatment of patients with pulmonary embolism. Arch Intern Med 2000;160:229.
95. Kovacs MJ, Anderson D, Morrow B, et al. Outpatient treatment of pulmonary embolism with dalteparin. Thromb Haemost 2000;83:209.
96. Bick RL. Therapy for venous thrombosis: guidelines for a competent and cost-effective approach. Clin Appl Thromb Haemost 1999;5:2.
97. Harrison L, McGinnis J, Crowther M, et al. Assessment of outpatient treatment of deep-vein thrombosis with low-molecular-weight heparin. Arch Intern Med 1998;158:2001.
98. Wells P, Kovacs M, Bormanis J, et al. Expanding eligibility for outpatient treatment of deep venous thrombosis and pulmonary embolus with low-molecular-weight heparin: a comparison of self-injection with homecare injection. Arch Intern Med 1998;158:1809.

Hydroxyapatite-Coated Femoral Arthroplasties: A Long-Term Study Through 29 Corail® Prostheses Explanted During a Ten-Year Survey

DOMINIQUE C.R. HARDY, M.D.
SENIOR ORTHOPAEDIC SURGEON
DEPARTMENT OF ORTHOPAEDIC SURGERY
UNIVERSITY HOSPITAL SAINT-PIERRE
BRUSSELS, BELGIUM

PATRICK FRAYSSINET, M.D., PH.D.
DEPARTMENT OF HISTO-CYTOLOGY
UNIVERSITY OF TOULOUSE-RANGUEIL
TOULOUSE, FRANCE

In our department, all the patients over 65 years of age with a displaced intracapsular fracture of the upper femur (type III and IV of the Garden's classification[1]) are treated with a femoral hemiarthroplasty (Figs. 1a & 1b). This practice is relatively universal among the European traumatologic centers. Two prospective and randomized trials, published in 2000,[2,3] reported a high rate of reoperation when treating these fractures with osteosynthesis (36% and 38% of the cases), thus indicating arthroplasty may be preferred.

Until 1988, we used cemented implants suitable in the vast majority of the cases; nevertheless, when we reviewed our results, an abnormally high perioperative mortality rate was noted. As did many other authors, we noted several instances in which the patients died of cardiac failure during cementation or the first postoperative week. When reviewing the preoperative cardiac assessment of these patients, they were noted to have a relatively good cardiac function. These patients were overhydrated intraoperatively by the anesthesiologist to prevent a cardiogenic shock during cementation, often associated with hypotension. A slight impairment of the cardiac function, usual in elderly patients, was the reason for such a major cardiac failure to occur after this overhydration. Therefore, we decided to use uncemented femoral implants.

In this particular context, hydroxyapatite (HA) seemed attractive for its superior properties of osteoconduction, but at the end of the 1980s no one knew if it was efficient when implanted in elderly patients.

Since April 1988, we use the Corail®

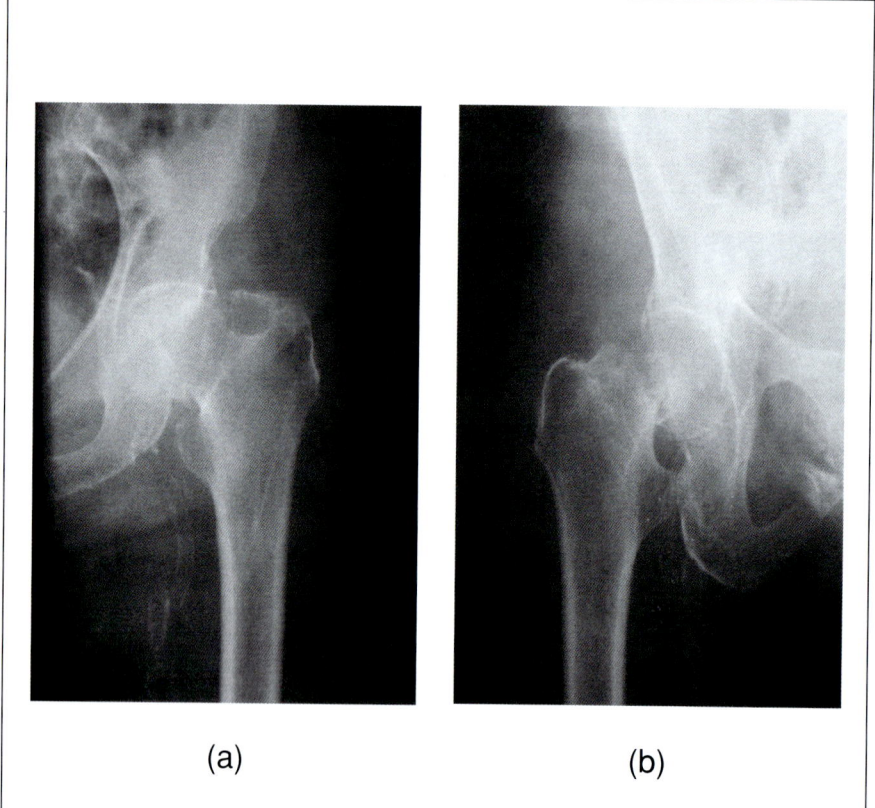

Figure 1. a) Garden IV type fracture in an 87-year-old patient. b) Corail® femoral arthroplasty with a bipolar head.

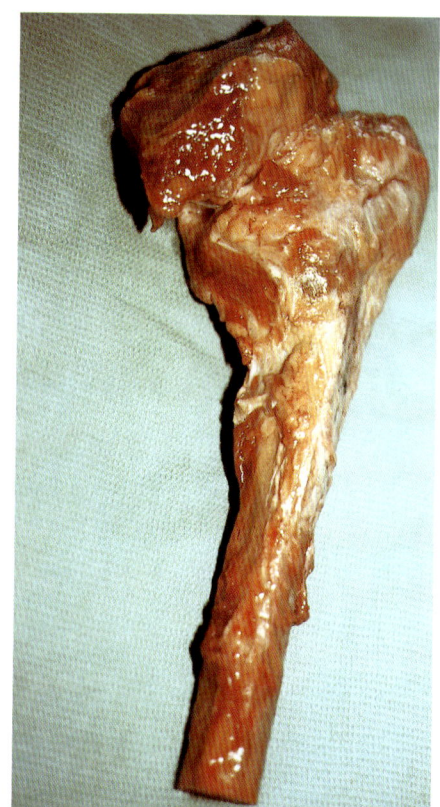

Figure 3. Fresh specimen obtained during autopsy of a 89-year-old-female. Delay of implantation was 24 months.

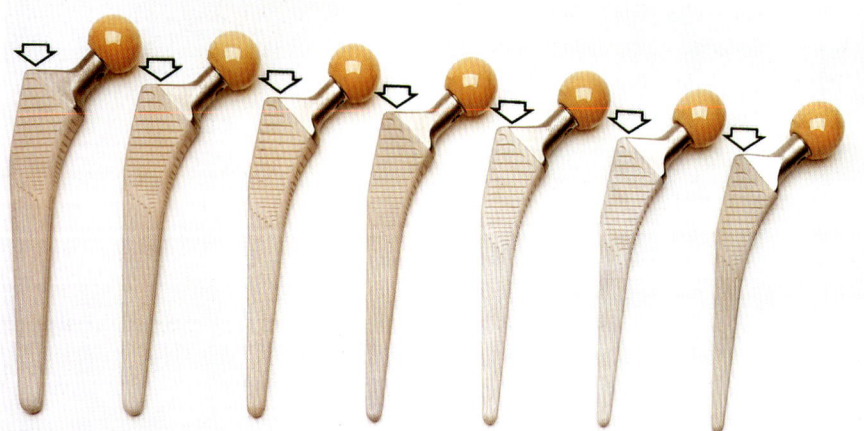

Figure 2. Corail arthroplasties exists in 8 sizes, from 9 to 16 (9 size is not represented).

stem, provided with a bi-articulated femoral head (Multipolar® head, Zimmer, Warsaw, USA) (Fig. 2).

As the "natural" mortality rate encountered in this group of patients is high (±25 % at one year), we decided to perform autopsies of the patients when they died after surgery to retrieve their prosthesis and the implanted femur. This article reports on our findings during these autopsies, and provides an overview of the natural history of osseointegration of these prostheses.

MATERIAL AND METHODS

Donors

Twenty-nine femurs implanted with a Corail® femoral arthroplasty were retrieved during systemic autopsies. These patients died for reasons unrelated to the surgery, except for the five-day implanted patient who died of cardiac failure in the postoperative period. Consent of the patients, their families, or their general practitioners was obtained for each patient.

Specimens

During autopsy, the hip was approached through the old scar and the femur stripped of its surrounding muscles and removed in its entirety, except for the first 13 specimens, in which the femur was transected several centimeters below the tip of the prosthesis. The joint was freed from the pelvi-trochanteric muscles and the entire acetabulum separated from the pelvic bones by three saw cuts. This procedure provided a one-piece specimen obtained without entering the joint or applying force to the implant. The femur was replaced with a telescopic rod and the soft tissues closed properly.

The fresh specimen was photographed (Fig. 3), radiographed under various orientations (Fig. 4), and fixed immediately in Karnowsky's solution (cacodylate buffer containing 2% formaldehyde and 2% glutaraldehyde) for 72 hours, then in phosphate buffer solutions for several weeks. After fixation (Fig. 5), the specimens were dehydrated in graduated ethanol solutions, cleared in xylol, and embedded in methylmethacrylate. Two-millimeter-thick sections were cut with a low-speed, cooled diamond saw and

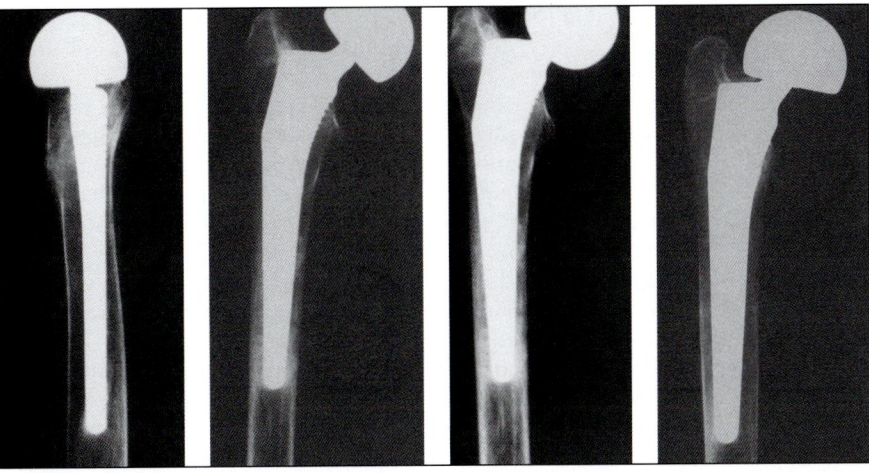

Figure 4. Specimen #25 obtained after 18 months in a 93-year-old patient. a) AP view, b) ¾ view, c) profile view, d) ¾ view.

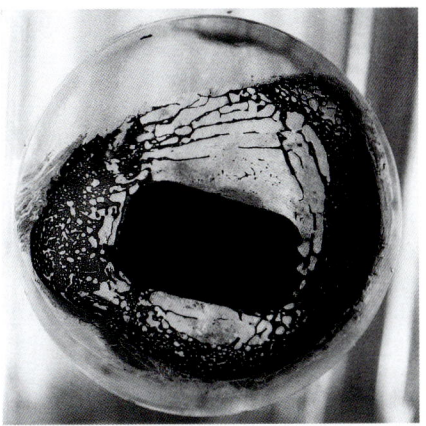

Figure 6. Macroscopic view of the proximal part of a prosthesis (specimen #12). The slide is re-embedded at the surface of a polystyrene-containing block.

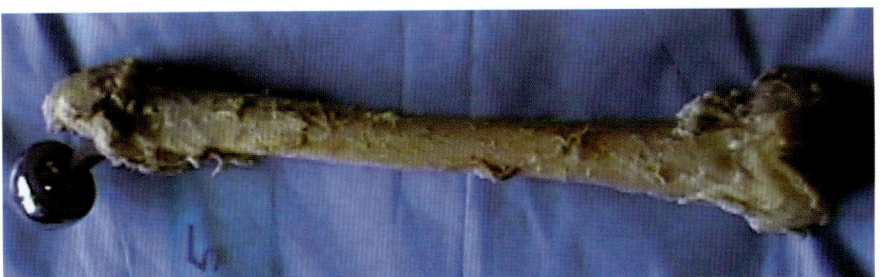

Figure 5. Photograph of a specimen after fixation in Karnovsky's fixative (specimen #29).

Table 1. Data of the 29 human explants obtained in this study

N°	Age	Sex	Walking ability score (Parker, 1994)	Implantation period
1	83	F	2	6 months
2	81	F	5	6 weeks
3	74	F	0	6 months
4	80	F	3	7 months
5	85	F	2	26 months
6	89	F	8	24 months
7	83	F	2	3 months
8	65	M	0	3 weeks
9	90	M	2	9.5 months
10	75	M	0	5 days
11	80	F	1	3 months
12	75	M	9	52 months
13	76	F	7	6 months
14	82	F	4	13 months
15	70	F	1	10 months
16	81	F	1	4 months
17	84	F	9	11 months
18	94	F	5	34 months
19	91	F	7	16 months
20	69	F	4	38 months
21	76	F	1	68 months
22	75	F	2	76 months
23	84	F	8	13 months
24	76	F	5	37 months
25	93	F	4	18 months
26	74	F	0	9 days
27	88	M	0	16 months
28	90	F	5	3 months
29	90	F	0	112 months

re-embedded at a surface of a block made of cold-setting, styrene-based polymer (Fig. 6). They were then polished down to a 50-μm thickness, and surface stained with a Fuschin-Toluidine solution after they were etched for 2 minutes in 2% formic acid solution and 2 hours in a 20% methanol solution. From 6 to 20 sections were prepared at various levels of the specimens. These sections were observed under either transmission or reflected light microscope (Reichert, Polyvar). A detailed account of this procedure was published by Frayssinet et al.[4] and Hardy et al.[5]

We have obtained 29 femoral explants. Table 1 summarizes the main clinical data of these patients.

RESULTS

Different Steps of This Osteointegration

Phase I: Bone Formation

Five days after implantation, the cells and extracellular matrix form a loose, connective tissue attached weakly to the coating. Some cells of this loose connective tissue differentiate into osteoblasts three or four weeks after implantation and synthesize osteoid substance.[6]

After two months of implantation, the coating is in contact with a mixture of osteoblasts, stromal cells, and bone marrow cells. Immobilization of osteoblasts was noted on the coating as well as on trabecular bone within the periprosthetic gap. These osteoblasts synthesize an osteogenic extracellular matrix that ossifies (Fig. 7). Progress of this bone formation process results in formation of lamellar bone onto the surface of the host bone, as well as onto the outer surface of the HA coating (Fig. 8).

At approximately the third month after surgery, coalescence between different fronts of osteogenesis occur. Immature trabecular bone is formed between the lamellar bone present on the surface of the coating and various ossification foci formed in the periprosthetic gap. An anatomic continuity results, responsible for the so-called "osseointegration process" (Fig. 9). This continuity is first present in the areas in which the periprosthetic gap is the narrowest. Gaps of up to 4 mm or 5 mm can be filled with newly formed bone in this fashion (Fig. 10). Where the gap is wider, only a thin lamellar bony apposition is present, unconnected to the host bone. Therefore, these bone sleeves are of minimal importance from a mechanical standpoint (Fig. 11).

Phase II: Bone Remodeling

Disposition of the interfacial bone tissue is similar in all the specimens obtained after one year. This similarity may be explained by a similar pattern of stress distribution in the periprosthetic bone. Morphologic adaptation of the bone to the local stresses is known under the general designation of Julius Wolff's laws. If these laws are founded, a similarity in the stress distribution results in a similar anatomy of the interfacial bone.

Anatomy of the interfacial bone in four zones are: trochanteric zone (zone I of Gruen, Amstutz and McNeice), calcar zone (zone VII), diaphyseal zone (zones II, III, V, & VI), and tip zone (zone IV) (Fig. 12).

In Zone I, radially-oriented trabeculae are noted in every specimen obtained after six months of implantation. These trabeculae are connected on one side with the trochanteric cancellous bone, and on the other side come into contact with the HA coating. Their length is surprising, as they may reach 6.5 cm in length (Fig. 13). These trabeculae cause a considerable interest regarding a mechanical point of view.

1. With a fully-coated prosthesis, an important stress shielding may be expected, which means a dramatic decrease in mechanical stimulation of the proximal femur, together with a hypertrophy of the femur at the level of the tip of the stem, due to an over-solicitation. The reality is entirely different. The proximal area, and particularly the greater trochanter, maintains a high

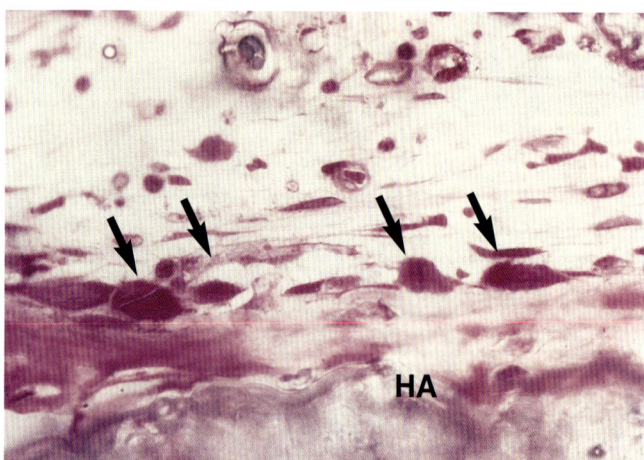

Figure 7. Osteoid matrix (appearing as pink amorphous deposit) on the surface of HA and synthetized by osteoblasts (black arrows).

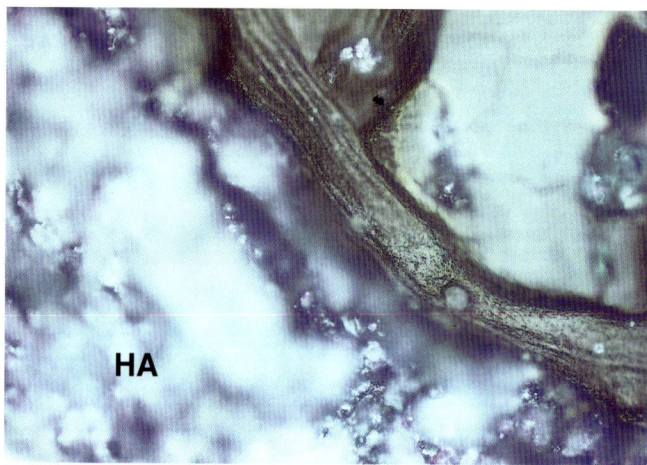

Figure 8. Lamellar bone formed on the surface of HA, without any intervening fibrous tissue (at the level of light microscopy).

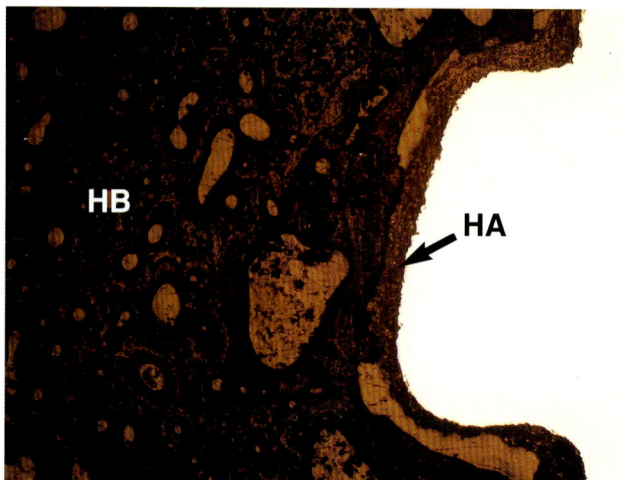

Figure 9. Formation of bone between the HA-coated implant (HA) and the host bone (HB). Note that partial degradation of the coating is visible (black arrow).

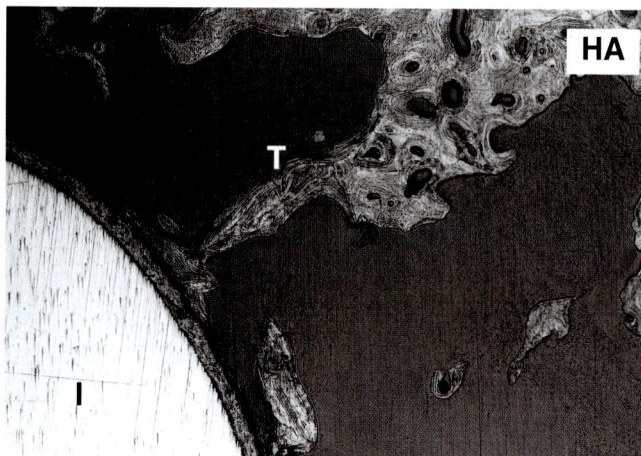

Figure 10. Formation of a bone trabecula (T) in the periprosthetic gap (several millimeters), establishing an anatomic continuity between the implant (I) and host bone (HB).

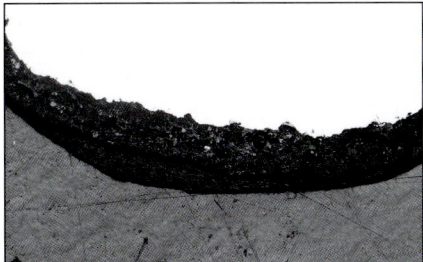

Figure. 11 Presence of a thin bone sleeve (of lamellar structure) on the HA surface. This sleeve is not connected to the host bone (not shown).

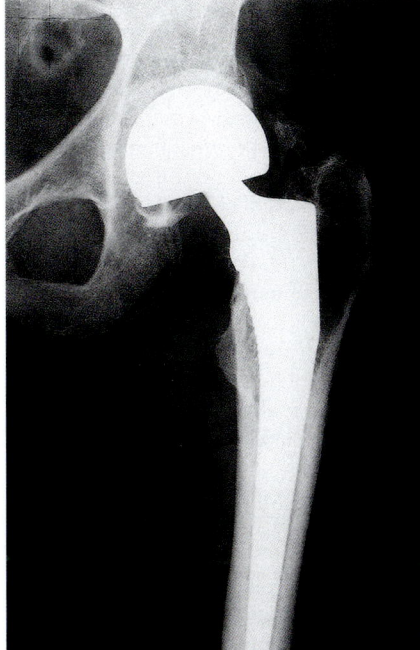

Figure 12. Zones of Gruen.

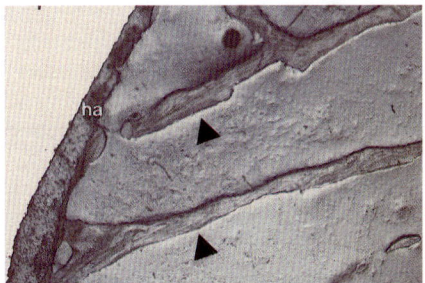

Figure 13. Long, thin bone trabeculae (arrows) radially oriented between the prosthesis and the trochanteric shell.

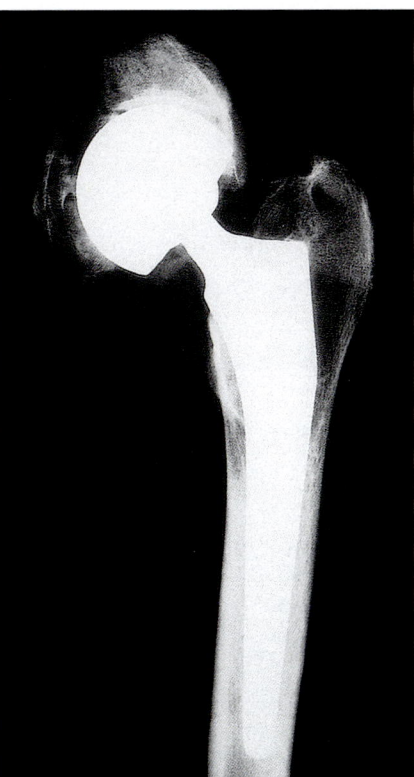

Figure 14. The greater trochanter areas is far from being osteopenic.

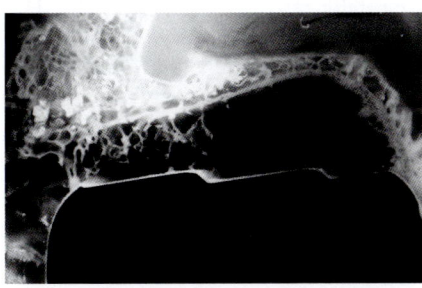

Figure 15. Bone trabeculae are preferentially present on the top of peaks and reliefs of the prosthesis, presumably due to a local, stress riser effect.

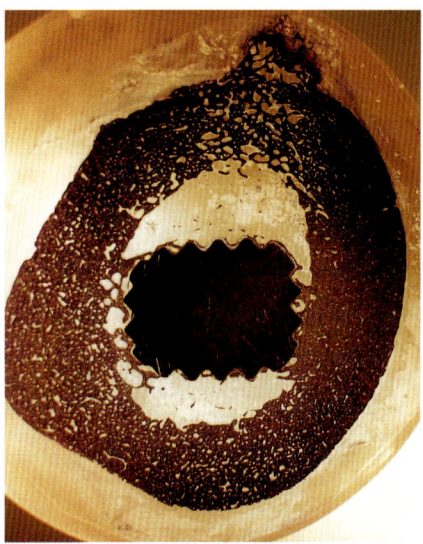

Figure 16. Diaphyseal section. Major bone formation is present on the medial and lateral aspects of the prosthesis, whereas the anterior and posterior aspects are simply covered by a thin layer of lamellar bone.

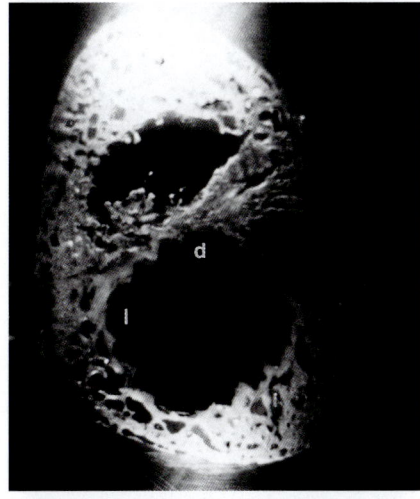

Figure 17. Rounded, thick trabeculae are clearly identified at the corners of the Corail® stem, presumably due to local, stress riser effect.

level of trophicity (Fig. 14).

2. Moreover, the location of these radially oriented trabeculae implies they are submitted to a tensile stress and few examples exist, if any, where long- and thin-bone trabeculae are submitted to traction.

3. Finally, if these trabeculae are submitted to traction, they are attached firmly to the HA coating, and the HA coating is fixed firmly to the underlying metallic substrate.

The importance of the grooves on the surface of the prosthesis is illustrated in Figure 15, showing that bone is mainly present at their level.

In Zone VII, a cancellous bone often appears between the implant and inner cortex. This cancellous bone is dense and formed with interconnected, round-shaped trabeculae. Their presence is more pronounced at the corners of the prosthesis. Cancellization of the inner cortex is constant.

In Zones II, III, V, and VI, in the diaphyseal segment of the stem, obliquely oriented trabeculae are visible between the prosthesis and endosteal bone.

These trabeculae are relatively thick and are present mainly at the inner and outer aspects of the prosthesis (Fig. 16). As mentioned previously for the proximal area, the anterior and posterior aspects of the prostheses are covered with a simple bony sleeve made of a thin lamellar bone. This sleeve is often unconnected with the surrounding host bone, except at the anterior aspect if the prosthesis is seated not too far from the anterior femoral cortex.

Rounded and thick trabecular bone is prominent at the level of the corners of the stem (Fig. 17).

In the areas where the implant is seated in close contact with the cortical haversian bone, haversian structurally

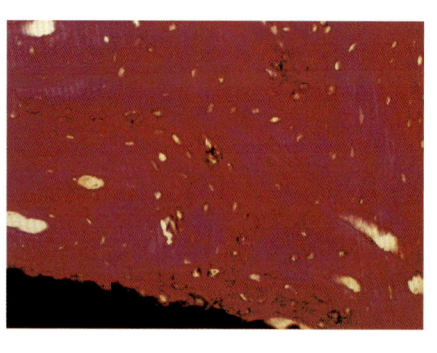

Figure 18. (a) Haversian structured bone (dark pink) is present between the original cortical bone (light pink) and the HA coating; (b) high cellularity of this bone is evident.

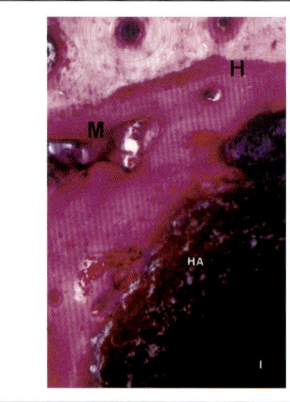

Figure 19. Cancellous bone (dark brown) is formed in the periprosthetic gap at the tip of the stem.

new bone is noted in the interfacial area (Fig. 18).

In Zone IV, at the tip of the implant, skeletal anchorage of the implant to the bone is usually firm. A dense cancellous bone tissue surrounds the implant and is largely interconnected with the endosteal layer of the femur all around (Fig. 19).

Phase III: Resorption

Resorption of the HA coating is observed in all the human explants obtained after 11 months of implantation. The HA coating may be partially or totally resorbed. Theoretically, HA can degrade in two ways: (1) solution-mediated dissolution, with progressive solubilization of the coating according to its physicochemical properties; and (2) cell-mediated resorption, in which osteoclasts and macrophages resorb the coating.

Quantitatively, the first one is the least important regarding our material. An average of 5 μm per year is accepted as the normal dissolution rate of a HA coating. The cell-mediated resorption is more important and areas of total resorption (150 μm) of HA may appear after 12 months.

Morphologically, interesting to note is that the HA coating uncovered with bone is more frequently resorbed entirely and rapidly, whereas the parts of the HA coating covered with bone remain intact longer. Exposure of the coating to the bone marrow seems important in the resorption process, because this process is mediated by cells that originate from the bone marrow.

To better understand this process, one must consider the normal turnover of bone. Bone undergoes transformations during its entire life. This turnover consists of four successive steps:

1. Resorption phase, in which bone is resorbed by the activated osteoclasts.
2. Reversal phase, in which remnants of acellular bone are resorbed by macrophages.
3. Reconstruction phase, in which osteoblasts fill the gap with newly formed bone.
4. Resting phase, in which the situation remains unchanged, waiting for a new resorption process.

This functional unit is known as the Bone Morphogenic Unit (Fig. 20).

HA coatings appear to undergo the same resorption process:

1. Resorption phase, in which activated osteoclast-like cells (named "ceramoclasts" by some authors) dig some lacunae in the surface of the HA coating (Fig. 21).
2. Reversal phase, in which macrophages phagocyte the numerous ceramic fragments released by the action of osteoclast-like cells (Fig. 22).
3. Reconstruction phase, in which osteoblasts (lining cells) rebuild new bone onto the remnants of the ceramic layer (Fig. 23).
4. Resting phase, in which the situation remains unchanged (Fig. 22).

Repetition of this resorption-reconstruction process lead to resorption of HA and progressive substitution of this coating with bone. The numerous cement lines (= arrest-lines) appearing in the newly formed bone indicate bone has formed at different times (Fig. 24).

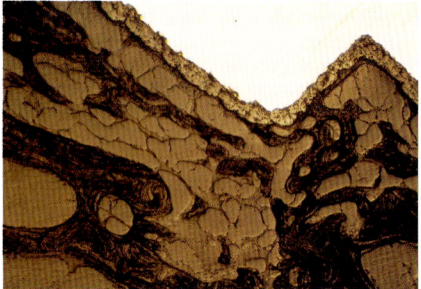

Figure 20. The four steps of the Bone Morphogenic Unit.

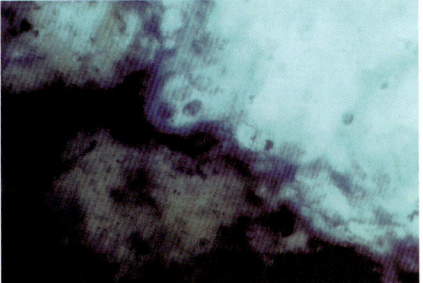

Figure 21. Osteoclast-like cells (dark arrow) create cutting cones into the HA coating.

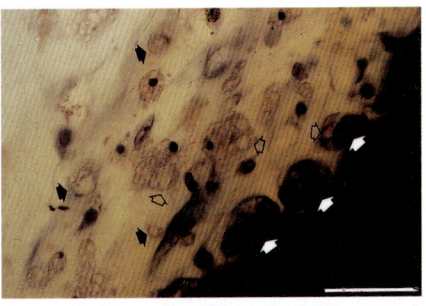

Figure 22. Macrophage-like cells (white arrows) resorb the numerous HA fragments resulting from the action of the osteoclasts. Note the presence of numerous ceramic fragments within the cytoplasmic compartment of the cells (dotted arrows) which appear free in the extracellular compartment (black arrows).

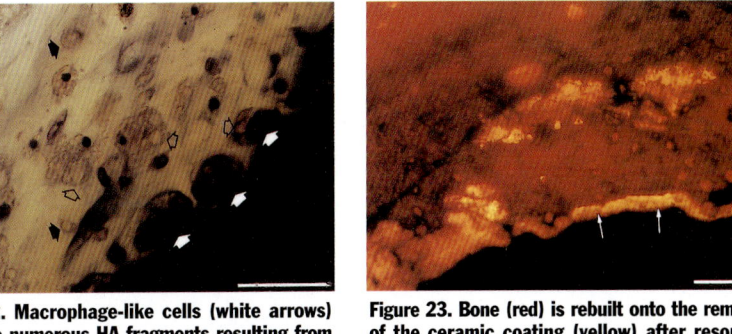

Figure 23. Bone (red) is rebuilt onto the remnants of the ceramic coating (yellow) after resorption has occurred. Numerous fragments appear embedded within the newly reformed bone

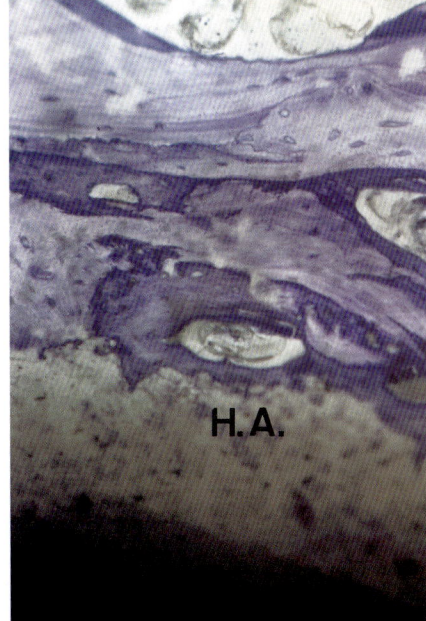

Figure 24. Numerous cement lines appear within the newly formed bone, indicating arrest in the osseointegration process.

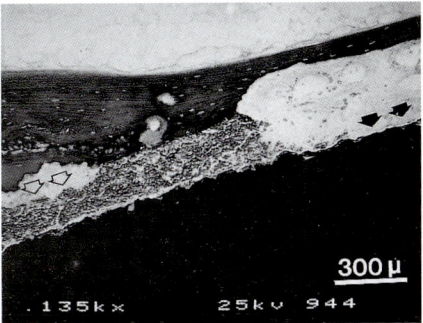

Figure 25. Resorption of the coating may be partial (dotted arrows) or complete (dark arrows). None occurs when bone prevents cells of the bone marrow from having access to the coating.

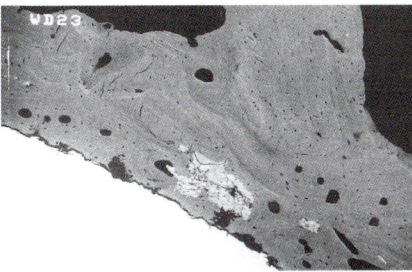

Figure 27. Reconstruction of the bone on the prosthetic surface after coating resorption. Some fragments appear engulfed within the newly formed bone.

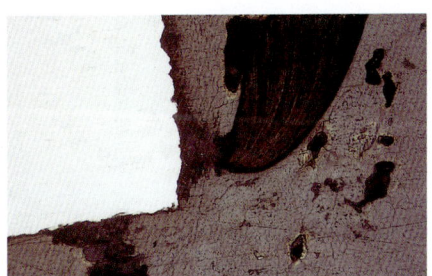

Figure 26. Resorption is nearly complete, except under the end of the bone trabeculae where a "cone" of coating remains morphologically unchanged.

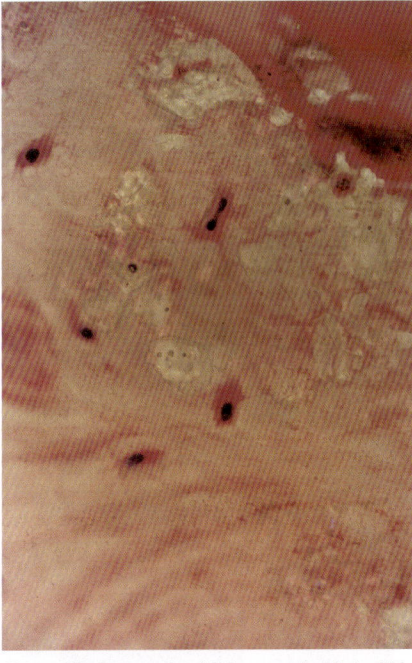

Figure 28. Fragments of HA are embedded within the newly formed bone. Osteocytes are able to send cytoplasmic extensions toward these fragments.

Resorption may be partial or total (Fig. 25). When partial, the prosthesis is left coated with an irregularly shaped remnant of ceramic; when total, the metallic substrate is in contact with the bone marrow (Fig. 26). In both instances, reconstruction of bone may be observed. When reconstruction has occurred, debris of the HA layer appear embedded within the newly re-formed bone (Figs. 27 & 28). The size of these flakes of HA coating are small in the majority of instances.

The Final Result
The Bone Affinity Index (BAI). Coverage of the prosthesis with bone may be quantified using the bone affinity index (BAI). This ratio is obtained by dividing the length of the coating covered with bone by total perimeter of the prosthesis in a given section. The result (expressed as a percentage) provides information regarding the mechanisms of bone formation in a given location. The graft (Fig. 29) shows the average BAI for six prostheses implanted for more than two years and for which histomorphometric studies have been done.

The Coating Resorption Index (CRI). Coating is resorbed progressively. This process initiates early in the life of the coating. It is noted as early as 11 months post implantation. Evaluation of the CRI may be done by measuring the thickness of the ceramic remnant every 500 µm on the entire perimeter of the prosthesis at a given level. Averaging the different values for a given section allows one to assess the importance of the phenomenon. The graft

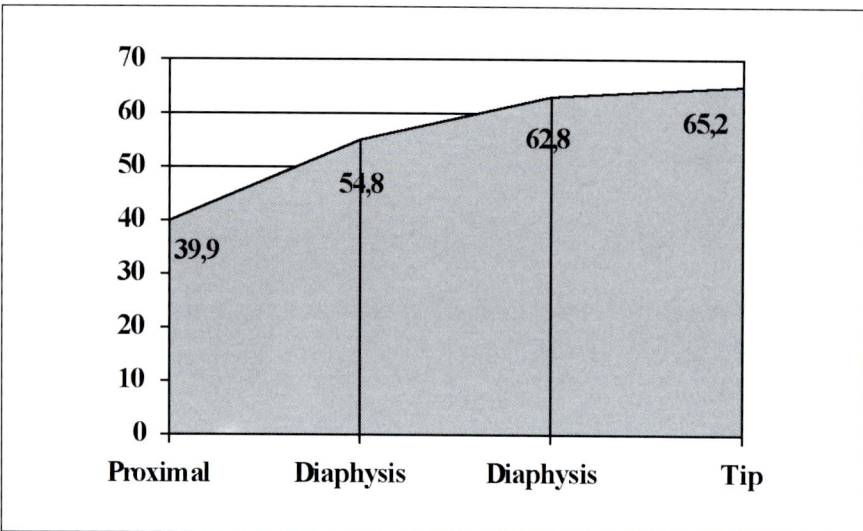

Figure 29. Bone Affinity Index (BAI) quantifies the coverage of the prosthesis by bone; the average BAI is shown for six prostheses implanted for more than two years.

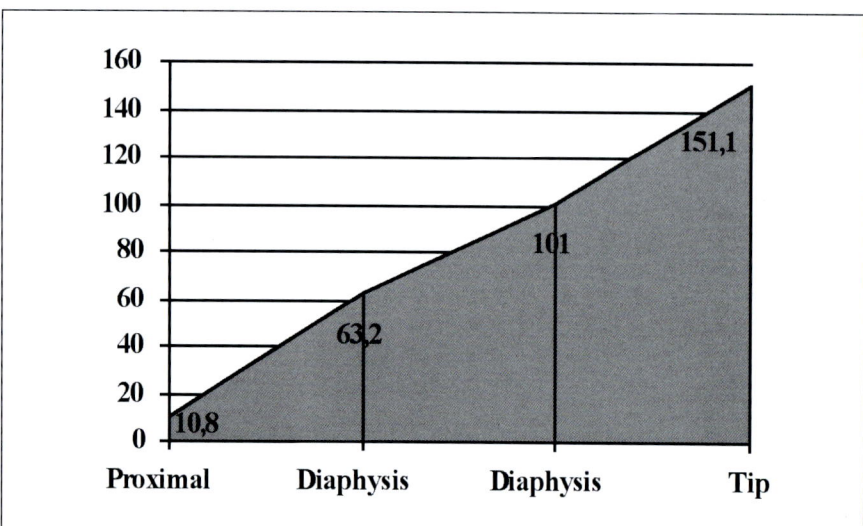

Figure 30. Coating Reabsorption Index (CRI) measures the rate of prosthesis coating reabsorption; the CRI for six prostheses implanted for more than two years is shown.

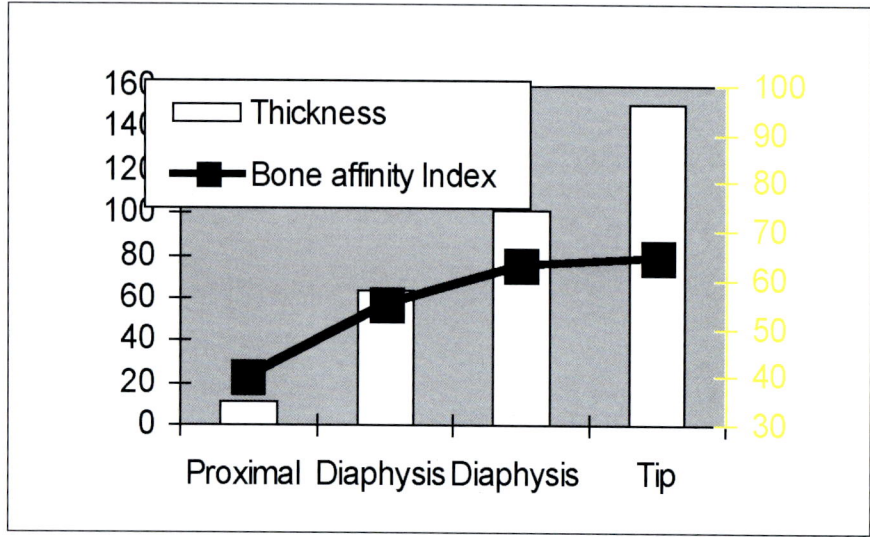

Figure 31. Overlay of the BAI and CRI demonstrates that the BAI and CRI occur at approximately the same rate.

(Fig. 30) shows the CRI for six prostheses implanted for more than two years and for which histomorphometric studies have been done.

MIXING THE TWO GRAFTS (BAI AND CRI) When the two graphs (BAI and CRI) are overlapped (Fig. 31), it appears clearly that the two curves are parallel, which may be explained hypothetically by the mechanisms of activation of the osteoclasts. A relative stress protection exists in the upper femur, which results in an activation of osteoclastic activity. These osteoclasts are responsible for bone loss at this area, and resorption of the newly formed bone in the unstressed areas, such as the anterior or posterior aspects of the implant—consistent with reduction of the BAI in the upper femur. Activated osteoclasts also are active on the HA coating, as it is similar chemically to natural HA. Thus, HA is resorbed progressively in the areas in which osteoclasts are activated preferentially, shown by the higher amount of HA resorption in the proximal area.

These findings indicate HA is effective in enhancing skeletal fixation, even in the presumably difficult context of geriatric patients, but resorption of HA remains a matter of concern. Loosening of the stem, due to the disappearance of the ceramic layer and migration of particles of HA inside the joint space, are the two usually reported pitfalls.

To our knowledge, until now, and despite a meticulous search, no loosening could be demonstrated. The HA coating disappears in the areas with expected low-stress transfer, as in the anterior and posterior aspects of the prosthesis proximally. In the other areas, where stress transfer is evident, HA becomes replaced progressively with bone, maintaining an optimal fixation of the prosthesis. In no instance were micromotion chambers evidenced. .

For the second problem related to HA resorption (i.e., migration of HA particles within the joint space), we have carefully examined 18 of the 29 bipolar heads of our series. Using scanning electron microscopy (SEM), we have looked for foreign bodies at the surface of the polyethylene insert. No HA particles were noted at the distance of the implant, nor in the joint tissues or on the weight-bearing surface of the polyethylene liner. Our material is different, as it consists of bipolar heads, in well-functioning implants, obtained from low-demanding patients. These findings cannot be transposed to total hip arthroplasties.

REFERENCES

1. Garden RS. Low-angle fixation in fractures of the femoral neck. J Bone Joint Surg 1961;43-B:647-63.
2. Parker MJ, Pryor GA. Internal fixation or arthroplasty for displaced cervical hip fractures in the elderly. A randomised controlled trial of 208 patients. Acta Orthop Scand 2000; 71(5) 440-6.
3. Johansson T, Jacobsson SA, Ivarsson I, et al. Internal fixation versus total hip arthroplasty in the treatment of displaced femoral neck fractures. A prospective randomized study of 100 hips. Acta Orthop Scand 2000;71(6): 597-602.
4. Frayssinet P, Tourenne F, Primout I, et al. A study of structure and degradation of non-polymeric biomaterials implanted in bone using reflected and transmitted light microscopy. Biotech Histochem 1993;68(6): 333-41.
5. Hardy DCR, Frayssinet P, Guilhem A, et al. Bonding of hydroxyapatite-coated femoral prostheses. Histopathology of specimens from four cases. J Bone Joint Surg 1991;73-B:732-40.
6. Frayssinet P, Hardy DCR, Conte P, et al. Analyse histologique de l'interface os/prothèse après implantation humaine de prothèses de hanche revêtues d'hydroxyapatite par projection plasma. Rev Chir Orthop, 1993;79:177-84.
7. Hardy DCR, Frayssinet P, Delincé P. Osteointegration of hydroxyapatite-coated stems of femoral prostheses. European J Orthop Surg Trauma 1999;9:75-81.
8. Frayssinet P, Tourenne F, Primout I, et al. A study of structure and degradation of non-polymeric biomaterials implanted in bone using reflected and transmitted light microscopy. Biotechnic Histochem 1993; 68:333-41.
9. Frayssinet P, Rouquet N, Tourenne F, et al. Cell-degradation of calcium phosphate ceramics. Celles Mater 1993;3 :383-94.
10. Frayssinet P, Hardy D, Rouquet N, et al. New observations on middle term hydroxyapatite-coated titanium alloy hip prostheses. Biomaterials 1992;13:668-74.
11. Hardy DCR, Frayssinet P, Guilhem A, et al. Bonding of hydroxyapatite-coated femoral prostheses. Histopathology of specimens from four cases. J Bone Joint Surg 1991;73-B:732-40.
12. Hardy DCR, Frayssinet P, Bonel G, et al. Two-years outcome of hydroxyapatite-coated prostheses. Two femoral prostheses retrieved at autopsy. Acta Orthop Scand 1994;65:253-7.
13. Hardy DCR, Frayssinet P, Krallis P, et al. Histopathology of a well-functioning hydroxyapatite-coated femoral prosthesis after 52 months. Acta Orthop Belg 1999;65(1):72-82.

NEW INDICATION

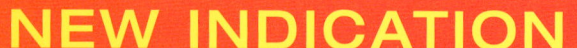

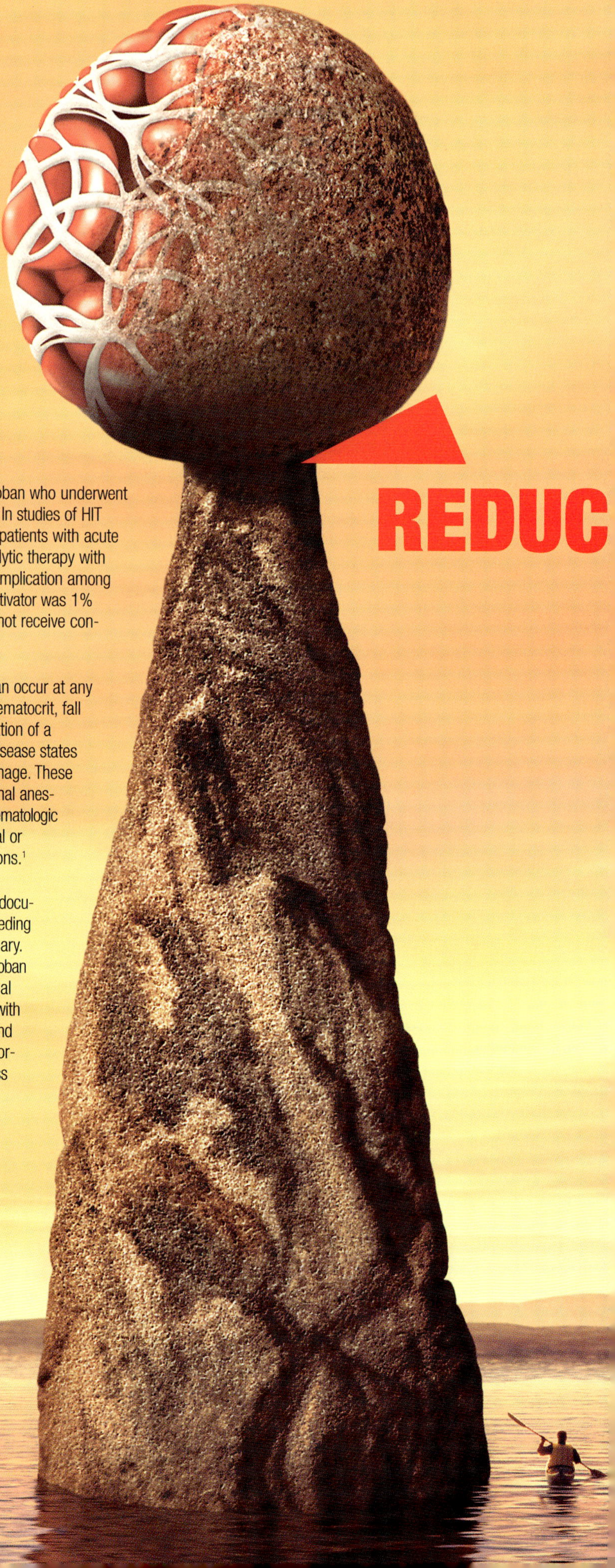

REDUC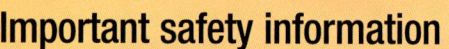

Important safety information

Intracranial bleeding did not occur in any HIT patient treated with Argatroban who underwent percutaneous coronary intervention (PCI) during initial or repeat treatment. In studies of HIT patients who did not undergo PCI, intracranial bleeding only occurred in patients with acute myocardial infarction who were started on both Argatroban and thrombolytic therapy with streptokinase. The overall frequency of this potentially life-threatening complication among patients receiving Argatroban and streptokinase or tissue plasminogen activator was 1% (8/810). Intracranial bleeding was not observed in 317 subjects who did not receive concomitant thrombolysis.[1]

As with all anticoagulants, bleeding is a serious concern. Hemorrhage can occur at any site in the body in patients receiving Argatroban. An unexpected fall in hematocrit, fall in blood pressure, or any unexplained symptom should lead to consideration of a hemorrhagic event. Argatroban should be used with extreme caution in disease states or other circumstances in which there is an increased danger of hemorrhage. These include severe hypertension; immediately following lumbar puncture; spinal anesthesia; major surgery, especially involving the brain, spinal cord, or eye; hematologic conditions associated with increased bleeding tendencies such as congenital or acquired bleeding disorders; and gastrointestinal lesions such as ulcerations.[1]

Argatroban is contraindicated in patients with overt bleeding or those with documented hypersensitivity to the product or any of its components. Major bleeding events observed with Argatroban included gastrointestinal and genitourinary. Intracranial bleeding was not observed in the 568 patients treated with Argatroban for HIT (with or without thrombosis). One patient experienced intracranial bleeding 4 days after discontinuation of Argatroban and following therapy with urokinase and oral anticoagulation. In patients receiving both Argatroban and thrombolytics for myocardial infarction, the incidence of intracranial hemorrhage was 1%. The most common non-hemorrhagic side effects regardless of treatment include dyspnea, hypotension, and fever.[1]

Reference: 1. Argatroban prescribing information, Texas Biotechnology Corporation and GlaxoSmithKline.

Please see brief summary of prescribing information on adjacent page.

GlaxoSmithKline

When patients are at risk and heparin is no longer an option due to heparin-induced thrombocytopenia (HIT)…

THE RISK OF THROMBOSIS

- Argatroban is NOW approved as anticoagulant therapy in patients who have or are at risk for HIT undergoing percutaneous coronary intervention (PCI)[1]
- Argatroban is the ONLY direct thrombin inhibitor approved for both the prophylaxis and treatment of thrombosis associated with HIT[1]

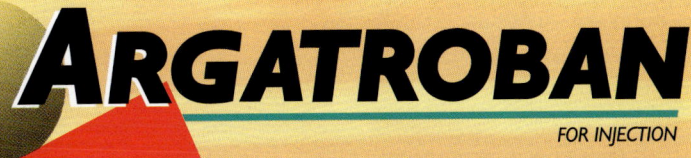

ARGATROBAN
FOR INJECTION

Antithrombin Anticoagulant

Argatroban Injection

Brief Summary: For full prescribing information, see package insert.

INDICATIONS AND USAGE: Argatroban is indicated as an anticoagulant for prophylaxis or treatment of thrombosis in patients with heparin-induced thrombocytopenia.

Argatroban is indicated as an anticoagulant in patients with or at risk for heparin-induced thrombocytopenia undergoing percutaneous coronary interventions (PCI).

CONTRAINDICATIONS: Argatroban is contraindicated in patients with overt major bleeding, or in patients hypersensitive to this product or any of its components (see WARNINGS).

WARNINGS: Argatroban is intended for intravenous administration. Discontinue parenteral anticoagulants before administration of Argatroban. **Hemorrhage:** Hemorrhage can occur at any site in the body in patients receiving Argatroban. An unexplained fall in hematocrit, fall in blood pressure, or any other unexplained symptom should lead to consideration of a hemorrhagic event. Use Argatroban with extreme caution in disease states and other circumstances in which there is an increased danger of hemorrhage: severe hypertension; immediately following lumbar puncture; spinal anesthesia; major surgery, especially involving the brain, spinal cord, or eye; hematologic conditions associated with increased bleeding tendencies such as congenital or acquired bleeding disorders and gastrointestinal lesions such as ulcerations.

PRECAUTIONS: Hepatic Impairment: Use caution when administering Argatroban to patients with hepatic disease, by starting with a lower dose and carefully titrating until the desired level of anticoagulation is achieved. Also, upon cessation of Argatroban infusion in the hepatically impaired patient, full reversal of anticoagulant effects may require longer than 4 hours due to decreased clearance and increased elimination half-life of Argatroban (see DOSAGE AND ADMINISTRATION in complete prescribing information). Avoid using high doses of Argatroban in PCI patients with clinically significant hepatic disease or AST/ALT levels >3 times the upper limit of normal. Such patients were not studied in PCI trials.

Laboratory Tests: Anticoagulation effects associated with Argatroban infusion at doses up to 40 μg/kg/min correlate with increases of the activated partial thromboplastin time (aPTT). Although other global clot-based tests including prothrombin time (PT), the International Normalized Ratio (INR) and thrombin time (TT) are affected by Argatroban, the therapeutic ranges for these tests have not been identified for Argatroban therapy. Plasma Argatroban concentrations also correlate well with anticoagulant effects (see CLINICAL PHARMACOLOGY in complete prescribing information). In clinical trials in PCI, the activated clotting time (ACT) was used for monitoring Argatroban anticoagulant activity during the procedure. The concomitant use of Argatroban and warfarin results in prolongation of the PT and INR beyond that produced by warfarin alone. Alternative approaches for monitoring concurrent Argatroban and warfarin therapy are described in DOSAGE AND ADMINISTRATION in complete prescribing information.

Drug Interactions: ***Heparin:*** Since heparin is contraindicated in patients with heparin-induced thrombocytopenia, the co-administration of Argatroban and heparin is unlikely for this indication. However, if Argatroban is to be initiated after cessation of heparin therapy, allow sufficient time for heparin's effect on the aPTT to decrease prior to initiation of Argatroban therapy. ***Aspirin/Acetaminophen:*** Pharmacokinetic or pharmacodynamic drug-drug interactions have not been demonstrated between Argatroban and concomitantly administered aspirin (162.5 mg orally given 26 and 2 hours prior to initiation of Argatroban 1 μg/kg/min over 4 hours) or acetaminophen (1000 mg orally given 12, 6 and 0 hours prior to, and 6 and 12 hours subsequent to, initiation of Argatroban 1.5 μg/kg/min over 18 hours). ***Oral anticoagulant agents:*** Pharmacokinetic drug-drug interactions between Argatroban and warfarin (7.5 mg single oral dose) have not been demonstrated. However, the concomitant use of Argatroban and warfarin (5-7.5 mg initial oral dose followed by 2.5-6 mg/day orally for 6-10 days) results in prolongation of the prothrombin time (PT) and International Normalized Ratio (INR) (see CLINICAL PHARMACOLOGY and DOSAGE AND ADMINISTRATION in complete prescribing information). ***Thrombolytic agents:*** The safety and effectiveness of Argatroban with thrombolytic agents have not been established (see ADVERSE REACTIONS, Intracranial Bleeding). ***Glycoprotein IIb/IIIa antagonists:*** The safety and effectiveness of Argatroban with glycoprotein IIb/IIIa antagonists have not been established. ***Co-administration:*** Concomitant use of Argatroban with antiplatelet agents, thrombolytics, and other anticoagulants may increase the risk of bleeding (see WARNINGS). Drug-drug interactions have not been observed between Argatroban and digoxin or erythromycin (see CLINICAL PHARMACOLOGY, Drug-Drug Interactions in complete prescribing information).

Carcinogenesis, Mutagenesis, Impairment of Fertility: No long-term studies in animals have been performed to evaluate the carcinogenic potential of Argatroban. Argatroban was not genotoxic in the Ames test, the Chinese hamster ovary cell (CHO/HGPRT) forward mutation test, the Chinese hamster lung fibroblast chromosome aberration test, the rat hepatocyte and WI-38 human fetal lung cell unscheduled DNA synthesis (UDS) tests, or the mouse micronucleus test. Argatroban at intravenous doses up to 27 mg/kg/day (0.3 times the recommended maximum human dose based on body surface area) was found to have no effect on fertility and reproductive performance of male and female rats.

Pregnancy. Teratogenic Effects. Pregnancy Category B: Teratology studies in rats with intravenous doses up to 27 mg/kg/day (0.3 times the recommended maximum human dose based on body surface area) and rabbits at intravenous doses up to 10.8 mg/kg/day (0.2 times the recommended maximum human dose based on body surface area) have revealed no evidence of impaired fertility or harm to the fetus due to Argatroban. There are, however, no adequate and well-controlled studies in pregnant women. Because animal reproduction studies are not always predictive of human response, use Argatroban during pregnancy only if clearly needed.

Nursing Mothers: Argatroban is detected in rodent milk. It is not known whether this drug is excreted in human milk. Because many drugs are excreted in human milk and because of the potential for serious adverse reactions in nursing infants from Argatroban, a decision should be made whether to discontinue nursing or to discontinue the drug, taking into account the importance of the drug to the mother.

Geriatric Use: In the clinical studies of adult patients with HIT or HITTS, the effectiveness of Argatroban was not affected by age.

Pediatric Use: The safety and effectiveness of Argatroban in patients below the age of 18 years have not been established.

ADDITIONAL INFORMATION: ***Cardiac Therapy:*** The safety and effectiveness of Argatroban for cardiac indications outside of percutaneous coronary intervention in patients with HIT have not been established.

Reexposure and Lack of Antibody Formation: Plasma from 12 healthy volunteers treated with Argatroban over 6 days showed no evidence of neutralizing antibodies. Repeated administration of Argatroban to more than 40 patients was tolerated with no loss of anticoagulant activity. No change in the dose is required.

ADVERSE REACTIONS: Adverse Events Reported in HIT/HITTS Patients: The following safety information is based on all 568 patients treated with Argatroban in Study 1 and Study 2, compared with 193 historical controls in which the adverse events were collected retrospectively. The adverse events include all hemorrhagic and non-hemorrhagic events. Major bleeding was defined as overt bleeding associated with a hemoglobin decrease ≥2 g/dL, that led to a transfusion of ≥2 units, or that was intracranial, retroperitoneal, or into a major prosthetic joint. Minor bleeding was overt bleeding that did not meet the criteria for major bleeding.

These are the most frequently observed hemorrhagic events among Argatroban-treated HIT/HITTS patients, presented separately by major and minor bleeding.

Major Hemorrhagic Events in HIT/HITTS Patients*

	Argatroban-treated patients (n=568) %	Historical Control (n=193) %
Overall Bleeding	5.3	6.7
Gastrointestinal	2.3	1.6
Genitourinary and hematuria	0.9	0.5
Decrease in hemoglobin and hematocrit	0.7	0
Multisystem hemorrhage and DIC	0.5	1
Limb and BKA stump	0.5	0
Intracranial hemorrhage	0†	0.5

Minor Hemorrhagic Events in HIT/HITTS Patients*

	Argatroban-treated patients (n=568) %	Historical Control (n=193) %
Gastrointestinal	14.4	18.1
Genitourinary and hematuria	11.6	0.8
Decrease in hemoglobin and hematocrit	10.4	0
Groin	5.4	3.1
Hemoptysis	2.9	0.8
Brachial	2.4	0.8

*Patients may have experienced more than one adverse event.

†One patient experienced intracranial hemorrhage 4 days after discontinuation of Argatroban and following therapy with urokinase and oral anticoagulation.

DIC = disseminated intravascular coagulation.

BKA = below the knee amputation.

The following is a list of the most frequently observed (≥2%) non-hemorrhagic events among 568 Argatroban-treated patients vs. 193 historical controls: dyspnea 8.1% vs. 8.8%; hypotension 7.2% vs. 2.6%; fever 6.9% vs. 2.1%; diarrhea 6.2% vs. 1.6%; sepsis 6.0% vs. 12.4%; cardiac arrest 5.8% vs. 3.1%; nausea 4.8% vs. 0.5%; ventricular tachycardia 4.8% vs. 3.1%; pain 4.6% vs. 3.1%; urinary tract infection 4.6% vs. 5.2%; vomiting 4.2% vs. 0%; infection 3.7% vs. 3.6%; pneumonia 3.3% vs. 9.3%; atrial fibrillation 3.0% vs. 11.4%; coughing 2.8% vs. 1.6%; abnormal renal function 2.8% vs. 4.7%; abdominal pain 2.6% vs. 1.6%; cerebrovascular disorder 2.3% vs. 4.1%. Patients may have experienced more than one adverse event.

Adverse Events Reported in HIT/HITTS Patients Undergoing PCI: The following safety information is based on 91 patients initially treated with Argatroban and 21 patients subsequently re-exposed to Argatroban for a total of 112 PCIs with Argatroban anticoagulation. The adverse events include hemorrhagic and non-hemorrhagic events.

Major bleeding was defined as bleeding that was overt and associated with a hemoglobin decrease ≥5 g/dL, that led to a transfusion of ≥2 units, or that was intracranial, retroperitoneal, or into a major prosthetic joint.

The rate of major bleeding events and intracranial hemorrhage in the PCI trials was 1.8% and in the placebo arm of the EPILOG trial (placebo plus standard dose, weight-adjusted heparin) was 3.1%.

These are the most frequently observed hemorrhagic events among Argatroban-treated HIT/HITTS patients undergoing PCI, presented separately by major and minor bleeding.

Major Hemorrhagic Events in HIT/HITTS patients undergoing PCI*

	Argatroban-treated Patients (n=112)† %
Retroperitoneal	0.9
Gastrointestinal	0.9
Intracranial Hemorrhage	0

Minor Hemorrhagic Events in HIT/HITTS patients undergoing PCI*

	Argatroban-treated Patients (n=112)† %
Groin (bleeding or hematoma)	3.6
Gastrointestinal (includes hematemesis)	2.6
Genitourinary (includes hematuria)	1.8
Decrease in hemoglobin and/or hematrocrit	1.8
CABG (coronary arteries)	1.8
Access site	0.9
Hemoptysis	0.9
Other	0.9

*Patients may have experienced more than one adverse event.

†91 patients who underwent 112 interventions.

CABG = coronary artery bypass graft.

The following is a list of the most frequently observed non-hemorrhagic events (>2%) among Argatroban-treated PCI patients (91 patients underwent 112 interventions) vs. 2226 controls: chest pain 15.2% vs. 9.3%; hypotension 10.7% vs. 10.3%; back pain 8.0% vs. 13.7%; nausea 7.1% vs. 11.5%; vomiting 6.3% vs. 6.8%; headache 5.4% vs. 5.5%; bradycardia 4.5% vs. 3.5%; abdominal pain 3.6% vs. 2.2%; fever 3.6% vs. < 0.5%; myocardial infarction 3.6% vs. not reported. Controls from EPIC (Evaluation of c7E3 Fab in the Prevention of Ischemic Complications), EPILOG (Evaluation in PTCA to Improve Long-Term Outcome with Abciximab GP IIb/IIIa Blockade Study) and CAPTURE (Chimeric 7E3 Antiplatelet Therapy in Unstable angina Refractory to standard treatment). Patients may have experienced more than one adverse event.

There were 22 serious adverse events in 17 Argatroban-treated HIT/HITTS patients undergoing PCI (19.6% in 112 interventions): chest pain 1/112 (0.9%), fever 1/112 (0.9%), retroperitoneal hemorrhage 1/112 (0.9%), angina pectoris 2/112 (1.8%), aortic stenosis 1/112 (0.9%), coronary thrombosis 2/112 (1.8%), arterial thrombosis 1/112 (0.9%), myocardial infarction 4/112 (3.5%), myocardial ischemia 2/112 (1.8%), occlusion coronary 2/112 (1.8%), gastrointestinal hemorrhage 1/112 (0.9%), gastrointestinal disorder (GERD) 1/112 (0.9%), cerebrovascular disorder 1/112 (0.9%), lung edema 1/112 (0.9%), vascular disorder 1/112 (0.9%). Individual events may also have been reported elsewhere (see hemorrhagic and non-hemorrhagic events). Some patients may have experienced more than one event.

Adverse Events Reported in Other Populations: The following safety information is based on a total of 1,127 individuals who were treated with Argatroban in clinical pharmacology studies (n=211) or for various clinical indications (n=916). **Intracranial Bleeding:** Intracranial bleeding only occurred in patients with acute myocardial infarction who were started on both Argatroban and thrombolytic therapy with streptokinase. The overall frequency of this potentially life-threatening complication among patients receiving both Argatroban and thrombolytic therapy (streptokinase or tissue plasminogen activator) was 1% (8 out of 810 patients). Intracranial bleeding was not observed in 317 subjects or patients who did not receive concomitant thrombolysis (see WARNINGS). **Allergic Reactions:** 156 allergic reactions or suspected allergic reactions were observed in 1,127 individuals treated with Argatroban in clinical pharmacology studies or for various clinical indications. About 95% (148/156) of these reactions occurred in patients who concomitantly received thrombolytic therapy (e.g., streptokinase) for acute myocardial infarction and/or contrast media for coronary angiography. Allergic reactions or suspected allergic reactions in populations other than HIT patients include (in descending order of frequency): Airway reactions (coughing, dyspnea): 10% or more; Skin reactions (rash, bullous eruption): 1 to <10%; General reactions (vasodilation): 1 to 10%.

Manufactured by **Abbott Laboratories**, North Chicago, IL 60064

Distributed by **GlaxoSmithKline**, Research Triangle Park, NC 27709 for **Texas Biotechnology Corporation**, Houston, TX 77030

BRS-AR:L3

©2002 The GlaxoSmithKline Group of Companies
All rights reserved. ARG019R0

Advances in Deep-Vein Thrombosis Treatment

JAMES EDWIN MUNTZ, M.D., F.A.C.P.

CLINICAL ASSOCIATE PROFESSOR OF INTERNAL MEDICINE
BAYLOR COLLEGE OF MEDICINE, HOUSTON, TEXAS
AND
UNIVERSITY OF TEXAS AT HOUSTON HEALTH SCIENCE CENTER

CLINICAL ASSOCIATE PROFESSOR OF ORTHOPEDIC SURGERY
BAYLOR COLLEGE OF MEDICINE, HOUSTON, TEXAS

Venous and arterial thromboses account for some of the most common causes of morbidity and mortality amongst patients in the United States and many other Western societies. Clotting disorders and hypercoagulable states are no longer just treated by hematologists, but by multiple specialties including internal medicine, family practice, critical care physicians and most recently, hospitalists. In more than 75% of cases, the cause of the thrombotic episodes can be identified. More than one-half of the patients with thrombosis harbor either congenital propensity to develop a thrombosis, or have an acquired event that precipitates a pro-thrombotic state.[1]

The purpose of this article is to review the developments in the following four topics as related to thrombosis: (1) approaches in diagnosis; (2) side effects associated with heparin, notably heparin-induced thrombocytopenia; (3) developments in the use of existing drugs and newer agents; and (4) advances in our understanding of the proper duration of treatment of DVT and PE.

DIAGNOSTIC APPROACHES AND MODALITIES

The "gold standard" method for detecting deep vein thrombosis (DVT) has been contrast venography, whereas, the diagnostic imaging method used most frequently in the United States is ultrasonography.[2] Contrast venography is decreasingly utilized because it is painful for the patient, can cause side effects, is relatively expensive, and time consuming. Additionally, in about 20 to 30% of cases, the test cannot reliably differentiate acute recurrent DVT from old non-acute DVT in patients with prior history of thrombosis.[3,4] Real-time B-mode ultrasonography with compression and pulsed wave Doppler flow analysis, using a combination of color Doppler flow images is accepted as being highly sensitive and specific between the pelvis and knees in patients with localized signs and symptoms and no prior history of DVT in the affected extremity. However, this method is much less accurate below the knee and in patients without localized signs or symptoms, or in patients with a prior history of DVT.[5]

New Developments

D-dimer testing became a very popular test in the last decade. Its most promising clinical benefit is associated with its benefit of possessing a high negative predictive value.[6] The assays initially were latex agglutination, which progressed into whole blood agglutination testing[7,8] and most recently advances have been made with the ELSA D-dimer testing.[9] Recently, at the British Thoracic Society Winter meeting,[10] researchers presented findings regarding the impact of D-dimer testing on management of suspected DVT and PE. These researchers compared a series of 88 patients with a negative D-dimer result with a cohort of 95 matched historical controls. The results demonstrated the negative predictive value of the D-dimer test was 100% for DVT with a sensitivity of 100% and specificity of 81 to 82%. The negative predictive value of D-dimer testing for PE was reported to be 81% with a sensitivity of 20%.[10] One of the most important impacts of D-dimer testing is the resultant decrease in the utilization of Doppler ultrasounds. This decrease has approached 25% in our institution, Methodist Hospital, Houston, Texas, with the apparent reduction in charges of approximately $400 per study.

In addition to the emergence of D-dimer testing, is an innovative nuclear medicine scan introduced within the last 5 years—Apcitide (Acutect®, Berlex Laboratories, Montville, NJ). This scan is a useful noninvasive test for the detection of DVT not only in the lower extremities, but also in the upper extremities and in the veins of the neck. Technetium Apcitide, formerly known as 99mTc-P280, is a radiolabelled peptide that binds with high affinity and specificity to the glycoprotein IIb/IIIa receptors.[11] The receptors reside on activated platelets that are involved in acute thrombosis.

Apcitide results have been compared to standard adjudicated venograms. The sensitivity between the two modalities was between 65-69% (Table 1). This diagnostic modality could be useful in patients with a prior history of DVT when venography might be indeterminate, however, more studies are needed to identify its position in the hierarchy of diagnostic testing.

A method for detection of DVT with a technetium 99m labeled peptide (DMP 444) was recently reported.[12] This compound also binds to the glycoprotein IIb/IIIa receptors on activated platelets. Although only a small number of patients have been studied, the preliminary human studies show that the compound initially appears to be safe and may be of value in the diagnosis of DVT. Shortcomings of the study were the comparator, ultrasound and a positive D-dimer; in lieu of venography. It is expected that the technique of diagnosis will be further validated in the upcoming PIOPED trial.[13,14]

The usefulness of performing indirect computerized tomographic venography after pulmonary CT angiography for detection of DVT in patients suspected of having a PE has also been described.[15] In this particular trial, 541 consecutive patients from 7 institutions underwent pulmonary CT angiography for suspected PE. Using a protocol that optimizes venous enhancement without additional contrast material injection, contiguous images from the pelvis to the popliteal fossa were obtained. The results showed that DVT was found by indirect CT venography in 45 patients or 8%, and PE was found at pulmonary CT angiography in 17% of 541 patients. Among 45 patients with DVT, it was noted that the DVT occurred in 16 patients who had no PE at pulmonary CT angiography, which increased the diagnostic positivity for thromboembolic disease by almost 20%. The investigators concluded that a substantial number of patients had DVT in the absence of PE by CT angiography. Combining the pulmonary CT angiography with indirect CT venography can increase accuracy in the diagnosis of venous thromboembolism. Due to the

Table 1. Apcitide vs. Venograms: Primary and Secondary Efficacy Endpoints

	Agreement Rate		
	Trial A	Trial B	Combined
Primary Endpoints Blind-Read 99mTc-apcitide vs Blind Read Venography	73.5%* (65.7%[1]; n=113)	59.3% (51.5%[1]; n=123)	66.1%* (60.7%[1]; n=236)
Blind-Read 99mTc-apcitide versus Hamilton Read Venography	68.2%* (60.0%[1]; n=110)	70.0%* (62.3%[1]; n=120)	69.1* (63.7%[1]; n=230)
Secondary Endpoint Blind-Read 99mTc-apcitide vs Institutional-Read Venography	69.6%* (61.7%[1]; n=113)	69.1%* (61.5%[1]; n=123)	69.3%* (64.0%[1]; n=238)
Institutional-Read 99mTc-apcitide vs Institutional-Read Venography	79.8* (71.1-86.3%)[2] (n=114)	68.6* (59.4-76.4%)[2] (n=121)	74.0* (67.9-79.4%)[2] (n=235)

[1]Lower bound of one-sided 95% confidence interval

[2]95% confidence intervals

* Statistically significantly greater than or equal to 75% (lower bound of one-sided 95% confidence interval is greater than or equal to 60%), p<0.05

fact that extra dye is not utilized, this may indeed be a useful research tool as well as have practical applications.[15]

HEPARIN-INDUCED THROMBOCYTOPENIA

An additional major advance made in the area of thrombosis management is our understanding of heparin-induced thrombocytopenia (HIT). This dreaded entity can be a major life- and limb-threatening complication of heparin and low-molecular-weight heparin treatment.[16] It may be seen during treatment of an acute thrombosis when the patient has an unexplained platelet drop or has propagation of a fairly well treated DVT or PE. Deterioration of the patient's condition during treatment with heparin or low-molecular- weight heparin should prompt full investigation and should include immediate measurement of the platelet count. Generally, HIT occurs 5 to 14 days after initiating heparin therapy and is independent of route of administration.[17] Heparin and heparin-based therapies continue to be one of the most commonly administered parenteral treatments in a hospital setting. Over 1 trillion units of heparin are used per year in the United States alone[18] and approximately 12 million patients are exposed to heparin each year.[19] While HIT is generally uncommon, more significantly it is under-recognized and under-diagnosed when it does occur.

Immediate consideration of HIT is essential to the accurate diagnosis and effective treatment of patients.[20-24] HIT should be as strongly suspected in cases of new or progressive thrombotic events. Immediate discontinuation of all forms of heparin is essential and is to be followed by initiation of alternative anticoagulation therapy. Newer diagnostic tests are available for HIT and thrombosis, but clinical suspicion is of paramount importance. A platelet count of less than 150,000 or a 50% drop in the platelet count from baseline should alert the clinician to the possibility of this particular complication.[25]

A detailed review of the diagnostic tests for HIT are beyond the scope of this particular publication, but the tests now are divided into functional assays and into the heparin PF4 ELISA assay. Advantages of the enzyme-linked immunoassay include the fact that it is a very sensitive test, normal platelets are not required, and it is easier to perform a fairly large number of tests quite easily.[26] The disadvantages are that one cannot assess cross reactivity, and there are frequently false positive tests without symptoms of HIT in the patient.[27]

Before direct thrombin inhibitors were approved for the treatment of HIT other therapeutic strategies included administration of IgG immunoglobulins and plasmapheresis.[27] Most of these situations were case reports, and therapies were anecdotal. Warfarin treatment immediately initiated following the discontinuation of heparin treatment, which theoretically would seem to help, actually made many of these patients worse. The progression of DVT with warfarin treatment leading to venous limb gangrene has been described.[28] This was due to hypercoagulable conditions; one being related to HIT, and the other is due to an acquired depletion of protein C and protein S levels which are involved in the vitamin K dependent pathway. Therefore, it is recommended that the treatment of HIT begin with thrombin inhibition before administration of warfarin.

Two direct thrombin inhibitors have been approved by the FDA for the treatment of HIT. The initial one lepirudin (Refludan®, Hoescht Marion Roussel, Kansas City, MO,[29] is indicated for treatment of HIT and more recently Argatroban® (Glaxo SmithKline, Research Triangle Park, NC),[30] has been approved for both prophylaxis and treatment of HIT. A third type of parenteral medication often used in HIT and thrombosis is danaparoid. The active components of danaparoid (Orgaran®, Organon Inc., West Orange, NJ) are isolated from porcine intestinal mucosa and include heparan sulfate 83%, dermatan sulfate 12% and chondroitin sulfate 5%.[31] This particular drug is an indirect thrombin inhibitor and its antithrombotic effect is exerted principally through antithrombin III. Danaparoid is generally excreted by the kidneys, and this drug is not approved for prevention or treatment of HIT but has been used on a compassionate usage basis. In vitro studies demonstrated 10% to 20% cross-reactivity with heparin-induced antibodies, but whether or not this is significant in vivo remains to be seen.[31]

ADVANCES IN PHARMACOLOGICAL MANAGEMENT

A recent article by Hirsh and Bates reviewed the influence clinical trials have on the treatment of venous thromboembolism.[32] The literature is inundated with numerous articles on the significant benefits of low-molecular-weight heparins.[33-35] Product usage has continued to increase throughout North America and we have witnessed new FDA approvals and new indications. Most recently, the low-molecular-weight heparin - enoxaparin (Lovenox®, Aventis Pharmaceuticals, Bridgewater, NJ), received FDA approval in December 2000 for the prevention of VTE in the medically ill patient.[36]

Questions about optimal dosing and fixed dosing drive new research. During the December 2000 annual meeting of the American Society of Hematology, researchers presented findings that certoparin (Sandoparin®, Novartis, Basel, Switzerland) is as efficacious as adjusted dose intravenous unfractionated heparin for the initial treatment of proximal DVT. The investigators concluded that fixed-dose, body-weight independent LMWH is as efficacious and safe as intravenous aPTT adjusted unfractionated heparin in the treatment of acute proximal DVT. The study involved a cohort of 1,220 patients, approximately half split into the LMWH group and the other half into the adjusted unfractionated heparin group, and then initial anticoagulation was followed by oral anticoagulation for 6 months in a multicenter prospective study. More recently in the Annals of Internal Medicine, results of an enoxaparin trial showed the efficacy of once a day versus twice a day LMWH, (enoxaparin versus unfractionated heparin).[37] Although the outcomes in each group were essentially similar, if one were to evaluate the subgroups of patients with obesity, cancer and iliofemoral vein thrombophlebitis, these patients did better with twice daily dosing than with once daily dosing. In summary, issues are still at hand about weight extreme patients and optimal dosing with LMWH.

Attempts remain to find an alternative to oral anticoagulant therapy with less bleeding complications in long-term treatment of DVT. In a recent trial 100 consecutive elderly patients 75 years of age or greater with venographically demonstrated proximal DVT were included in a randomized fashion.[38] All patients were treated for 10 days with adjusted doses of intravenous heparin and then randomly allocated to receive vitamin K antagonists targeting an INR of 2.0 to 3.0 or subcutaneous enoxaparin once a day for 3 months. All patients were followed clinically and venographically for a 1-year period of time. In comparison with oral anticoagulants the findings were inconclusive due to the wide confidence intervals for different screening outcomes; however, the outcomes suggest there may have been fewer bleeding complications in the LMWH group, and efficacy was similar between the 2 groups.[38]

Further novel approaches to prophylaxis in DVT have come under observation with the release of new drugs. Phase two trials involving ORG31540/SR90107A (pentasaccharide) versus LMWH were published.[39] Pentasaccharide is a completely synthesized novel compound with pure anti-X_a effects. This was a dose finding trial that involved five different doses of pentasaccharide — two of which were discontinued for safety reasons.[39] The findings in this trial set the groundwork for the optimal dose ranging for the phase 3 trials that have subsequently been presented at the ASH meeting in December 2000 in San Francisco, comparing the pentasaccharide compound with LMWH in hip replacement, knee replacement and hip fracture patients. Also presented at the American Society of Hematology was a study involving melagatran (Astra-Zeneca, Wilmington, DE), a new compound being studied in orthopedic surgery patients in the prevention of DVT and PE.[40] The obvious advantages in an oral direct thrombin inhibitor such as melagatran is that it is delivered as a prodrug. There are essentially no drug-to-drug interactions and no monitoring is required. The chemical name of the thrombin inhibitor melagatrin, H376-95, is currently undergoing investigation in knee replacement trials as well as prophylaxis in total hip arthroplasty.

THERAPEUTIC ADVANCES IN DURATION OF THERAPY

Conventional wisdom has led clinicians to continue anticoagulation therapy in patients with venous thromboembolism for approximately 3 months.[41] Some clinicians initially have tried 6 weeks of therapy only to return to 3 months to 6 months of continued treatment. Patients with recurrent venous thrombosis and those with idiopathic venous disease are generally treated for a longer period of time.[42] A well-designed study comparing 6 weeks to 6 months of oral anticoagulant therapy in recurrent DVT patients showed that there was a significantly lower recurrence rate in the patients treated for 6 months.[43] Kearon et. al., performed a multicenter double blind randomized trial in which patients with idiopathic DVT were assigned to 3 months of anticoagulation versus 2 years of treatment with Warfarin (Bristol Myers Squibb, Princeton, NJ).[43] The trial was terminated prematurely due to the fact the recurrence rate was 27% in the group treated for 3 months as opposed to only 2% in the patients that remained on continued treatment.

When evaluating the duration of therapy, the clinician must compare the risk of bleeding versus the risk of recurrent venous disease. When weighing the situation, one must specify location and subsequently stratify patients into distal clot versus proximal clot and decisions about length of therapy and intensity of therapy. Also, importance needs to be attached to whether this is a first-time clot or recurrent clot. Idiopathic venous thromboembolism seems to require a longer period of treatment as well as does recurrent DVT and PE. All of these are well documented with recommendations per the recent ACCP Chest supplement published in January of 2001.[44]

CONCLUSIONS

The prophylaxis and treatment of thromboembolic disease continues to remain in the forefront of medical research and other efforts to better equip physicians with tools for diagnosis and the pharmaceuticals to either prevent or treat thrombosis. The need for this research is obvious—thromboembolism remains one of the leading causes of mortality and morbidity in the world. The approach to diagnosis is growing with the uptake of D-Dimer testing and newer nuclear medicine scans. The former method may obviate the need for the many of the venographic and ultrasound techniques[45], whereas, the latter, requires additional study. One of the basic tenets of medicine is to do no harm to the patient. Our understanding of the etiology and management of heparin-induced thrombocytopenia has grown tremendously, and more importantly, being incorporated into the decision schemes of practitioners. The educational requirement to always remain vigilant for this life-threatening complication remains strong and further efforts in this area are warranted.

The armamentarium of pharmaceuticals and indications for use of existing pharmaceuticals also continues to grow. The emergence of LMWH as a standard of therapy in many thrombotic conditions, as well as the emergence of newer agents, will require the conscious efforts to evaluate all these agents for use in patient populations. Careful consideration of incorporating prophylaxis in medical patients particularly will grow in the next few years, as well as the further use of agents outside of the hospital.

Finally, the actual period a patient is at risk of developing a DVT or PE following a pro-thrombotic condition will require further research. Evidence indicates, for instance, that our previous concept of the risk period probably underestimates true risk. As these threads of research and development come together—our overall goal of cost-conscious, safe, and effective management of thrombosis—will be achieved.

REFERENCES

1. Bick R. Syndromes of thrombosis and hypercoagulability. Med Clinics of NA. 1998; 82: 409-458.
2. Lensing AWA, Hirsh J, Büller HR; Diagnosis of Venous Thrombosis. In: Colman RW, Hirsh J, Marder VJ, eds. Hemostasis and Thrombosis: Basic principles and clinical practices, Third Edition Philadelphia: J P Lippincott Company; 1994: 1297-1302.
3. Hirsh J, Hoak J. Management of deep vein thrombosis and pulmonary embolism. Circulation. 1996. 993: 2212-2245.
4. Anand SS, Wells PS, Hunt D, et al. Does the patient have deep vein thrombosis? JAMA. 1998: 279; 1094-1099.
5. Cronan JJ: Venous thromboembolic disease: the role of ultrasound. Radiology. 1993; 186:619-630.
6. Bounameaux H, Cirafici P, DeMoerlose P, et al. Measurement of D-Dimer as diagnostic aide in suspected pulmonary embolism. Lancet. 1991; 337:196-200.
7. Ginsberg JS, Wells PS, Brill-Edwards P, et al. Application of a novel and rapid whole blood assay for D-Dimer in patients with clinically-suspected pulmonary embolism. Thrombosis Hemostasis. 1995; 73:35-38.
8. Wells PS, Brill-Edwards P, Stevens P, et al. A novel and rapid whole blood assay for D-Dimer in patients with clinically-suspected deep vein thrombosis. Circulation. 1995; 91:2184-2187.

9. Bounameaux H, De Moerloose P, Pierrier A, Roeber G. Plasma measurement of D-Dimer as diagnostic aid in suspected venous thromboembolism: an overview. Thrombosis Hemostasis. 1994; 71: 1-7.
10. Fountzopolus E, Jones C, Richards R. The impact of D-Dimer testing on the management of suspected deep vein thrombosis in pulmonary embolism. Presented at the British Thoracic Society Winter Meeting 2000, December 13-15, 2000. London. Abstract.
11. Muto P, Lastoria S, Varella P, et al. Detecting deep venous thrombosis with technetium 99m-label synthetic peptide P280. J Nuclear Medicine. 1995; 36: 1384-1391.
12. Klem JA, Schafer JV. J Nuclear Cardiology. 2000; 7:359-364.
13. The PIOPED Investigators. Value of the ventilation/perfusion scan and acute pulmonary embolism. Results of the prospective investigation of pulmonary embolism diagnosis (PIOPED). JAMA. 1990; 263: 2753-9.
14. Oser RF, Zukerman DA, Gutierrez SR, Brink JA. Anatomic distribution of pulmonary emboli at pulmonary angiography: Implications for cross sectional imaging. Radiology. 1996; 199: 31-5.
15. Cham MD, Yankelevitz DF, Shaham D, et al. Deep venous thrombosis: detection by using indirect CT venography. Radiology. 2000;216:744-751.
16. Warkentin TE, Levine MN, Hirsh J, et al. Heparin induced thrombocytopenia in patients treated with low-molecular-weight heparin or unfractionated heparin. NEJM. 1995;332:1330-1335.
17. Warkentin TE. Seminars in Hematology. 1998; 35 (4): 9-16.
18. Fehey DA: Heparin Induced Thrombocytopenia. Journal of Vascular Nursing. 1995; 13: 112-116.
19. Kelton JG and Warkentin TE. Current Therapy and Hematology Oncology. Fifth Edition. New York, Mosby. 1995:149-152.
20. Warkentin TE, Kelton JG. A fourteen-year study of heparin induced thrombocytopenia. Am J Med. 1996; 101: 502-507.
21. Brieger DB, Mak KH, Topel E. Heparin-induced thrombocytopenia. J Am Coll of Cardiol. 1998; 1449-1459.
22. Lee DH, Warkentin TE. Frequency of heparin-induced thrombocytopenia. In: Warkentin TE, Greinicher A. Heparin-Induced Thrombocytopenia. New York: Marcell Dekker, 2000; 81-112.
23. Warkentin TE, et al. Impact of patient population on the risk of HIT. Blood. 2000; 96: 1703-1708.
24. Warkentin TE, Kelton JG. Heparin and Platelets. Hematology Oncology Clinics of NA. 1990; 4: 243-264.
25. Warkentin TE, Levine MN, Hirsh J, et al. Heparin-induced thrombocytopenia in patients treated with low-molecular-weight heparin or unfractionated heparin. NEJM. 1995; 332: 1330-1335.
26. College of American Pathologists Consensus. Arch of Path Lab Med. 1998; 122: 782-798.
27. Personal Communication with Warkentin TE. Miami, Florida. February 2001.
28. Warkentin TE, Chong BH, Greinacher A. Heparin-induced thrombocytopenia: toward consensus. Thrombosis Hemostasis. 1998; 79: 1-7.
29. Warkentin TE, Elavathil LJ, Hayward CP, et al. The pathogenesis of venous-limb gangrene associated with heparin-induced thrombocytopenia. Ann of Int Med. 1997; 127: 804-812.
30. Press Release. Anticoagulant Argatroban Available In The United States. Smith-Kline Beecham. 2000.
31. Magnani HN. Orgaran (Danaparoid sodium). Use in heparin-induced thrombocytopenia. Platelets. 1997; 8: 74-81.
32. Hirsh J, Bates S, Clinical trials that have influenced the treatment of thromboembolism: a historical perspective. Ann of Int Med. 2001; 134: 409-417.
33. Prandoni P, Lensing AW, Büller HR, et al. Comparison of subcutaneous low-molecular-weight heparin with intravenous standard heparin and proximal deep venous thrombosis. Lancet. 1992; 339: 441-5.
34. Levine M, Hirsh J, Leclerc J, Anderson D, et al. A comparison of low-molecular-weight heparin administered primarily at home with unfractionated heparin administered in the hospital for proximal deep vein thrombosis. NEJM. 1996; 334: 677-81.
35. Columbus Investigators. Low-molecular-weight heparin in the treatment of patients with venous thromboembolism. NEJM. 1997; 337: 657-62.
36. Samama MM, Cohn AT; Comparison of enoxaparin with placebo for the prevention of venous thromboembolism in acutely ill medical patients. NEJM. 1999;341(11): 793-800.
37. Merli G, Spiro T, Olsson CG, et al. Subcutaneous enoxaparin once- or twice-daily compared with unfractionated heparin for treatment of thromboembolic disease. Ann Int Med. 2001;134:191-202.
38. Veiga, F. Escriba A. Low-molecular-weight heparin (enoxaparin) versus oral anticoagulant therapy. Thrombosis Hemostasis. 2000; 84: 559-564.
39. Turpie AG, Gallus A, Hoek J, et al. A synthetic pentasaccharide for the prevention of deep-vein thrombosis after total hip replacement. NEJM. 2001;344: 619-625.
40. Frances CW, Davidson BL, Berkowitz SD. Randomized, double-blind, comparative study of H376/95, an oral direct thrombin inhibitor, and warfarin to prevent venous thromboembolism (VTE after total-knee arthroplasty). Submitted for publication and presentation at the International Society for Thrombosis Hemostasis July 2001. Abstract.
41. Hirsh J. Optimal duration of anticoagulant therapy for venous thrombosis. NEJM. 1995; 332: 1710-1.
42. Schulman S, Lockner D, Juhlin-Dannfelt A. The duration of oral anticoagulation for deep venous thrombosis. a randomized trial. Medica Scandinavia. 1985; 217: 547-52.
43. Kearon CM, Hirsh J, Weitz J, et al. A comparison of three months of anticoagulation with extended anticoagulation for a first episode of idiopathic venous thromboembolism. NEJM. 1999; 340: 901-7 91-7.
44. Sixth ACCP Consensus Conference on Antithrombotic Therapy. Chest. 2001;119:1-370.
45. European Heart Journal Task Force Report. Guidelines on Diagnosis and Management of Acute Pulmonary Embolism. Eur Heart J 2000;21:1301-36.

Surgical Advances for the New Millenium

- **Updates on Recent Innovations in Surgery**
- **Peer Reviewed by Expert Specialty Surgeons**
- **Indexed on MEDLINE**

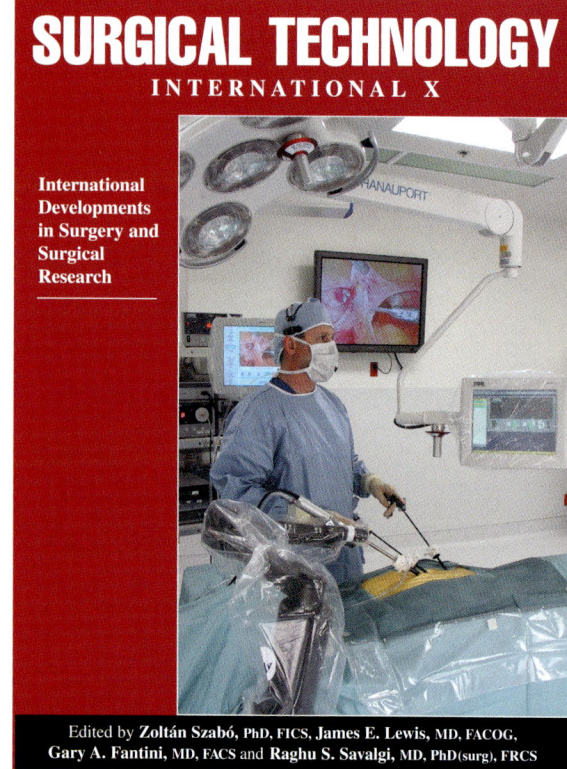

"Surgical Technology International does a splendid job of showcasing the many aspects of recent surgical achievement and innovation that have been possible as we hurtle forward into the new millenium."
—M. David Tilson, M.D.
Professor of Surgery
Columbia University, New York

"The authors are to be congratulated on the latest edition of what is essential reading for surgeons in every discipline."
—Tom Bates, F.R.C.S.
Consultant Surgeon
The William Harvey Hospital
Ashford, Kent, England, UK

ISBN No. 1-890131-06-7

Order a 3-year subscription now and get 50% off the bookstore price!

Yes, please enter my subscription to Surgical Techonology International for:

☐ 3 years (6 Issues) $285   ☐ 2 years (4 Issues) $215   ☐ 1 year (2 Issues) $145   ☐ Individual Copy ($95)

Please add 10% per year for shipping & handling on U.S. orders.

Please add $46 per year for shipping & handling for international orders.   ISBN No.: 1-890131-06-7

☐ Special Back Issue Set STI III - STI X - $685 US, $755 overseas - (Includes shipping)
☐ AMEX   ☐ MasterCard   ☐ VISA   ☐ Check enclosed*   ☐ Bill me

Card Number: ☐☐☐☐ ☐☐☐☐ ☐☐☐☐ ☐☐☐☐

Signature: _____   Expiration Date: _____
Name: _____   Institution: _____
Address: _____
City: _____   State: _____   Zip: _____
Country: _____   Phone/Fax: _____
                              Email: _____

Please send to: Universal Medical Press, Inc., 2443 Fillmore Street, #229, San Francisco, CA 94115, USA,
or FAX YOUR ORDER TO: 1-415-436-9791. / Telephone: 1-415-436-9790 / E-mail: info@ump.com / Website: www.ump.com

*Make checks payable to **Universal Medical. Press, Inc.** California residents, please add applicable state sales tax.

Treatment of Articular Cartilage Defects with the Autologous Chondrocyte Transplantation (ACT)

ANDREAS BURKART, M.D.
CONSULTANT SURGEON

ANDREAS BALTHASAR IMHOFF, M.D.
CHAIRMAN AND PROFESSOR OF SURGERY

DEPARTMENT OF ORTHOPEDIC SPORTS MEDICINE
TECHNICAL UNIVERSITY OF MUNICH
MUNICH, GERMANY

Symptomatic chondral lesions in the knee remain a problem for young sportsmen and pose a difficult management issue for orthopedic surgeons and patients alike. Damaged articular cartilage has a limited potential for healing and can lead to premature arthritis.[1-3] Articular defects larger than 2 mm to 4 mm in diameter rarely heal.[4,5] Neither articular cartilage possesses a lymphatic drainage, a sufficient blood supply, nor neural elements. Also, they are sheltered even from immunological recognition, because of the extracellular matrix surrounding the chondrocyte.[4,5]

Cartilage damage limited to the cartilage itself—without penetration of the subchondral bone—stimulate only a slight reaction in the adjacent chondrocytes.[6] If a penetration of the subchondral bone is present, one can observe a healing response and fill the defect with new tissue, normally with fibrocartilage. Fibrocartilage consists primarily of type I collagen and lacks the mechanical characteristics required for long-term durability.[7] According to Minas and Nehrer,[8] this treatment results in an initially successful outcome followed by return of symptoms and the eventual need for further surgery after two to five years. That repair tissue often succumbs to mechanical stresses, with premature degeneration and delamination.[8] Treatment options include restoration, replacement, relieving, and resection. Restoration means healing or regeneration of the joint surface; replacement can be accomplished with use of an allograft or prosthesis, and an osteotomy can relieve a damaged joint surface.[6] Techniques such as drilling,[9] arthroscopic abrasion arthroplasty,[10] or microfracture technique[6] are not able to develop a durable, high-demand repair tissue for larger chondral lesions.[11,12]

New techniques, like the osteochondral autograft transplantation or posterior condyle transfer, are as promising.[13-16]

The focus of this article is on restoration of articular cartilage with transplantation of autologous chondrocytes. This technique was developed by Grande and colleagues,[17] and more recently by Brittberg and co-workers.[18] Chondrocytes taken from biopsy specimens of cartilage were grown in a monolayer culture to increase the cell population. After released enzymatically from culture, these cells were suspended in a liquid medium and placed beneath a periosteal graft sewn over the defect. The periosteal graft was transplanted with the cambium layer facing down into the defect.

INDICATIONS

Autologous chondrocyte transplantation (ACT) is indicated for a symptomatic, full-thickness cartilage defect of the femoral articular surface in a physiologically young patient. Osteochondritis dissecans is also an indication for grade III or IV according to the Outerbridge classification. Bipolar chondral injuries and osteoarthritis are contraindications.[8] Preoperative x-rays and magnetic resonance imaging (MRI) for determining the extent of a cartilage lesion are useful. The determination of whether a patient is a candidate for ACT is obtained by arthroscopy.

MATERIALS AND METHODS

From November 1996 to November 1999, the authors performed autologous chondrocyte transplantation in ten patients with 14 full-thickness defects. The study group included seven men and three women, whose ages ranged from 24 to 45 (average: 36) years. The medial femoral condyle was the most frequent defect site, with seven followed by the lateral femoral condyle (4) and trochlea (3). The average size of the chondral lesions was 6.3 cm^2 (4 cm^2 to 12 cm^2). Patients had undergone, on average, two prior surgical procedures that addressed the chondral lesions (Table 1). Pre- and postoperatively (3, 6, and 12 months), the

Table 1. Patients Characteristics

Patient	Age (Years)	Diagnosis	Defect-Size (cm)	Operations Before ACT
N.A.	24	ACL-rupture, cartilage damage medial FC	2.7 x 1.8	Meniscal surgery, Drilling, ACL-reconstruction
A.H.	45	Traumatic cartilage damage med./lat. FC, Trochlea	1 x 2.2 3 x 2 4 x 2	Drilling, Debridement
B.A.	31	Osteochondrosis dissecans lateral FC	2 x 2	Spongiosaplasty, Refixation of OD
K.K.	35	ACL-rupture, cartilage damage medial FC	2 x 1.5	ACL-reconstruction
S.J.C.	33	Osteonecrosis medial FC, cartilage damage Trochlea, med./lat. FC	5 x 3 2 x 2 2 x 2	Drilling, Debridement osteochondral Transfer Trochlea, Condyle transfer Med. FC
S.J.	34	Osteonecrosis med. FC, cartilage damage lateral FC	3 x 4	Condyle transfer medial FC
S.U.	40	Cartilage damage medial FC	2 x 3	ACL-reconstruction
K.Cl.	37	Cartilage damage medial FC	3.5 x 1.5	Removal of loose bodies, Drilling
S.M.	40	Trochlea	2 x 2	
F.J.	39	Cartilage damage medial FC	2 x 2	ACL-reconstruction, Meniscal surgery

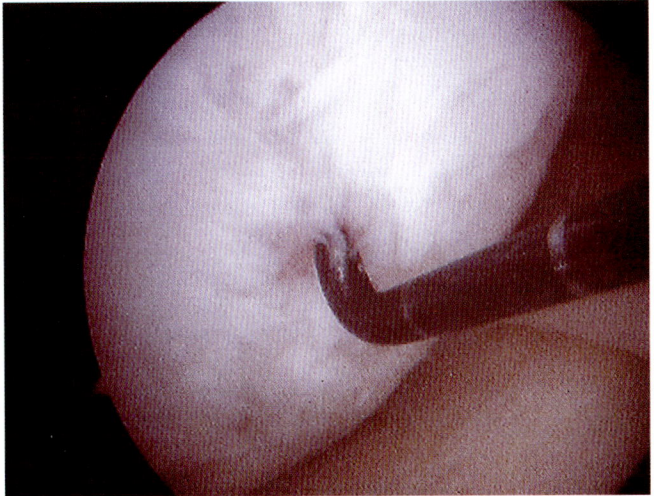

Figure 1. Preoperative MRI from patient, K.K., coronar and sections demonstrating a cartilage damage at the medial femoral condyle (T1-FFE: TR 28, TE 13, Flip 45).

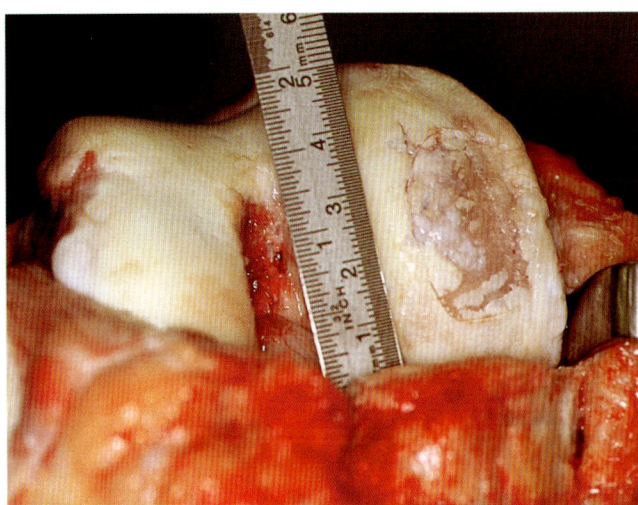

Figure 2. Corresponding arthroscopic picture to Figure 1.

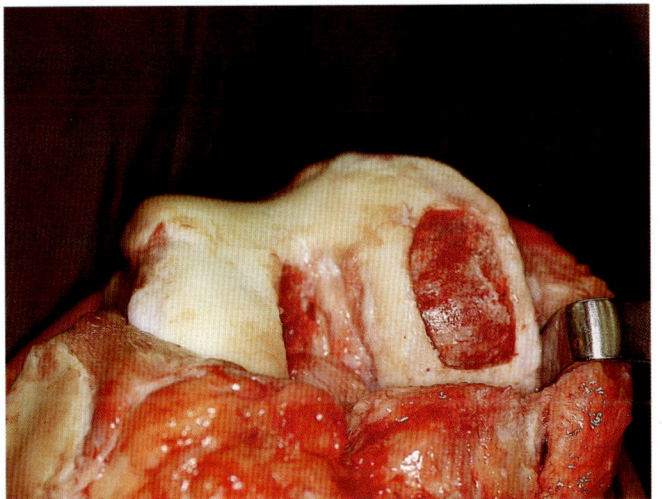

Figure 3a. Cartilage damage at the medial femoral condyle, patient, S.U.
Figure 3b. After surgical debridement, preparing the transplantation site.

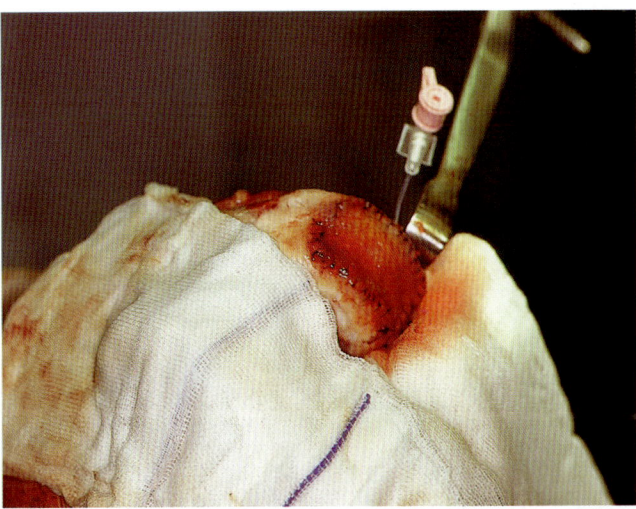

Figure 4. Sutured periosteal flap, testing water-tight integrity with a gauge.

authors performed a MRI for evaluation of the transplantation site (size of the defect, surrounding cartilage, changes in bone structure, synovitis, erosions, signal irregularities) (Fig. 1) with the following sequences: De3d, T1- and T2-weighted, T1 with intravenous Gadolinium (Hardware: Siemens, 1.0 Tesla + Artoscan [Esaote]). Clinical evaluation was done according to the Lysholm score.

Technique of ACT

First, an arthroscopic assessment of the cartilage damage, length and width, and quality of the surrounding articular cartilage was performed (Fig. 2). Healthy cartilage should be available for periosteum suturing. If the lesion was considered appropriate, a small biopsy of cartilage tissue was harvested from a non-weight-bearing portion of the knee (mostly the superior medial edge of the trochlea, approximately 5 mm wide by 1 cm in length) and sent for laboratory culture, which took approximately three weeks for culturing. Biopsy instruments included curette or sharp gouges.

Predisposing factors to chondral injury should be either corrected in a staged or concomitant fashion with ACT, which means corrective osteotomy in a varus or valgus malalignment, correction of patellofemoral malalignment, and assessment of ligamentous or bone insufficiency.

For implantation, the authors perform an arthrotomy, usually through a midline incision or longitudinal parapatellar incision.

One should perform a radical debridement of all fissured and undermined articular cartilage to viable borders of surrounding cartilage (Figs. 3a & 3b). Caution has to be taken to not violate the subchondral bone. If one perforates the subchondral bone plate, a mixed stem-cell population fills in the chondral defect in addition to the end-differentiated chondrocytes that have grown in vitro.[19] The defect is measured in its length and width. A periosteal flap distal to the pes anserinus insertion is then taken. The outside of the periosteum is marked with a pen so it is not placed upside down when implanted. It is sutured with a 6/0 bioabsorbable suture (Prolene) to the cartilage. To avoid hypertrophy of the transplant, the periosteal flap has to be the same size as the

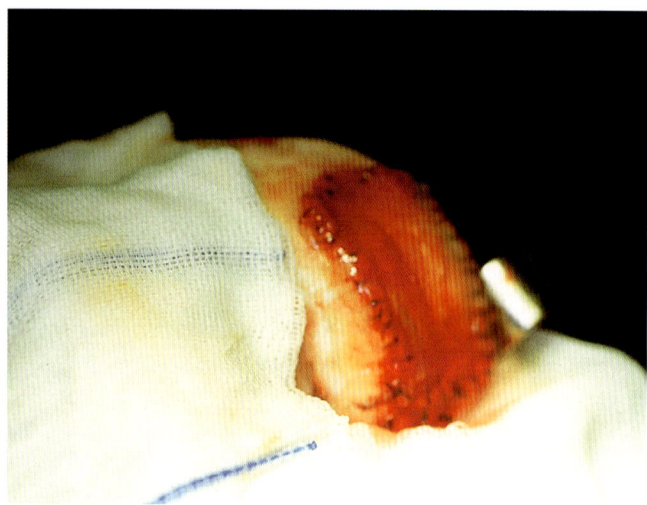

Figure 5. After ACT with sutured periosteal flap.

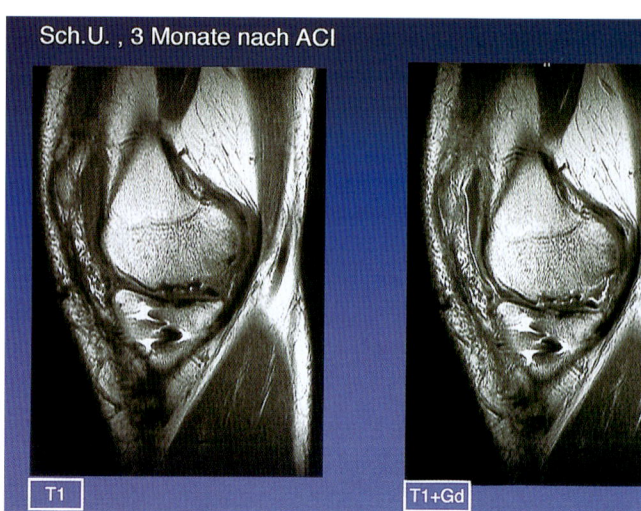

Figure 6. MRI from patient, S.U., three months after ACI:
a) T1-weighted (TR 722,0; TE 20.0/1; Spinecho): Notice signal irregularities at the transplantation site. b) T1-weighted with intravenous Gadolinium: Notice partial GD-uptake at the transplantation site.

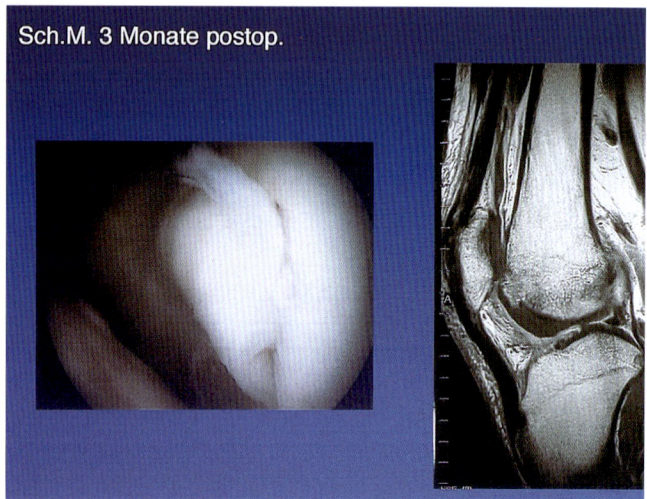

Figure 7. MRI from patient, S.M., three months after ACT.
a) Hypertrophy of the transplant at the trochlea site. b) Corresponding arthroscopic picture.

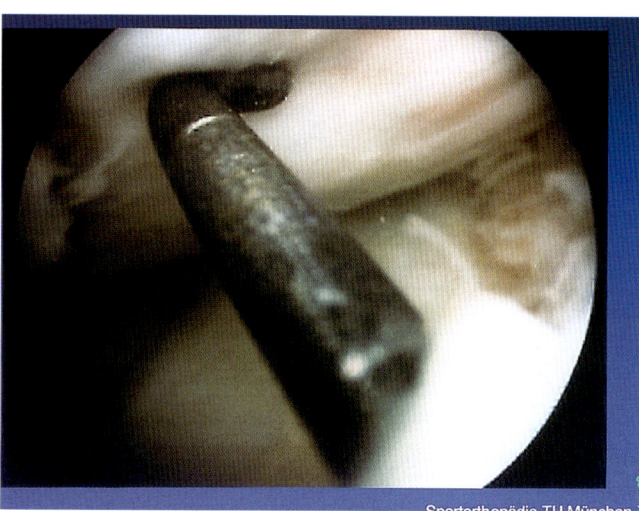

Figure 8. Arthroscopic picture, three months after ACT. Notice the spongy transplantation site.

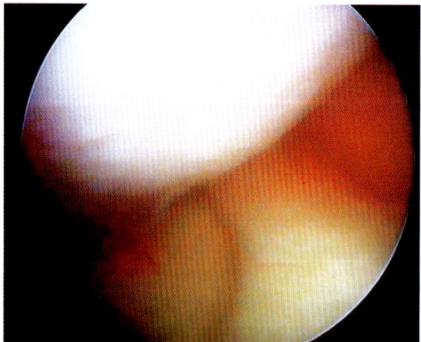

Figure 9. Arthroscopic picture from patient, K.K., one year after ACI.

defect. Periosteum water-tight integrity testing is assessed by using a plastic gauge. By filling the defect with saline, any leakage can be seen easily (Fig. 4). If water integrity cannot be obtained by suture technique, a fibrin sealant is used. After aspiration of the saline chondrocyte suspension is injected under the periosteal flap, several sutures are used to close the remaining defect. Fibrin glue can be used to ensure peripheral water tightness (Fig. 5). The wound is then closed in layers.

To decrease the likelihood of intra-articular adhesion, continuous passive motion (CPM) should start on the next day. The aim is to regain as full a range of motion as the patient tolerates. To prevent the likelihood of periosteal overload and central degeneration of delamination of the graft, the patient is kept non-weight-bearing for six weeks after surgery, increasing to full body weight by 12 weeks postoperatively. Isometric muscle exercises are allowed postoperatively.

RESULTS

Magnetic Resonance Imaging (MRI)

In all patients, an interruption of the broad band of hypointensity was present. Mainly in the first three months postoperatively, one could see signal irregularities with Gadolinium-uptake at the surface and in the bone (Figs. 6a,b). Hypertrophy of the transplant were well visualized in the MRI in two patients at the trochlea site (Figs. 7a,b). Up to 12 months postoperatively, signal irregularities

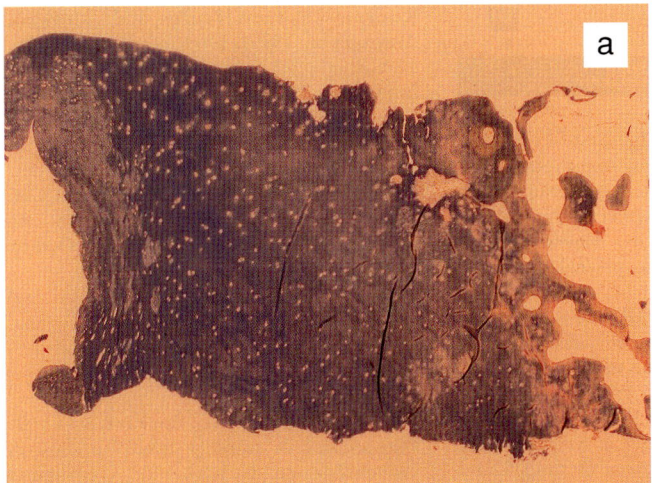
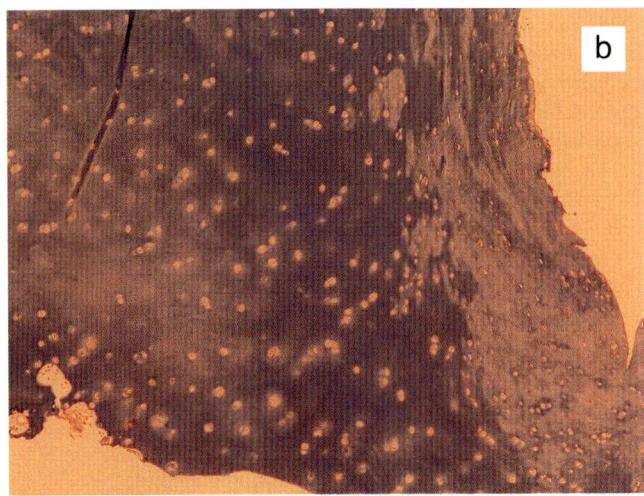
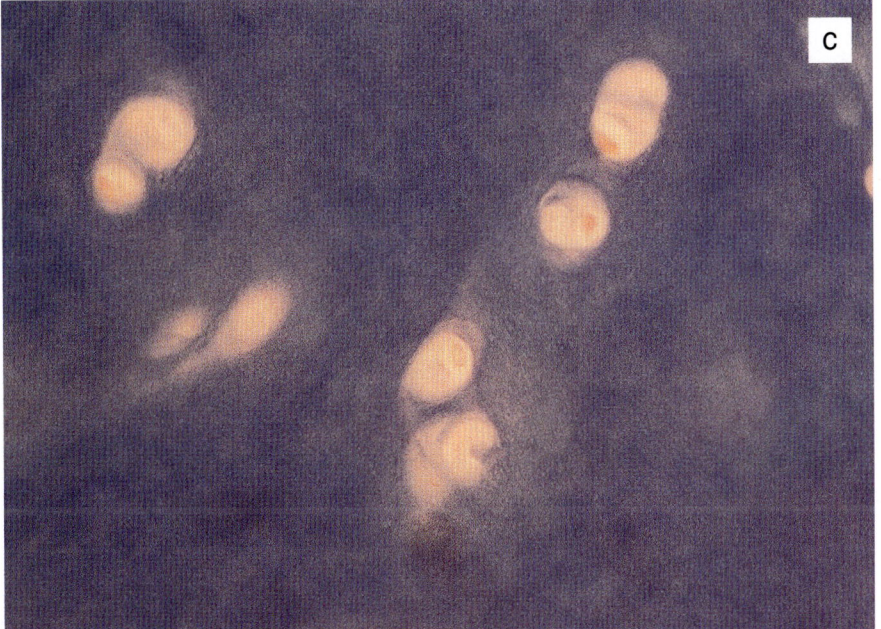

Figure 10. Biopsy from patient, K.K, one year after ACT: a) Overview of the biopsy (staining: Azan). b) Notice columnar appearance of the cells of the hyalin-like repair tissue (staining: Azan). c) Rounded cells and mitotic-like activity, cluster formation (staining: Azan).

were decreased and no additional Gadolinium-uptake was present.

Arthroscopy

Three months postoperatively, the boarders of the transplant were visible and the transplant itself was spongy when probed (Fig. 8). Color and texture were similar to the surrounding bone. Twelve months postoperatively, the transplant was stiffer and smooth, so one could hardly separate it from the surrounding cartilage (Fig. 9). Two complications were seen at the trochlea site and patients had to be reoperated by smoothening the hypertrophy (Fig. 7b).

Histology

In six patients, hyaline-like cartilage taken from the transplantation site 4, 7, and 12 months postoperatively was detected. A columnar appearance of the cells was present at the base. Cells were rounded, but one also could see cluster-formation and a mitotic-like activity (Figs. 10a, b, c).

Clinical Examination

All patients reported reduced pain and swelling. Two patients with a hypertrophy of the transplant complained of crepitus and pain until the revision arthroscopy. Lysholm-score improved from preoperatively 78 to postoperatively 92.

DISCUSSION

Articular cartilage lesions frequently result in pain, swelling, and mechanical symptoms. They often reduce the patient's quality of life dramatically. In an effort to produce more durable hyaline repair tissue, the autologous chondrocyte implantation technique was developed. Brittberg and colleagues[18] reported promising results in 23 patients, with a follow up from 16 to 66 months. Eighty-eight percent of the patients with femoral condylar defects had good-to-excellent results. Peterson[20] presented the two- to ten-year outcomes of 219 patients. The best results were shown on the femoral condyle. Moreover, he demonstrated the examination of 38 patients followed for more than five years (mean: 7.4) in 96% good/excellent results. In the patellar region, 31% of the patients had poor results; in the trochlea, 42%; and in more than one lesion, 25%. In 14 patients, he performed an arthroscopy postoperatively with mechanical testing of the transplant. The hyaline-like repair tissue demonstrated near-normal stiffness compared to the fibrocartilaginous tissue. In 19 biopsies taken from the transplantation site, he reported hyaline-like repair tissue in 74%, with an 86% correlation between the presence of hyaline-like tissue and clinical improvement. Minas and Nehrer[8] reported on their experience in 50 patients. They noted a gradual time-related improvement in patients' symptoms. By 12 months, a 90% improvement was reported, and by 18 months, a near-complete resolution of the pain. These data corresponded to the findings at second-look arthroscopy from an indentable softer tissue at three to six months to a firm nonindentable tissue at 18 months. The Cartilage Repair Registry periodic reported results from 1067 implantations in 1051 patients.[21] Compared to baseline, a statistically significant improvement was noted in overall condition and patient symptomatology at 12, 24, and 36 months postoperatively; 73.5% showed an improvement after 36 months.

Adhesions/fibroarthrosis in 2.8% and hypertrophic changes in 1.9% were the most frequent complications. Our results also were as promising.[1,22] Hypertrophy of the transplant in the trochlea region was the only complication in our study. Studies in the literature report the best indications for ACT are symptomatic cartilage defects in the femoral condyle.[1,22] It seems that, with time, the transplant becomes stiffer with improvement in patients' symptoms.

Treatment of cartilage defects by marrow-stimulation techniques, by penetrating the subchondral bone plate to provide mesenchymal stem cells within the fibrin clot, have demonstrated only fair- to-poor, long-term results. It appears with the ACT one can provide hyaline-like repair tissue with corresponding improvement in the histologic, biomechanical, and durability characteristics. Future treatments will likely involve implantation of tissues and cells that respond to local stimuli, by growing and differentiating into mature chondrocytes capable of producing extracellular matrix that integrate into surrounding tissue.

REFERENCES

1. Burkart A, Imhoff AB. Erste Ergebnisse nach autologer Chondrozytenimplantation unter Berücksichtigung kernspintomographischer und histologischer Untersuchungen. In: Imhoff AB, Burkart A, eds. Knieinstabilität-Knorpelschaden. Steinkopffverlag, Darmstadt; 1999. p 75-82.
2. Furukawa T, Eyre DR, Koide S, et al. Biochemical studies on repair cartilage resurfacing experimental defects in the rabbit knee. J Bone Joint Surg 1980;62A:79-89.
3. Messner K, Maletius W. The long term prognosis for severe damage to weight bearing cartilage in the knee. Acta Orthop Scand 1996;67:165-8.
4. Buckwalter JA, Mankin HJ. Articular cartilage. Part I: Tissue design and chondrocyte-matrix interaction. J Bone Joint Surg 1997;79A:600-11.
5. Buckwalter JA, Mankin HJ. Articular cartilage. Part II: Degeneration and osteoarthritis, repair, regeneration, and transplantation. J Bone Joint Surg 1997;79A:612-32.
6. O'Driscoll SW. Current concepts review: the healing and regeneration of articular cartilage. J Bone Joint Surg 1998;80-A:1795-812.
7. Nehrer S, Spector M, Minas T. Tissue retrieved from revised articular cartilage repair procedures reflects mechanisms of failure. Presented at the Annual Meeting of the American Academy of Orthopedic Surgeons, San Francisco, CA, February 12-15, 1997.
8. Minas T, Nehrer S. Current concepts in the treatment of articular cartilage defects. Orthopedics 1997;20:525-38.
9. Tippet JW. Articular cartilage drilling and osteotomy in osteoarthritis of the knee. In: McGinty JB, ed. Operative arthroscopy. New York, NY: Raven Press; 1991. p 325-39.
10. Johnson LL. Arthroscopic abrasion arthroplasty. In: McGinty JB, ed. Operative arthroscopy. New York, NY: Raven Press; 1991. p 341-60.
11. Burkart A, Imhoff AB. Therapie des Knorpelschadens-Heute und Morgen. Arthroskopie 1999;12:4-17.
12. Gillogly SD. Autologous chondrocyte implantation: current state of the art. In: Imhoff AB, Burkart A, eds. Knieinstabilität-Knorpelschaden. Steinkopffverlag, Darmstadt; 1999. p 60-6.
13. Convery FR, Akeson WH, Keown GH. The repair of large osteochondral defects. An experimental study in horses. Clin Orthop 1972;82:253-62.
14. Imhoff AB, Öttl G. Arthroscopic and open techniques for transplantation of osteochondral autografts and allografts in different joints. Surg Technol Inter VIII; 1999. p 249-52.
15. Imhoff A, Öttl G, Burkart A, et al. Osteochondrale autologe transplantation an verschiedenen Gelenken. Orthopäde 1999;28:33-44.
16. Imhoff A, Burkart A, Öttl G. Der posteriore kondylentransfer: erste ergebnisse mit einer salvage-operation. Orthopäde 1999;28:45-54.
17. Grande DA, Pitman MI, Peterson L, et al. The repair of experimentally produced defects in rabbit articular cartilage by autologous chondrocyte transplantation. J Orthop Res 1989;7:208-18.
18. Brittberg M, Lindahl A, Nilsson A, et al. Treatment of deep cartilage defects in the knee with autologous chondrocyte transplantation. New Engl J Med 1994;331:889-95.
19. Rodrigo JJ, Steadman RJ, Silliman JF, al. Improvement of full-thickness chondral defect healing in the human knee after debridement and microfracture using continuous passive motion. Am J Knee Surg 1994;7:109-16.
20. Peterson L. Autologous chondrocyte transplantation: 2-10 year follow-up in 219 patients. Presentation Abstract, AAOS, New Orleans, LA, March 1998.
21. Cartilage Repair Registry (Volume 5), Cambridge, MA. Genzyme Tissue Repair; 1999.
22. Burkart A, Imhoff AB. MRI findings after autologous chondrocyte transplantation in correlation with histology and arthroscopy. Boston: International Cartilage Repair Society; 1998. p 16.-8.

Bone Grafts

MATTHEW J. W. HUBBLE, M.B., B.S., F.R.C.S. (ORTH)
LECTURER IN ORTHOPAEDIC AND TRAUMA SURGERY
UNIVERSITY OF BRISTOL
BRISTOL, ENGLAND, U.K.

VISITING FELLOW
DEPARTMENT OF ORTHOPAEDIC SURGERY
THE ALFRED HOSPITAL
MELBOURNE, AUSTRALIA

Bone grafts are used in musculoskeletal surgery to restore structural integrity and enhance osteogenic potential. The demand for bone graft for skeletal reconstruction in bone tumor, revision arthroplasty, and trauma surgery, coupled with recent advances in understanding and application of the biology of bone transplantation, has resulted in an exponential increase in the number of bone-grafting procedures performed over the last decade. It is estimated that 1.5 million bone-grafting procedures are currently performed worldwide each year, compared to a fraction of that number 20 years ago. Major developments also have resulted in the harvesting, storage, and use of bone grafts and production of graft derivatives, substitutes, and bone-inducing agents.

HISTORY

Apart from the case described in Genesis 2:22, the first bone-grafting procedure is attributed to St. Damian and St. Cosmos, who in the third century A.D., are reputed to have performed a cadaveric lower-limb allograft transplantation for the benefit of a faithful church warden suffering from a tumor of the leg.[1,2] The first xenograft bone transplantation is attributed to the use of dog bone to successfully cover human skull defects, reported by Baha'-ul-Douleh in 1501 and later by van Meekeren in 1668.[3] In more modern times, Lexer in 1908[4], MacEwen in 1909[5], and Albee in 1915[6] described several cases of allograft bone transplantation with variable success.[3-6] In the 1930s, Orell reported the successful use of purified xenograft bone (os purum) in 49 cases[7], and by the 1940s autogenous bone grafting, particularly in maxillofacial surgery, was commonplace. In the 1950s, Herndon and Chase reported that freezing reduced the immunogenicity of allograft bone[8] and the United States Navy Tissue Bank was established in 1951.[9] Marshall Urist first demonstrated the osteoinductive properties of demineralized bone matrix in 1965.[10] However, not until the 1980s and 1990s did allograft bone-banking facilities, free vascularized autograft transfer, and production of synthetic bone-graft alternatives and of bone-inducing agents by tissue engineering become widespread. The estimate is that 426,000 bone-grafting procedures were performed in the United States in 1996 compared to only 5,000 to 10,000 in 1985.[11]

BIOLOGY

Bone transplantation may occur from one site to another within the same person (autograft), or between two different people of the same species (allograft). In addition, bone from animals of different species can be used (xenograft), and a number of synthetically manufactured bone-graft substitutes, derivatives, and additives are currently available. Autograft bone is the "gold standard" bone-grafting material; it is non-immunogenic and contains viable osteoinductive proteins and osteoprogenitor cells, and as such has, at least in part, an ability to directly form viable new bone (osteogenic).

Conversely, transplanted allograft and xenograft bone, in an untreated form, can be highly immunogenic, sometimes stimulating a potent incompatibility reaction.[12] This immunogenicity can be modified, however, by a variety of treatment and processing procedures, including freezing, freeze drying, gamma irradiation, and chemical means.[11] The resultant grafts, although less immunogenic, have little or no direct osteogenic capacity. They act primarily as a microporous framework, or scaffold, upon which new host bone is laid down (osteoconductive). One increasing area of investigation is in the role of substances that, although not bone grafts themselves, cause bone formation by host tissues (osteoinductive), rather than being directly osteogenic. These substances include bone marrow aspirate, and proteins of the transforming growth factor beta (TGF-B) and bone morphogenetic protein (BMP) families.[13]

Graft incorporation is a complex process that varies significantly depending on the source (auto, allo, xeno, or synthetic graft) and form (dense cortical bone or more porous cancellous bone) of the graft, and is also greatly influenced by vascularity of the host tissues and mechanical environment in which it is placed. However, incorporation of all bone-graft types involve the five common stages of hemorrhage, inflammation, revascularization, substitution, and remodeling[14]. Transplanted autogenous cancellous bone remains the most commonly used bone-grafting material, incorporation of which is a model for other graft types. Hemorrhage and inflammation occur rapidly after insertion of graft into the host bed. The vast majority of transplanted cells in the graft die in the transplantation process, particularly osteocytes within trabecular lacunae, but surface osteoblasts do survive and contribute to new bone formation. Due to the compatible porosity of cancellous bone, vascular ingrowth by host vessels, and ingress of host osteoblast and osteoclast precursors, is facilitated and occurs as early as 48 hours from the time of surgery. This process is promoted by the presence within the graft of a number of osteoinductive proteins, including growth factors, morphogenetic proteins, and cytokines. As the neovascularization process occurs, from the periphery toward the center of each graft fragment, host osteoblasts are deposited on the dead trabeculae of the graft. These lay down seams of new osteoid on the dead graft. The combined trabeculae of new host and dead donor bone are then resorbed by osteoclasts and replaced by further new host bone. The entire process is known as 'creeping substitution', beginning at the periphery and progressing painstakingly toward the centre of the graft. Remodeling then continues during the process of graft incorporation; the entire process takes many months to complete.

Autogenous cancellous bone, because of its lack of immunogenicity, its directly osteogenic and osteoinductive properties, and having an ideal structure to promote osteoconduction, is an optimum grafting material from a biologic perspective, although it has little structural integrity or mechanical strength. All other graft types incorporate less well. Dense cancellous bone, without a trabecular meshwork to promote osteoconduction, incorporates slowly, and often never fully incorporates. Allograft and xenograft bone, if unprocessed, may incite a brisk immunogenic response leading to graft resorption, and processed grafts have little inductive or osteogenic properties and act primarily as an osteoconductive scaffold, as do the synthetic graft substitutes.

IMMUNOLOGY

The immunology of bone grafting is less well understood than that of transplanted parenchymal tissues, and is available data relates more to animal than human studies. However, the response of the host to allograft or xenograft bone is known to be primarily a cell-mediated response to cell surface antigens in the foreign bone, particularly class I and II antigens encoded by the major histocompatibility complex (MHC) genes. These antigens are primarily recognized by T lymphocytes of the killer/suppressor phenotype, and exposure promotes their proliferation. Rejection may incorporate antibody-mediated, cell-mediated or antibody-dependent, cell-mediated, cytotoxicity.[12,15] The process of rejection is variable, ranging from graft resorption, to incomplete incorporation, fracture, or non-union. These responses to fresh allograft or xenograft bone have been shown to be reduced by freezing, and further reduced by freeze-drying and irradiation. Processing grafts to minimize their cellular content and matching of MHC antigens have also been shown to correlate with greater biologic and clinical success.[16]

BIOMECHANICS

In addition to its biologic properties, any bone-grafting material must be appropriate for the mechanical environment in which it is placed, and capable of tolerating the loads placed upon it. Also, bone-graft remodeling occurs in response to mechanical load; both excessive and inadequate loads can result in graft resorption or failure, whereas a beneficial mechanical environment promotes graft incorporation.

The mechanical properties of a bone graft are dependent on its material properties (strong compact cortical bone versus weak porous cancellous bone) and its cross-sectional geometry. The mechanical properties of a graft are of variable significance, some being used primarily for their biologic properties, such as morcellized autogenous cancellous bone, and others primarily for their mechanical properties, such as a proximal femoral replacement cortical allograft. In addition, bone grafts are used frequently in combination with prostheses or internal fixation systems, which support or protect the graft.[17] The mechanical properties of the graft also vary with time, reducing by resorption after initial implantation, and then increasing as new bone formation and remodeling occurs. Long-term mechanical competence of the graft is dependent on at least a degree of biologic incorporation.

The mechanical characteristics of a bone graft can be altered significantly by many of the processing procedures used to treat the grafts. Freezing bone has a minimal effect on its physical properties, which is not the case for freeze drying that impairs a graft's mechanical properties.[18] Autoclave sterilization and irradiation both cause a dose-dependent decrease in graft strength, and demineralization greatly reduces a graft's compressive strength.[19]

AUTOGRAFT

Autogenous bone makes the best graft and it remains the type of bone graft used most commonly, usually as small fragments or wedges. Advances in the field of microsurgery have made it possible to transfer autogenous bone grafts on vascular pedicles, including segments of fibula, rib, ilium and radius, often as composite grafts with attached soft tissues.[1,20] Harvesting of both vascularized and non-vascularized autograft, however, entails an additional incision, increased morbidity, and weakening of the donor bone.[21,22] The choice of donor sites and amount that can be harvested is limited. Attempts to circumvent these limitations has led to use of allograft and xenograft bone, and investigation of graft alternatives.

ALLOGRAFT

Allograft bone is currently widely used and increasingly available. It is used in the form of small fragments, bulk, strut, segmental, and osteochondral grafts, which can be obtained from both living and cadaveric donors. Femoral head allografts, obtained from appropriate donors at the time of hip arthroplasty surgery, are the most readily available source of graft. Cadaveric donors are used to obtain larger segmental or strut grafts and osteochondral grafts. Bulk grafts are used particularly for limb and joint reconstruction in revision arthroplasty and tumor surgery.

BONE BANKING

Bone banks now exist around the world at both a local and regional level, although there has been an increasing trend to centralization and standardization in recent years. In the United Kingdom, for example, the working party of the British Orthopaedic Association has published recommendations concerning administration of services, screening of donors, harvesting and sterilization of allograft.[23] These include centralisation and administration by the Blood Transfusion Service, exclusion of donors with systemic or infective disease, screening for human immunodeficiency virus (HIV), hepatitis B and C, and syphilis, and ensuring rhesus compatibility in women of childbearing age. In the United States similar protocols have been established by the Food and Drug Administration (FDA) and American Association of Tissue Banks, and in Europe by the Association of Musculoskeletal Transplantation (EMAST).[24-26] Processing includes washing the grafts in a variety of agents, principally alcohol, to remove blood and marrow, which reduces graft immunogenicity as well as minimizing the chance of viral transmission, before storage at -70°C. At least four cases of HIV transmission from bone transplantation have been recorded in the United States in addition to bacterial contamination of grafts, despite sterile harvesting techniques.[27-30]

As a result, many bone banks currently undertake 'secondary sterilization' using gamma irradiation or ethylene oxide. Both, in addition to freezing, reduce allograft immunogenicity, but also alter the mechanical properties of the graft that may be of relevance to its subsequent use.[31,32] There have also been reports of occult malignant tumors being present in tissue that would have been suitable for bone-bank donation, and histologic examination of donor tissues has been proposed.[33-34] Processing procedures are becoming more advanced and many banks now offer prepared struts, wedges, threaded dowels, and rods of allograft for a variety of specialized purposes in addition to morcellized chips and bulk grafts.

XENOGRAFTS

The cost and logistic problems of procuring and preparing human allograft, and free availability of animal tissue, use of xenograft bone as an alternative has been explored extensively because of the rapidly increasing demand for bone graft. Initial studies were hampered by the high immunogenicity of the xenograft tissue. However recent advances in the processing of xenogenic bone has led to production of partially deproteinized, defatted derivatives with low antigenicity and mechanical properties similar to human bone. Combined with autogenous bone marrow to make composite grafts, they have achieved success in a variety of applications.[35,36] Currently, three commercially produced purified xenografts are available, *Kiel bone*, *Surgibone* and *Lubboc*. All three are bovine in origin. Animal tissue is also not without the potential risk of disease transmission, and emergence of bovine spongiform encephalopathy (BSE) has raised the specter of prion transmission by xeno-transplantation.

BONE-GRAFT SUBSTITUTES

An ever-increasing number of artificial bone-graft substitutes are undergoing investigation as alternatives to autogenic or allogenic bone.[37] These are all solely osteoconductive, although they can be augmented by the addition of autogenous bone marrow or other inducing agents. They depend on their porosity, both in terms of pore size (ideally 100 to 600 microns) and pore density (in the region of 75% to 80%), and their chemical structure to promote bone ingrowth and remodeling. Substitutes currently in use include porous ceramics, corals, and collagen derivatives.

Porous ceramics of hydroxyapatite and tricalcium phosphate have the ability to bond to bone (osteotropic), are inert and are resorbed, tricalcium phosphate quickly and hydroxyapatite slowly. A combined preparation, *Triosite* (40% tricalcium phosphate and 60% hydroxyapatite), has recently completed favorable clinical trials as an autograft alternative in spinal fusion surgery.[38] Interest is increasing regarding the use of calcium phosphate cements, which can be prepared as a liquid and then harden into a crystalline phase with compressive strengths similar to cancellous bone. These cements can be injected into fracture sites or bone defects with a syringe, which then harden into material that cause little or no foreign-body reaction and are readily remodeled by osteoclasts. They have already been shown to be useful in treatment of distal radial fractures and show promise in a variety of other fields.[39,40]

Certain South Pacific corals (madreporic corals), such as the genus *Porites* and *Gonipora*, have a porous calcium carbonate exoskeleton architecturally similar to cancellous bone, with a pore size ranging from 150 to 600 microns. The calcium carbonate structure can be converted into mechanically superior porous hydroxyapatite by the hydrothermal replamineform process without altering the internal architecture. Marketed commercially as *Biocoral* since 1988, and more recently in a hydroxyapatite form as *Interpore*, corals have demonstrated ingrowth and active new bone formation and remodeling.[41] However, the use of coralline implants has been hampered by their poor initial strength and handling properties.

Decalcified bone consists principally of collagen that, in turn, has a structure conducive to mineral deposition and binding of non-collagenous matrix proteins. In isolation, collagen functions poorly as a grafting material, but if combined with tricalcium phosphate (TCP) or hydroxyapatite (HA) and inducing agents such as bone marrow or BMP, does promote new bone formation. Composites of bovine type 1 collagen with TCP and HA (*Collagraft*™), Collagraft Bone Graft Matrix Strip, NeuColl Incorporated, Palo Alto, CA) have undergone multicenter studies in the treatment of fracture non-unions and spinal fusions.[42] Although promoting union, they have not been as effective as autograft in most situations and lack the structural strength required for many skeletal applications.

BONE INDUCTION

Bank allograft, xenograft, and bone substitutes, unlike fresh autograft, have little or no direct osteogenic or osteoinductive capacity. They can, however, be made osteogenic if mixed with autologous marrow to make a composite graft, the marrow providing a rich source of osteoprogenitor cells and inductive agents.[43] The discovery by Urist that demineralized bone matrix (DMB) can induce the transformation of primitive mesenchymal cells into mature osteoblasts, in turn resulting in bone formation, has stimulated the search for other osteoinductive agents.[10] Bone matrix has since been shown to contain a group of proteins, the bone morphogenetic proteins (BMPs), members of the TGF-B superfamily. BMP 2 and 7 have been shown to be, by themselves, capable of inducing the formation of bone and cartilage in vivo and can now be synthesized by recombinant deoxyribonucleic acid (DNA) technology. The possibility of 'super charging' bone grafts or substitutes to enhance their osteogenic potential by combining them with BMP, coating prosthetic components to enhance bone ingrowth and skeletal fixation, and direct application of BMP to stimulate fracture healing, are all currently being explored.[44-46]

THE FUTURE

Due to the rapid expansion in use of bone grafts for skeletal reconstruction, demand for allograft bone now exceeds supply.[47] The search for a readily available, cheap, safe and effective alternative is underway. A suitable graft must be porous to promote osteoconduction, have sufficient strength for skeletal application, and be biocompatible. The ideal graft is likely to be a composite, augmented by addition of a genetically engineered-inducing agent to enhance its osteogenic potential.

REFERENCES

1. Guelinckx PJ, Sinsel NK. The 'Eve" procedure. The transfer of vascularised seventh rib, fascia, cartilage and serratus muscle to reconstruct difficult defects. Plast Reconstr Surg 1993; 97(3): 527-35.
2. Mankin HJ, Doppelt S, Tomford W. Clinical experience with allograft implantation. Clin Orthop 1983; 174: 69-86.
3. Umana HR. Grafting of bone from a dog into the human skull: an historical note. Plast Reconstr Surg 1995; 96(6): 1481.
4. Lexer E. Die Verwendung der freien knochenplastic nebst versuchen uber gelenkversteifung unt gelenk-transplantation. Arth Klin Chir 1908; 86: 939-66
5. MacEwen W. Intrahuman bone grafting and reimplantation of bone. Ann Surg 1909; 50: 959-68.
6. Albee FH. The fundamental principles involved in the use of bone graft in surgery. Am J Med Sci 1915; 149: 313-25.
7. Orell S. Surgical bone grafting with os purum, os novum and boiled bone. J Bone Joint Surg [Br] 1937; 19: 873-85.
8. Chase SW, Herndon CH. The fate of autogenous and homogenous bone grafts. J Bone Joint Surg [Am] 1955; 37A: 809-41.
9. Hyatt GW, Turner TC, Bassett CAL et al. New methods for preserving bone, skin and blood vessels. Post Grad Med 1952; 12: 239-54.
10. Urist MR. Bone formation by autoinduction. Science 1965; 150: 893-9.
11. Boyce T, Edwards J, Scarborough N. Allograft bone. The influence of processing on safety and performance. Orthop Clin N Am 1999; 30(4): 571-81.
12. Stevenson S., Horowitz M. Current concepts review. The response to bone allografts. J Bone Joint Surg [Am] 1997; 74A: 939-50.
13. Ludwig SC, Boden SD. Osteoinductive bone graft substitutes for spinal fusion. Orthop Clin North Am 1999; 30(4): 635-45.
14. Stevenson S. Biology of bone grafts. Orthop Clin North Am 1999; 30(4): 543-52.
15. Strong DM, Friedlander GE, Tomford WW, et al. Immunologic responses in human recipients of osseous and osteochondral allografts. Clin Orthop 1996; 326: 107-14.
16. Stevenson S, Li XQ, Martin B. The fate of cancellous and cortical bone after the transplantation of fresh and frozen tissue antigen matched and mismatched osteochondral allografts in dogs. J Bone Joint Surg [Am] 1991; 73A. 1143-56.
17. Eldridge JD, Smith EJ, Hubble MJ et al. Massive subsidence following femoral impaction bone grafting in revision total hip arthroplasty. J Arthroplasty 1997; 12(5): 535-40.
18. Conrad EU, Ericksen DP, Tencer AF, et al. The effects of freeze drying and rehydration on cancellous bone. Clin Orthop 1993; 290: 279-84.
19. Hamer AJ, Strachan JR, Black MM, et al. Biomechanical properties of cortical allograft bone using a new method of bone strength measurement:a comparison of fresh, fresh-frozen and irradiated bone. J Bone Joint Surg [Br] 1996; 78B: 363-86.
20. Han CS, Wood MB, Bishop AT, et al.. Vascularised bone transfer. J Bone Joint Surg Am 1992; 74A: 1441-9.
21. Goulet JA, Senunas LE, DeSilva GL, et al. Autogenous iliac crest bone graft. Complications and functional assessment. Clin Orthop 1997; 339: 76-81.
22. Vail TP, Urbaniak JR. Donor site morbidity with the use of vascularised autogenous fibular grafts. J Bone Joint Surg 1996; 78A: 204-11.
23. British Orthopaedic Association. The collection and storage of bone allografts. Report of the allograft bone bank working party. London. British Orthopaedic Association, 1992.
24. Department of Health and Human Services (FDA): Human tissue intended for transplantation. Fed Reg 1997; 62: 40429-47.
25. American Association of Tissue Banks: Standards for Tissue Banking. McLean VA. American Association of Tissue Banks. 1996.
26. European Association for Musculoskeltal Transplantation. Common standards for musculoskeletal tissue banking. European Association for Musculoskeletal Transplantation. 1997.
27. Buck BE, Malinin TI, Brown MD. Bone transplantation and human immunodeficiency virus. Clin Orthop 1989; 240: 113-21.
28. Conrad EU, Gretch DR, Obermeyer KR, et al. Transmission of hepatitis C virus by tissue transplantation. J Bone Joint Surg [Am] 1995; 77A: 214-24.
29. Tomford WW. Transmission of disease through transplantation of musculoskeletal allografts. J Bone Joint Surg [Am] 1995; 77A: 1742-54.
30. Deijkers RL, Bloem RM, Petit PL et al. Contamination of bone allografts: analysis of incidence and predisposing factors. J Bone Joint Surg [Br] 1997; 79B: 161-6.
31. Fideler BM, Vangsness CT, Moore T, et al. Effects of gamma irradiation on the human immunodeficiency virus. A study in frozen human bone-patellar ligament-bone grafts obtained from infected cadavera. J Bone Joint Surg [Am] 1994; 76A: 1032-5.
32. Thoren K, Aspenberg P. Ethylene oxide sterilization impairs allograft incorporation in a conduction chamber. Clin Orthop 1995; 318: 259-64.
33. Palmer SH, Gibbons CL, Athanasou NA. The pathology of bone allograft. J Bone Joint Surg [Br] 1999; 81B: 333-5.
34. Sugihara S, van Ginkel AD, Jiya TU et al. Histopathology of retrieved allografts of the femoral head. J Bone Joint Surg [Br] 1999;

81B: 336-41.
35. Salama R. Xenogeneic bone grafting in humans. 1983; Clin Orthop 174: 113-21.
36. Hubble MJ, Goodship AE, Learmonth ID. Xenograft bone for impaction grafting in revision THR. An in vivo pilot study. J Bone and Joint Surg [Br] 1997; 79B: (IV Suppl), 468S.
37. Perry CR. Bone repair techniques, bone graft and bone graft substitutes. Clin Orthop 1999; 360: 71-86.
38. Ransford AO, Morley T, Edgar P, et al. Synthetic porous ceramic compared with autograft in scoliosis surgery. J Bone Joint Surg [Br] 1998; 80B: 8-13.
39. Jupiter JB, Winters S, Lowe C, et al. Repair of five distal radius fractures with an investigational cancellous bone cement. J Orthop Trauma 1997; 11: 110-6.
40. Moore DC, Frankenburg EP, Goulet JA, et al. Hip screw augmentation with an in-situ setting calcium phosphate cement. J Orthop Trauma 1997; 11: 577-83.
41. Shors EC. Coralline bone graft substitutes. Orthop Clin North Am 1999; 30(4): 599-613.
42. Kocialkowski A, Wallace WA, Burwell RG. Collagraft combined with autogenic bone marrow: experimental and clinical results. In: Urist MR, O'Connor BT, Burwell RG, eds. Bone grafts, derivatives and substitutes. Oxford: Butterworth Heinman, 1994. p 271-99.
43. Burwell RG. The function of bone marrow in the incorporation of a bone graft. Clin Orthop 1985; 200: 124-41.
44. Sumner DR, Turner TM, Purchio AF, et al. Enhancement of bone ingrowth by transforming growth factor beta. J Bone Joint Surg [Am] 1995; 77A: 1135-47.
45. Kienapfel H, Sprey C, Wilke A, et al. Implant fixation by bone ingrowth. J Arthroplasty 1999; 14(3): 355-68.
46. Einhorn TA. Enhancement of fracture healing J Bone Joint Surg [Am] 1995; 77A: 940-56.
47. Galea G, Kopman D, Graham BJ. The supply and demand of bone allograft for revision hip surgery in Scotland. J Bone Joint Surg [Br] 1998; 80B:4: 595-9.

Percutaneous Microdecompressive Endoscopic Thoracic Discectomy for Herniated Thoracic Discs

JOHN C. CHIU, M.D., F.R.C.S., F.A.C.S.
CHIEF, NEUROSPINE SURGERY

THOMAS J. CLIFFORD, M.D.
NEUROSURGICAL CONSULTANT, NEUROSPINE SURGERY

ROMULO SISON, O.P.A.-C., C.S.T.
PHYSICIAN ASSISTANT, NEUROSPINE SURGERY

CALIFORNIA CENTER FOR MINIMALLY INVASIVE SPINE SURGERY
THOUSAND OAKS, CALIFORNIA

Spinal surgeons have long sought to find a procedure of choice by which to treat thoracic disc herniations.[1-4] The threat of cord injury has stimulated many attempted approaches including posterior laminectomy (abandoned currently as too likely to result in neurologic loss), costotransversectomy, trans-thoracic trans-pleural, postero-lateral, trans-pedicular and, more recently, transthoracic endoscopic.[5-11] Commonly, surgery is not contemplated unless significant cord compression and neurologic deficit is present.[9, 12-15]

A significant number of patients complain of thoracic spine pain, intercostal pain, chest wall, upper abdominal pain, and occasionally low back pain due to smaller thoracic disc protrusions in the absence of severe neurologic deficit or dramatic radiologic abnormalities (Figs. 1a & 1b). With improved diagnostic methods such as magnetic resonance imaging (MRI) scans, computed tomography (CT) scans and CT-myelograms, the diagnosis of such smaller thoracic disc protrusions is now far more common.[6] Usually, these patients receive some period of physical therapy and analgesics, and, if not cured, are expected to live with their discomfort because severe postoperative complications are feared if open surgical treatment is attempted.

The purpose of this paper is to describe the technique, safety, and efficacy of a method for treating these patients by outpatient percutaneous microdecompressive endoscopic thoracic discectomy.[8, 16]

MATERIAL AND METHODS

Beginning in early 1996, 100 consecutive patients with a total of 152 contained thoracic disc protrusions demonstrated on MRI from T1 through T12 and appropriate to their pain level, and who had failed at least 12 weeks of conservative therapy, and had positive intraoperative thoracic discograms,[17] (Fig. 2) pain-provocation disc injection tests, or both, and were treated by this procedure. The study group of 100

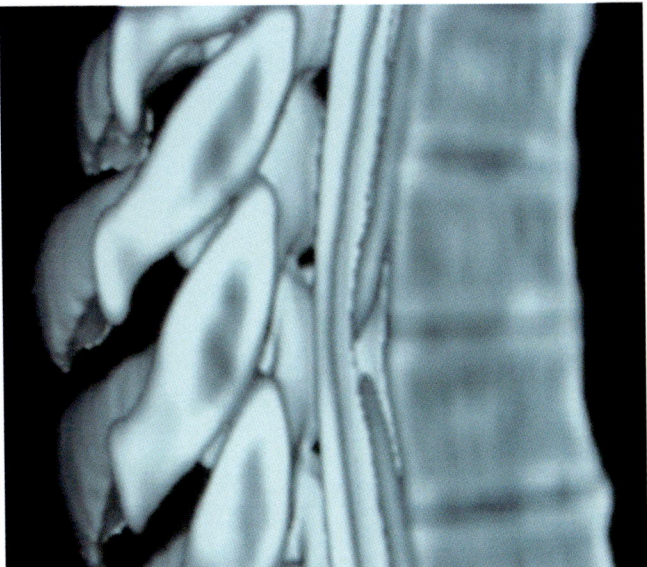
Figure 1a. Helical computed tomography showing disc herniation.

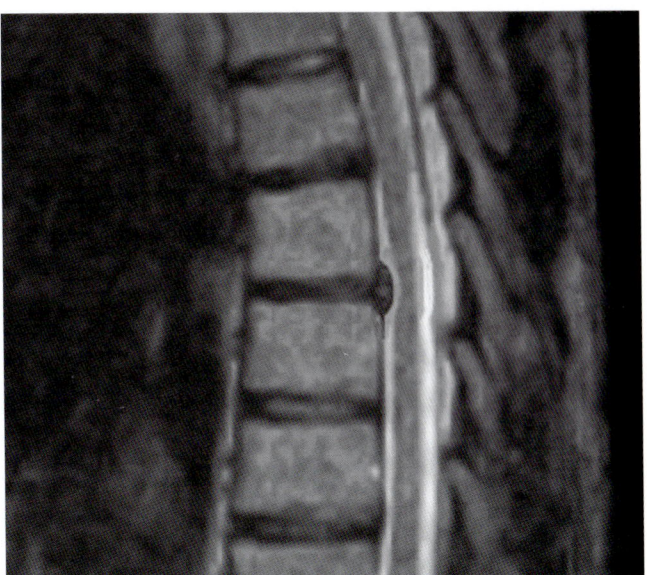
Figure 1b. Magnetic resonance imaging showing thoracic protrusion.

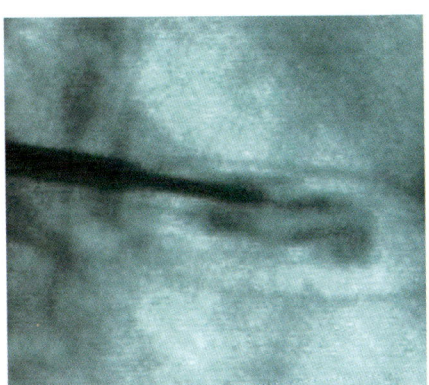
Figure 2. Abnormal thoracic discogram.

patients included 57 men and 43 women, with an average age of 43 (33 to 71) years. Follow up was 4 to 54 (average: 44) months.

INDICATIONS

Pain in the thoracic spine, radiating to the chest wall, possibly with numbness and paresthesia, in an intercostal distribution due to thoracic disc.

Positive MRI or CT scan or myelogram for a fully contained thoracic disc herniation.

No relief after at least 12 weeks of conservative therapy.

Positive intraoperative discogram, pain provocation disc injection test, or both.[3]

CONTRAINDICATIONS

Evidence of acute or progressive degenerative spinal cord disease.

Evidence of neurologic or vascular pathologies mimicking a herniated disc.

Evidence of advanced spondylosis (significant bone spurs) with severe disk space narrowing, diffuse annular bulging, and other spine irregularities.

Evidence of significant bony spurs that could block entry into the disc space.

Severe cord compression.

Any evidence of spinal pathology other than soft contained protruded disc.

TECHNIQUE [5,6]

Selected patients are treated in an operating room under local anesthesia. They are placed prone on the table with a radiolucent 20% angled sponge under the symptomatic side of the chest angling it into an oblique position. The Anesthesiologist maintains mild sedation, but the patient is able to respond. The back is prepped and draped. With a C-arm, the abnormal level is identified.

Under local anesthesia, a beveled 18-gauge, 3½-inch spinal needle is introduced 4 to 5 cm from the midline over the rib at the desired level. The needle is advanced incrementally under C-arm control at approximately a 35° to 45° angle to the skin, aiming toward the center of the disc between the interpedicular line medially and rib head at the costovertebral border laterally. After the annulus is punctured, the needlepoint is advanced to the middle of the disc. Isovue contrast is injected, observing the ease and volume of injection, fluoroscopic appearance in anterior-posterior (AP) and lateral projections, and the patient's description of any pain produced, its location, and intensity.[4] If the discogram and pain provocation tests are confirmatory, surgery is performed.

The stylette of the spinal needle is removed and a 12-inch plain guidewire is passed through it into the center of the disc. The needle is then removed. A small skin incision is made. The discectomy cannula with its contained dilator is passed over the guidewire. Position is checked frequently by fluoroscopy.

Positioned under C-arm control and with endoscopic magnification, the disc is decompressed with curettes (Figs. 3 & 4) micro-forceps (Figs. 5 & 6), and the discectome. Small osteophytes can be removed with micro-curettes and forceps. Removal is aided by a rocking excursion of the cannula in a 25 arc, a "fan sweep" motion from side to side, that creates an oval cone-shaped area of removed disc totaling up to 50. A Holmium: YAG laser is used to ablate some disc (500 joules, 8.5 watts, 10 Hz, 5 seconds on-5 seconds off) and then, at a lower power setting (300 joules, 5 watts), to shrink and contract the disc further.[16] This procedure also may cause Sino-vertebral neurolysis. The discectome is again used briefly to remove charred debris. The disc space is again visualized by endoscopy to ensure removal is satisfactory; the probe and cannula are then removed. Marcaine (0.25%) is infiltrated subcuta-

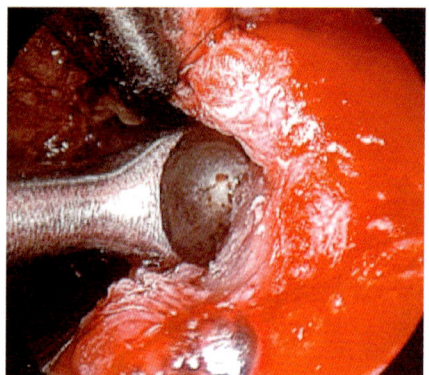

Figure 3. Endoscopic view of microcurette.

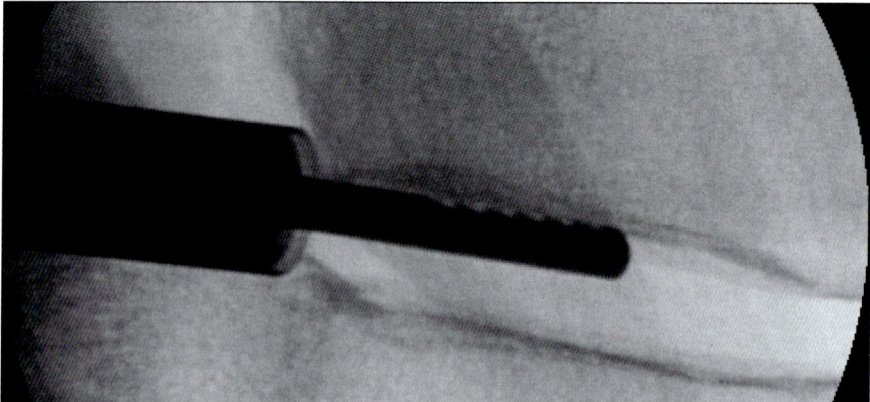

Figure 4. Fluoroscopic view of rasp.

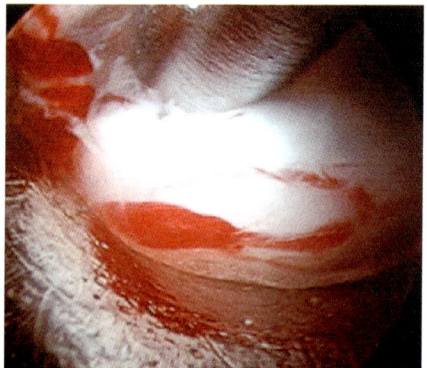

Figure 5. Endoscopic view of exposed nerve root.

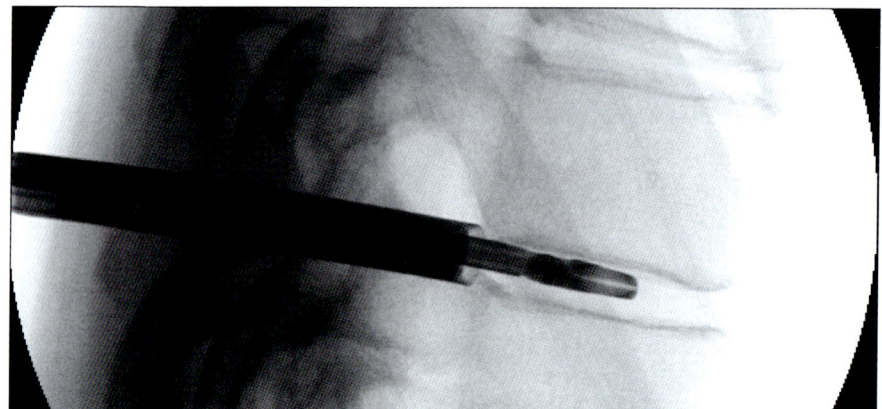

Figure 6. Fluoroscopic view of forceps.

neously about the wound. A band-aid is applied to the wound.

The patient is checked neurologically before leaving the operating room. Chest x-ray done in the Recovery Room rules out a pneumothorax. At the beginning of the procedure, patients receive Ancef (2 g) and Decadron (20 mg) given intravenously.

RESULTS

Average postoperative follow up of 44 (4 to 54) months demonstrates 96% of patients are excellent-to-good (Tables 1a & 1b). No operative complications have been noted. Four (4%) patients had persistent thoracic pain and paresthesia, although their pain improved 80% overall. The average time before returning to work has ten days for non-workmen's compensation patients. All patients received non-ablative, lower-energy Holmium laser applications to the disc to shrink and tighten the disc perimeter (thermodiskoplasty).

DISCUSSION

Like all percutaneous minimally

Table 1a. Results (Symptomatic Improvements)

Symptom	Pre-Op - # Patients	Post-Op - # Patients
Severe spine pain	100 (100%)	0 (0%)
Mild spine pain	0 (0%)	4 (4%)
Required analgesics	100 (100%)	4 (4%)
Muscle weakness	51 (51%)	2 (2%)
Muscle spasm	91 (91%)	2 (2%)
Persistent numbness	68 (68%)	4 (4%)

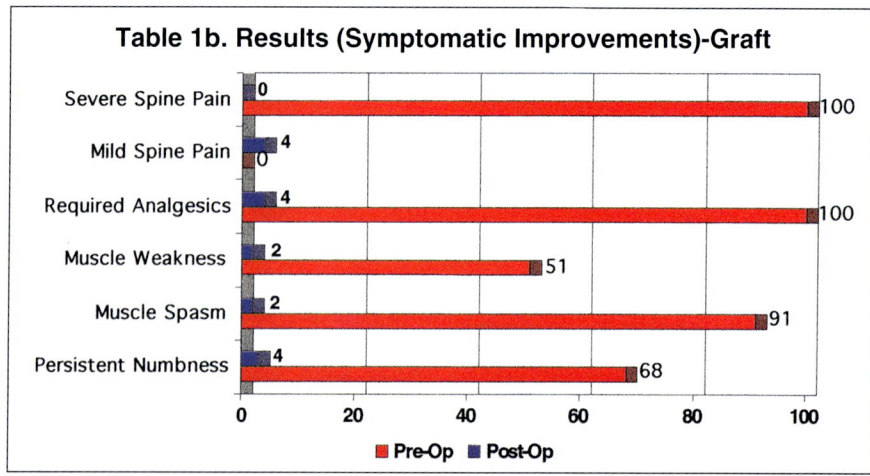

Table 1b. Results (Symptomatic Improvements)-Graft

invasive procedures, this thoracic discectomy does not interfere with the bones or joints of the spine, nor requires manipulation of the nerve roots or spinal dura. Insertion of the micro-instruments through the skin and muscle makes a 2.5-mm diameter track as the only wound, so there can be no injury to, or postoperative scarring around, the nerves. It is an outpatient procedure. Morbidity is negligible and promotes a rapid return to normal levels of activity.[6]

Successful thoracic discectomy requires full appreciation of the surgical anatomy involved and relationships of the rib head, pedicles, disc space, and spinal cord. A probe placed too close to the midline may cause neurologic injury; if too anterior, there may be injury to the major vessels, or sympathetic chain, as well as a possible pneumothorax.

Good results also depend on the general principles of microdiscectomy discussed elsewhere, such as achieving the triad of debulking the disc, decreasing intradiscal pressure, and by thermodiskoplasty-a shrinking of disc material to further reduce the profile of the disc. The procedure also treats possible toxic disc syndrome by removing an area of the central disc and continuous irrigation of the interspace throughout the operation. Use of multiple modalities[6] such as micro-instrumentation, a more powerful discectome, use of the Holmium laser (Trimedyne) side firing probe, sometimes for disc ablation at higher energies and always for thermodiskoplasty at lower energies,[5,16] and endoscopy to guide therapy and evaluate its effectiveness is essential for a good result.

CONCLUSION

Percutaneous endoscopic decompressive discectomy done for symptomatic thoracic herniated nucleus pulposus with added laser "tightening" of the disc (thermodiskoplasty),[5,16] is an easy, safe, and efficacious way to treat contained protruded thoracic discs. This type of minimally invasive and less traumatic outpatient procedure leads to less morbidity, rapid recovery, and significant economic savings. Patients who obtain a good result initially appear to remain pain free.

ACKNOWLEDGMENT

Holmium laser probe (side firing) is a product of Trimedyne, P.O. Box 57001, Irvine, California 92619

REFERENCES

1. Arseni C, Nash F. Protrusion of thoracic intervertebral disc. Acta Neurochir 1963;11:1-33.
2. Carson J, Gumper J, Jefferson A. Diagnosis and treatment of thoracic intervertebral disc protrusions. J Neurol Neurosurg Psychiat 1971;134:68-77.
3. Stillerman CB, Weiss MH. Principles of surgical approaches to the thoracic spine. Neurosurgical Clinics of North America, January 1996.
4. Nicholas T, Curtis AD. Current management of thoracic disc herniation. Contemp Neurosurg 1996;18(19): 1-7.
5. Chiu JC, Clifford TJ, Negron F, et al. Microdecompressive percutaneous discectomy: spinal discectomy with new laser thermodiskoplasty for non-extruded herniated nucleus polposus. Surg Technol Int VIII 1999;343-51.
6. Chiu J, Clifford T. Percutaneous thoracic discectomy. In: Savitz M, Chiu J, Yeung T, eds. The practice of minimally invasive spinal technique, 1st ed. Richmond, VA: AAMISMS Education, LLC; 2000. p 211-6.
7. Dickman C, Mican C. Thoracoscopic approaches for the treatment of anterior thoracic spinal pathology. BNJ Quart 1996;12:4-12.
8. Dietze D, Fessler R. Thoracic disc herniations. Neurosurg Clin N Am 1993;4:75-9.
9. Love JG, Schorn VG.. Thoracic disc protrusions. JAMA 1965;191:627-31.
10. Perot PL, Munro DD. Transthoracic removal of midline thoracic disc protrusion causing spinal cord compression. J Neurosurg 1963;31:452-8.
11. Tovi D, Strang RR. Thoracic intervertebral disc protrusions. Acta Chir Scand (Suppl) 1960;267:1-41.
12. Hawk WA. Spinal compression caused by ecchondrosis of the intervertebral fibro-cartilage: with a review of the recent literature. Brain 1936;59:204-24.
13. Hulme A. The surgical approach to thoracic intervertebral disc protrusions. J Neurol Neurosurg Psychiat 1960;23:133-7.
14. Key CA. On paraplegia depending on the ligaments of the spine. Guys Hosp Rep 1838;3:17-34.
15. Logue V. Thoracic intervertebral disc prolapse with spinal cord compression. J Neurol Neurosurg Psychiat 1952;15:227-41.
16. Chiu, J, Clifford T, Richley R, et al. Low energy, non-ablative holmium laser thermodiskoplasty for intervertebral disk shrinkage with a tightening effect J Neurol Orthopaed Surg 1999;19(1):34-8.
17. Schellhas K.P, Pollei, SR, Dorwart RH. Thoracic discography: a safe and reliable technique. Spine 1994;18:2103-9.

SPLAR & SPLAR Foundation

Division of Distant Medicine, Surgery & Allied Sciences

www.splar.com

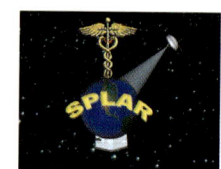

How You Can Benefit From SPLAR

◆ Do you want to globalize yourself and mix with diverse communities around the world?

◆ Do you want recognition for your goodwill and wisdom?

◆ Do you want to participate in SPLAR humanitarian activities locally & globally?

◆ Do you want to give a helping hand to needy people in the developing countries?

◆ There is a place for everybody in SPLAR programs. Please inform us (Info@SPLAR.com), your name, address, and tel & fax no. We will get in touch with you soon.

SPLAR Foundation: CO-PHET Movement

◆ Care for the Orphans, Physically Handicapped, Health care for the poor, Elderly & Terminally Ill

◆ Donations payable to 'SPLAR Foundation', PO Box 3208, New Haven CT 06515, USA

SPLAR Activities in Developing Countries

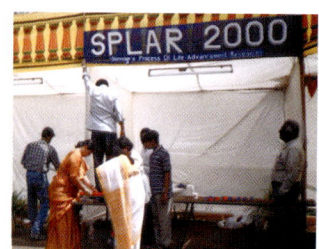
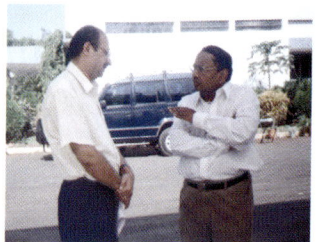
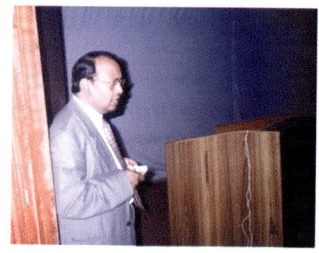

Raghu Savalgi
MD, PhD(Surg), MBA, APC(IT), LRCP, MRCS, FRCS
Chairman, SPLAR & SPLAR Foundation, P.O.Box 3208, New Haven, CT 06515, USA
Tel: 001 203 397 8700 , 1 877 ME SPLAR; Fax: 001 203 397 8701; Info@SPLAR.COM;
WWW.SPLAR.COM

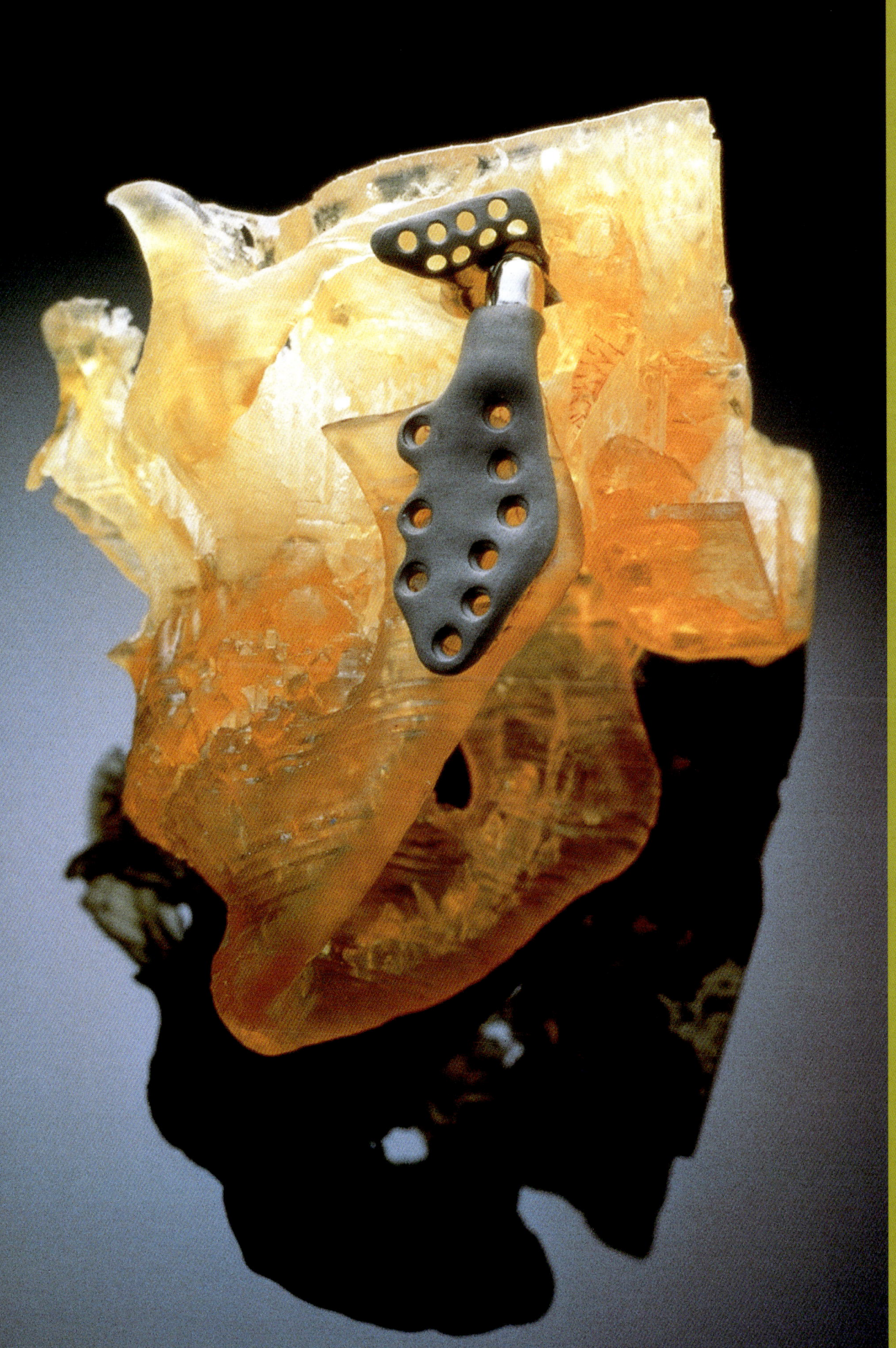

Plastic & Reconstructive Surgery

TMJ IMPLANTS, INC.

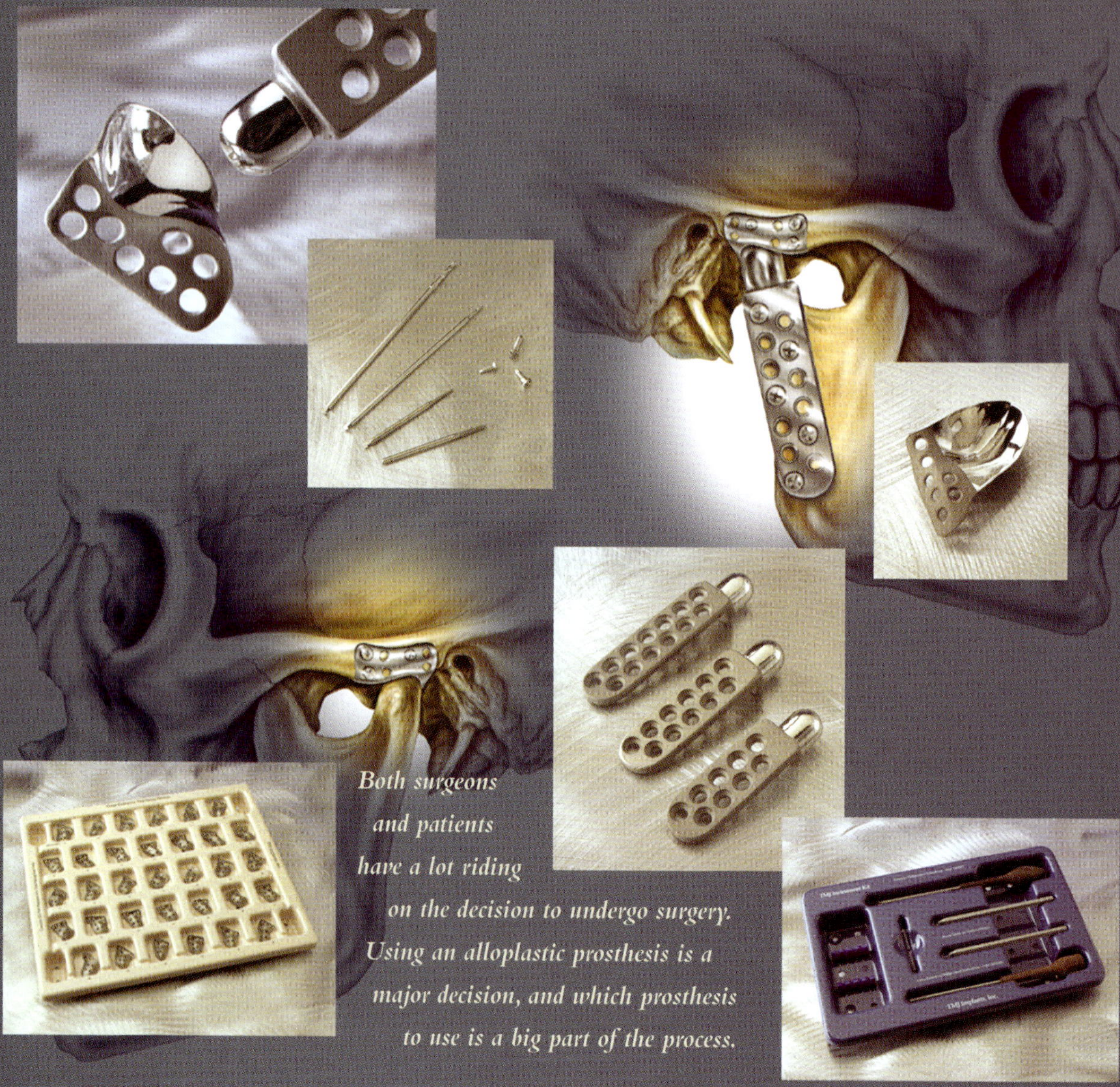

Both surgeons and patients have a lot riding on the decision to undergo surgery. Using an alloplastic prosthesis is a major decision, and which prosthesis to use is a big part of the process.

A JOINT DECISION

TMJ IMPLANTS, INC. MAKES THE DECISION EASIER!

ONE OF A KIND
TMJ Implants, Inc. is the only temporomandibular implant manufacturer who:

- Offers a comprehensive system of choice for advanced management of TMJ disorders
- Supplies a total and partial "stock" device, and a Patient-Specific™ device
- Offers the optimum wear-performance characteristics of a metal/metal total joint.

STATE OF THE ART
The Christensen TMJ Prostheses Systems are time-tested systems which have combined cutting edge technology with established orthopaedic materials and manufacturing processes. The wide range of options available through the Christensen TMJ Prostheses Systems means that patients and surgeons can reach a joint decision suitable to the patient's needs.

SAFE AND EFFECTIVE
Field performance of nearly 40 years attest to the durability and effectiveness of the device.* Clinical data compiled for thousands of patients demonstrate that the Christensen TMJ Partial and Total Prostheses Systems are safe and effective for the reduction of pain and improvement in function.**

REGISTERED AND APPROVED
The Christensen TMJ Prostheses Systems have been reviewed by three significant regulatory agencies resulting in approvals from the U.S. Food and Drug Administration (FDA), CE Mark (approval for marketing in Europe) and the Ministry of Health Canada. In addition, TMJ Implants, Inc. is certified and registered to EN-ISO9001/EN46001 international quality system standards.

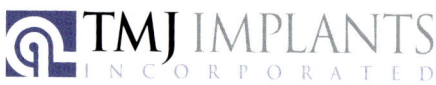

www.tmj.com   303.277.1338

©2001 TMJ Implants, Inc. A Joint Decision is a service mark of TMJ Implants, Inc.
* Data on file. ** TMJ Registry Tracking 1993 to present.

Use of the Christensen TMJ Fossa-Eminence Prosthesis™ System: A Retrospective Clinical Study

CARRIE BRITTON, B.S.
TMJ IMPLANTS, INC.
GOLDEN, CO

ROBERT W. CHRISTENSEN, D.D.S.
ADJUNCT PROFESSOR OF BIOENGINEERING, CLEMSON UNIVERSITY
CLEMSON, SC

JAMES T. CURRY, D.D.S.
PRIVATE OMS PRACTICE
HIGHLAND RANCH, CO

Disc displacements develop from alterations in the structural integrity of the condyle-disc complex. A definitive treatment that may be considered for such derangements is surgical correction. The goal of surgery is to return the disc to normal functional relationship with the condyle, or replace the disc with an alloplast. Surgery, is, therefore, considered when conservative therapy fails to adequately resolve the symptoms, progression of the disorder occurs, or both.[1]

A partial TMJ Fossa-Eminence joint reconstruction is indicated for use in cases where chronic, non-reducing disc displacement or meniscal perforation is involved.[2] Researchers have never been able to show, after a perforation has occurred, that spontaneous repair can take place.[3,4] Protecting these bone surfaces by a layer of dense fibrous connective tissue or fibrocartilage is imperative to have normal and pain-free function.[4] The treatment of temporomandibular joint disease (TMD) with the TMJ Fossa-Eminence Prosthesis™ is designed to provide a smooth surface for articulation with the natural condyle in a partial joint replacement procedure. The extremely thin profile of the implant (0.5 mm) allows minimal remodeling to the diseased joint.

The target population for a partial joint replacement for which a TMJ Fossa-Eminence Prosthesis™ is indicated includes those patients for whom smooth and asymptomatic articulation of the natural condyle against the natural fossa is not possible due to internal derangement (perforated or damaged meniscus), inflammatory arthritis, trauma, recurrent fibrosis or bony ankylosis, previously failed implant surgery, or any other pathologic disorder that has been unresponsive to other modalities of treatment.[5]

Partial surface replacement represents a significant development in the evolution of TMJ arthroplasty. The TMJ Fossa-Eminence Prosthesis™ was first described in 1963, and has been in use since 1961.[5] It has been estimated that more than 16,500 partial and total Christensen TMJ Prostheses™ systems have been implanted by hundreds of surgeons since their introduction in the early 1960s. Some surgeons believe the

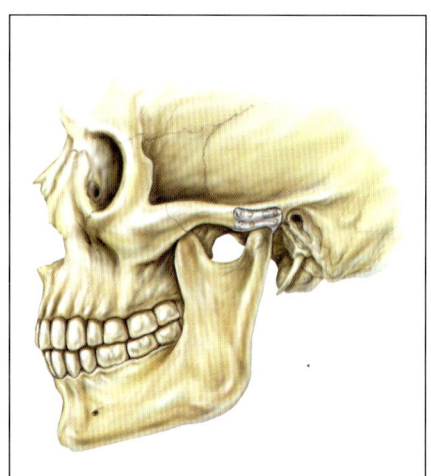

Figure 1. Schematic drawing of the Christensen TMJ Fossa-Eminence Prosthesis™.

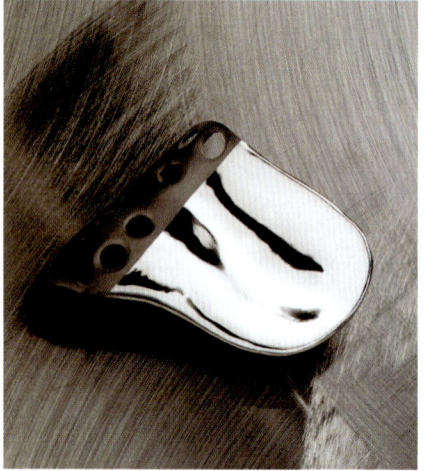

Figure 2. Photograph of a Christensen TMJ Fossa-Eminence Prosthesis™.

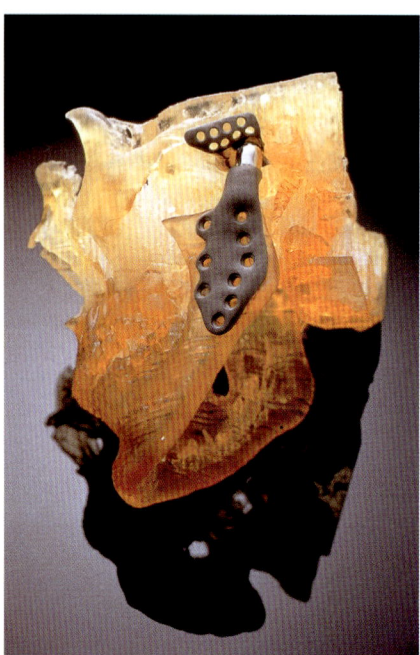

Figure 3. Photograph of a Christensen Patient-Specific™ Prosthesis.

likelihood of developing severe bony deterioration, ankylosis, and fibrous adhesions can be reduced following discectomy by placing an interpositional material between the head of the natural condyle and glenoid fossa.[6,7] Severe complications, including destructive lesions of the mandibular condyle following the use of some alloplastic implant materials, have led to a bias against using any alloplastic material as an interpositional implant within the TMJ.[8] Dolwick and Audemorte[9] Ryan,[10] and others have documented foreign body, radiographic, and clinical failures have soured surgeons to the prospect of "permanent" replacement of the disc following arthroplasty with discectomy. Christensen reported on the use of Cobalt-Chromium Alloy TMJ Fossa-Eminence Prosthesis™ inserted between the head of the mandibular condyle and glenoid fossa in 1963.[11] Eleven years later, Christensen reported good long-term results with the use of a metal glenoid fossa-eminence prosthesis, with no reported problems involving destruction of the natural mandibular condyle or foreign-body reaction.[7]

The Christensen TMJ Fossa-Eminence Prosthesis™ is designed to provide a smooth surface for articulation with the natural condyle in a partial joint replacement or hemiarthroplasty application (Fig. 1). Co-Cr alloy has had a long history of use in orthopedic applications.[12] The American Society for Testing and Materials (ASTM) stated that this material "...has been shown to produce a well characterized level of local biological response following long term clinical use..."[13] The target population for a hemiarthroplasty using a TMJ Fossa-Eminence Prosthesis™ as a partial TMJ replacement system includes patients exhibiting diseased TMJs that have proved to be non-responsive to other treatment options, including various non-surgical modalities or invasive procedures and where the natural condyle is healthy or salvageable.

The current study reports retrospective clinical data on the use of a highly polished cobalt-chromium alloy (Co-Cr) Fossa-Eminence Prosthesis™ used by itself, composed of a Co-Cr framework (Fig. 2). This cast Co-Cr prosthesis covers the entire glenoid fossa, articular eminence, and lateral rim of the zygomatic process.[14] It is secured to the base of the skull with four Co-Cr screws. The prosthesis, and screws with which it is secured to the skull, are manufactured from surgical Co-Cr-Mo alloy (ASTM F75/ASTM F799).

The precision fitting of the TMJ Patient Specific™ Prosthesis (TMJ Implants, Inc., Golden, CO) (Fig. 3) is offered in custom anatomical models and implants. The technology is stereolithography (SLA). A computed tomography (CT) scan is taken and a three-dimensional model is fabricated showing both external and internal anatomy. The model is accurate to within approximately 1 mm,[15] creating a conforming prosthesis to the patient's anatomy as well as creating an instrumental study model for the surgeon to plan, rehearse, and perform a more precise surgery. This model is useful to the surgeon operating on a patient with an extremely deformed or mutilated TMJ.

MATERIALS AND METHODS

Clinical Study—Patient Selection

Patient selection for partial joint replacement for which the TMJ Fossa-Eminence Prosthesis™ is indicated includes those patients who have a need for smooth and asymptomatic articulation of the natural condyle against the natural glenoid fossa, and it is not possible due to internal derangement (perforated or damaged meniscus), inflammatory arthritis, trauma, recurrent fibrosis or bony ankylosis, previously failed implant surgery, or any other pathologic disorder, that has been unresponsive to other modalities of treatment.[16]

In one such study, patients were selected based on duration and implant type. The records reviewed in this study included all patients identified as a partial joint candidate (TMJ Fossa-Eminence Prosthesis™ only), with a minimum of three years' implant duration, and whose records contained a preoperative and minimum of three-year postoperative radiograph.

The surgical approach to the TMJ, for placement of the Fossa-Eminence Prosthesis™, is a relatively simple and safe procedure. At surgery, the most accurate fitting prosthesis is inserted, using the Christensen TMJ System. Eighty-eight different sizes and shapes are available, 44 for the right side and 44 for the left side. With the availability of variations in size and shapes of fossas

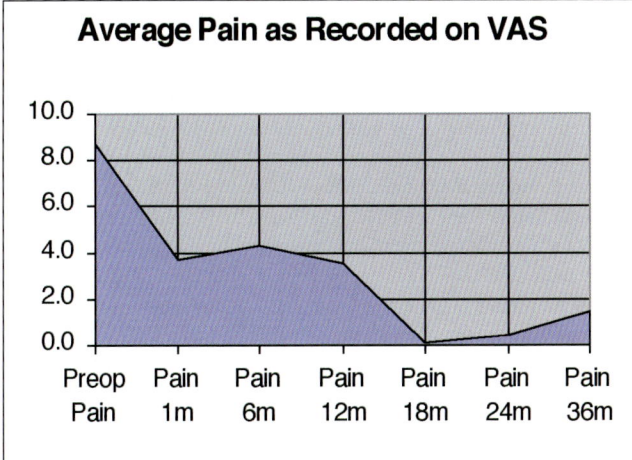

Figure 4. Prospective clinical average pain levels measured on Visual Analog Scale (VAS).

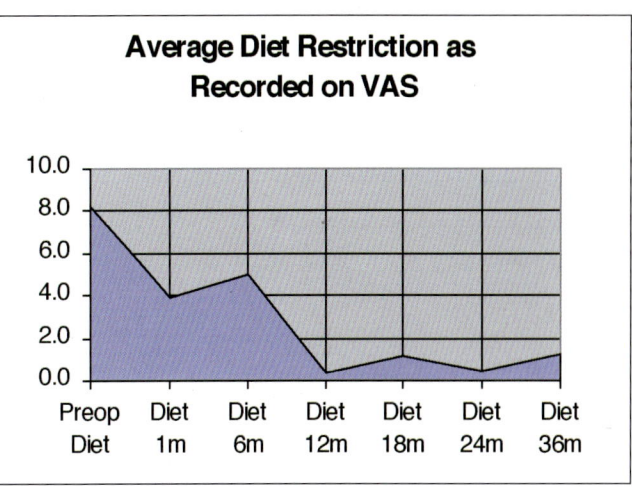

Figure 5. Prospective clinical average diet restriction levels measured on Visual Analog Scale (VAS).

and eminences TMJ Implants, Inc. makes available, one has no difficulty in selecting a proper fitting prosthesis for a given patient. The system has trial-sizing templates that correspond in size and shape to the available prostheses. The sizers also are made of Co-Cr and can be reused after steam sterilization. The sizers have a series of holes on their surface to allow the surgeon to determine the "best fit" of the prostheses provided before placement of the final, sterile prosthesis. The standard system also includes Co-Cr bone screws and drill bits sized to the screws. The prosthesis is fixed to the base of the skull with Co-Cr bones screws.[17]

Co-Cr alloy has had a long history of use in orthopedic applications.[18] Having been used for surgical implant applications for nearly 65 years, ASTM states this material "...has been shown to produce a well characterized level of local biological response following long term clinical use..." and has been used as a controlled material as required by the International Organization for Standardization (ISO) and Food and Drug Administration (FDA) guidelines.[19] A recently accepted abstract at the Society for Biomaterials shows that the metal-on-metal TMJ Fossa-Eminence and Condylar Prostheses™, which has been used in approximately 1000 patients over the last decade, demonstrates clinical results that parallel the positive European orthopedic experience (100,000+ joints) with metal-on-metal hips.

Two recent studies have been conducted that support the safety and effectiveness of the TMJ Foss-Eminence Prosthesis™ systems. The first is the TMJ Implants, Inc. Registry; the second is a prospective clinical study, TMJ-96-001. The objectives of these studies were to demonstrate the TMJ Fossa-Eminence Prosthesis™ used alone (partial joint replacement) reduces TMJ pain significantly and improves intercisal opening. An additional objective of the prospective clinical study included a review of the incidence of the device related adverse events occurring during the study.

Pain measurements were recorded using a 10-cm Visual Analog Scale (VAS) (Fig. 4). The left side of the scale represented no pain, whereas the right side represented the most severe pain imaginable. The patients were instructed to mark a vertical line on the scale to indicate their perceived level of pain. At the point where this vertical line crossed the horizontal scale, a measure was recorded using a ruler graduated in millimeters. Interincisal opening was measured in millimeters using a Therabite™ scale (Therabite™ Corp., Newtown, PA). The intercisal opening was measured at the point at which the patient could not open his/her mouth any wider.

RESULTS

Demographic information from the registry provides a valuable overview of patients who receive partial TMJ prostheses. The average age of patients entering the registry is 40.5 (standard deviation: 12) years.

As of March 27, 2000, 2892 patients had received the bi-lateral or unilateral TMJ Fossa-Eminence™ joint replacements. Of these 2892 patients, 1358 had provided preoperative pain data using the 10-cm VAS. The 1358 recipients represented 1909 TMJ Fossa-Eminence Prostheses™ placed, and 88 patients with 121 devices in which data were available at each time for analysis. Of this group of patients, 79 (90%) were female, and 9 (10%) were male. Patients showed a reduction in pain (8.0 to 1.0) and improved intercisal opening (27.1 mm to 34.0 mm) from six months to five years post-surgery.

Urbanek[14] reported on 134 bi-lateral partial joints, 84 unilateral partial joints, for a total of 218 patients, and 383 total devices from September 1993 to June 2000. Of his patients, 195 (89%) were females and 23 (11%) were male. Data on the patients' ability to eat and level of pain were measured preoperatively and at regular postoperative intervals using a VAS. Intercisal opening was measured at the same times using a Therabite™ scale. In the patients who had received the Fossa-Eminence Prosthesis™, 94% showed significant improvement in their ability to eat and 96% showed significant decrease in pain six months to four years after surgery (Fig. 4). Intercisal opening improved from a mean value of 32.35 mm to 35.00 mm (Figs. 5 & 6). This study suggests that the TMJ Fossa-Eminence Prosthesis™ System is effective in reducing pain and improving function in patients who suffer from a number of different problems.

In another retrospective study, Curry reviewed records for 18 patients with the partial joint implant between January 1965 and July 1992. Fifteen of the patients were female-83%, three of

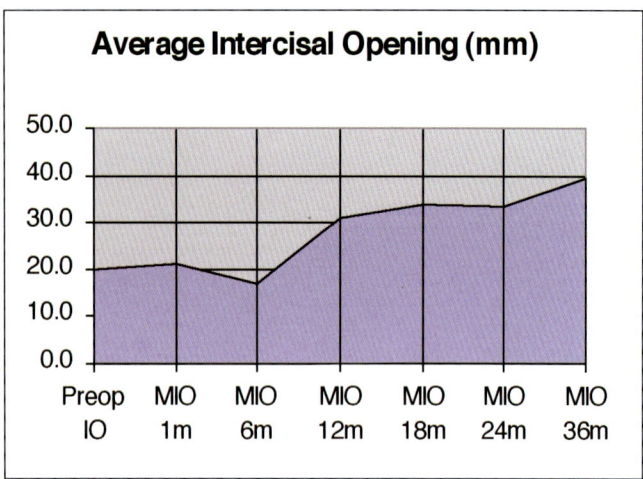

Figure 6. Prospective clinical average intercisal opening measured in millimeters.

the patients were male-17%. The average age of these patients at the time of implant placement was 35.4 years (Table 1). Fourteen patients received bilateral partial joint implants and four received unilateral partial joint implants (two left and two right). The indication for hemiarthroplasty with placement of TMJ Fossa-Eminence Prosthesis™ was internal derangement for 16 of the 18 patients. Degenerative joint disease with meniscal perforation was listed as the indication for surgery for two patients (Table 1). The charts indicate five of the patients reported that their TMJ symptoms began following motor vehicle accidents.

Two surgically related events were noted in the files. One event, a dislocation of the condyle, occurred immediately following surgery that required repositioning under anesthesia with no recurrence of the problem. The second event occurred when the head of a screw, used to fix the fossa implant to the zygoma, was sheared off during tightening. No problems have been reported because of this event and the device continues to function.

Additional surgery has been performed on four of the 18 (22%) patients. Three (17%) patients had the meniscus repositioned and retained at the time of implant placement and required an additional surgery to remove the damaged meniscus. One (6%) patient required a styloidectomy to relieve pain from an elongated styloid process. These additional procedures were not related to use of the partial joint implant, as the symptoms were relieved following meniscectomy with retention of the TMJ Fossa-Eminence Prosthesis™. None of the patients who required meniscectomy at the time of implant placement has required additional surgical intervention.

A review of the postoperative radiographs indicates no significant deleterious changes occurred in the natural condyles of these partial joint patients. Five patients were available for CT scans of their TMJs to provide a comparison of a panorex radiograph to a CT

Table 1. Data on 18 Patients Treated with Hemiarthroplasty.

Pt ID #	DOS	DOB	Age	Gender	Indication	Last PO X-ray	Duration (yrs)
1	12/23/1988	11/28/1970	18	F	ID	02/19/1994	5.2
2	12/28/1988	05/22/1975	14	F	ID	01/10/1995	6.0
3	02/02/1989	06/12/1954	35	F	ID	09/01/1992	3.6
4	02/09/1989	05/27/1960	29	F	ID	03/26/1999	10.1
5	09/08/1989	03/22/1951	38	F	ID/DJD/perf	06/26/1997	7.8
6	09/15/1989	03/04/1949	41	M	ID/perf	02/19/1994	4.4
7	10/12/1989	02/03/1941	49	F	ID	02/21/1994	4.4
8	03/10/1990	12/31/1957	32	M	ID	02/22/1994	4.0
9	03/09/1990	12/20/1960	29	F	ID/perf	02/22/1993	3.0
10	09/05/1990	04/26/1956	34	M	ID/trauma	10/21/1996	6.1
11	12/17/1990	10/04/1967	23	F	ID/osteoarth.	03/03/1997	6.2
12	12/18/1990	08/09/1944	46	F	ID/DJD	03/26/1999	8.3
13	12/28/1990	11/20/1956	34	F	ID/perf	01/08/1996	5.0
14	05/08/1991	05/25/1937	54	F	ID	07/16/1996	5.2
15	09/23/1991	12/26/1938	53	F	ID/perf	04/06/1999	7.5
16	04/15/1992	12/20/1962	29	F	ID	06/15/1998	6.2
17	07/09/1992	11/22/1961	31	F	DJD/perf	09/04/1996	4.2
18	01/01/1965	01/01/1917	48	F	ID	10/01/2000	35.8
		Mean	35.4				7.4
		SD	11.4				7.3
		Max	54.0				35.8
		Min	13.6				3.0

scan (Figs. 7-10). The files of three patients indicated slight bony changes had occurred from the preoperative radiographic status. Patient 9 exhibited advanced degenerative condylar disease at the time of implant placement and has not required additional treatment since hemiarthroplasty with placement of a fossa liner. Patient 11 also exhibited degenerative condylar disease at the time of implant placement that required initial condylar arthroplasty with no requirement for additional surgery to date (Fig. 11). The records indicate that total joint replacement was contemplated at the time of the original surgery; however, the more conservative approach, that of hemiarthroplasty, was used in an effort to preserve the patient's condyle, which appears to have been a prudent choice. Patient 5 exhibited moderate "degenerative" change in the right condyle when evaluated radiographically postoperatively. Additional follow up indicates this change represents adaptive remodeling rather than pathological degeneration.

A review of the pre- and postoperative interincisal opening measurements was conducted (Table 2). Three patients experienced a decrease in opening over time, two of whom had large incisal openings before surgery (67 mm and 52 mm). The interincisal measurement at last follow up for each of these patients was 52 mm and 40 mm (Fig. 12). The third patient experienced a slight decrease from 40 mm to 39 mm.

None of the 18 patients reported in this review have required removal of the device, nor have any required conversion to a total joint to address their symptoms.

Review of the postoperative radiographs indicates no deleterious changes in the natural condyle in these partial joint patients. The duration from implant of the last postoperative radiograph ranged from 3 to 35 (average = 7.3) years. No indications of degenerative changes were present due to placement of the partial joint. The review of radiographs is supported by the clinical findings, including bite and opening data, none of which indicate the partial TMJ Fossa-Eminence Prosthesis™ had contributed to a degradation of the joint. Any bony changes noted were indicative of progression of disease. The radiographs indicated that use of the partial joint had protected the bone

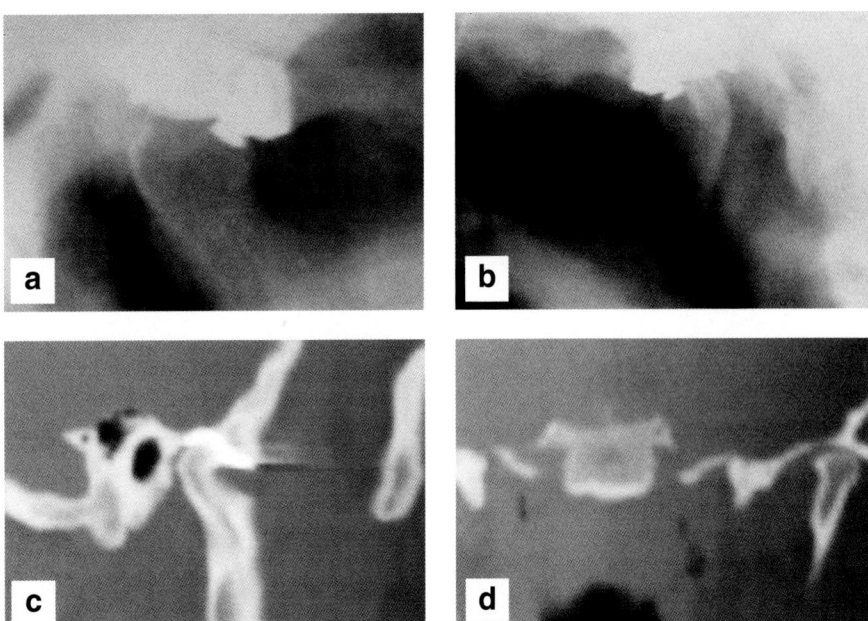

Figure 7. Comparison of preoperative and postopertive radiographs in patient #4's left temporomandibular joint with Stage III ID, 28 yr F. a) Post-op Panorex 3/94, 5 y 1 m - Pain: 0.0, Diet: 0.0, MIO 48 mm. b) Pre-op Panorex 2/89, Pain: 1.8, Diet: 4.8, MIO 31 mm. c, d) Post-op CT Scans 3/99, 10 y 1 m, Occlusion: Unchanged, Pain: 0.0, Diet: 0.0, MIO 48 mm.

Table 2. Comparative Data on 18 Patients Pre-op Opening and Post-op Opening.

Pt ID	Implant Date	Pre-op Opening	Post-Op Opening	Date Measured
1	12/23/88	33	40	3/2/98
2	12/28/88	43	44	1/23/97
3	2/2/89	33	35	3/1/96
4	2/9/89	32	56	2/29/96
5	9/8/89	31	45	8/19/97
6	9/15/89	67	52	9/8/96
7	10/12/89	39	45	9/1/96
8	3/10/90	52	40	6/8/90
9	3/9/90	22	30	3/26/91
10	9/5/90	29	41	4/22/99
11	12/17/90	43	63	10/7/96
12	12/18/90	40	39	3/26/99
13	12/28/90	30	33	3/4/96
14	5/8/91	20	34	7/16/96
15	9/23/91	40	42	4/6/99
16	4/15/92	32	39	8/28/97
17	7/9/92	27	46	9/4/96
18	1/1/65	35	45	10/1/00

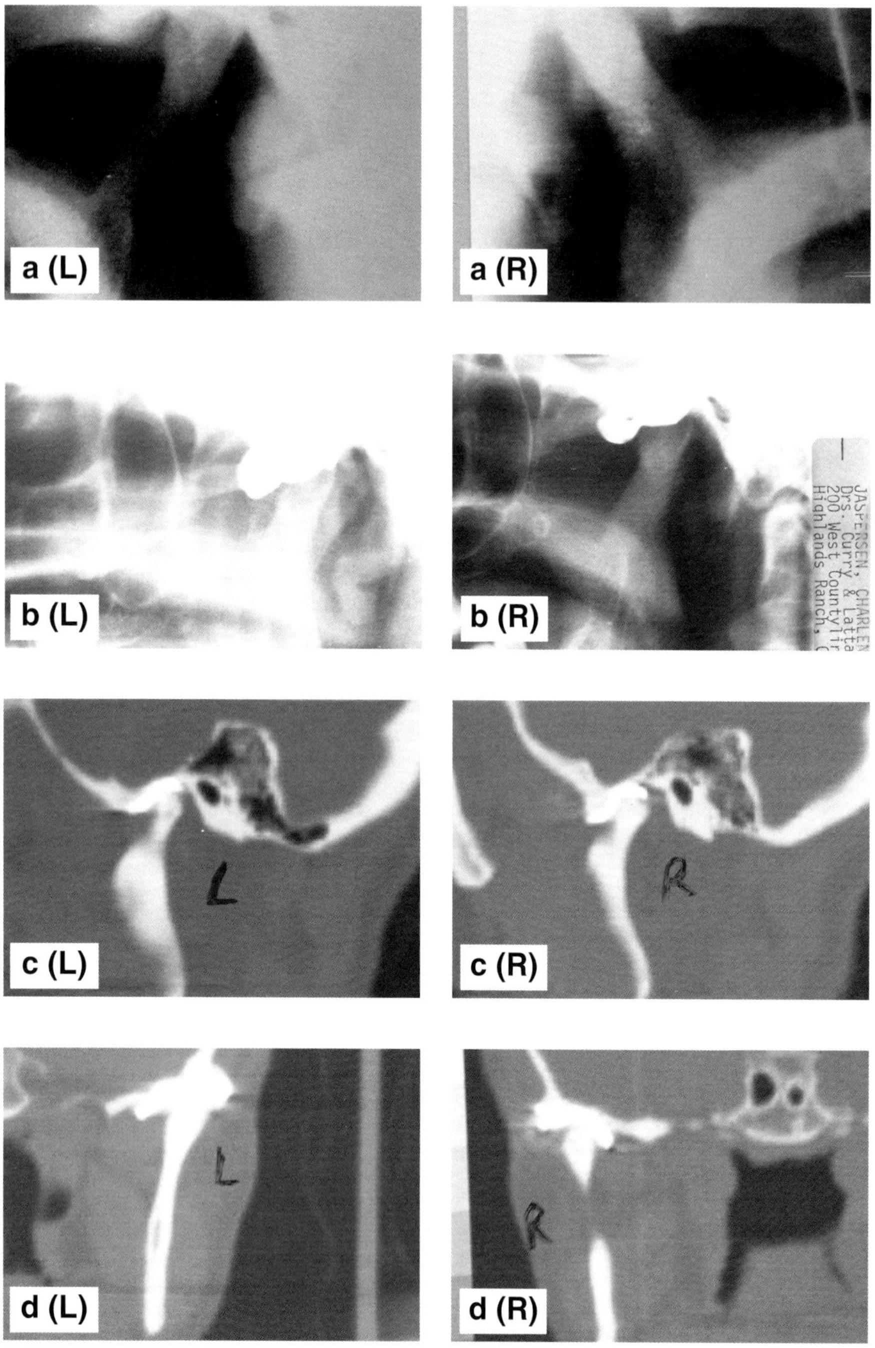

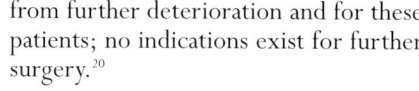

from further deterioration and for these patients; no indications exist for further surgery.[20]

Adverse Events

Clinical data compiled for thousands of patients demonstrate the TMJ Fossa-Eminence Prosthesis™ is safe, whether used individually or in combination with the TMJ Condylar Prosthesis™. Device-related adverse events occurred at an extremely low (< 0.5%) rate, and non-device-related adverse events experienced by the patients were as expected, based on the nature of TMD and the surgical procedure used. These data establish an absence of unreasonable risk of illness or injury associated use of the TMJ Fossa-Eminence and Condylar Prosthesis™.

DISCUSSION

This implant system, combined with modern precision manufacturing of metal articulating services, has piloted in a new era of partial joint reconstruction. Current data indicate the tissues around such an implant (metal/metal total) tolerate metallic wear debris much better than polyethylene.

Biocompatibility tests were conducted to confirm the compatibility of the implant materials used in these devices. Tests were conducted to confirm the devices, as manufactured by TMJ Implants, Inc., remain biocompatible. These confirmatory tests were *in-vitro* Cytoxicity, Genotoxicity, Mutagenicity, and Irritation and Intracutaneous reactivity, Systemic Toxicity, and Contact Sensitivity.

Results of a literature search also support the suitability of this material for the chosen application. An assessment of the effects of wear particles of cobalt-chrome on the TMJ space in 12 New Zealand rabbits has yielded no lasting inflammatory response. No for-

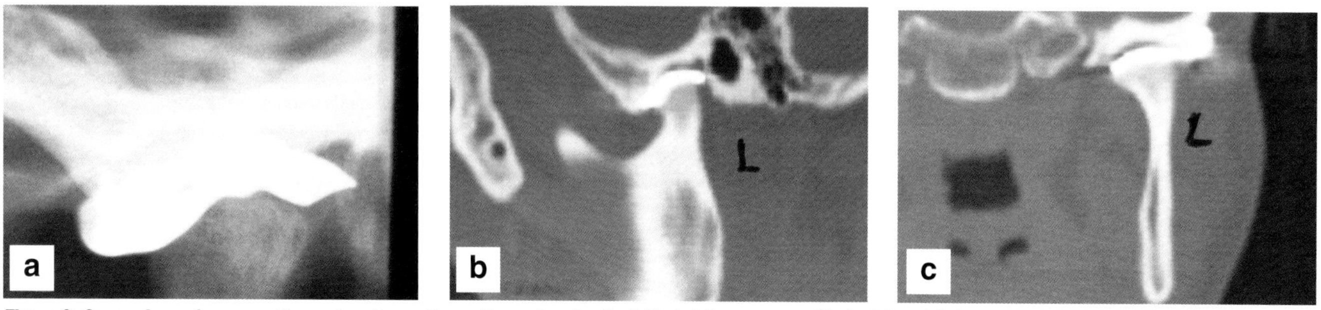

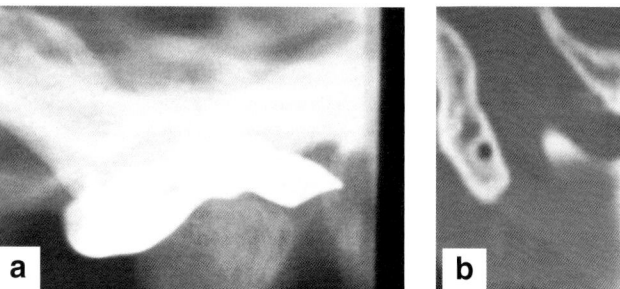

Figure 8. Comparison of preoperative and postoperative radiographs of patient #12's temporomandibular joints with Stage V ID, 46 yr F. a) Pre-op L/R Panorex 12/90, 46 yr F - Pain: 9.2, Diet: 10.0, MIO: 35 mm. b) Post-op L/R Panorex 1/96, 5 y 1 m - Pain: 0.0, Diet: 0.0, MIO: 39 mm. c, d) Post-op CT Scans L/R 3/99, 9 y 9 m - Pain: 0.0, Diet: 0.0, MIO: 39 mm.

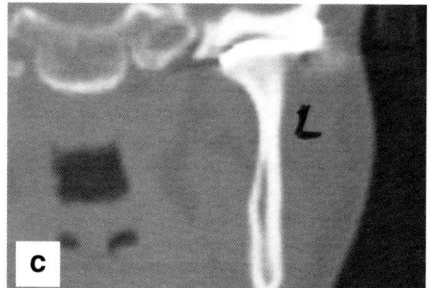

Figure 9. Comparison of preoperative and postoperative radiographs of patient #'s left temporomandibular joint with Stage IV ID, 31 yr F, DOS 1/93, Pre-op Pain: 9.0, Diet: 7.5, MIO 33 mm. a) Post-op Panorex, 9/00, Pain: 0.0, Diet: 0.0, MIO 47 mm. b) Post-op Sagittal CT, 3/99. c) Post-op Coronal CT, 3/99.

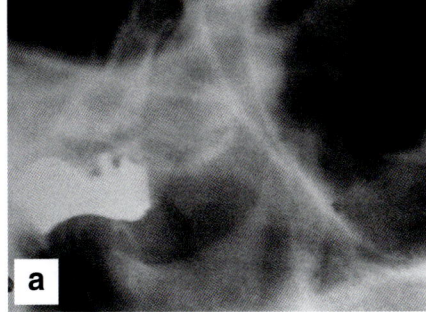
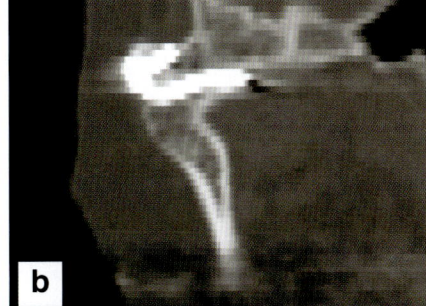
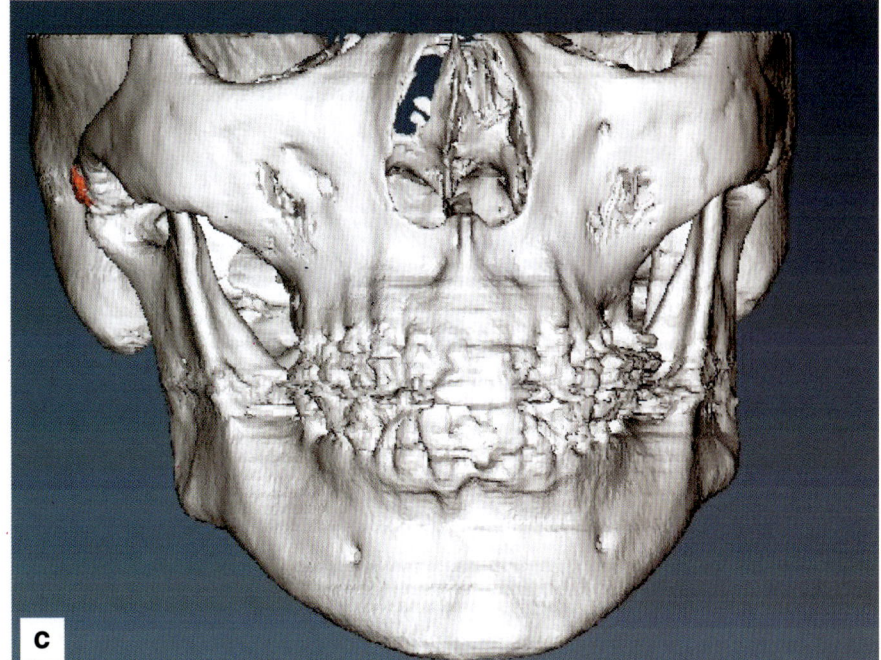
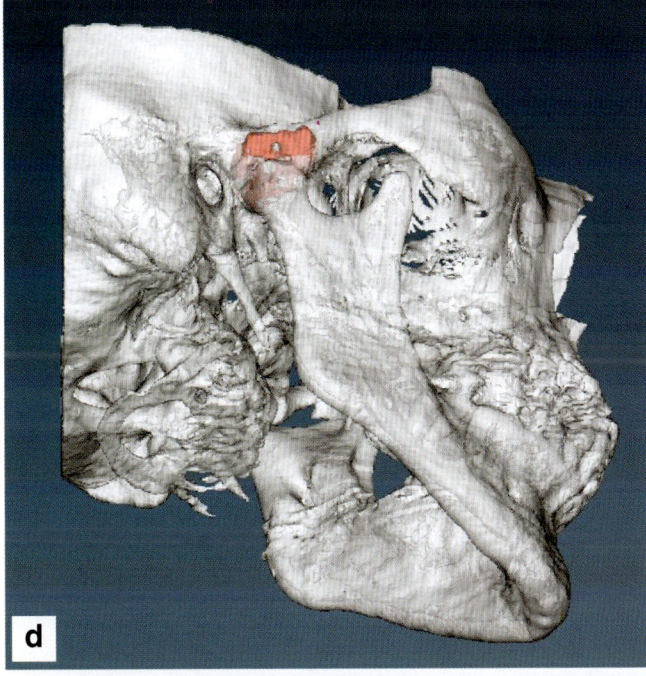
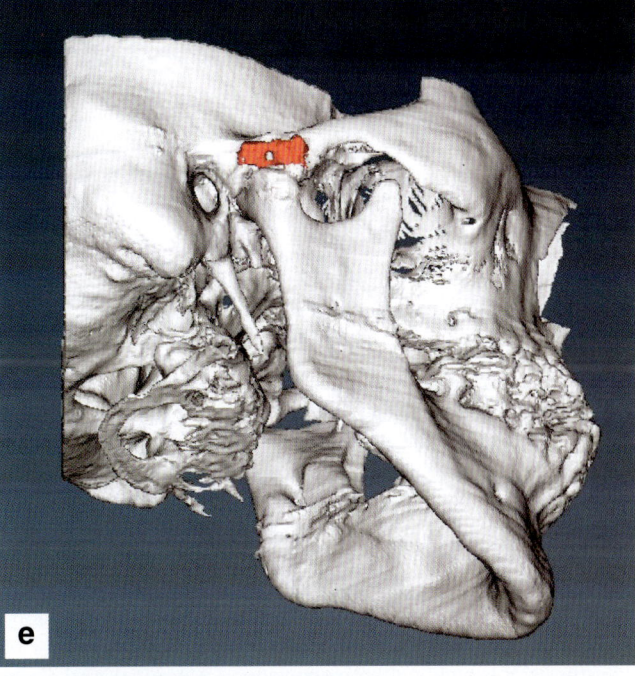

Figure 10. 35-year postoperative radiographs of patient #18's left temporomandibular joint with Stage VID, 48 yr F, DOS 1/65. a) 35-year Post-op Panorex 10/00, 35 y 10 m, MIO45 mm. b) 35-year Post-op CT scan, 9/00. c, d, & e) 35-year Post-op 3-dimensional reconstructed images of the CT scan image data received before creating a stereolithographic model, 9/00.

eign-body reaction was noted, and no giant cells were present at any time. All other organ pathologic findings were normal, as were the results of all blood studies.

The TMJ Fossa-Eminence Prosthesis™ is designed to provide a thin (0.5-mm), rigid, well-fitting prosthetic covering for the articulating surface of the TMJ composed of the glenoid fossa and articular eminence of the temporal bone. The articular surface of the prosthetic glenoid fossa and articular eminence is highly polished to minimize friction in joint movement.

The Christensen TMJ Fossa-Eminence Prosthesis™ is offered in "off-the-shelf" stock prostheses in a number of different sizes as well as the Christensen Patient-Specific™ Prostheses. The Patient-Specific™ Prostheses are used to fit the specific anatomical contours of a patient's glenoid fossa in such instances as trauma, and severe neoplastic or degenerative disease. The prosthesis, and screws with which it is to be secured to the skull, are manufactured from surgical Co-Cr-Mo alloy (ASTA F75/ASTM F799). These devices are intended for permanent implantation and are for single use only.

All components of the Fossa kit, including individual prosthesis, drills

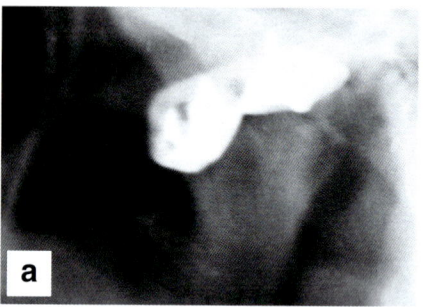 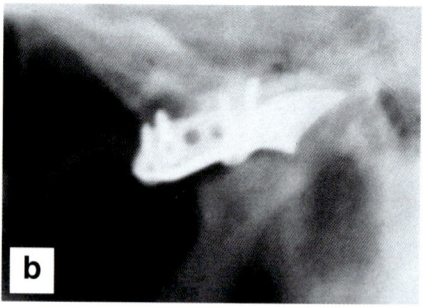

Figure 11. Represents the postoperative radiographs of patient #11's temporomandibular joints with Stage V ID, 24 yr F, DOS 12/90, Pre-op Pain: 7.9, Diet: 7.3, MIO 43 mm; Post-op Pain: 6.1, Diet: 5.9, MIO 42 mm. a) Post-op panorex L, 10/99. b) Post-op panorex R, 10/99. At the time of surgery, the patient opted for partial replacements rather than total. The slight change in the condylar head postoperatively has been read as adaptive rather that pathological.

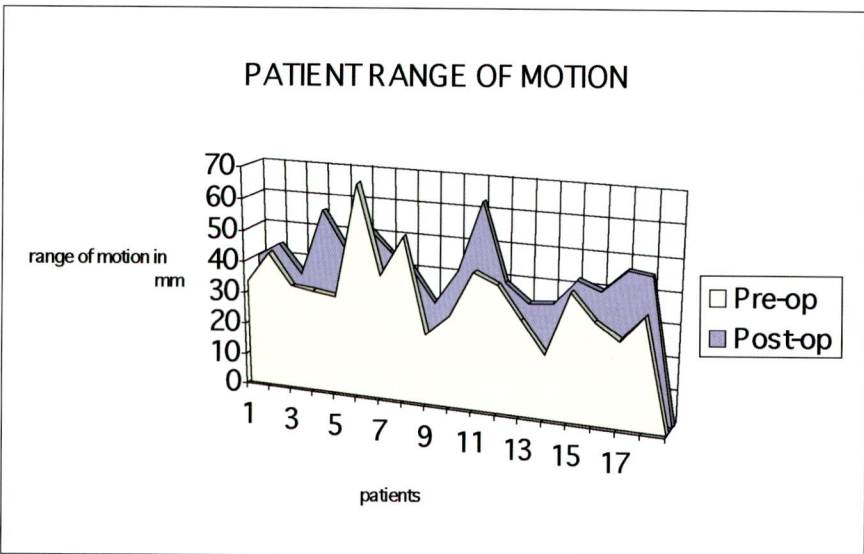

Figure 12. Comparison of pre- and postoperative range of motion.

and screws are sterilized by gamma-irradiation or e-beam radiation (2.5 Mrads), and are packaged in individual double-peel polyethylene terephthalate, glycol (PETG) modified and Tyvek containers.

The TMJ Implants, Inc. Registry data and Prospective Clinical Study data collected to date have clearly demonstrated that the TMJ Fossa-Eminence Prosthesis™ is highly effective in reduction of TMJ pain, reducing diet restrictions, and improving interincisal opening. Additionally, since 1992, the cumulative incidence rate of Medical Device Reports filed with the FDA is 0.57 of 1.0%. No evidence exists of degradation of the natural condyle because of the uses of the metal fossa liner. In more than 90% of the patients in the Registry since 1993, none show progression of the partial joint reconstruction to a total joint reconstruction.

Boering has addressed clinical and radiographic progression of TMD.[19] Progression appears to take on at least two forms, clinical and radiographic. The radiographic changes indicating progression were flattening, sclerosis, cyst, and osteophyte formation. Boering also noted a difference in length between the ascending ramus of the affected side when compared with the unaffected side. Progression of TMD can be severe to the point of being considered pathological and destructive in nature, or mild to the point of being considered physiologic and remodeling in nature. Pathologic condylar degeneration is often manifested by (1) clinically worsening symptoms, (2) development of a malocclusion with open bite, and (3) radiographic evidence of condylar deterioration.

This retrospective review has addressed these issues in an effort to determine whether the presence of a metal fossa liner can be expected to cause significant deleterious changes to the natural mandibular condyle. The authors believe many patients can benefit from hemiarthroplasty rather than total joint replacement if early intervention with this technique is used. Hemiarthroplasty has been used in orthopedic applications and is considered a well-accepted surgical procedure.[20] In an effort to preserve bone stock, orthopedic surgeons have at their disposal a technique that provides the benefits of hemiarthroplasty when the conditions are appropriate. Oral and Maxillofacial Surgeons have desired to preserve the bone and soft tissues of the TMJ when appropriate. Various techniques have been proposed over the last 20 years to "preserve" TMJ structures; these include disc repositioning by plication and arthroscopic techniques. A number of reports have been generated in peer-reviewed literature that indicate the futility of such efforts over time.[21,22] When partial TMJ reconstruction is contemplated, the memory of the disaster brought on by use of materials that showed a tendency to fragment over time causing serious destruction of bone and soft-tissue elements of the jaw joint makes one cautious. In this article, evidence has been presented that the bone of the mandibular condyle generally does not show signs of pathological degeneration after years of articulating against a cobalt/chrome liner. The clinical outcomes also indicate no unacceptable degenerative conditions occurred because of hemiarthroplasty with placement of a "permanent" implant. If the natural mandibular condyle is affected adversely following placement of a Christensen TMJ Fossa-Eminence Prosthesis™, radiographic evidence of pathological bony changes manifested by condylar deterioration and malocclusion should be evident in many of the patients who have been treated with this technique. It appears from previous reports,[23] as well as the clinical and radiographic review of these 18 patients, that pathological bony changes are not encountered frequently following placement of a metal fossa liner. The authors believe destructive pathological changes in the natural mandibular condyle occur because of progressive disease rather than as a process caused merely by articulation against a metal liner. Additional reports are encouraged to further evaluate the safety and efficacy of placing a metal fossa liner in a hemiarthroplasty application in the TMJ.

REFERENCES

1. Okeson JP. Treatment of disc-interference disorders. In: Reinhardt RW, ed. Management of temporomandibular disorder and occlusion 2nd ed. St. Louis: CV Mosby Co; 1989. p 357-9.
2. Holmlund AB, Gynther G, Axelsson S. Diskectomy in treatment of internal derangement of the temporomandibular joint: follow-up at 1, 3, and 5 years. Oral Surg Oral Med Oral Pathol 1993;76:266-71.
3. Sarnat BG, Laskin DM. The temporomandibular joint, 3rd ed. In: Sarnat BG, ed. Springfield, IL: Charles C Thomas Publisher; 1979. p 287.
4. Laskin DM. Etiology of the pain-dysfunction syndrome. J Am Dent Assoc 1969: 79: 147.
5. Christensen RW. Arthroplastic Implantation of the temporomandibular joint. In: Cranin AN. ed. Oral implantology 1st ed. Illinois: Charles C. Thomas; 1967, p 284-97.
6. Hellsing G, Holmlund A. Development of anterior disk displacement in the temporomandibular joint: an autopsy study. J Pros Dent 1985;53:397-401.
7. Christensen, RW. The temporomandibular joint prosthesis eleven years later. J Oral Implantol 1972;2:34-8.
8. Westesson PL, Eriksson, L, Lindstrom C. Destructive lesions of the mandibular condyle following diskectomy with temporary silicone implant. Oral Surg Oral Med Oral Pathol 1987;63:143-50.
9. Dolwick MF, Audemorte TB: Silicone-induced foreign body reaction and lymphadenopathy after temporomandibular joint arthroplasty. Oral Surg 1985;59:449-52.
10. Ryan DE: Temporomandibular disorders. Curr Opin Rheumatol 1993;(2):209-18.
11. Christensen RW. The correction of mandibular ankylosis by arthroplasty and insertion of a vitallium glenoid fossa prosthesis: a new technique. Am J Orthopedics 1963;48:28-34.
12. Muller ME. Lessons of 30 years of total hip arthroplasty. Clin Orthop 1992;274:12-21.
13. Lippincott AL, Chase DC, Christensen RW. Alternative total TMJ arthroplasty: metal-on metal for longevity in implant survivorship and patient satisfaction. In: San Francisco, CA: Surg Technol Inter VII, Universal Medical Press, Inc.; p 425-35.
14. Urbanek, A. TMJ Implants, Inc. Internal Report. Nov 2000.
15. Klimek L, Klein H, Schneider W, et al. Stereolithography modeling for reconstructive head surgery. Acta Otorhinolaryngol Belg 1993;47(3):329-34.
16. Robinson A, Russell R, Robinson A, et al. TMJ fossa-eminence prosthesis placement on the absence of the meniscus. J Dent Res 1993;72(Spec No):104-421.
17. Gerard D, Hudson J. The Christensen temporomandibular joint prosthesis system, an overview. In: Total temporomandibular joint reconstruction, oral and maxillofacial surgery. Clin North Am, 2000;12(1):134-5.
18. Curry JT. The effects of hemiarthroplasty utilizing a metal fossa prosthesis on the mandibular condyle: a retrospective review. TM Journal 2000:(1)6-12.
19. Boering G. Natural history of internal derangements. In: Current concepts of TM joint disease. Conference, Nashville, TN, March 1993.
20. Hartsock L, Estes WJ, Murray CA, et al. Shoulder hemiarthroplasty for proximal humeral fractures. Orthop Clin North Am 1998;29:467-75.
21. Westesson PL, Cohen JM, Tallents RH. Magnetic resonance imaging of temporomandibular joint after surgical treatment of internal derangement. Oral Surg Oral Med Oral Pathol 1991;(4)71:407-11.
22. Montgomery MT, Van Sickels JE, Harms SE. Success of temporomandibular joint arthroscopy in disc displacement with and without reduction. Oral Surg Oral Med Oral Pathol 1991;71:651-9.
23. Chase DC, Hudson JW, Gerard DA, et al. The Christensen prosthesis: a retrospective clinical study. Oral Surg Oral Med Oral Pathol 1995;80(3):273-8.

Visit our Website at www.ump.com

Search Engine

Article of the Month

Product Profile

Home Page

Product Profile

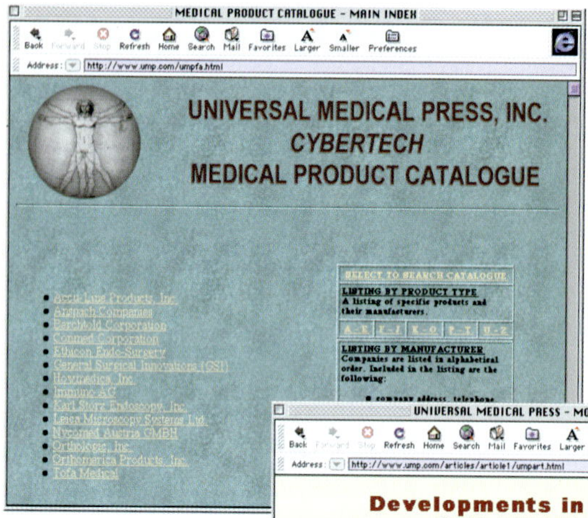

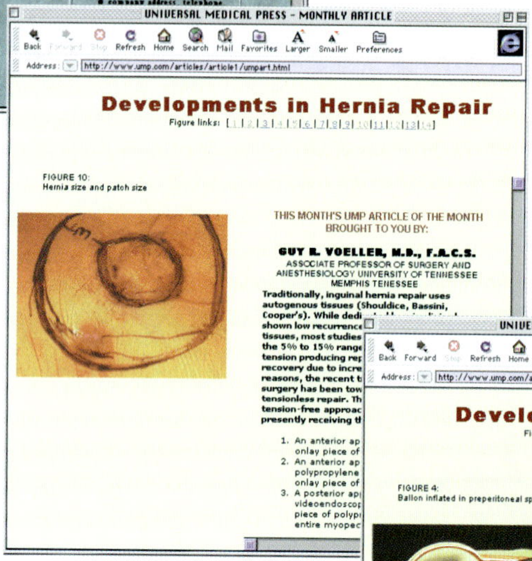

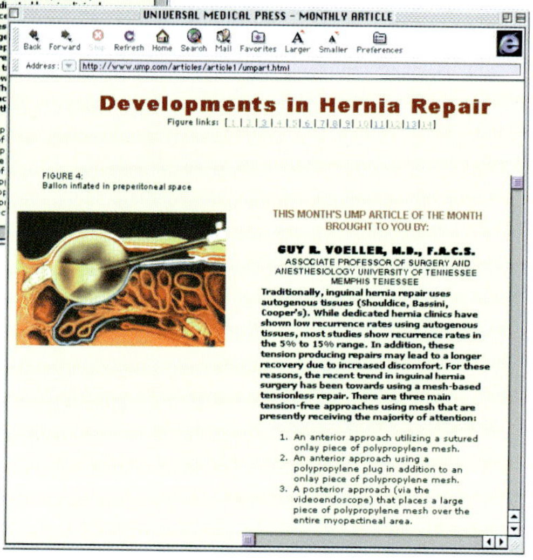

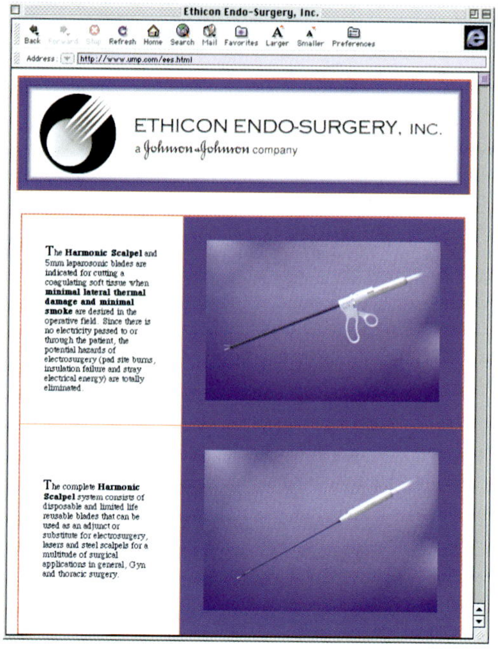

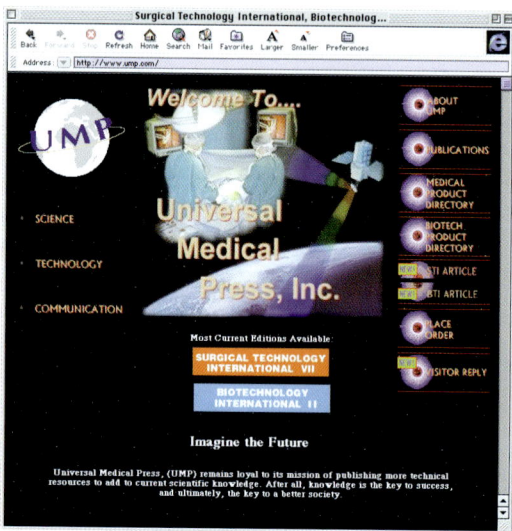

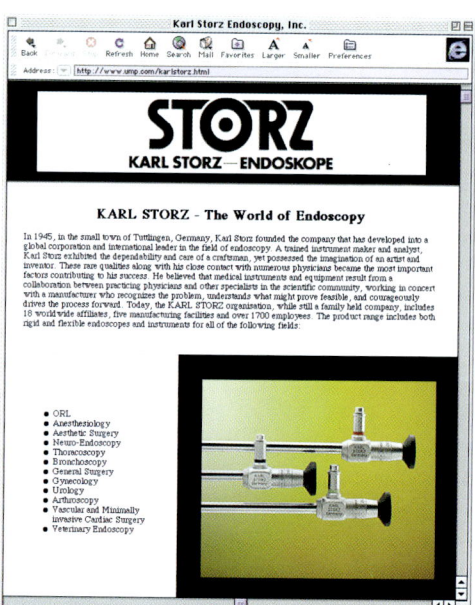

Subperiosteal Rejuvenation of The Forehead

JAY M. PENSLER, M.D.
ASSOCIATE CLINICAL PROFESSOR OF PLASTIC SURGERY
NORTHWESTERN UNIVERSITY MEDICAL SCHOOL
CHICAGO, IL

KAVEH ALIZADEH, M.D.
LONG ISLAND PLASTIC SURGICAL GROUP, GARDEN CITY, NY
ATTENDING, MANHATTAN EYE, EAR, AND THROAT HOSPITAL, NEW YORK

Subperiosteal rejuvenation of the forehead may be performed through several small incisions in the brow. Small incisions are placed in the hairline and within the hair-bearing portion of the brow. The procedure provides a safe and reliable way to improve the position of the brow. The addition of resorbable screw fixation improves the stability of the brow position postoperatively and facilitates healing in the desired location. Subperiosteal brow lift may be performed successfully by way of minimally invasive incisions with favorable results.

METHODS

The authors have established that a small incision placed directly in the brow can provide excellent exposure to the lower forehead, based on our extensive experience in craniofacial surgery. If the incision is beveled correctly and an atraumatic technique pursued during dissection and closure of the wound, the brow incision provides an excellent aesthetic result in all age groups. Subperiosteal dissection of the entire forehead, combined with removal of the corrugator supercilii and procerus muscles, facilitates predictable elevation of the forehead. Furthermore, based on our large series of craniofacial reconstructions using resorbable screw rigid-fixation, it became apparent that resorbable fixation would provide the optimal means of securing the soft tissue to the underlying bone without the potential risks of permanent screws and plates.

TECHNIQUE

A thorough physical examination is performed on the patient to identify the anatomy of the bony landmarks. After the supraorbital and supratrochlear notches on the foramen are marked, a brow incision is made immediately lateral to the foramen using a #11 scalpel blade, making sure to bevel the knife in the direction of the hair follicles. When the subperiosteal plane is entered, an endoscopic elevator is introduced and dissection is carried out in the subperiosteal plane to the level of the temporal fusion line and the forehead is, thus, released from all lateral attachments. If planned, a corrugator and procerus resection also can be carried out at this time.

After the forehead is released from all periosteal attachments, small stab incisions are made over the desired fixation points, or upper lid blepharoplasty incisions are used for placement of the resorbable screws (Lactosorb, Walter

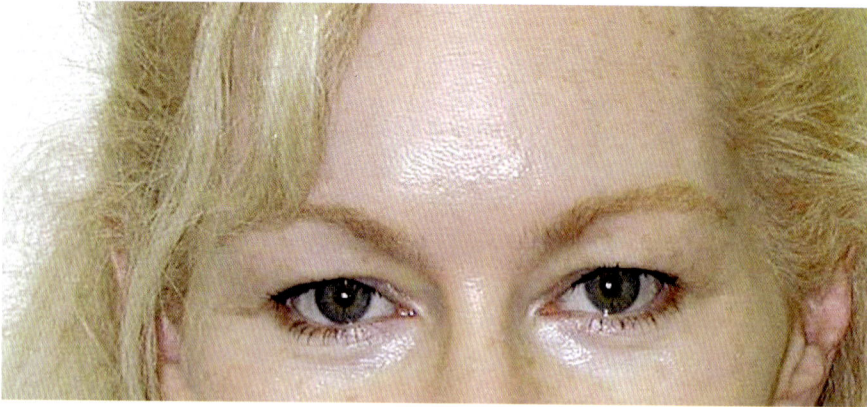

Figure 1. Preoperative photography of 59-year-old patient before brow lift and lower lid blepharoplasty.

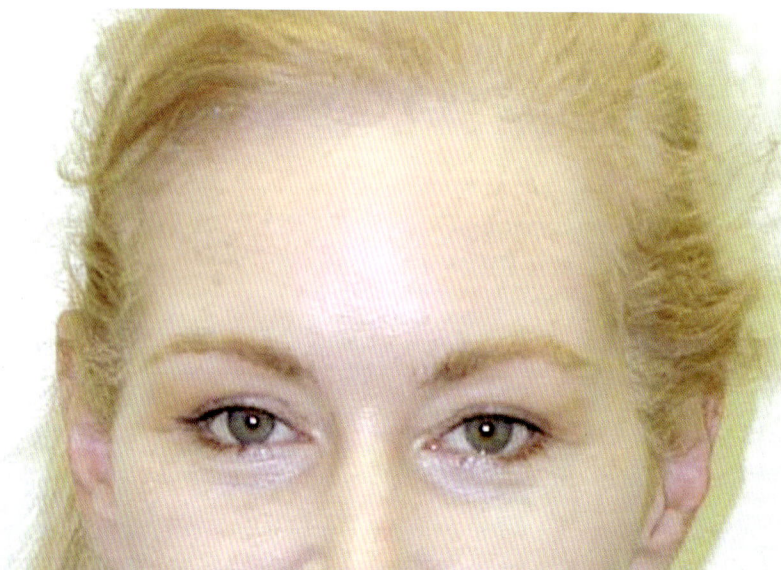

Figure 2. Postoperative appearance at six months following brow lift and lower lid blepharoplasty. Note improved position of brow.

Lorenz Surgical, Jacksonville, FL). This procedure is accomplished by use of the hand-held, self-drilling, and tapping device in a single maneuver (Walter Lorenz Surgical). The 7-mm long resorbable brow screws are then inserted. The suture is pulled tight, elevating the forehead to the desired position, and tied after completely seeding the screw into the bone. It is important to completely release the dermal attachments of the stab incision to prevent dimpling postoperatively. The wound beds are then irrigated and closed.

DISCUSSION

Forehead suspension has become an integral component of the rejuvenation of the upper third of the face (Fig.1).[1-5] When used properly, it raises the brows to the precisely desired position, and improves the appearance of the mid-forehead rhytids while minimizing the required upper lid skin excision (Fig.2).

Successful execution of the subperiosteal forehead lift is dependent on thorough knowledge of the anatomy of the forehead to avoid damage to the neurovascular bundles, coupled with proper soft-tissue fixation to diminish undue tension of the incisions. The supraorbital neurovascular bundles are identified. The vessels are noted as they exit the notch in the supraorbital rim and deflected inferiorly. Supraorbital vessels that exit by way of a foramen are freed with a small osteotome.

This technique allows excellent exposure to the subperiosteal plane and stable fixation of the soft tissues, thus minimizing incisional tension and scalp alopecia. Use of resorbable screws has added the advantage of stable fixation without concern of permanent indwelling devices that could migrate intracranially or exteriorize from the scalp.[6]

Forehead lifting has become an integral component in rejuvenation of the face. New techniques such as described here, which allow precision in soft-tissue placement, will have an increasingly critical role in future surgical procedures to enhance the results.

REFERENCES

1. Ramirez OM. The anchor subperiosteal forehead lift. Plast Reconstr Surg 1995;95(6):993-1003.
2. Isse NG. Endoscopic forehead lift. Evolution and update. Clin Plast Surg 1995;22(4):661-73.
3. Muller GH. Endoscopic forehead lift: the subperiosteal pulling stitch. Aesthetic Plast Surg 1996;20(4):297-301.
4. Kobienia BJ, Van Beek A. Calvarial fixation during endoscopic brow lift. Plast Reconstr Surg 1998;102(1):238-40.
5. Roberts TL III, Ellis LB. In pursuit of optimal rejuvenation of the forehead: endoscopic brow lift with simultaneous carbon dioxide laser resurfacing. Plast Reconstr Surg 1998;101(4):1075-84.
6. Pakkanen M, Salisbury AV, Ersek RA. Biodegradable positive fixation for the endoscopic brow lift. Plast Reconstr Surg 1996;98(6):1087-91.

Surgical Advances for the New Millenium

- **Updates on Recent Innovations in Surgery**
- **Peer Reviewed by Expert Specialty Surgeons**
- **Indexed on MEDLINE**

"**Surgical Technology International** does a splendid job of showcasing the many aspects of recent surgical achievement and innovation that have been possible as we hurtle forward into the new millenium."
—M. David Tilson, M.D.
Professor of Surgery
Columbia University, New York

"The authors are to be congratulated on the latest edition of what is essential reading for surgeons in every discipline."
—Tom Bates, F.R.C.S.
Consultant Surgeon
The William Harvey Hospital
Ashford, Kent, England, UK

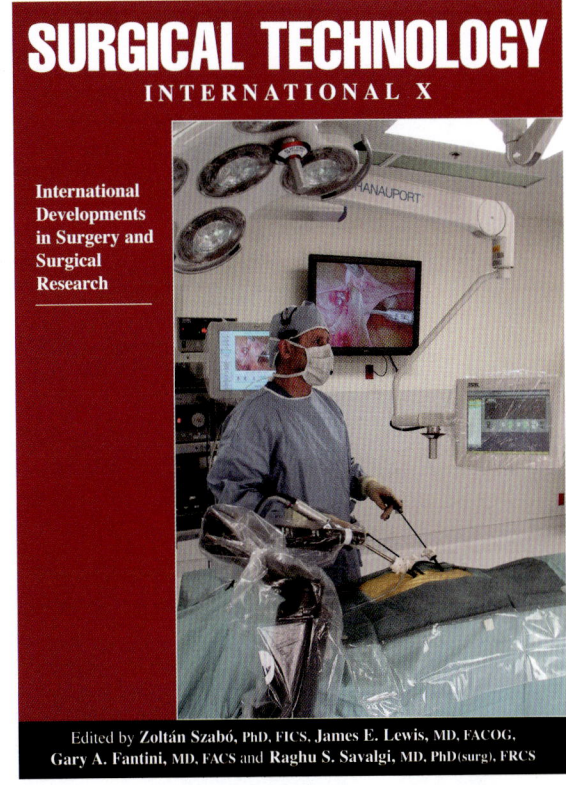

ISBN No. 1-890131-06-7

Order a 3-year subscription now and get 50% off the bookstore price!

Yes, please enter my subscription to Surgical Techonology International for:

☐ 3 years (6 Issues) $285 ☐ 2 years (4 Issues) $215 ☐ 1 year (2 Issues) $145 ☐ Individual Copy ($95)

Please add 10% per year for shipping & handling on U.S. orders.
Please add $46 per year for shipping & handling for international orders.

ISBN No.: 1-890131-06-7

☐ Special Back Issue Set STI III - STI X - $685 US, $755 overseas - (Includes shipping)
☐ AMEX ☐ MasterCard ☐ VISA ☐ Check enclosed* ☐ Bill me

Card Number: ☐☐☐☐ ☐☐☐☐ ☐☐☐☐ ☐☐☐☐

Signature: _____ Expiration Date: _____
Name: _____ Institution: _____
Address: _____
City: _____ State: _____ Zip: _____
Country: _____ Phone/Fax: _____
Email: _____

Please send to: Universal Medical Press, Inc., 2443 Fillmore Street, #229, San Francisco, CA 94115, USA,
or FAX YOUR ORDER TO: 1-415-436-9791. / Telephone: 1-415-436-9790 / E-mail: info@ump.com / Website: www.ump.com

* Make checks payable to **Universal Medical. Press, Inc.** California residents, please add applicable state sales tax.

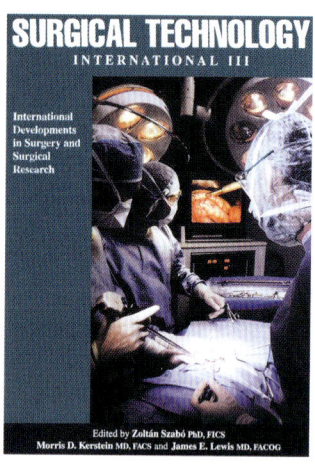
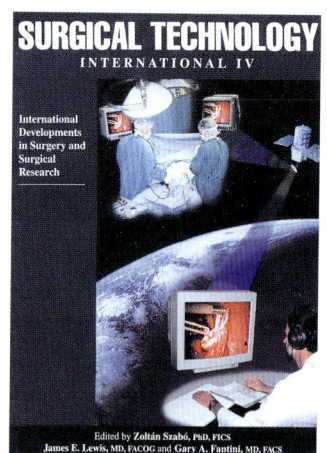
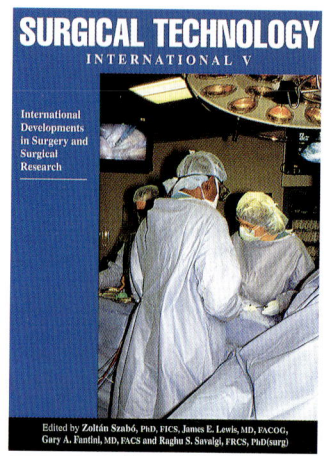
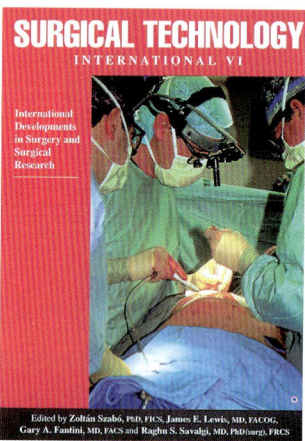
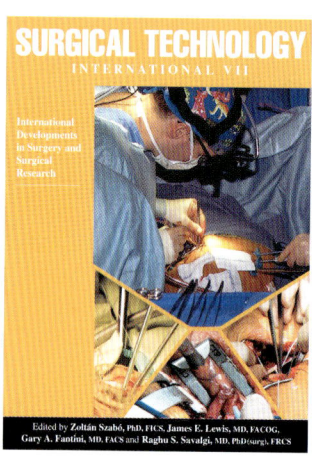
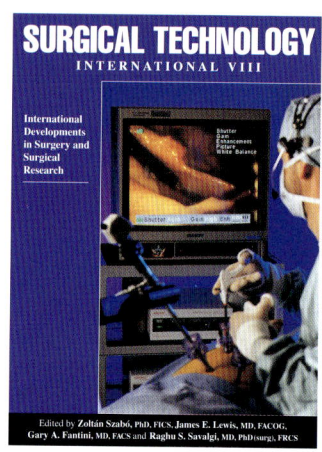
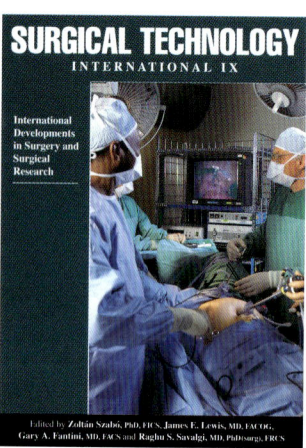
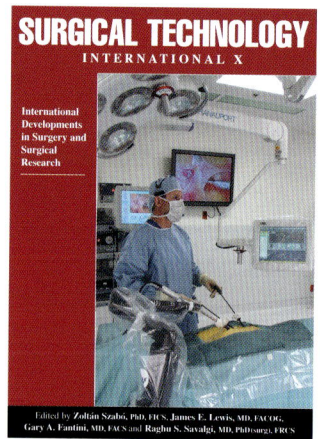

To order reprints please visit our website at http://www.ump.com or email us on Reprints@ump.com
Tel: 1-415-436-9790
Fax: 1-415-436-9791

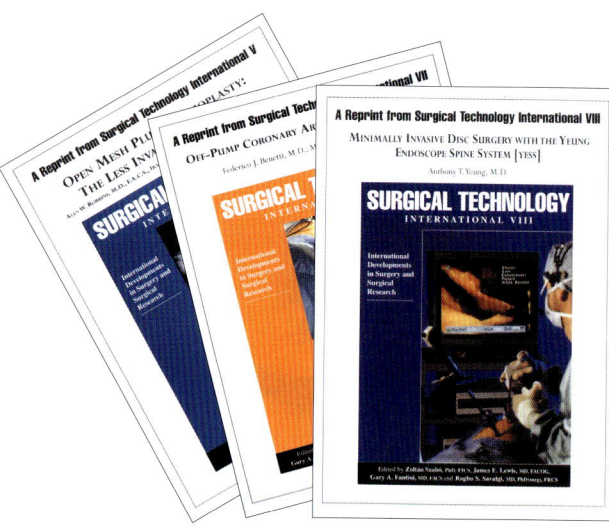
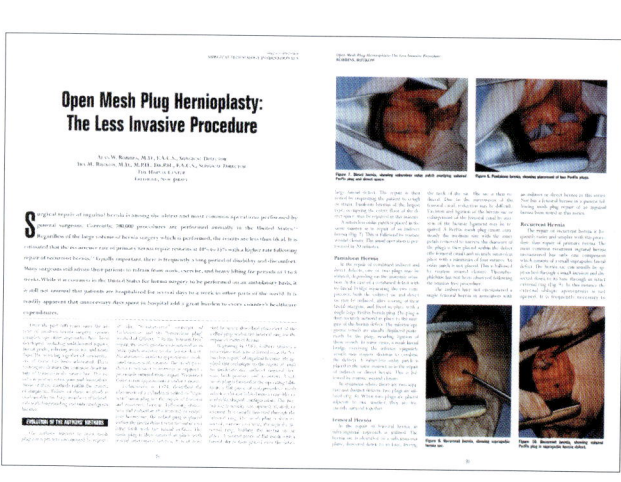

Visit our Website at
www.ump.com

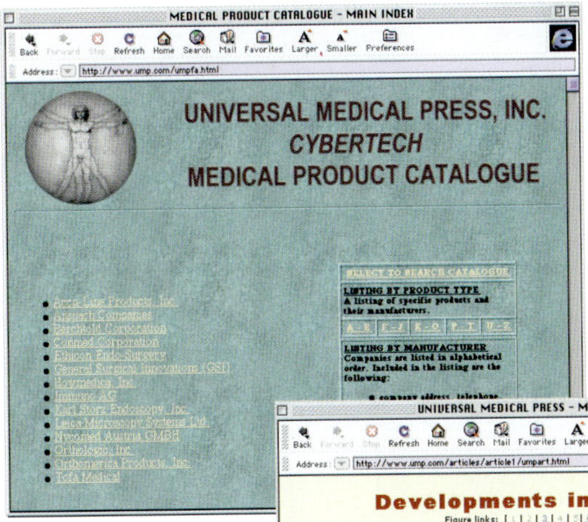

Search Engine

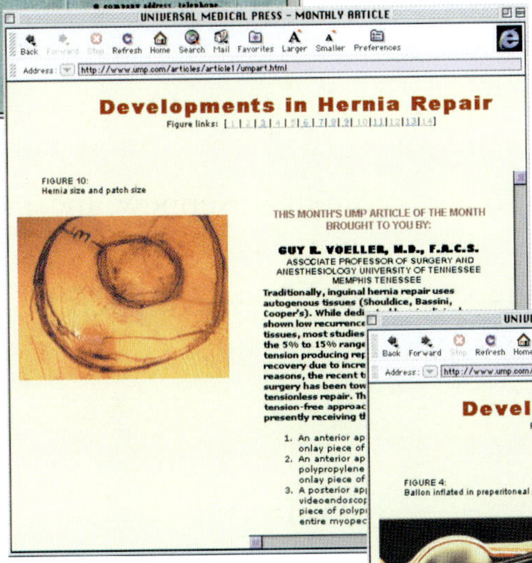

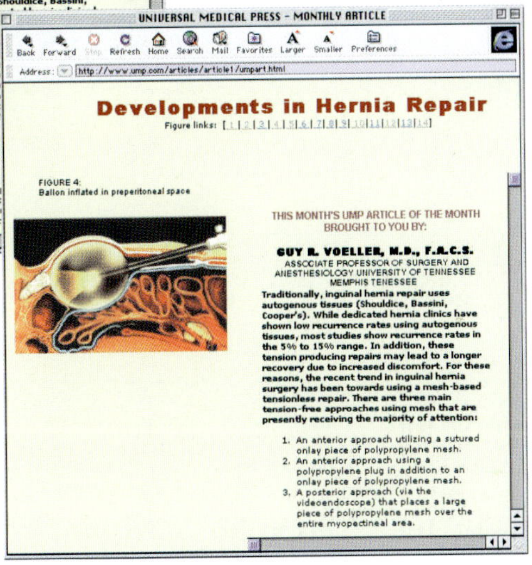

Article of the Month

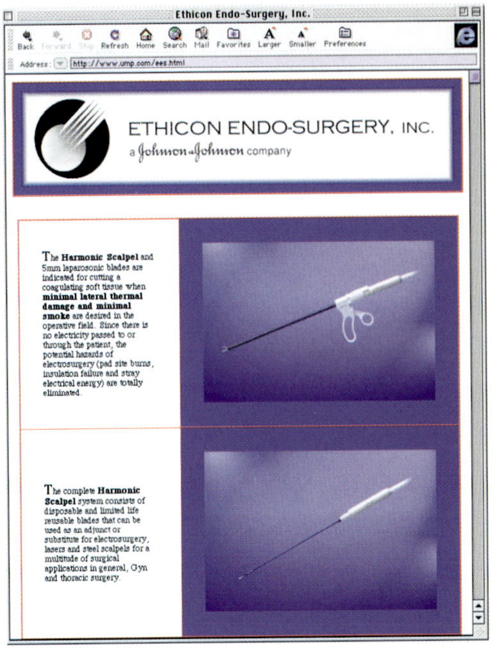

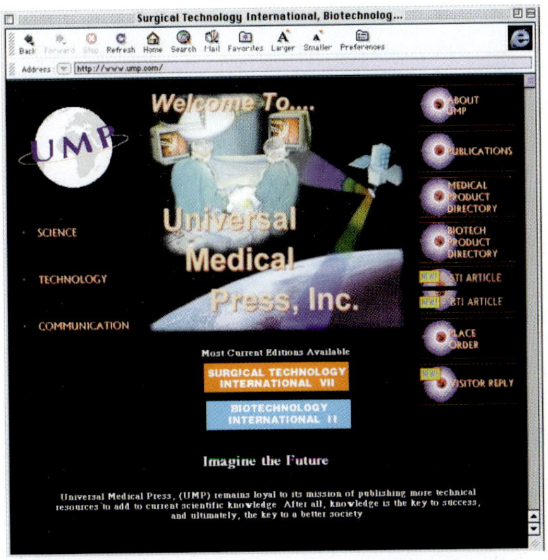

Home Page

Product Profile

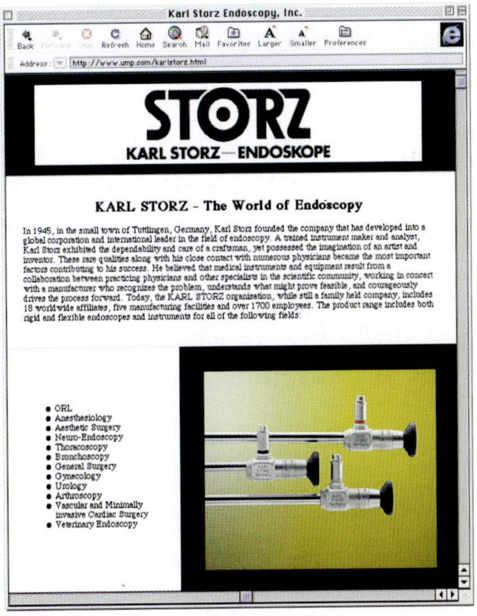

Product Profile

Advertisers Index

SURGICAL TECHNOLOGY INTERNATIONAL™ X

Argomedical 220

Biotechnology International 176

Cardiovations 118

Dornier Med Tech 88

Depuy, Inc. 192

Ethicon Endo-Surgery, Inc. 10

Ethicon Endo-Surgery, Inc./ Neoprobe.... 76

Glaxo SmithKline Pharmaceuticals.... 246-48

Karl Storz Endoscopy-America, Inc. ..IFC, 38, 66

MOET Institute 53

Novartis Pharmaceuticals.................... 22, 24

Richard Wolf GmbH........................... 12, 16

Schwarz Pharma.. 14

Smith & Nephew, Inc. .... 194, IBC

Sorin Biomedica S.p.A 150

SPLAR 270

STERIS Corp.. 6-7

St. Jude's Medical 120

TMJ Implants, Inc................................... 272

Valleylab/Tyco Healthcare...................... 54

Please visit our website at

www.ump.com

for further information

on products and manufacturers.

Send e-mail requests for information

to **productinfo@ump.com**